Exercise Physiology

Exercise Physiology

Edited by **Pablo De Souza**

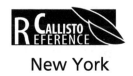

New York

Published by Callisto Reference,
106 Park Avenue, Suite 200,
New York, NY 10016, USA
www.callistoreference.com

Exercise Physiology
Edited by Pablo De Souza

© 2016 Callisto Reference

International Standard Book Number: 978-1-63239-629-7 (Hardback)

Contents

Preface

This book has been an outcome of determined endeavour from a group of educationists in the field. The primary objective was to involve a broad spectrum of professionals from diverse cultural background involved in the field for developing new researches. The book not only targets students but also scholars pursuing higher research for further enhancement of the theoretical and practical applications of the subject.

This book provides its readers with an advanced understanding of exercise physiology. It studies in detail the responses of the body to exercise and its corresponding impact. Exercise acts as a physical medicine that has the ability to remediate impairments and promote mobility, function, and quality of life through physical intervention. It emphasizes the acute and chronic effects of exercise on various physiological systems in adults and the integrative nature of these physiological responses. As this field is emerging at a rapid pace, the contents of this book will help the readers understand the modern concepts and applications of the subject. It aims to shed light on some of the unexplored aspects of exercise physiology and present the recent researches in this field.

It was an honour to edit such a profound book and also a challenging task to compile and examine all the relevant data for accuracy and originality. I wish to acknowledge the efforts of the contributors for submitting such brilliant and diverse chapters in the field and for endlessly working for the completion of the book. Last, but not the least; I thank my family for being a constant source of support in all my research endeavours.

Editor

TRPA1 mediates amplified sympathetic responsiveness to activation of metabolically sensitive muscle afferents in rats with femoral artery occlusion

Jihong Xing[1]*, Jian Lu[2] and Jianhua Li[2]*

[1] Department of Emergency Medicine, The First Hospital of Jilin University, Changchun, Jilin, China, [2] Pennsylvania State Heart and Vascular Institute, The Pennsylvania State University College of Medicine, Hershey, PA, USA

Edited by:
Donal O'Leary,
Wayne State University School of
Medicine, USA

Reviewed by:
Scott Alan Smith,
University of Texas Southwestern
Medical Center at Dallas, USA
Hanjun Wang,
University of Nebraska Medical
Center, USA

*Correspondence:
Jihong Xing,
Department of Emergency Medicine,
The First Hospital of Jilin University,
Changchun, Jilin 130021, China
jhxing79@gmail.com;
Jianhua Li,
Heart and Vascular Institute, Penn
State College of Medicine, 500
University Dr, Hershey, PA 17033, USA
jianhuali@hmc.psu.edu

Autonomic responses to activation of mechanically and metabolically sensitive muscle afferent nerves during static contraction are augmented in rats with femoral artery occlusion. Moreover, metabolically sensitive transient receptor potential cation channel subfamily A, member 1 (TRPA1) has been reported to contribute to sympathetic nerve activity (SNA) and arterial blood pressure (BP) responses evoked by static muscle contraction. Thus, in the present study, we examined the mechanisms by which afferent nerves' TRPA1 plays a role in regulating amplified sympathetic responsiveness due to a restriction of blood flow directed to the hindlimb muscles. Our data show that 24–72 h of femoral artery occlusion (1) upregulates the protein levels of TRPA1 in dorsal root ganglion (DRG) tissues; (2) selectively increases expression of TRPA1 in DRG neurons supplying metabolically sensitive afferent nerves of C-fiber (group IV); and (3) enhances renal SNA and BP responses to AITC (a TRPA1 agonist) injected into the hindlimb muscles. In addition, our data demonstrate that blocking TRPA1 attenuates SNA and BP responses during muscle contraction to a greater degree in ligated rats than those responses in control rats. In contrast, blocking TRPA1 fails to attenuate SNA and BP responses during passive tendon stretch in both groups. Overall, results of this study indicate that alternations in muscle afferent nerves' TRPA1 likely contribute to enhanced sympathetically mediated autonomic responses via the metabolic component of the muscle reflex under circumstances of chronic muscle ischemia.

Keywords: muscle afferent nerve, TRPA1, peripheral arterial disease, hindlimb ischemia

Introduction

Peripheral arterial disease (PAD) is atherosclerotic disease with a decrease in blood flow to the arteries of the lower extremities. In this disease, the most common symptom is intermittent claudication, which is worsened by exercise activity due to muscle ischemia but subsides at when the metabolic demand of the active muscles is decreased (Rejeski et al., 2008).

Exercise increases sympathetic nerve activity (SNA) (Mark et al., 1985; Victor et al., 1988; Sinoway et al., 1989), an effect which in turn increases arterial blood pressure (BP), heart rate

(HR), myocardial contractility and peripheral vascular resistance. Two mechanisms, namely central command and the exercise pressor reflex, evoke this exercise-induced increase in SNA. Central command postulates a parallel and simultaneous increase in sympathetic and alpha motoneuron discharge (Goodwin et al., 1972; Waldrop et al., 1996). The exercise pressor reflex postulates that thin fiber muscle afferent nerves (group III & IV) innervating skeletal muscles are activated by contraction-induced mechanical and metabolic stimuli to elicit a reflex increase in SNA (Mccloskey and Mitchell, 1972; Mitchell et al., 1983; Kaufman and Forster, 1996). It was observed that both systolic and diastolic BP rise significantly in the patients with PAD than in the normal subjects during walking (Baccelli et al., 1997). Furthermore, the exercise pressor reflex plays a crucial role in evoking the exaggerated BP response to walking in PAD patients (Baccelli et al., 1999).

Ligation of the femoral artery in rats serves as a useful model to study human PAD (Waters et al., 2004). Using this model, prior studies have shown that the SNA and BP responses to muscle contraction as well as to stimulation of several muscle metabolic receptors are enhanced in ligated rats compared with non-ligated rats (Li and Xing, 2012). Nonetheless, the precious mechanisms responsible for amplified responsiveness of SNA and BP during stimulation of muscle afferents in ligated animals still need to be determined.

Transient receptor potential channel A1 (TRPA1) is a member of branch A of the transient receptor potential (TRP) family of nonselective cation channels. This channel is expressed in the sensory (nerves) neurons and is involved in acute and inflammatory pain (Story et al., 2003; Bandell et al., 2004; Obata et al., 2005; Bautista et al., 2006; Katsura et al., 2006; Kwan et al., 2006; Macpherson et al., 2007). TRPA1 acts as a sensory receptor in response to pungent and reactive chemicals such as allylisothiocyanate (AITC, used as a TRPA1 agonist), allicin, cinnamaldehyde, formaldehyde, N-methylmaleimide, and α, β-unsaturated aldehydes (Story et al., 2003; Bandell et al., 2004; Jordt et al., 2004; Bautista et al., 2005). TRPA1 also serves as a sensor of cold temperature and mechanical deformation (Story et al., 2003; Nagata et al., 2005; Obata et al., 2005; Kwan et al., 2006; Kindt et al., 2007; Sawada et al., 2007; Trevisani et al., 2007). Besides pungent chemicals, endogenously generated molecules i.e., bradykinin, reactive oxygen species, and 4-hydroxynonenal that are produced during inflammation and oxidative stress, respectively, can activate TRPA1 (Bandell et al., 2004; Trevisani et al., 2007; Bessac et al., 2008).

A recent study has demonstrated that intra-arterial injection of AITC into the hindlimb muscle circulation of healthy rats led to increases in SNA and BP via a reflex mechanism (Koba et al., 2011). Also, this study has suggested that TRPA1 plays a role in activating the exercise pressor reflex and acid phosphate, bradykinin and arachidonic acid, which are accumulated in exercising muscle, are likely endogenous stimulants of TRPA1.

Thus, the purpose of this study was to determine the mechanisms by which afferent nerves' TRPA1 contributes to the regulation of the amplified sympathetic responsiveness in a rat model of femoral artery occlusion. Overall, our hypothesis was that the higher protein levels of TRPA1 in dorsal root ganglion

(DRG) neurons supplying metabolically sensitive afferent nerves of C-fiber (group IV) are induced with a restriction of blood flow directed to the hindlimb muscles, effects which in turn exaggerate the metabolic component of the exercise pressor reflex as a consequence.

Materials and Methods

The Institutional Animal Care and Use Committee of Pennsylvania State College of Medicine has approved all animal experimental procedures, which were complied with the National Institutes of Health (NIH) guidelines.

Ligation of Femoral Artery

Under inhalation of an isoflurane-oxygen mixture (2–5% isoflurane in 100% oxygen), the surgical procedures were performed in 86 male Sprague–Dawley rats (5–7 week old) as previously described (Xing et al., 2008; Liu et al., 2010; Lu et al., 2013). For the western blotting and ($n = 18$) immunofluorescence experiments ($n = 4$), the rat's femoral artery on one limb was surgically exposed, dissected, and ligated ~3 mm distal to the inguinal ligament; this served as "ligated limb." The same procedures were performed on the other limb except that a suture was placed below the femoral artery but was not tied; this served as "control limb." For the experiment of SNA and BP recording, the rats were divided between those that had the right femoral artery ligation ["ligated rats" ($n = 34$)] and those that had sham surgeries on the right hindlimb ["control rat" ($n = 30$)]. Then, 6 to 72 h were allowed for recovery before the experiments began.

Western Blot Analysis

Eighteen rats were used to examine expression of TRPA1 protein in lumbar (L4–L6) DRGs of control and limbs with 6, 24, and 72 h of femoral artery occlusion. Western blot methods were performed as previously described (Liu et al., 2010; Lu et al., 2013). In brief, DRGs of the rats were removed. All DRGs tissues from individual rats were sampled for western blot analysis. Total protein was then extracted by homogenizing DRG sample in ice-cold radioimmunoprecipitation assay buffer containing 25 mM Tris·HCl (pH 7.6), 150 mM NaCl, 1% Nonidet P-40, 1% sodium deoxycholate, and 0.1% sodium dodecyl sulfate (SDS) with protease inhibitor cocktail kit (Sigma-Aldrich, St. Louis, MO). The lysates were centrifuged at 15,000 g for 15 min at 4°C; the supernatants were collected for measurements of protein concentrations using a bicinchoninic acid assay reagent kit (Pierce Biotechnology, Rockford, IL) and then stored in −80°C for later use.

After being denatured by heating at 95°C for 5 min in an SDS sample buffer (Cell Signaling Technology, Danvers, MA), the supernatant samples containing 20 μg of protein was loaded onto 4–20% Mini-Protean TGX Precast gels (Bio-Rad Laboratories, Hercules, CA) and then electrically transferred to a polyvinylidene fluoride membrane (GE Water & Process Tech, Trevose, PA) (Liu et al., 2010; Lu et al., 2013). The membrane was blocked in 5% nonfat milk in 0.1% Tween-TBS buffer for 1 h and was then incubated overnight with primary antibody: rabbit anit-TRPA1 at 1:500 dilutions (Novus).

After being fully washed, the membrane was incubated with horseradish peroxidase-linked anti-rabbit secondary antibody at 1:1000 dilutions and visualized for immunoreactivity using an enhanced chemiluminescence system (Cell Signaling Technology). The membrane was stripped and incubated with mouse anti-β-actin (Sigma-Aldrich) to show equal loading of the protein in the western blot analysis. The bands recognized by the primary antibody were visualized by exposure of the membrane onto an X-ray film. Then, the film was scanned and the optical densities of TRPA1 and β-actin bands were determined using the NIH Scion Image Software (Liu et al., 2010; Lu et al., 2013).

Fluorescence Immunohistochemistry

As described in our previous work (Liu et al., 2010; Lu et al., 2012; Xing et al., 2012), the four rats were anesthetized by inhalation of an isoflurane-oxygen mixture and then transcardially perfused with 200 ml of ice-cold saline containing 1000 units heparin followed by 500 ml of 4% fresh prepared, ice-cold paraformaldehyde in phosphate-buffered saline (PBS, pH 7.4). L4–L6 DRGs of control limbs and limbs with 24 h of femoral occlusion were immediately dissected out and immersed in the same fixative at 4°C for 2 h. The tissues were then stored in PBS containing 30% sucrose overnight. Then, a cryostat was used to obtain 10 μm of DRG sections.

DRG sections were fixed in 4% of paraformaldehyde in PBS for 10 min at room temperature. After being washed with PBS, the tissue were permeabilized, blocked in 0.3% Triton X-100 in PBS supplemented with 5% goat serum for 1 h, and then incubated with rabbit anti-TRPA1 (1:200, Novus) antibody overnight at 4°C. After being washed in PBS, the sections were incubated with goat anti-rabbit fluorescein isothiocyanate (FITC) labeled secondary antibody (1: 200, Invitrogen) for 2 h at room temperature.

To examine localization of TRPA1 within DRG neurons supplying C-fiber and A-fiber, the sections were incubated with the second primary antibody (mouse anti-peripherin at 1:200, Sigma; and anti-NF200 at 1:200 Abcam) overnight (Liu et al., 2010; Lu et al., 2012; Xing et al., 2012). Peripherin and NF200 are used to label neurons with C-fiber and A-fiber, respectively. Briefly, after incubation, the sections were washed and incubated for 2 h at room temperature with secondary antibody (Alexa Fluor-594 conjugated goat anti-mouse IgG, dilution: 1:200). Then, the sections were washed in PBS, and coverslipped.

FITC- and Alexa Fluor-594-labeled DRG neurons were examined using a Nikon Eclipse 80i microscope with appropriate filters, and the images were stored digitally on a computer. As described previously (Liu et al., 2010), at least five sections containing L4–L6 DRGs per rat were randomly chosen for analysis of FITC and Alexa Fluor-594 staining intensity. Thus, the four rats used in this experiment provided a sufficient power to statistical analysis. A threshold value of staining intensity was set according to the mean staining intensity of background using the Nis-Elements software (Nikon, Co.). Cells with >1.75 times of background intensity were considered to be positive. The number of total TRPA1 immunostaining and peripherin/NF200

positive neurons was counted in each section (Liu et al., 2010). Percentages of double (FITC and peripherin /NF200)-labeled neurons were calculated: total number of double-labeled cells × 100/total number of peripherin/NF200 positive cells (Lu et al., 2012; Xing et al., 2012, 2013). Note that the majority of DRG neurons showed a clear nucleus and perimeter and they were counted. To minimize the possibility of counting a single DRG neuron more than once, DRG sections were collected on 5 glass slides in series, and tissues from one of slides were processed for immunocytochemical analysis.

Examination of the Exercise Pressor Reflex
Surgical Procedures

The 30 control rats and 34 rats with 24 h of femoral occlusion were anesthetized with a mixture of 2–5% isoflurane and oxygen and ventilated as describe previously (Xing et al., 2008; Liu et al., 2010; Lu et al., 2013). The right jugular vein and common carotid artery were cannulated to deliver fluids and to connect a pressure transducer for measurement arterial BP, respectively. A catheter (PE10) was then inserted into the distal side of the right femoral artery for injection of drugs into the arterial blood supply of the hindlimb muscles. During the experiments, baseline BP and fluid balance were maintained with a continuous infusion of saline. Body temperature was continuously monitored and maintained at 37.5–38.5°C with a heating pad and external heating lamps.

A laminectomy was performed to expose the lower lumbar and upper scaral portions of the spinal cord after the rats were placed in a spinal unit (Kopf Instruments) as described in the previous work (Smith et al., 2001; Lu et al., 2012). The spinal roots were exposed and the right L4 and L5 ventral roots visually identified with assistance of an anatomical microscope (Cooper Surgical, Inc.). The peripheral ends of the transected L4 and L5 ventral roots were then placed on bipolar platinum stimulating electrodes. A pool was formed by using the skin and muscle on the back and the exposed spinal region was filled with warmed (37°C) mineral oil.

In a subset group of experiments, a bundle of the renal nerves on the left side was carefully dissected from other connective tissues. A piece of laboratory film was placed under the isolated nerves, and two tips of a bipolar electrode used to record neural activity were placed between the nerves and the film; these were embedded in a silicone gel. Once the gel hardened, the silicone rubber was fixed to the surrounding tissue with a glue containing α-cyanoacrylate. The skin on the back was used to form a pool that was filled with warm (37°C) mineral oil. The renal SNA (RSNA) signal was amplified with an amplifier (P511, Grass Instruments) with a band-pass filter of 300 Hz in low-cut frequency and of 3 kHz in high-cut frequency and recorded as previously described (Xing et al., 2008; Liu et al., 2010; Lu et al., 2013).

Decerebration was performed as previously described (Smith et al., 2001; Xing et al., 2008; Liu et al., 2010; Lu et al., 2012) to avoid the confounding effects of anesthesia on the reflex pressor response. A transverse section was made anterior to the superior colliculus and extending ventrally to the mammillary bodies. All brain tissues from rostral to the section were removed. Following this procedure, the anesthesia was withdrawn from the rats. The calcaneal bone of right hindlimb was cut and its tendon was attached to a force transducer (Grass FT10), and the knee joints were secured by clamping the patellar tendon to a spinal unit. A recovery period of 60 min was allowed before the experiment began.

Experimental Protocols

A diagram of **Figure 1** illustrates experimental designs examining the exercise pressor reflex. In the first group of experiments, in order to determine the sympathetic, BP and HR responses to activation of metabolically sensitive TRPA1 in control rats and ligated rats. Three dosages of AITC (TRPA1 agonist) (10, 20, 40 μg/kg body) were injected into arterial blood supply of the right hindlimb muscles of control rats ($n = 12$) and rats with 24 h of femoral artery occlusion ($n = 14$). The concentrations of AITC were selected on the basis of the results of a prior study (Koba et al., 2011). The injection volume was adjusted to 0.1–0.2 ml according to rat's body weight. The duration of the injection was 1 min. At least 20 min were allowed between injections. In some experiments, sciatic and femoral nerves were cut and then 40 μg/kg of AITC was injected in control rats and ligated rats ($n = 5$ in each group). This allowed us to rule out the systemic effects of AITC.

In the second group of experiments, static muscle contractions in the right hindlimb were performed by electrical stimulation of the L4 and L5 ventral roots (30 s, 3-times motor threshold with a period of 0.1 ms at 40 Hz) in control rats ($n = 8$) and rats whose femoral artery was ligated for 24 h ($n = 8$). The purpose of this experiment was to examine if femoral artery occlusion altered the effects of blocking TRPA1 receptor on BP and HR responses evoked by stimulation of both mechanically and chemically sensitive muscle afferent nerves. Note that RSNA was not examined in this experiment due to electrical interference during the ventral root stimulation. Each static muscle contraction was performed 15 min after arterial injection of DMSO (control and recovery) and 3 mg of HC-030031 (TRPA1 antagonist) (Koba et al., 2011). Then, 20 min was allowed after contraction and before next injection. The injected volume was 0.25 ml and the duration of injections was 1 min. Thus, there was a ∼36-min resting period between bouts of muscle contraction. In addition,

3 mg of HC-030031 (0.25 ml over 1 min) was injected into jugular vein and then BP response to contraction was examined in six control rats. This allowed us to exclude the systemic effects evoked by arterial injection HC-030031.

In the third group of experiments, passive tendon stretch was performed in the right hindlimb of control rats ($n = 10$) and rats ($n = 12$) whose femoral artery was ligated for 24 h before the experiments. Passive tendon stretch (500 g of tension) was produced manually over ∼5 s by using a rack and pinion attached to the Achilles' tendon of control and ligated rats. Each bout of muscle stretch was maintained for 30 s after 500 g of tension was achieved. Muscle stretch was used to activate the mechanoreceptor component of the exercise pressor reflex. The purpose of this study was to examine if vascular insufficiency observed in ligated rats altered SNA, BP, and HR responses evoked by stimulation of mechanically sensitive muscle afferent nerves alone. Similar to the protocol used in the muscle contraction experiments, arterial injection of DMSO before muscle stretch was performed as control and recovery and arterial injection of 3 mg of HC-030031 was employed to block TRPA1.

Recording of Experimental Data

All measured data of RSNA, BP, HR and muscle tension were continuously recorded and stored on a computer with PowerLab system (Ad instruments, Castle Hill, Australia). As described previously (Xing et al., 2008; Lu et al., 2012, 2013), mean arterial pressure (MAP) was obtained by integrating the arterial signal with a time constant of 4 s. HR was calculated on a basis of beat to beat from the arterial pressure pulse. The peak responses of MAP and HR were determined by the peak change from the control value. The muscle tension response during the ventral root stimulation was also recorded. RSNA signals were transformed into absolute values, integrated over 1 s interval, and subtracted by 1 s of integrated background noise. To quantify RSNA response to AITC injection and passive tendon stretch (by loading ∼500 g of muscle tension), baseline values were obtained by taking the mean value for the 30 s immediately before each intervention and by ascribing the mean value of 100%, and relative change from baseline during the injection and stretch were then evaluated.

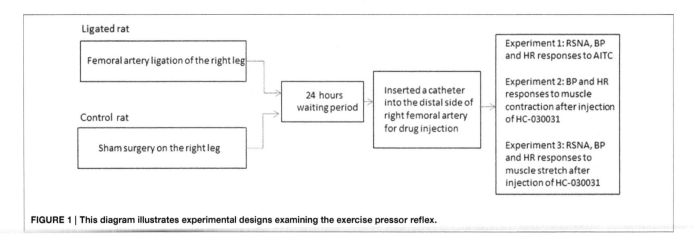

FIGURE 1 | This diagram illustrates experimental designs examining the exercise pressor reflex.

Data Statistical Analysis

One-Way repeated measures analysis of variance (ANOVA) was used to analyze data of Western Blot and immunohistochemistry, and Two-Way ANOVA was used to analyze data of RSNA, MAP, HR, and muscle tension. As appropriate, Tukey's *post-hoc* tests were used. All values were presented as mean ± SEM. For all analyses, differences were considered significant at $P < 0.05$. All statistical analyses were performed using SPSS for Windows version 20.0.

Results

TRPA1 Expression in DRG Neurons

The expression of TRPA1 proteins in L4–L6 DRG neurons of control and ligated limbs was examined using western blot analysis. Typical bands and average data of **Figure 2** show that the protein levels of TRPA1 are significantly increased 24 and 72 h ($n = 6$ in each group) after femoral artery ligation. Nevertheless, 6 h of femoral artery ligation ($n = 6$) did not significantly increase TRPA1 expression as compared with control. In addition, there were insignificant differences in the protein levels of TRPA1 24 and 72 h after the ligation. Thus, 24 h of femoral artery ligation was used for other groups of experiments in this report.

TRPA1 Distributions within DRG Neurons with Different Phenotypes

In this experiment, we further determined if TRPA1 exists within DRG neurons that supply C- and/or A-fiber afferent nerves. The dual immunofluorescence techniques were used to examine co-localization of fluorescent TRPA1 and peripherin/NF200 immunoreactivity in the DRG neurons of control limbs and ligated limbs. The appearance of TRPA1 and peripherin/NF200 within DRG neurons is characterized by fluorescent green and red color, respectively (**Figures 3A,B**). Note that there was no significant difference in number of peripherin- and NF200-positve DRG neurons between both experimental groups.

The photomicrographs in **Figure 3A** show that the most TRPA1 staining appears in C-fiber of DRG neurons in both control and ligated groups. The percentage of double-labeled neurons with TRPA1 and peripherin was significantly greater in the ligated limbs than that in control limbs. They were 39 ± 2% in control limbs ($n = 4$) and 52 ± 3% ($P < 0.05$ vs. control) in ligated limbs ($n = 4$). In contrast, the photomicrographs in **Figure 3B** show that few A-fiber of DRG neurons include TRPA1 staining in both control and ligated groups. The percentage of double-labeled neurons with TRPA1 and NF200 was similar in both groups. These double-labeled neuron were <5% in controls ($n = 4$) and in the ligation group ($n = 4$) ($P > 0.05$ vs. control).

Engagement of TRPA1 in the Exercise Pressor Reflex
RSNA, BP, and HR Responses to Stimulation of TRPA1

Baseline values for MAP and HR before arterial injections of AITC are 93 ± 4 mmHg and 396 ± 16 beats/min in control rats ($n = 12$); and 91 ± 3 mmHg and 403 ± 19 beats/min in ligated

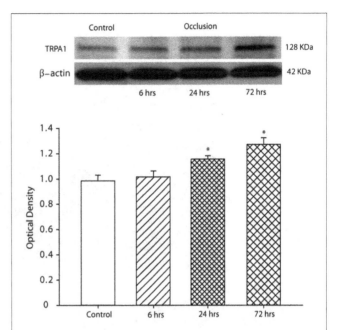

FIGURE 2 | Effects of femoral artery occlusion on TRPA1 expression at different time courses. Western blot analysis was used to examine the protein levels of TRPA1 in DRG tissues. **Top**: representative bands of TRPA1 expression. Bands of β-actin are used as control for an equal protein loading. **Bottom**: average data. The optical density is expressed in arbitrary units normalized against a control sample. Data in histograms represent means ± SEM; $n = 6$ in each group. *$P < 0.05$ vs. control.

rats ($n = 14$), respectively. There were no significant differences in basal MAP and HR before injections. Typical and average data of **Figure 4** illustrates the effects of increasing concentrations (10, 20, and 40 μg/kg body wt) of AITC injected into the hindlimb muscles on RSNA, MAP, and HR in control rats and ligated rats. Arterial injection of AITC evoked dose-related increases in RSNA and MAP in both groups. Those responses induced by 40 μg/kg of AITC were significantly amplified in ligated rats compared with responses in control rats. The RSNA and MAP responses to arterial injection of AITC (40 μg/kg body wt) were 61 ± 5% and 31 ± 5 mmHg in 12 control rats; and 89 ± 8% and 44 ± 3 mmHg in 14 ligated rats ($P < 0.05$ ligation vs. control), respectively. Note that there was no significant difference in HR responses evoked by an arterial injection of AITC in both groups. In addition, MAP response to arterial injection of 40 μg of AITC was 4 ± 1 mmHg in control rats ($n = 5$) and 5 ± 1 mmHg in ligated rats ($n = 5$) after section of the sciatic and femoral nerves ($P > 0.05$ vs. their respective baseline).

BP and HR Responses to Muscle Contraction after Blocking of TRPA1

Baseline MAPs and HRs were 96 ± 3 mm Hg and 393 ± 11 bpm in control rats ($n = 8$); and 95 ± 2 mm Hg and 391 ± 12 bpm in rats whose femoral artery was ligated for 24 h ($n = 8$) ($P > 0.05$ vs. control). Typical traces and average data in **Figure 5** show 24 h of femoral occlusion significantly increased the responses of MAP and HR evoked by muscle contraction. Moreover, **Figure 5** shows MAP and HR responses to muscle contraction

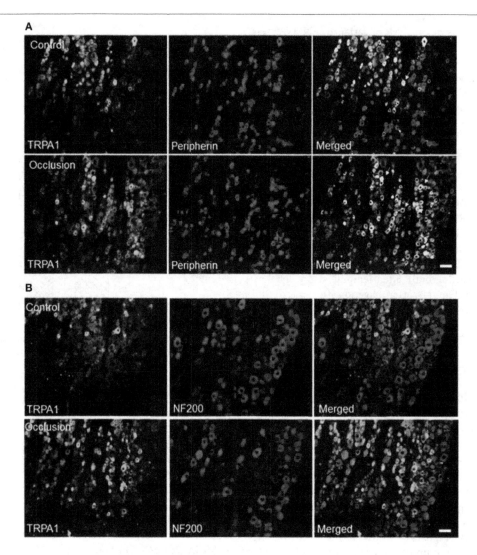

FIGURE 3 | Immunofluorescence was employed to examine double-labeling for TRPA1 and peripherin and NF200. Peripherin was used to label DRG neurons that supply thin C-fibers afferent nerves. NF200 was used to identify A-fibers of DRG neurons. **(A)** Representative photomicrographs show TRPA1 and peripherin staining in DRG neurons of a control limb (top) and a ligated limb (bottom). Arrows indicate representative cells positive for both TRPA1 and peripherin after they were merged. The number of double labeled DRG neurons is greater in ligated limbs than in control limbs. Scale bar = 50 μm. **(B)** Photomicrographs are representative to illustrate staining of TRPA1 and NF200 in DRG neurons of a control limb (top) and a ligated limb (bottom). There were few DRG neurons containing both TRPA1 and NF200 staining in both groups. No differences in the number of double-stained TRPA1 and NF200 were observed in DRG neurons of the control and ligated limbs. Scale bar = 50 μm.

after blocking TRPA1 with arterial injection of 3 mg of HC-030031 in control rats and ligated rats. HC-030031 significantly inhibited MAP and HR responses induced by muscle contraction in control and ligated rats. In control rats, the MAP and HR responses were 16 ± 2 mmHg and 19 ± 3 bpm with saline injection; and 10 ± 2 mmHg and 10 ± 1 bpm with HC-030031 treatment ($P < 0.05$, HC-030031 treatment vs. saline control for both MAP and HR responses). In ligated rats, the MAP and HR responses were 27 ± 3 mmHg and 32 ± 3 bpm with vehicle injection; and 11 ± 2 mmHg and 11 ± 4 bpm with HC-030031 treatment ($P < 0.05$, HC-030031 treatment vs. vehicle control for both MAP and HR responses). The attenuating effects of HC-030031 were greater in ligated rats than in control rats (MAP

and HR: 59 and 67% in ligated rats vs. 38 and 49% in control rats, $P < 0.05$. $n = 8$ in each group). No significant difference was observed in tension response in two groups. In six control rats, intravenous injection of HC-030031 failed to attenuate BP response to contraction (MAP response: 18 ± 3 mmHg before HC-030031 and 17 ± 2 mmHg after HC-030031, $P > 0.05$).

RSNA, BP, and HR Responses to Passive Tendon Stretch after Blocking of TRPA1

There were no significant differences in baseline values for MAP and HR in control rats ($n = 10$) and ligated rats ($n = 12$). Baseline MAPs and HRs were 97 ± 5 mm Hg; 387 ± 12 bpm in control rats; and 95 ± 5 mm Hg; 392 ± 10 bpm in ligated rats

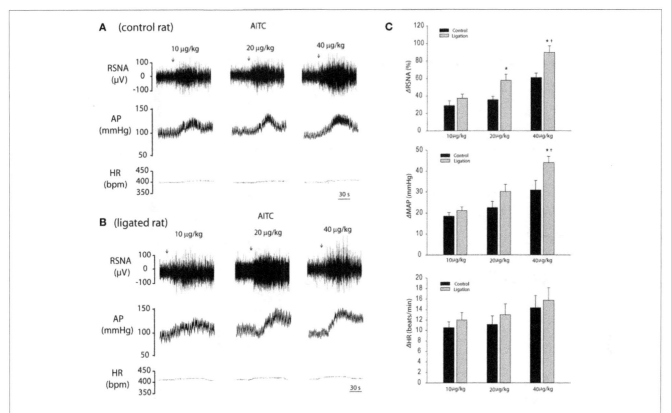

FIGURE 4 | Changes in RSNA, MAP and HR in response to stimulation of TRPA1 with arterial injection of AITC (TRPA1 agonist). (A,B) Typical traces obtained from a control rat and ligated rat. Arrows indicate a start of injections. **(C)** Average data. Three dosages of AITC (10, 20, 40 μg/kg body) were injected into the arterial blood supply of the hindlimb muscles of control rats ($n = 12$) and rats with 24 h of femoral artery occlusion ($n = 14$). No significant difference was observed in baseline MAP and HR. Values are means ± SEM. *$P < 0.05$, compared with control. †$P < 0.05$ indicates significant differences among different dosages.

($P > 0.05$ vs. control). Typical traces and average data in **Figure 6** demonstrate RSNA, MAP, and HR responses to muscle stretch during each intervention. Before blocking TRPA1, significantly higher RSNA and MAP responses were observed in the ligated rats vs. the control rats. No significant HR responses were seen in the two groups during stretch. Blocking TRPA1 with arterial injection of 3 mg of HC-030031 did not elicit significant changes in RSNA, MAP and HR responses during muscle stretch in either the control rats or the ligated rats. i.e., in ligated rats, RSNA, and MAP responses induced by ~500 g of muscle tension were 49 ± 3% and 22 ± 3 mm Hg in control, and 48 ± 4% and 21 ± 3 mmHg ($P > 0.05$ vs. control) after 3 mg of HC-030031.

Discussion

The purpose of the present study was to determine whether TRPA1 on primary muscle afferent nerves contributes to the enhanced sympathetic responsiveness elicited by femoral artery ligation. The results of this study have shown that that 24 and 72 h of femoral artery occlusion significantly amplifies the protein levels of TRPA1 in lumbar DRGs of ligated limbs, and that increased expression of TRPA1 selectively appears within DRG neurons that supply C-fiber afferents but not A-fiber afferents. In addition, stimulation of TRPA1 with injection of AITC into the arterial blood supply of the hindlimb muscles

evokes greater increases in RSNA and BP in ligated rats than in control rats. This result further supports the idea that femoral artery occlusion upregulates the expression of TRPA1 in muscle afferents nerves. Moreover, our data demonstrate that blocking TRPA1 attenuates BP and HR responses during muscle contraction to a greater degree in ligated rats than those responses in control rats. In contrast, blocking TRPA1 fails to attenuate SNA and BP responses during passive tendon stretch in both groups. Accordingly, the findings of this study suggest that enhanced TRPA1 in muscle afferent nerves plays a role in regulating amplified sympathetic responsiveness after femoral artery occlusion via the metabolic component of the exercise pressor reflex.

Our prior work has suggested that femoral artery ligation increases expression of metabolite receptors (i.e., ASIC3 and P2X3) in DRG and there are insignificant differences in the levels of these receptors in rats with 24 h of ligation and in rats with 72 h of ligation (Liu et al., 2010, 2011). Likewise, the magnitudes of BP response to muscle contraction were observed to reach at a similar degree in rats with 24 h of ligation and in rats with 72 h of ligation (Tsuchimochi et al., 2010; Lu et al., 2012). Accordingly, in the current study we examined the effects of 24 h of ligation on the SNA, BP, and HR responses to AITC and to muscle contraction/stretch. However, it should be noted that TRPA1 expression in DRG of rats with 72 h of ligation appears

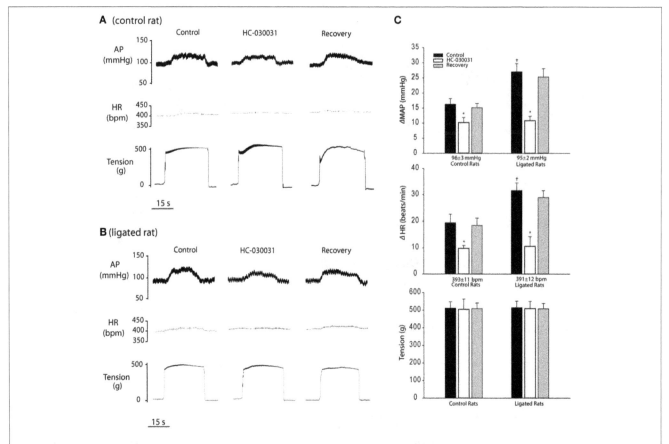

FIGURE 5 | Changes in MAP, HR and muscle tension in response to static contraction after an inhibition of TRPA1 by 3 mg of HC-030031 (TRPA1 antagonist). Muscle contraction was evoked by electrical stimulation of the L4 and L5 ventral roots. Blocking TRPA1 significantly attenuated the MAP and HR responses to muscle contraction in control rats and rats with 24 h of femoral artery ligation. **(A,B)** Typical traces obtained from a control rat and ligated rat. **(C)** Average data. The attenuating effects of HC-030031 were greater in ligated rats (MAP and HR: 59 and 67%. $P < 0.05$ vs. control rats, $n = 8$) than in control rats (MAP and HR: 38 and 49%, $n = 8$). No significant difference was observed in baseline MAP and HR, and muscle tension responses in two groups. Values are means ± SEM. *$P < 0.05$ vs. vehicle control. †$P < 0.05$ indicates ligated rats vs. control rats.

to be slightly greater as compared with 24 h of ligation in the current study. It would be very likely to obtain optimal results if we have examined the reflex experiments 72 h post ligation. Another possibility is that an increased TRPA1 activity after 24 h of the femoral ligation is independent of its protein expression. Nonetheless, results of our current study have demonstrated that 24 h of ligation has greater effects on the reflex responses to arterial injection of AITC and HC-030031.

The current data show that 24 h femoral artery occlusion increased the protein levels of TRPA1 and amplified the SNA and BP responses to stimulation of AITC as compared with controls. One potential mechanism by which TRPA1 plays a regulatory role is a functional interaction of proteinase-activated receptor-2 (PAR2) and TRPA1 in DRG neurons. Co-localization of TRPA1 with PAR2 has been found in rat DRG neurons and the activation of PAR2 has been reported to increase TRPA1 induced currents in DRG neurons (Dai et al., 2007). In addition, a prior study has shown that the mRNA expression of PAR2 increased by 1.9-fold in adductor muscles of mice whose femoral artery was ligated for a day (Milia et al., 2002).

In a prior study using the patch clamp methods, AITC from 10 to 1000 μM were successively applied to the same DRG neuron and the data of this study demonstrated that EC50 value for AITC is 173 μM and the saturating concentration is about 1 mM (Raisinghani et al., 2011). Brief application (20–50 s) of AITC at 200 μM has been shown to induce responses that were readily reversible, but continuous application of higher concentrations (>500 μM) of AITC induced a complete desensitization of the current response (Raisinghani et al., 2011). A recent study has also shown that in healthy decerebrated rats, intra-arterially injection of AITC (10–50 μg/kg body weight) into the hindlimb muscle circulation led to increases in SNA via a reflex pathway (Koba et al., 2011). Also, a dose-response relation was observed after those dosages of AITC were injected into the femoral artery (Koba et al., 2011). Considering that AITC was dissolved in the 0.2 ml of saline and its molecular weight is 99.15, the concentrations of AITC used in this *in vivo* study were ~0.5–2.5 mM (Koba et al., 2011). Because AITC injected into the muscle tissue via femoral artery can be partly metabolized we assumed that 10–50 μg/kg of AITC were effective to stimulate

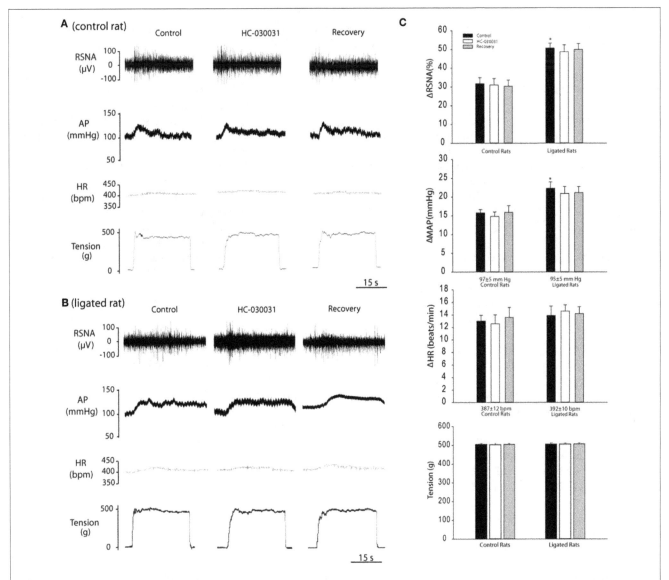

FIGURE 6 | Changes in RSNA, MAP and HR in response to passive tendon stretch after an inhibition of TRPA1 by 3 mg of HC-030031 (TRPA1 antagonist). Passive tendon stretch was evoked by loading ~500 g of muscle tension on the triceps surae muscle. **(A,B)** Typical traces obtained from a control rat and ligated rat. **(C)** Average data. After blocking TRPA1, responses of RSNA, MAP and HR to muscle stretch were observed in control rats ($n = 10$) and rats whose femoral artery was ligated for 24 h ($n = 12$). Note that blocking TRPA1 failed to attenuate the RSNA, MAP, and HR responses to muscle stretch in both control rats and ligated rats. Values are means ± SEM. *$P < 0.05$ indicates ligated rats vs. control rats.

TRPA1 with minimal desensitization. Furthermore, this prior study has demonstrated that TRPA1 plays a role in regulating SNA via stimulating the metabolic component of the exercise pressor reflex. Therefore, in the current study, the similar dosages AITC was selected to stimulate TRPA1 on muscle afferent nerves and our results show that greater SNA and BP response are evoked in ligated rats after arterial injection of the same dosage of AITC into the hindlimb muscles than those responses in control rats. However, it is noted that femoral ligation did not significantly amplified HR response to AITC. This is consistent with our previous results showing that HR response to activation of other metabolic receptors (i.e., ASIC3 and P2X3)

is not significantly altered by femoral ligation (Liu et al., 2010, 2011).

In addition, prior studies have demonstrated that TRPA1 knockout mice displayed behavioral deficits in sensing noxious cutaneous mechanical pain (Kwan et al., 2006, 2009). TRPA1 is considered to likely play a role in mediating mechanical hypersensitivity (Brierley et al., 2011). Given that thin fiber muscle afferent nerves (group III & IV) innervating skeletal muscles are activated by contraction-induced mechanical and metabolic stimuli to elicit reflex increases in SNA and BP during the exercise pressor reflex (Mitchell et al., 1983; Kaufman and Forster, 1996), we also examined the effects of blocking TRPA1 on the SNA, BP and HR responses evoked by static muscle contraction and passive tendon stretch. Our data show that femoral ligation significantly amplified BP and HR responses to muscle contraction (stimulation of both mechanically and metabolically sensitive muscle afferent nerves). Furthermore, blocking TRPA1 attenuated BP and HR responses to muscle contraction to a greater degree in ligated rats than those responses in control rats. It is speculated that a larger level of TRPA1 was likely attenuated after injection of HC-030031 into the hindlimb. This is consistent with results demonstrating that expression of TRPA1 in DRG neurons appeared to be greater in ligated rats than that in control rats. On the other hand, blocking TRPA1 failed to attenuate SNA, BP, and HR responses during passive tendon stretch (stimulation of mechanically sensitive muscle afferent nerves) in both groups. Thus, it would appear that stimulation of TRPA1 does not activate the mechanical component of the exercise pressor reflex.

What are endogenous muscle metabolites within contracting muscles to stimulate TRPA1 still needs to be determined. In addition to pungent chemicals found in nature, endogenously generated molecules such as bradykinin, reactive oxygen species, and 4-hydroxynonenal that are produced during inflammation and oxidative stress, respectively, can activate TRPA1 (Bandell et al., 2004; Trevisani et al., 2007; Bessac et al., 2008). Acid phosphate, bradykinin and arachidonic acid, which are accumulated in contracting muscles, are considered as potential endogenous stimuli engaged in the exercise pressor reflex (Koba et al., 2011). Furthermore, recent studies from our laboratory and others support the concept that muscle metabolites can sensitize mechanically sensitive afferents and increase mechanoreflex-mediated SNA response (Li and Sinoway, 2002; Koba et al., 2007; Cui et al., 2008; Gao et al., 2008). Sensitization of the mechanoreflex would not occur during passive muscle stretch as metabolites are not accumulated during this maneuver. This would account for why blockade of TRPA1 was ineffective at attenuating the response to stretch but might still play a role in the sensitization of the mechanoreflex during contraction (when metabolites accumulate). Bradykinin has been reported to modulate the exercise pressor reflex via kinin B2 receptor (Pan et al., 1993). Femoral artery occlusion amplifies SNA and BP responses to stimulation of stimulation of mechanically sensitive muscle afferent nerves and increased responses are attenuated by blocking kinin B2 receptor (Leal et al., 2013; Lu et al., 2013). Thus, we speculate that some muscle metabolites and their respective receptors such as bradykinin/kinin B2 receptor may play a role in regulating the exercise pressor reflex via TRPA1 engagement as stimulus as well as modulator after femoral artery occlusion.

TRPA1 has a similar structure to TRPV1 receptor, but with numerous ankyrin repeats in its amino (N) terminal (Jaquemar et al., 1999). TRPA1 has been shown to be co-expressed with TRPV1 (Story et al., 2003). Many agonists have been identified to activate both TRPA1 and TRPV1 receptors (Koizumi et al., 2009; Okumura et al., 2010). AITC can activate porcine TRPV1 (Ohta et al., 2007). Note that application of AITC in the micromolar range did not significantly affect currents recorded in TRPV1-transfected HEK293 cells. However, TRPV1 contributes to the DRG neuron responses to 3 mM of mustard oil (Everaerts et al., 2011). Likewise, a previous study has shown that cell membrane staining of TRPA1 increased upon 1 min treatment of 1 μM of capsaicin (Schmidt et al., 2009). Also, this prior study has demonstrated that activation of TRPV1 by capsaicin that was accompanied with localized calcium influx acutely increased TRPA1 membrane surface expression while TRPV1 levels were unchanged (Schmidt et al., 2009). Our published work showed that a higher density of TRPV1 immunostaining was induced within DRG neurons of rats with 24 h of femoral artery occlusion when compared with that in control rats, and that the arterial occlusion insult induced greater peak of inward current amplitudes in DRG neurons to capsaicin (Xing et al., 2008). Thus, we speculate that artery occlusion-enhanced expression and responses of TRPV1 in DRG neurons likely induced a greater calcium influx and increased TRPA1 membrane surface expression in engagement in the role played by TRPA1 observed in our current study.

In summary, the data of the present study have shown that the femoral artery occlusion significantly increases the levels of TRPA1 protein in lumbar DRG neurons. The enhanced expression of TRPA1 is specifically observed in DRG neurons supplying C-fiber muscle afferent nerves. Stimulation of TRPA1 in DRG neurons with AITC evokes greater increases in SNA and BP in rats with femoral occlusion. In addition, blocking TRPA1 in muscle afferent nerves significantly attenuates SNA and BP responses evoked by stimulation of metabolically sensitive muscle afferent nerves, but not by stimulation of mechanically sensitive muscle afferent nerves. Overall, our findings suggest that TRPA1 in muscle afferent nerves plays an important role in augmented sympathetic responsiveness via the metabolic component of the exercise pressor reflex when blood supply to the hindlimb muscles is insufficient as observed in PAD.

Grant Support

This study was supported by NIH P01 HL096570 & NIH R01 HL090720 and American Heart Association Established Investigator Award 0840130N.

References

Baccelli, G., Reggiani, P., Mattioli, A., Corbellini, E., Garducci, S., and Catalano, M. (1999). The exercise pressor reflex and changes in radial arterial pressure and heart rate during walking in patients with arteriosclerosis obliterans. *Angiology* 50, 361–374. doi: 10.1177/0003319799050 00502

Baccelli, G., Reggiani, P., Mattioli, A., Corbellini, E., Garducci, S., Catalano, M., et al. (1997). Hemodynamic changes in the lower limbs during treadmill walking in normal subjects and in patients with arteriosclerosis obliterans. *Angiology* 48, 795–803. doi: 10.1177/000331979704800906

Bandell, M., Story, G. M., Hwang, S. W., Viswanath, V., Eid, S. R., Petrus, M. J., et al. (2004). Noxious cold ion channel TRPA1 is activated by pungent compounds and bradykinin. *Neuron* 41, 849–857. doi: 10.1016/S0896-6273(04)00150-3

Bautista, D. M., Jordt, S.-E., Nikai, T., Tsuruda, P. R., Read, A. J., Poblete, J., et al. (2006). TRPA1 mediates the inflammatory actions of environmental irritants and proalgesic agents. *Cell* 124, 1269–1282. doi: 10.1016/j.cell.2006.02.023

Bautista, D. M., Movahed, P., Hinman, A., Axelsson, H. E., Sterner, O., Högestätt, E. D., et al. (2005). Pungent products from garlic activate the sensory ion channel TRPA1. *Proc. Natl. Acad. Sci. U.S.A.* 102, 12248–12252. doi: 10.1073/pnas.0505356102

Bessac, B. F., Sivula, M., Von Hehn, C. A., Escalera, J., Cohn, L., and Jordt, S.-E. (2008). TRPA1 is a major oxidant sensor in murine airway sensory neurons. *J. Clin. Invest.* 118, 1899–1910. doi: 10.1172/JCI34192

Brierley, S. M., Castro, J., Harrington, A. M., Hughes, P. A., Page, A. J., Rychkov, G. Y., et al. (2011). TRPA1 contributes to specific mechanically activated currents and sensory neuron mechanical hypersensitivity. *J. Physiol.* 589, 3575–3593. doi: 10.1113/jphysiol.2011.206789

Cui, J., Mascarenhas, V., Moradkhan, R., Blaha, C., and Sinoway, L. I. (2008). Effects of muscle metabolites on responses of muscle sympathetic nerve activity to mechanoreceptor(s) stimulation in healthy humans. *Am. J. Physiol. Regul. Integr. Comp. Physiol.* 294, R458–R466. doi: 10.1152/ajpregu.00475.2007

Dai, Y., Wang, S., Tominaga, M., Yamamoto, S., Fukuoka, T., Higashi, T., et al. (2007). Sensitization of TRPA1 by PAR2 contributes to the sensation of inflammatory pain.[Erratum appears in J Clin Invest. 2007 Oct; 117(10):3140]. *J. Clin. Invest.* 117, 1979–1987. doi: 10.1172/JCI30951

Everaerts, W., Gees, M., Alpizar, Y. A., Farre, R., Leten, C., Apetrei, A., et al. (2011). The capsaicin receptor TRPV1 is a crucial mediator of the noxious effects of mustard oil. *Curr. Biol.* 21, 316–321. doi: 10.1016/j.cub.2011.01.031

Gao, Z., Koba, S., Sinoway, L., and Li, J. (2008). 20-HETE increases renal sympathetic nerve activity via activation of chemically and mechanically sensitive muscle afferents. *J. Physiol.* 586, 2581–2591. doi: 10.1113/jphysiol.2008.150730

Goodwin, G. M., Mccloskey, D. I., and Mitchell, J. H. (1972). Cardiovascular and respiratory responses to changes in central command during isometric exercise at constant muscle tension. *J. Physiol. (Lond.)* 226, 173–190. doi: 10.1113/jphysiol.1972.sp009979

Jaquemar, D., Schenker, T., and Trueb, B. (1999). An ankyrin-like protein with transmembrane domains is specifically lost after oncogenic transformation of human fibroblasts. *J. Biol. Chem.* 274, 7325–7333. doi: 10.1074/jbc.274.11.7325

Jordt, S.-E., Bautista, D. M., Chuang, H.-H., Mckemy, D. D., Zygmunt, P. M., Högestätt, E. D., et al. (2004). Mustard oils and cannabinoids excite sensory nerve fibres through the TRP channel ANKTM1. *Nature* 427, 260–265. doi: 10.1038/nature02282

Katsura, H., Obata, K., Mizushima, T., Yamanaka, H., Kobayashi, K., Dai, Y., et al. (2006). Antisense knock down of TRPA1, but not TRPM8, alleviates cold hyperalgesia after spinal nerve ligation in rats. *Exp. Neurol.* 200, 112–123. doi: 10.1016/j.expneurol.2006.01.031

Kaufman, M. P., and Forster, H. V. (1996). "Reflexes controlling circulatory, ventilatory and airway responses to exercise. Chapter 10," in *Handbook of Physiology - Section 12, Exercise: Regulation and Integration of Multiple Systems*, eds L. B. Rowell and J. T. Shepherd (New York, NY: Oxford University Press), 381–447.

Kindt, K. S., Viswanath, V., Macpherson, L., Quast, K., Hu, H., Patapoutian, A., et al. (2007). Caenorhabditis elegans TRPA-1 functions in mechanosensation. *Nat. Neurosci.* 10, 568–577. doi: 10.1038/nn1886

Koba, S., Hayes, S. G., and Sinoway, L. I. (2011). Transient receptor potential A1 channel contributes to activation of the muscle reflex. *Am. J. Physiol. Heart Circ. Physiol.* 300, H201–H213. doi: 10.1152/ajpheart.00547.2009

Koba, S., Xing, J., Sinoway, L. I., and Li, J. (2007). Differential sympathetic outflow elicited by active muscle in rats. *Am. J. Physiol. Heart Circ. Physiol.* 293, H2335–H2343. doi: 10.1152/ajpheart.00469.2007

Koizumi, K., Iwasaki, Y., Narukawa, M., Iitsuka, Y., Fukao, T., Seki, T., et al. (2009). Diallyl sulfides in garlic activate both TRPA1 and TRPV1. *Biochem. Biophys. Res. Commun.* 382, 545–548. doi: 10.1016/j.bbrc.2009.03.066

Kwan, K. Y., Allchorne, A. J., Vollrath, M. A., Christensen, A. P., Zhang, D.-S., Woolf, C. J., et al. (2006). TRPA1 contributes to cold, mechanical, and chemical nociception but is not essential for hair-cell transduction. *Neuron* 50, 277–289. doi: 10.1016/j.neuron.2006.03.042

Kwan, K. Y., Glazer, J. M., Corey, D. P., Rice, F. L., and Stucky, C. L. (2009). TRPA1 modulates mechanotransduction in cutaneous sensory neurons. *J. Neurosci.* 29, 4808–4819. doi: 10.1523/JNEUROSCI.5380-08.2009

Leal, A. K., Stone, A. J., Yamauchi, K., Mccord, J. L., and Kaufman, M. P. (2013). Blockade of B2 receptors attenuates the responses of group III afferents to static contraction. *Neurosci. Lett.* 555, 231–236. doi: 10.1016/j.neulet.2013.09.013

Li, J., and Sinoway, L. I. (2002). ATP stimulates chemically sensitive and sensitizes mechanically sensitive afferents. *Am. J. Physiol. Heart Circ. Physiol.* 283, H2636–H2643. doi: 10.1152/ajpheart.00395.2002

Li, J., and Xing, J. (2012). Muscle afferent receptors engaged in augmented sympathetic responsiveness in peripheral artery disease. *Front. Physiol.* 3:247. doi: 10.3389/fphys.2012.00247

Liu, J., Gao, Z., and Li, J. (2010). Femoral artery occlusion increases expression of ASIC3 in dorsal root ganglion neurons. *Am. J. Physiol. Heart Circ. Physiol.* 299, H1357–H1364. doi: 10.1152/ajpheart.00612.2010

Liu, J., Li, J. D., Lu, J., Xing, J., and Li, J. (2011). Contribution of nerve growth factor to upregulation of P2X(3) expression in DRG neurons of rats with femoral artery occlusion. *Am. J. Physiol. Heart Circ. Physiol.* 301, H1070–H1079. doi: 10.1152/ajpheart.00188.2011

Lu, J., Xing, J., and Li, J. (2012). Role for NGF in augmented sympathetic nerve response to activation of mechanically and metabolically sensitive muscle afferents in rats with femoral artery occlusion. *J. Appl. Physiol.* 113, 1311–1322. doi: 10.1152/japplphysiol.00617.2012

Lu, J., Xing, J., and Li, J. (2013). Bradykinin B2 receptor contributes to the exaggerated muscle mechanoreflex in rats with femoral artery occlusion. *Am. J. Physiol. Heart Circ. Physiol.* 304, H1166–H1174. doi: 10.1152/ajpheart.00926.2012

Macpherson, L. J., Dubin, A. E., Evans, M. J., Marr, F., Schultz, P. G., Cravatt, B. F., et al. (2007). Noxious compounds activate TRPA1 ion channels through covalent modification of cysteines. *Nature* 445, 541–545. doi: 10.1038/nature05544

Mark, A. L., Victor, R. G., Nerhed, C., and Wallin, B. G. (1985). Microneurographic studies of the mechanisms of sympathetic nerve responses to static exercise in humans. *Circ. Res.* 57, 461–469. doi: 10.1161/01.RES.57.3.461

Mccloskey, D. I., and Mitchell, J. H. (1972). Reflex cardiovascular and respiratory responses originating in exercising muscle. *J. Physiol.* 224, 173–186. doi: 10.1113/jphysiol.1972.sp009887

Milia, A. F., Salis, M. B., Stacca, T., Pinna, A., Madeddu, P., Trevisani, M., et al. (2002). Protease-activated receptor-2 stimulates angiogenesis and accelerates hemodynamic recovery in a mouse model of hindlimb ischemia. *Circ. Res.* 91, 346–352. doi: 10.1161/01.RES.0000031958.92781.9E

Mitchell, J. H., Kaufman, M. P., and Iwamoto, G. A. (1983). The exercise pressor reflex: its cardiovascular effects, afferent mechanisms, and central pathways. *Annu. Rev. Physiol.* 45, 229–242. doi: 10.1146/annurev.ph.45.030183.001305

Nagata, K., Duggan, A., Kumar, G., and Garcia-Anoveros, J. (2005). Nociceptor and hair cell transducer properties of TRPA1, a channel for pain and hearing. *J. Neurosci.* 25, 4052–4061. doi: 10.1523/JNEUROSCI.0013-05.2005

Obata, K., Katsura, H., Mizushima, T., Yamanaka, H., Kobayashi, K., Dai, Y., et al. (2005). TRPA1 induced in sensory neurons contributes to cold hyperalgesia after inflammation and nerve injury.[Erratum appears in J Clin Invest. 2010 Jan; 120(1):394]. *J. Clin. Invest.* 115, 2393–2401. doi: 10.1172/JCI25437

Ohta, T., Imagawa, T., and Ito, S. (2007). Novel agonistic action of mustard oil on recombinant and endogenous porcine transient receptor potential V1 (pTRPV1) channels. *Biochem. Pharmacol.* 73, 1646–1656. doi: 10.1016/j.bcp.2007.01.029

Okumura, Y., Narukawa, M., Iwasaki, Y., Ishikawa, A., Matsuda, H., Yoshikawa, M., et al. (2010). Activation of TRPV1 and TRPA1 by black pepper components. *Biosci. Biotechnol. Biochem.* 74, 1068–1072. doi: 10.1271/bbb.90964

Pan, H. L., Stebbins, C. L., and Longhurst, J. C. (1993). Bradykinin contributes to the exercise pressor reflex: mechanism of action. *J. Appl. Physiol.* 75, 2061–2068.

Raisinghani, M., Zhong, L., Jeffry, J. A., Bishnoi, M., Pabbidi, R. M., Pimentel, F., et al. (2011). Activation characteristics of transient receptor potential ankyrin 1 and its role in nociception. *Am. J. Physiol. Heart Circ. Physiol.* 301, C587–600. doi: 10.1152/ajpcell.00465.2010

Rejeski, W. J., Tian, L., Liao, Y., and Mcdermott, M. M. (2008). Social cognitive constructs and the promotion of physical activity in patients with peripheral artery disease. *J. Cardiopulm. Rehabil. Prev.* 28, 65–72. doi: 10.1097/01.HCR.0000311512.61967.6e

Sawada, Y., Hosokawa, H., Hori, A., Matsumura, K., and Kobayashi, S. (2007). Cold sensitivity of recombinant TRPA1 channels. *Brain Res.* 1160, 39–46. doi: 10.1016/j.brainres.2007.05.047

Schmidt, M., Dubin, A. E., Petrus, M. J., Earley, T. J., and Patapoutian, A. (2009). Nociceptive signals induce trafficking of TRPA1 to the plasma membrane. *Neuron* 64, 498–509. doi: 10.1016/j.neuron.2009.09.030

Sinoway, L., Prophet, S., Gorman, I., Mosher, T., Shenberger, J., Dolecki, M., et al. (1989). Muscle Acidosis during Static Exercise Is Associated with Calf Vasoconstriction. *J. Appl. Physiol.* 66, 429–436.

Smith, S. A., Mitchell, J. H., and Garry, M. G. (2001). Electrically induced static exercise elicits a pressor response in the decerebrate rat. *J. Physiol.* 537, 961–970. doi: 10.1113/jphysiol.2001.012918

Story, G. M., Peier, A. M., Reeve, A. J., Eid, S. R., Mosbacher, J., Hricik, T. R., et al. (2003). ANKTM1, a TRP-like channel expressed in nociceptive neurons, is activated by cold temperatures. *Cell* 112, 819–829. doi: 10.1016/S0092-8674(03)00158-2

Trevisani, M., Siemens, J., Materazzi, S., Bautista, D. M., Nassini, R., Campi, B., et al. (2007). 4-Hydroxynonenal, an endogenous aldehyde, causes pain and neurogenic inflammation through activation of the irritant receptor TRPA1. *Proc. Natl. Acad. Sci. U.S.A.* 104, 13519–13524. doi: 10.1073/pnas.0705923104

Tsuchimochi, H., Mccord, J. L., Hayes, S. G., Koba, S., and Kaufman, M. P. (2010). Chronic femoral artery occlusion augments exercise pressor reflex in decerebrated rats. *Am. J. Physiol. Heart Circ. Physiol.* 299, H106–H113. doi: 10.1152/ajpheart.00141.2010

Victor, R. G., Bertocci, L. A., Pryor, S. L., and Nunnally, R. (1988). Sympathetic nerve discharge is coupled to muscle cell pH during exercise in humans. *J. Clin. Invest.* 82, 1301–1305. doi: 10.1172/JCI113730

Waldrop, T. G., Eldridge, F. L., Iwamoto, G. A., and Mitchell, J. H. (1996). "Central neural control of respiration and circulation during exercise. Chapter 9," in *Handbook of Physiology - Section 12, Exercise: Regulation and Integration of Multiple Systems*, eds L. B. Rowell and J. T. Shepherd (New York, NY: Oxford University Press), 333–380.

Waters, R. E., Terjung, R. L., Peters, K. G., and Annex, B. H. (2004). Preclinical models of human peripheral arterial occlusive disease: implications for investigation of therapeutic agents. *J. Appl. Physiol.* 97, 773–780. doi: 10.1152/japplphysiol.00107.2004

Xing, J., Gao, Z., Lu, J., Sinoway, L. I., and Li, J. (2008). Femoral artery occlusion augments TRPV1-mediated sympathetic responsiveness. *Am. J. Physiol. Heart Circ. Physiol.* 295, H1262–H1269. doi: 10.1152/ajpheart.00271.2008

Xing, J., Lu, J., and Li, J. (2012). Acid-sensing ion channel subtype 3 function and immunolabelling increases in skeletal muscle sensory neurons following femoral artery occlusion. *J. Physiol.* 590, 1261–1272. doi: 10.1113/jphysiol.2011.221788

Xing, J., Lu, J., and Li, J. (2013). Augmented P2X response and immunolabeling in dorsal root ganglion neurons innervating skeletal muscle following femoral artery occlusion. *J. Neurophysiol.* 109, 2161–2168. doi: 10.1152/jn.01068.2012

Conflict of Interest Statement: The authors declare that the research was conducted in the absence of any commercial or financial relationships that could be construed as a potential conflict of interest.

Gas analyzer's drift leads to systematic error in maximal oxygen uptake and maximal respiratory exchange ratio determination

Ibai Garcia-Tabar[1], Jean P. Eclache[2], José F. Aramendi[1] and Esteban M. Gorostiaga[1]*

[1] *Studies, Research and Sports Medicine Center, Government of Navarre, Pamplona, Spain,* [2] *Laboratory of Performance, Sport-Occupational Activities-Biology-Association, Lyon-Chassieu, France*

The aim was to examine the drift in the measurements of fractional concentration of oxygen (FO_2) and carbon dioxide (FCO_2) of a Nafion-using metabolic cart during incremental maximal exercise in 18 young and 12 elderly males, and to propose a way in which the drift can be corrected. The drift was verified by comparing the pre-test calibration values with the immediate post-test verification values of the calibration gases. The system demonstrated an average downscale drift ($P < 0.001$) in FO_2 and FCO_2 of −0.18% and −0.05%, respectively. Compared with measured values, corrected average maximal oxygen uptakevalues were 5–6% lower ($P < 0.001$) whereas corrected maximal respiratory exchange ratio values were 8–9% higher ($P < 0.001$). The drift was not due to an electronic instability in the analyzers because it was reverted after 20 min of recovery from the end of the exercise. The drift may be related to an incomplete removal of water vapor from the expired gas during transit through the Nafion conducting tube. These data demonstrate the importance of checking FO_2 and FCO_2 values by regular pre-test calibrations and post-test verifications, and also the importance of correcting a possible shift immediately after exercise.

Keywords: exercise testing, maximal oxygen consumption, gas exchange, calibration, verification

Edited by:
Kimberly Huey,
Drake University, USA

Reviewed by:
Kenneth Harrington McKeever,
Rutgers, The State University of
New Jersey, USA
Jordan A. Guenette,
University of British Columbia, Canada

*Correspondence:
Esteban M. Gorostiaga
esteban.gorostiaga.ayestaran@
ofnavarra.oo

INTRODUCTION

Maximal oxygen uptake ($\dot{V}o_{2max}$) is defined as the highest rate at which oxygen can be taken up and utilized by the body during exercise. In laboratory settings, $\dot{V}o_{2max}$ is commonly measured during incremental exercise to exhaustion, during which expired air is analyzed. The key variables needed to calculate $\dot{V}o_{2max}$ are the ventilator flow and the inspired and the expired fractional concentrations of oxygen (F_IO_2 and F_EO_2, respectively) and carbon dioxide (F_ICO_2 and F_ECO_2, respectively) (Hodges et al., 2005; Gore et al., 2013).

One of the main potential sources of error in the calculation of $\dot{V}o_{2max}$ using automated systems is related to the stability of F_EO_2 and F_ECO_2 measurements, because the electronic oxygen (O_2) and carbon dioxide (CO_2) analyzers are prone to drift over time (Winter, 2012; Gore et al., 2013). To our knowledge, there is surprisingly relatively little information available on the stability of O_2 and CO_2 analyzing systems over time during incremental exercise (Hodges et al., 2005; Salier Eriksson et al., 2012). In virtually all the publications that have measured $\dot{V}o_{2max}$, the authors have mentioned performing a pre-test calibration. As it has been pointed out in a recent Editorial (Winter, 2012), in the majority of these studies it is rare to see, however, equivalent post-test verifications. For instance, after reviewing more than 50 studies measuring $\dot{V}_{O2max}$ published between 1973 and 2012, we have found only 8 studies (~16%) in which the authors mentioned that the analyzers' drift at the completion of exercise was assessed (Wilmore et al., 1976; Armstrong and Costill, 1985; Prieur et al., 1998; McLaughlin et al., 2001; Rietjens et al., 2001; Day et al., 2003; Gore et al., 2003; Bowen et al., 2012). Only 4 of these 8 studies reported the average numerical drift values in O_2% and CO_2% (Wilmore et al., 1976; Armstrong and Costill, 1985; Prieur et al., 1998; Rietjens et al., 2001), which ranged from 0.02 to 0.22%. These reported drift values, according to the equations governing gas concentrations (Beaver et al., 1973; Wasserman et al., 1994a), would have caused an error in $\dot{V}_{O2max}$ up to 8–9% in standard laboratory conditions (~20°C of temperature, ~40% of relative humidity and ~720 mmHg of barometric pressure). Furthermore, none of these 4 studies gave any criterion for the maximum drift error that can be accepted. It is still unknown whether the drift magnitude is related to some physical or physiological exercise variables and how long any particular drift remains after the end of exercise. It is also unclear how the drift readings should be adjusted or corrected to overcome the inaccuracy due to the drift (Winter, 2012).

Clearly, it seems that the process of post-test verification tends to be overlooked and there is insufficient data available on how stable specific gas analysis systems are during exercise conditions (Atkinson et al., 2005; Salier Eriksson et al., 2012). This issue may be particularly relevant in several modern analyzers, in which the exhaled gas is not dried but is equilibrated with the laboratory environment by the use of a length of semi-permeable Nafion tubing (Medbø et al., 2002; Larsson et al., 2004). The purpose of the present study was, therefore, to examine the drift over time of a Nafion-using O_2 and CO_2 analyzing system during maximal incremental exercise in experienced athletes and elderly sedentary males. By including sedentary elderly and young athletic subjects, as well as short and long-duration exercise protocols, a large range of metabolic responses and exercise durations were examined and the influence of the drift on oxygen uptake ($\dot{V}_{O2}$), CO_2 output ($\dot{V}_{CO2}$) and respiratory exchange ratio (RER) assessment was determined. This study also proposed a way in which the error might be reduced.

MATERIALS AND METHODS

Subjects

Eighteen male amateur athletes (young group) and twelve older men (elderly group) volunteered to participate in the study. Athletes were recruited from various regional Sports Federations (Swimming, Athletics, Basketball, Basque-Ball, Paddle Tennis, Mountainccring and Climbing, Karate, Taekwondo, Judo, and Boxing). Athletes' mean (± SD) age, height, body mass, and percentage of body fat were 22 ± 6 years, 182 ± 7 cm, 79.3 ± 8.3 kg and 10.4 ± 3.1%, respectively. Participants in the elderly group were recruited from a Physical Activity Program for persons over 55. Mean (± SD) age, height, body mass, and percentage of body fat of the participants constituting the elderly

group were 69 ± 6 years, 167 ± 7 cm, 85.9 ± 13.3 kg and 27.3 ± 4.3%, respectively. A detailed medical history was taken on the day of the study. No subject reported a history of abnormal dyspnea on exertion or of angina.

Written informed consent was obtained from all volunteers prior to their participation. The study was approved by the Institutional Review Committee of the Instituto Navarro del Deporte y Jueventud (Government of Navarre, Spain), according to the requirements of the Declaration of Helsinki.

Exercise Trials

Two different maximal incremental exercise protocols, with different exercise stage duration, were used for each population to examine whether the drift is influenced by the duration of the test. All testing sessions within each group were performed at the same time of the day in an air-controlled and well ventilated laboratory with a volume of 1121 m³. Young and elderly individuals reported to the laboratory at least 2 h after their last meal and having refrained from caffeine, alcohol, and strenuous or non-habitual exercise for 24 h before testing. Participants were habituated to the exercise testing equipment and procedures, as they were previously tested in the same laboratory using similar testing procedures.

Young Exercise Trials

Participants were habituated to the exercise testing equipment and procedures, as they were previously tested in the same laboratory using similar testing procedures. $\dot{V}_{O2max}$ was determined by a continuous maximal graded exercise test while sitting on a mechanically braked cycle-ergometer (Monark, Ergomedic 839-E, Varberg, Sweden). The exercise started at 20 W and the load was increased by 20 W every 2 min until volitional exhaustion. This exercise protocol was designed to reach volitional exhaustion within 23–33 min. It has been shown that relatively short (8–12 min) or long (~30 min) protocols do not affect attainment of $\dot{V}_{O2max}$ in highly motivated athletes (Gore et al., 2013). Participants maintained a constant cycling pedaling cadence of 60 rpm. Exhaustion was defined as the subject not being able to maintain the required pedaling cadence, despite vigorous verbal encouragement during the last min of exercise.

Elderly Exercise Trials

$\dot{V}_{O2max}$ was determined by a continuous incremental maximal exercise test on a treadmill ergometer (Kuntaväline, Hyper Treadmill 2040, Finland). The exercise test started at 5.5 km· h⁻¹, after one min the speed was increased to 6.1 km· h⁻¹ for another min, and thereafter grade was increased 1.1% every min until volitional exertion. Exhaustion was defined as the subjects not being able to maintain the required exercise intensity or they wished to stop.

At least two of the following criteria had to be met to determine $\dot{V}_{O2max}$ in both groups (American College of Sports Medicine, 2009): (1) no increase in $\dot{V}_{O2}$ despite increased workload, defined as a $\dot{V}_{O2}$ increment of less than 120 ml· min⁻¹ per stage in the young group or a $\dot{V}_{O2}$ increment of less than 1.75 ml· kg⁻¹· min⁻¹ per stage in the elderly group. This criterion implies that any increment lower than 50% of the metabolic demand of these protocols' stages was accepted as a $\dot{V}o_2$ plateau (Taylor et al., 1955). (2) A maximal respiratory exchange ratio (RER_{max}) greater than 1.10 (Robergs et al., 2010); (3) peak blood lactate concentration greater than $8\,mmol\cdot L^{-1}$, and (4) peak heart rate exceeding 90% of age predicted maximum (220-age). Heart rate (Polar Electro Oy, RS800CX, Kempele, Finland) was monitored throughout the exercise in both groups. Capillary blood samples from hyperemic earlobe were obtained at rest, on completion of the trial and at the 1st and 3rd min of recovery. After cleaning and puncturing, the single-use enzyme-coated electrode test strip was directly filled by a $5\,\mu l$ whole-blood sample and blood lactate concentration was amperometrically determined (Arkray KDK Corporation, Lactate Pro LT-1710, Shiga, Japan).

Collection of Respiratory Gases

Participants were fitted with an appropriately sized mouth and nasal breathing mask (Series 7930, Hans Rudolph, Kansas City, MO, USA) adjusted with a headgear (Vacu-Med, Ventura, CA, USA). Metabolic data was continuously collected using a Vista Mini-CPX (Vacu-Med, Silver Edition 17670, Ventura, CA, USA) computer-integrated metabolic system. The Vista Mini-CPX is a high precision mass flowmeter instrument composed of a turbine flow sensor and O_2 and CO_2 analyzers designed to measure the flow of the exhaled gases and the concentrations in the O_2 and CO_2 gases on-line. At the start of each test, room temperature ($_RT$), barometric pressure (P_B), and relative room humidity ($_RH$) were measured (Precision Barometer, Lufft, Fellbach, Germany) and these data were entered manually into the computer. The environmental laboratory conditions were kept within the recommended values (18–23°C with a relative humidity lower than 70%) (Gore et al., 2013) by means of a heating system.

Minute expired ventilation ($\dot{V}_E$) is calculated by a signal generated by the volume transducer of the turbine flow sensor. F_EO_2 is measured at $_RH$ through a disposable galvanic fuel cell (Teledyne Analytical Instruments, R-22MED Oxygen Sensor, Industry, CA, USA). F_ECO_2 is measured at $_RH$ through a nondispersive infrared system (Servomex, Ir1507 CO_2 infrared transducer, Crowborough, UK). According to the manufacturer, the CO_2 and O_2 analyzers have zero drift (<1.5 Torr in 1 h for the CO_2 analyzer and 0.3% a week at constant temperature for the O_2 analyzer) and their response times are 90 to 130 ms (CO_2 analyzer) and 5 s (O_2 analyzer). This time delay is automatically assessed and the length of the airline is taken into account according to the manufacturer's specifications. From these measurements the metabolic cart's computer calculates the mass flow of $\dot{V}o_2$ (in liters per minute), $\dot{V}co_2$ (in liters per minute), and the ratio of $\dot{V}o_2$ to $\dot{V}co_2$ (RER) with an accuracy (according to the manufacturer) of ±1% in measures of F_EO_2 and F_ECO_2, of ±2% in measures of $\dot{V}_E$, and of ±3% in measures of $\dot{V}o_2$ and $\dot{V}co_2$.

This metabolic system uses a proportional sampling approach in the process of mixing the exhaled gases. Thus, the flow rate of this sampling is closely related to the flow of exhalation at ~0.5% of its rate, and directs the exhaled gases in three steps

TABLE 1 | Room environmental conditions (mean ± SD) during the exercise and non-exercise trials.

	Young exercise trials (N = 18)	Young non-exercise trials (N = 18)	Elderly exercise trials (N = 12)	Elderly non-exercise trials (N = 12)
Temperature (°C)	21.0 ± 1.2	20.4 ± 0.5	20.4 ± 0.5	20.1 ± 0.3
Humidity (%)	27 ± 6	28 ± 4	28 ± 4	24 ± 1
Pressure (mmHG)	726 ± 5*	716 ± 4	716 ± 4	715 ± 4

*Significantly different from the simulated trials; P < 0.01.

into the O_2 and CO_2 gas analyzers connected in parallel: (1) through a capillary tube, into a miniature mixing chamber, (2) through a built-in Nafion gas dryer humidifier conducting 180 tube (29 cm long × 1 mm inner diameter), and (3) through a capillary tube system with the same configuration of sampling tube length, diameter and pump flow rate for both analyzers. The Nafion tube is a semi-permeable membrane to water vapor made of copolymer of tetrafluoroethylene (Teflon®) and perfluoro-3,6-dioxa-4-methyl-7-octene-sulfonic acid, highly selective in the removal of water from the vapor phase. The Nafion tube allows water vapor to pass in and out of the tube by absorption and conveys the exhaled gases to the gas analyzers once an equilibrium is reached with the ambient humidity (Macfarlane, 2001). According to the Nafion manufacturer, during exercise the water vapor tension of the aspirated gas sample (relative humidity ~100%) (Bageant, 1976; Macfarlane, 2001; Atkinson et al., 2005) is reduced in milliseconds to the level of $_RH$ of the laboratory environment (~27%, **Table 1**) by moving the water through the Nafion membrane wall and evaporating it very quickly into the surrounding air. Conversely, the typically dry calibration gas is humidified by the Nafion tubing to the level of $_RH$. This system provides a constant value of water vapor tension of the exhaled and calibration gases just prior to the entry of the samples into the gas analyzers. The Nafion tube was replaced at least every 3 years according to the manufacturer. All tests were carried out within the 18 months following the last Nafion tube replacement.

The metabolic measurement software supplied with the analyzer (Vacu-Med, TurboFit 5, Ventura, CA, USA) was set to report mean metabolic data over a 30 s time period and to adjust the volume of the expired air to standard conditions (STPD) for temperature (0°C), pressure (760 mmHg), and dry (absence of water vapor). $\dot{V}o_{2max}$ was defined as the highest 30-s $\dot{V}o_2$ value averaged over two consecutive readings, and its time-corresponding values of $\dot{V}co_2$, $\dot{V}_E$ and RER were considered as $\dot{V}co_{2max}$, $\dot{V}_{E_{max}}$, and RER_{max}, respectively.

Pre-test Calibration and Post-test Verification Processes

The instrument was warmed up for at least 2 h prior to every exercise test to minimize any possible electrical drift. Calibration of the O_2 and CO_2 analyzers was performed immediately prior to every test using two-point calibration with two precision-analyzed gas mixtures. One calibration point was room air (O_2:

20.93%; CO_2: 0.00%) Non-hygroscopic soda lime CO_2 absorbent (Vacu-Med, Ventura, CA, USA) was used for maximum precision of ambient CO_2 measurement. Thus, fractional concentrations of room air were assumed to be 20.93% O_2 and 0.00% CO_2. The second point was a high-precision certified calibration tank gas containing 15.05% O_2, 5.99% CO_2 and balanced nitrogen. This high-precision gas was determined gravimetrically, was obtained from a reliable gas supplier (Praxair, Madrid, Spain) and had a claimed accuracy of ±0.02%. Turbine flow calibration was determined using a high-precision 3-L calibration syringe (Vacu-Med, Calibringe 1092, Ventura, CA, USA), in a five-pump series. A series of complete pumps of the syringe and of gas calibrations were repeated until the difference between the current and the previous calibration was less than 0.05 L for volume and less than 0.02% for O_2 and CO_2. When the calibration process was finished, the gas sample line was connected to the subject's mask.

Within 15 s of the completion of each exercise trial the sample line was removed from the connection to the face mask/turbine and the after trial verification of FO_2, FCO_2 and turbine flow measurements was performed. Both calibration gases (room air and tank gas) were run through the metabolic system to check for the drift of the analyzer over the course of the measurement period. Verification readings of the calibration gases and the flow sensor were noted down and compared with the calibration references.

Correction of Metabolic Data

Post-test verifications readings were used to correct the metabolic data measured by the Vista Mini-CPX. Corrected $\dot{V}_E$ ($\dot{V}_{EC}$) in STPD condition was calculated as follows:

$$\dot{V}_{EC} = 3 \cdot \dot{V}_{E_{me}} \cdot [Cal + (Ver - Cal)]^{-1}$$
$$\dot{V}_{EC} = 3 \cdot \dot{V}_{E_{me}} \cdot [Ver]^{-1}$$

where "3" was the volume (L) of the syringe used to calibrate the flow sensor, "$\dot{V}_{E_{me}}$" was the minute ventilation (L· min^{-1}) in STPD condition measured by the metabolic cart, "Cal" was the calibration readout (L) recorded before the exercise and "Ver" was the verification readout (L) recorded after the exercise.

Correction of FO_2 is illustrated in **Figure 1**. During the pre-test calibration process we adjusted the gain settings of the span potentiometers to the corresponding voltage outputs, so that readings of O_2% (tank gas: y_1 = 15.05%; room air: y_2 = 20.93%) equaled real O_2% (x_1 = y_1; x_2 = y_2). The equation of the pre-test calibration regression line is therefore:

$$Y = X$$

During the post-exercise verification process we used the same pre-test calibration gases (x_1 = 15.05% O_2; x_2 = 20.93% O_2), but the %O_2 values read (y'_1 and y'_2) were different from the O_2% read during the pre-test calibration process. In this case, the equation of the post-test verification regression line is:

$$Y = A' \cdot X + B'$$

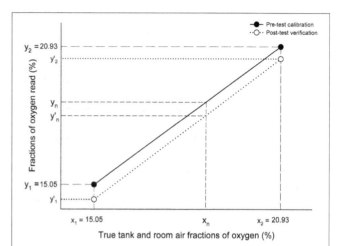

FIGURE 1 | Correction of fractional concentrations of oxygen. x_1 and x_2, true tank (x_1 = 15.05%) and room air (x_2 = 20.93%) fractions of oxygen; y_1 and y_2, fractions of tank (y_1 = 15.05%) and room oxygen (y_2 = 20.93%) read by the analyzer during the pre-test calibration process when the true tank (x_1) and room air (x_2) gases were aspirated by the analyzers; y'_1 and y'_2, fractions of tank (y'_1), and room oxygen (y'_2) read by the oxygen analyzer during the post-test verification process when true tank (x_1) and room air (x_2) gases were aspirated by the analyzers.

Being:

$$A' = (y'_2 - y'_1)/(x_2 - x_1)$$
$$B' = y'_2 - (A' \cdot x_2)$$

For a given value of (y'_n) measured at $\dot{V}o_{2max}$ during exercise, we can calculate the corresponding value of x (x_n) from the equation of the post-test verification line (Y = A'X + B') as follows:

$$y'_n = A' \cdot x_n + B'$$
$$x_n = (y'_n - B')/A'$$

Therefore, the corrected F_EO_2 value at $\dot{V}o_{2max}$ (y'_n) in the pre-test calibration line (Y = X) is:

$$y'_n = x_n$$

F_ECO_2 was corrected using this same procedure. Once the corrected F_EO_2, F_ECO_2, and $\dot{V}_{EC}$ were obtained, formulas provided by the manufacturer [see Beaver et al. (1973) or Wasserman et al. (1994a) for further detail] were employed to correct $\dot{V}o_2$ and $\dot{V}co_2$ as follows:

$$\dot{V}co_2 = (F_ECO_2 - FiCO_2) \cdot \dot{V}_{EC} \cdot HF$$
$$\dot{V}o_2 = [FiO_2 \cdot FeN_2 \cdot (FiN_2)^{-1} - F_EO_2] \cdot \dot{V}_{EC} \cdot HF$$

where $FiCO_2$, FiO_2, and FiN_2 are fractions of inspired carbon dioxide, oxygen and nitrogen respectively, F_ECO_2, F_EO_2, and FeN_2 are fractions of corrected expired carbon dioxide, oxygen and nitrogen respectively, $\dot{V}_{EC}$ is the corrected minute ventilation

(L·min^{-1}) in STPD condition, and HF is the humidity factor defined as:

$$HF = P_B - PH_2O(\text{at } _RT, _R H) \cdot (P_B)^{-1}$$

where P_B is the barometric pressure (mmHg) and PH_2O is the pressure of water (mmHg) at room temperature ($_RT$) and humidity ($_RH$). Standard tables provided by the manufacturer, also presented by Wasserman et al. (1994b), were used to determine PH_2O.

The metabolic system calculates FiN_2 and FeN_2 using the next two formulas:

$$FiN_2 = 0.79 \cdot HF$$
$$FeN_2 = HF - F_EO_2 - F_ECO_2$$

where it is assumed that FiN_2 is constant and FeN_2 is the remaining fractional gas of HF, F_EO_2 and F_ECO_2.

All corrections were performed off-line using specific routines developed in a commercial software package (The MathWorks Inc., MATLAB R2008a, Natick, MA, USA).

Non-exercise Trials

To check the stability of the analyzers, each exercise test was pair-matched on duration, time of the day and number of pre-test calibrations and post-test verifications assessed, with a non-exercise trial, accounting for a total of 30 non-exercise trials (one per subject). These non-exercise trials consisted of performing the identical calibration and verification processes of the gas analyzers over the same time interval to that used during each exercise trial. Between the calibrations and verifications, the metabolic system worked throughout but no subject was connected to the metabolic cart. No flow or volume measures were recorded.

Recovery Trials

The pattern of change in FO_2 and FCO_2 during the first 30 min of recovery after the completion of the exercise trials, and after disconnecting the gas sample line from the mask, was investigated immediately after 9 exercise trials. These recovery trials consisted of performing the post-test verifications of the gas analyzers within 15 s of the completion of each exercise trial, but also at 3, 5, 10, 15, 20, and 30 min of recovery from each exercise trial.

Statistics

Standard statistical methods were used for the calculation of means, standard deviations (SD), standard errors of the estimates (SEE), and confidence intervals (CI). Data were analyzed using parametric statistics following confirmation of normality, homoscedasticity, and when appropriate sphericity. Gas measure readings after the trials (verification readings) were compared with the concentrations of the standard calibration gases (calibration readings) using two-tailed one-sample Student's t-tests. Two-tailed Student's paired t-tests were used to analyze differences between verification readings of the exercise trials

and their paired non-exercise trials, as well as between the non-corrected (measured) and corrected values of the respiratory parameters. Respiratory values of the elderly and young groups were compared by two-tailed independent samples t-tests, with Levene's tests used to assess equality of variances. Relationships between variables of interest were assessed by linear regression analyses. Pearson product-moment correlation coefficients (r) were used to indicate the magnitude and direction of each linear relationship. The slopes of the regression lines in elderly and young groups were compared using analysis of covariance (ANCOVA). Differences between pre- and post-test values in FO_2 and FCO_2 during the recovery period were analyzed using one factor ANOVA with repeated measures. When significance was found, Student's t-test with Bonferroni correction for multiple comparisons was used to locate the significance. Significance was set at $P < 0.05$. Statistical analyses were performed using SPSS 17.0 (SPSS Inc., Chicago, USA). Data in the text, tables and figures are reported as mean $\pm$ SD.

RESULTS

Exercise Trials

As designed, the duration of the young cycling exercise trials ($26:53 \pm 3$ min) was higher ($P < 0.001$) than the duration of the elderly treadmill exercise trials ($9:29 \pm 3$ min). Maximal power output reached by young athletes was 294 ± 34 W (3.74 ± 0.54 W·kg^{-1}). Maximal grade attained by elderly individuals at 6.1 km·h^{-1} was $8.5 \pm 3.9\%$. Young athletes attained significantly higher ($P < 0.001$) peak heart rate and peak blood lactate concentration values (195 ± 11 b·min^{-1} and 10.3 ± 2.2 mmol·L^{-1}) compared to elderly individuals (144 ± 24 b·min^{-1} and 6.6 ± 1.7 mmol·L^{-1}, respectively).

The pre-test calibration and post-test verification values of FO_2 and FCO_2 of the room air and tank gases assessed within 15 s of the completion of each exercise trial in the whole group of subjects are presented in **Table 2**. The system showed a downscale drift ($P < 0.001$) in FO_2 and FCO_2 from pre- to post-test values in the exercise trials. Mean absolute differences between pre- and post test values were -0.18% (room air) and -0.14% (tank gas) in O_2 and 0.00% (room air) and -0.05% (tank gas) in CO_2. Expressed as a percentage of the average pre-test calibration values, the magnitude of the downscale drift was similar ($\sim0.9\%$) in both analyzers. There was no statistical difference ($P = 0.08$; 95% CI: -0.00 to 0.01 L) in the registered air volumes between post-test verification (2.99 ± 0.01 L) and pre-test calibration values (2.99 ± 0.01 L). This means that the calibration factor for ventilation volume was essentially constant throughout the test period.

Figure 2 presents the relationships in the total sample between the individual values of $\dot{V}_{Emax}$ and the individual post-test verification values of FO_2 and FCO_2 of both calibration gases (room air and tank gas). Regression analyses indicated significant negative correlations between $\dot{V}_{Emax}$ and post-test verification values of room air FO_2 in the total sample ($r = -0.48$; $P = 0.007$; SEE = 0.056%; 95% CI: 20.77–20.91%) and in the young group ($r = -0.49$; $P = 0.03$; SEE = 0.057%; 95% CI:

TABLE 2 | Calibration (pre-test) and verification (post-test) readings of the exercise and non-exercise trials.

	Fractional oxygen concentration (%)				Fractional carbon dioxide concentration (%)			
	Room air		Tank gas		Room air		Tank gas	
	Pre	Post	Pre	Post	Pre	Post	Pre	Post
EXERCISE TRIALS, N = 30								
Mean	20.93	20.75**	15.05	14.91**	0.00	0.00**	5.99	5.94**
SD	N/A	0.06	N/A	0.07	N/A	0.01	N/A	0.02
RANGE								
Min	N/A	20.61	N/A	14.82	N/A	0.00	N/A	5.89
Max	N/A	20.91	N/A	15.05	N/A	0.02	N/A	5.97
NON-EXERCISE TRIALS, N = 30								
Mean	20.93	20.93††	15.05	15.05††	0.00	0.01*†	5.99	6.00*††
SD	N/A	0.01	N/A	0.01	N/A	0.01	N/A	0.01
RANGE								
Min	N/A	20.90	N/A	15.03	N/A	0.00	N/A	5.99
Max	N/A	20.95	N/A	15.07	N/A	0.02	N/A	6.02

Pre, pre-test calibration readings; Post, post-test verification readings.
*Significantly different from Pre: *$P < 0.01$, **$P < 0.001$.*
Significantly different from the exercise trials: †$P < 0.01$, ††$P < 0.001$.

20.75–21.04%). The gradients of the rest of the relationships presented in **Figure 2** were not different from zero ($P < 0.05$). According to the ANCOVA results, the slopes of the regression lines were not different among groups ($P > 0.05$). No significant relationships were observed between test duration and post-test verification values of FO_2 and FCO_2 ($P > 0.05$). No other relevant significance was found between respiratory parameters and post-trial readings.

Non-exercise Trials

During the non-exercise trials, the drift over time in the electronic gas analysis system was minimal because FO_2 and FCO_2 remained very stable throughout the time (**Table 2**). The highest individual difference in the post-test verification during the non-exercise trials was only of 0.03% in FO_2 and of 0.02% in FCO_2.

Measured and Corrected Respiratory Values

Measured F_EO_2 values reached at $\dot{V}_{O_{2max}}$ during exercise by the young and elderly groups were 17.39 ± 0.29% and 17.18 ± 0.52%, respectively. When these values were corrected with the proposed correction equation, the corresponding F_EO_2 values at $\dot{V}_{O_{2max}}$ were 17.54 ± 0.32% and 17.32 ± 0.53% for the young and elderly groups, respectively. Measured F_ECO_2 values reached at $\dot{V}_{O_{2max}}$ by the young and elderly groups were 3.77 ± 0.28% and 4.00 ± 0.51%, respectively. When these values were corrected, the corresponding F_ECO_2 values at $\dot{V}_{O_{2max}}$ were 3.80 ± 0.29% and 4.03 ± 0.50% for the young and elderly groups, respectively. Inasmuch as no drift was observed in the calibration factor for ventilation volume during exercise, there were no differences between corrected and measured values of $\dot{V}_{E_{max}}$ in any of the groups ($P > 0.05$). Average $\dot{V}_{E_{max}}$ was 88% higher ($P < 0.001$;

95% CI 49 to 80 L·min^{-1}) in the young group compared with the elderly group (137 vs. 73 L·min^{-1}).

The corrected F_EO_2 and F_ECO_2 values resulted in systematic significant changes in $\dot{V}_{CO_{2max}}$ and $\dot{V}_{O_{2max}}$ values. Measured $\dot{V}_{CO_{2max}}$ values reached by the young and elderly groups were 4.93 ± 0.57 L·min^{-1} and 2.82 ± 0.61% L·min^{-1}, respectively. When these values were corrected, the average $\dot{V}_{CO_{2max}}$ values (5.07 ± 0.59 L·min^{-1} and 2.98 ± 0.62 L·min^{-1} for the young and elderly groups respectively) were 3–5% higher ($P < 0.001$) than the corresponding measured values. The measured average $\dot{V}_{O_{2max}}$ values in the young and elderly groups were 4.64 ± 0.56 L·min^{-1} and 2.62 ± 0.50 L·min^{-1}, respectively. Corrected average $\dot{V}_{O_{2max}}$ values (4.35 ± 0.46 and 2.50 ± 0.47 L·min^{-1} for the young and elderly groups, respectively) were 5–6% lower ($P < 0.001$) than the corresponding measured values. The individual overestimation of the measured $\dot{V}_{O_{2max}}$ values ranged from 0.3 to 11%. **Figure 3A** shows the average and the individual measured and corrected $\dot{V}_{O_{2max}}$ values, expressed relative to kilogram of body mass, in the young and elderly subjects. Average corrected $\dot{V}_{O_{2max}}$ values were 3.6 ml·kg^{-1}·min^{-1} (young) and 1.4 ml·kg^{-1}·min^{-1} (elderly) lower ($P < 0.001$) than the average measured $\dot{V}_{O_{2max}}$ values. In every subject, the corrected $\dot{V}_{O_{2max}}$ value was lower than the measured value.

Figure 3B shows the average and the individual measured and corrected RER$_{max}$ values in the young and elderly subjects. The average measured RER$_{max}$ values were 1.06 ± 0.05 in the young group and 1.07 ± 0.05 in the elderly group. When these values were corrected, the average RER$_{max}$ values (1.16 ± 0.06 and 1.15 ± 0.06 for the young and elderly groups, respectively) were 8–9% higher ($P < 0.001$) than the corresponding measured values. In every subject, the corrected RER$_{max}$ value was higher than the measured value.

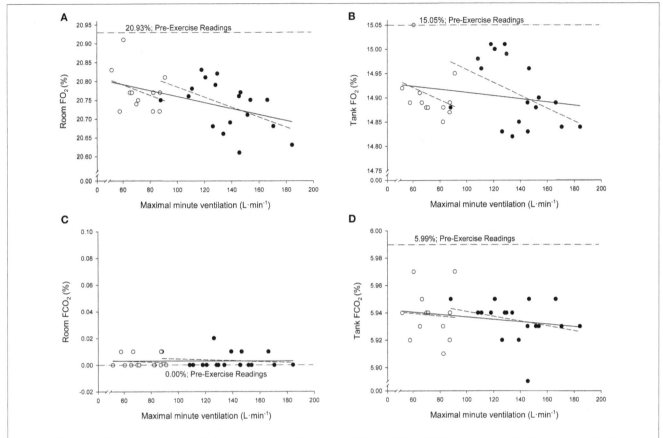

FIGURE 2 | Relationships between the individual values of maximal minute ventilation and the individual post-test verification values of fractional concentrations of oxygen (FO_2; A,B) and carbon dioxide (FCO_2; C,D) when both calibration gases (room air and tank gas) were run through the metabolic system after maximal exercise. Open circles: elderly sedentary subjects. Filled circles: young athletes.

When the measured values were taken into account, 14 out of the 18 young subjects (78%) and 9 out of the 12 old subjects (75%) satisfied at least two of the criteria established to verify attainment of $\dot{V}o_{2max}$. When the RER_{max} and the $\dot{V}o_{2max}$ values were corrected, the ratio of the subjects who met these criteria increased to 89 and 83% in the young and elderly groups respectively.

Recovery Trials

Figure 4 shows the average and individual FO_2 changes observed in 9 subjects when the post-test verification process was repeated several times during the first 30 min of recovery after the completion of the exercise trials, and after disconnecting the gas sample line from the subjects' mask. During the first 5 min of recovery the average FO_2 remained similar to the significantly diminished values ($P < 0.001$) read immediately after the end of the exercise trials. From that time on, the FO_2 reading values increased progressively and linearly over the time. The disappearance of the drift was completed after 20 min of recovery, although at this time the average FO_2 readings still tended to be slightly lower than the pre-test calibration values ($P = 0.20$). Similar patterns were observed for the time course of FCO_2 changes (data not shown).

DISCUSSION

The main finding of this study is that the pre-test calibration and the post-test verification values of O_2 and CO_2 demonstrated a downscale drift in the O_2 and CO_2 readings. The drift was observed in all the exercise tests and was higher than the absolute accuracy of at least $\pm0.03\%$ (Gore et al., 2013) and $\pm0.05\%$ (Jones, 1988) that laboratories should strive to attain for electronic O_2 and CO_2 analyzers. This indicates that the present metabolic system systematically underestimates F_EO_2 and F_ECO_2 values during maximal exercise.

Several potential sources of error, working separately or together, could explain the F_EO_2 and F_ECO_2 downscale drifts during maximal exercise (Robergs et al., 2010). One potential source of error may be due to an electrical instability in the analyzers over time (Kannagi et al., 1983). Evidence of this mechanism, however, has not been provided. When a series of calibrations were assessed during the non-exercise pair-matched trials without any subject being connected to the metabolic system, the O_2 and CO_2 readings remained unchanged over the course of the period (**Table 2**). This suggests that no baseline drift of the analyzers occurred due to an electronic error,

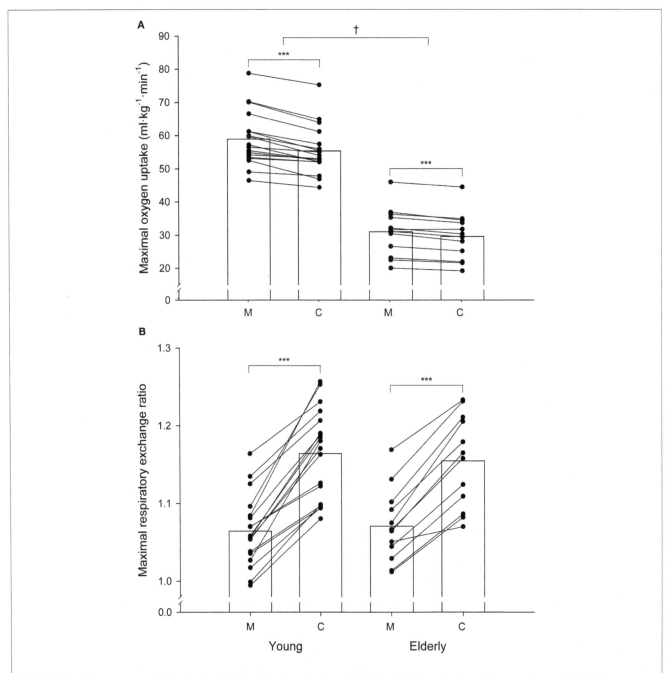

FIGURE 3 | Individual measured (M) and corrected (C) values of maximal oxygen uptake (A) and maximal respiratory exchange ratio (B) in the young and elderly groups. Maximal oxygen uptake is expressed in ml·kg·min^{-1}. The *bars* indicate mean values. ***Significant difference between the corrected and the corresponding measured values ($P < 0.001$). †Significant difference between groups ($P < 0.05$).

indicating that the analyzers were electrically stable for a long period of time.

The most likely factor explaining the reduction in O_2 and CO_2 percentages may be associated with how water vapor is handled in the aspirated gas by the analyser. The metabolic system used in the present study sends the exhaled gas to the O_2 and CO_2 gas analyzers through a built-in Nafion gas dryer humidifier conducting tube. This tube provides a constant value of water vapor tension of the exhaled and the calibration gases just prior to the entry of the samples into the gas analyzers. It is possible that the observed downscale drift could be partly explained by an incomplete removal of the water vapor tension of the aspirated gas by the analyser to equilibrate the partial water vapor pressure (PH_2O) into and out of the Nafion tube wall. Since the O_2 and CO_2 analyzers are partial pressure sensors that measure gas fractions of the total gas volume including water vapor, and

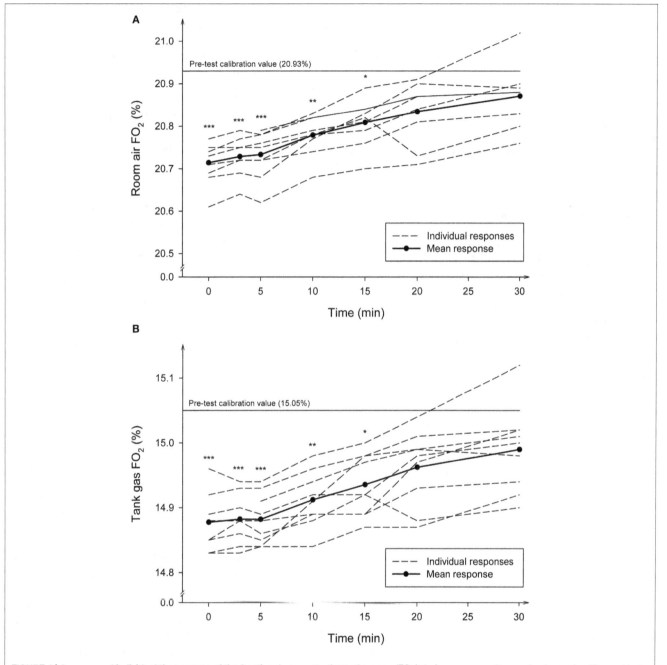

FIGURE 4 | Average and individual time course of the fractional concentrations of oxygen (FO₂) during recovery after maximal exercise. The post-test verification values read by the gas analyzers using the room air **(A)** and the tank gas **(B)** were measured at 20 s, 3, 5, 10, 15, 20, and 30 min of recovery. The number of observations made at each time-point was 9. ***Significantly different from pre-test ($P < 0.001$); **Significantly different from pre-test ($P < 0.01$); *Significantly different form pre-test ($P < 0.05$).

they are sensitive to the presence of water vapor molecules, the passage of excessive water vapor to the gas analyzers could raise the PH_2O of the sample. A rise in PH_2O would reduce O_2 and CO_2 fractions by the factor $[(P_B - PH_2O \text{ excess}) \cdot (P_B)^{-1}]$ or $[(1 - FH_2O)]$ (Gore et al., 2013) and the analyzer would read lower concentration values (Auchincloss et al., 1970). The observation that the O_2 and CO_2 drifts were almost completely reversed in a few min after exercise by simply disconnecting the

sampling line from the flow-meter and the subject's mask, and by flushing the system with room air (**Figure 4**), supports the notion that some failure in the drying process occurred during exercise.

Under the assumption of an incomplete removal of the water vapor, it is possible to estimate the average extra amount of PH_2O at a given temperature that was not removed by the Nafion tube to equilibrate the aspirated gas by the analyzers to the level of ambient humidity during exercise. This can be calculated from the average drift values observed in the O_2 (from 20.93 to 20.75% and from 15.05 to 14.91%) and CO_2 analyzers (from 5.99 to 5.94%) (**Table 2**) using the following formula (Bageant, 1976; Gore et al., 2013):

$$\text{Read } O_2\% = [\text{True } O_2\% \cdot (P_B - PH_2O)] \cdot (P_B)^{-1}$$

where read $O_2\%$ is the oxygen percentage read during the post-test verification, true $O_2\%$ is the oxygen percentage read during the pre-test calibration, and P_B is ambient barometric pressure (in our case: ~724 mmHg).

In that case, the estimated average PH_2O that could not be removed was 6.2 mmHg (range 0.7–11 mmHg) for the O_2 calibration with room air, 6.7 mmHg (range: 0–11 mmHg) for the O_2 calibration with the tank, and 6.0 mmHg (range: 2.4–12.1 mmHg) for the CO_2 calibration with the tank. Inasmuch as the PH_2O of the exhaled gas leaving the body is ~47 mmHg (on the basis of ~100% of relative humidity, at body temperature) (Bageant, 1976), an incomplete average removal of around 6.3 mmHg of water vapor corresponds to ~13% of excess in relative humidity ($6.3 \cdot 100 \cdot 47^{-1}$) that cannot be cleared from the circuit, with individual values ranging from 2 to 24%.

The reason why the Nafion tube could not fully equilibrate the gas being conveyed to the analyzers with the ambient humidity is unknown. However it can be related to:

(1) A saturation process that reduces active surface area in the Nafion tubing. It is known that some saturation process occurs in the Nafion tubing since the wall of the tubing always retains some residual water, because the sulphonic acid groups within the Nafion polymer will never give up all their water (Mauritz and Moore, 2004). When the dryer becomes progressively physically wet over time, a failure to dry occurs. This failure to dry may be more relevant when the exhaled air flow is high and, therefore, when the aspirated gas sample's flow rate (0.5% of the exhaled flow rate) and its water vapor content are high. For example, in the young exercise trials the amount of water vapor content to be removed out of the Nafion tube can be 16 times higher at maximal exercise (exhaled flow gas: 190 L·min^{-1}; aspired gas: 950 ml·min^{-1}) than at rest (exhaled flow gas: 12 L·min^{-1}; aspired gas: 60 ml·min^{-1}). This is in agreement with the significant linear negative correlation observed in this study between $\dot{V}_{E_{max}}$ and the magnitude of the drift in FO_2 (**Figure 2**). This strongly suggests that the higher the $\dot{V}_E$ and the amount of water vapor to be removed, the higher the absolute magnitude of the drift.

(2) The inability of the system to maintain a very low water pressure outside, in the air surrounding the Nafion tube wall. An excess of condensate water vapor may be surrounding the Nafion tube as a consequence of the release of the excess of moisture out of the tube. This process may be more pronounced when the Nafion tube is located inside the metabolic measurement cart, such as in the metabolic system used in this study. In such a case, the fan of the metabolic cart cannot remove this excess water vapor condensed inside the metabolic cart.

(3) Factors like the accumulation of sweat, saliva, foreign bodies and condensation generated by the subject can enter the internal lumen of the sampling line; a portion of exhaled air is drawn and, therefore, a change in the resistance of the delivery tubing or in the gas sampling rate can occur. This could contribute to a decrease in the gas flow rate and pressure in the sampling tube, leading to irregular results (Atkinson et al., 2005; Gore et al., 2013).

The present results support the above theoretical possibilities that cause an incomplete removal of water vapor of the aspired gas transported from the mouth to the analyzers before the gas enters the analyzers. This would explain the significant downscale drift in the O_2 and CO_2 analyzers that occurs during continuous measurement during human exercise.

The practical question to consider is the influence of the analyzers' drifts on $\dot{V}_{O_{2max}}$. The correction used for the difference between the pre- and post-test conditions indicated that the corrected $\dot{V}_{O_{2max}}$ values were on average 3.6 ml·kg^{-1}·min^{-1} (young subjects) and 1.4 ml·kg^{-1}·min^{-1} (older subjects) lower than those of the measured values. When expressed relative to the individual $\dot{V}_{O_{2max}}$ values, the average difference between the measured and the corrected $\dot{V}_{O_{2max}}$ values was similar (5–6%) in the young and the elderly subjects. This suggests that, in relative terms, there is a systematic and considerable overestimation in the measurement of $\dot{V}_{O_{2max}}$ that is uniform over a full range of $\dot{V}_{O_{2max}}$ values regardless of exercise duration. The average technological error of 5–6% may be considered unacceptable because it is larger than the ±0.5 to ±3% (technological error) or the ±2.2 to ±4% (technological plus biological variation) accuracy standards accepted for the precision of $\dot{V}_{O_{2max}}$ measurement by most certifying organizations that supervise the accreditation process of the metabolic systems (American Thoracic Society, 1987; Gore et al., 2013). The present results may explain, at least partly, the reason why a measurement error of 5% in $\dot{V}_{O_{2max}}$ between laboratories and metabolic systems is nowadays a difficult goal to achieve, owing to the combined technical error and the biological variation (Hodges et al., 2005).

A question raised is the comparison of the corrected $\dot{V}_{O_{2max}}$ and RER_{max} data with published values. When compared to the measured values, the average corrected $\dot{V}_{O_{2max}}$ values in the elderly group (29.6 ml·kg^{-1}·min^{-1}) and the average corrected $\dot{V}_{O_{2max}}$-to cycling work rate values in the young group (14.7 ml O_2·W^{-1}) are lower than the measured values (31.0 ml·kg^{-1}·min^{-1} and 15.7 ml O_2·W^{-1}), and compare favorably with those estimated for the elderly group (29.5 ml·kg^{-1}·min^{-1}) using the formula of the American College of Sports Medicine (2009) and with the average ratio (14.1 ml O_2·W^{-1}; range: 12.1–18.6) reported by other investigators using different metabolic systems during long duration (15–27 min) incremental maximal cycling tests (Pollock et al., 1982; Armstrong and Costill, 1985; Storer et al., 1990; American College of Sports Medicine, 2009; Bowen et al., 2012; Petot et al., 2012; Adami et al., 2013). The average corrected RER_{max} was 9% higher than the measured RER_{max} in the young group (1.16 vs. 1.06) and 8% higher in the elderly group (1.15 vs. 1.07). When RER_{max} values were not corrected, only 17% of the young and

25% of the elderly subjects reached a RER_{max} greater than 1.10, the most widely used secondary criterion to verify attainment of $\dot{V}_{O2max}$ (Howley et al., 1995; American College of Sports Medicine, 2009). A major effect of correcting the RER_{max} values was that the ratio of the subjects reaching a RER_{max} greater than 1.10 was increased to 72% in the young group and to 75% in the elderly group. The difference between the corrected and measured RER_{max} values suggests that some inconsistencies and failures found in several studies to satisfy RER_{max} criterion for achievement of $\dot{V}_{O2max}$ may be largely due to an artifact related to technological error (Bowen et al., 2012). This indicates that correction of $\dot{V}_{O2max}$ and RER_{max} values, on the basis of the F_EO_2 and F_ECO_2 drifts observed, produced more reasonable and satisfactory values than the measured ones.

This study has several limitations. The major drawback comes from the fact that we did not corroborate the validity of the correction method suggested. There is also a lack of consensus on which method is the most appropriate to assess the reliability and validity of $\dot{V}_{O2}$ measures (Salier Eriksson et al., 2012). The conventional Douglas bag procedure has been regarded as the gold standard method to validate metabolic measurement systems (McLaughlin et al., 2001; Rietjens et al., 2001). This method remains, however, very limited (Salier Eriksson et al., 2012). In any case, in close agreement with our corrected values, Medbø et al. (2002) and Larsson et al. (2004) found that a commercial metabolic system (Metamax II), utilizing a built-in Nafion conducting tube, significantly overestimated $\dot{V}_{O2}$ by 4–13% and underestimated RER by 6% compared to the Douglas bag method. However, other validation studies have produced more varied results (Versteeg and Kippersluis, 1989; Bassett et al., 2001; McLaughlin et al., 2001). An alternative method to validate $\dot{V}_{O2}$ and RER measures is to use a metabolic calibrator system. However, the external validity of such a test is limited since it often uses dry gases and does not involve challenging factors such as humidified gases and irregular breathing patterns (Macfarlane, 2001). In the absence of a reliable gold standard method, the rationale for the analyzer's drift correction method used in this study is that the time point at $\dot{V}_{O2max}$, which was reached close to the end of the test, is close to the time point at which the post-test verification was undertaken (within 15 sec of the end of each test). It seems, therefore, justifiable to remove and correct the variations observed in F_EO_2 and F_ECO_2 at $\dot{V}_{O2max}$ by adjusting the analyzer pre-exercise base-line values to the post-exercise verification values.

Another limitation of this study is that we used a single metabolic system. Therefore, the generalizability of our findings is constrained to the metabolic cart and the analyzers used. However, four studies reporting the average numerical downscale drifts in O_2 immediately after exercise using other metabolic systems have found values ranging from −0.02 to −0.22% (Wilmore et al., 1976; Armstrong and Costill, 1985; Prieur et al., 1998; Rietjens et al., 2001). This indicates that an absolute downscale drift also occurs in other metabolic systems. If the main source of the error is related to the built-in Nafion gas dryer humidifier conducting tube, a lower error (or none) should occur when gas fractions are measured as fractions of dry gas, when ambient relative humidity is higher than in the present study (e.g., 60%) or when the condensate water vapor surrounding the Nafion tube is more efficiently removed. A wider study is needed to extend the present findings to the wide metabolic systems' population.

CONCLUSION AND PERSPECTIVES

In conclusion, the present experiment indicates that, under controlled laboratory conditions, a physiologically significant downscale drift in FO_2 and FCO_2 was observed over time at the end of maximal exercise in elderly sedentary and young athletes using a metabolic cart equipped with a built-in Nafion conducting tube. The most likely explanation for the drift is an accumulation of excess water vapor in the sample line which could not be completely removed during transit through the Nafion conducting tube. The correction method proposed indicates that ignoring the effects of the drift would induce an average $\dot{V}_{O2max}$ overestimation of 5–6% and a RER_{max} underestimation of 8–9%, with errors ranging up to 11–12% ($\dot{V}_{O2max}$) and up to 15–16% (RER_{max}). Therefore, ignoring the drift can have an important influence on the accurate calculation of these variables. The disagreement between the measured and the corrected $\dot{V}_{O2max}$ and RER_{max} values observed in this particular metabolic system is not acceptable to test athletes, to prescribe exercise intensities, to calculate the fat oxidation rate from RER values, or to use the respiratory values for some other clinical purposes, such as to guide treatment in patients with chronic heart failure (Bowen et al., 2012), to enter in cardiac transplantation listing, to indicate the health status or to predict prognosis and mortality (Myers et al., 2002; Mehra et al., 2006). The implications of the present study point to the necessity to check FO_2 and FCO_2 values by carefully calibrating the pre-test calibration gases and verifying a possible shift immediately after exercise, as well as to correct the respiratory data in situations where the drift in O_2 and CO_2 analyzers occurs. Special care must be taken in studies where a Nafion conducting tube is used. Further research in this area is certainly warranted to establish valid correction factors for each device.

AUTHOR CONTRIBUTIONS

EG, IG, and JE conceived and designed the experiments; EG, IG, and JA contributed to the acquisition and analysis of the data; EG, IG, JE, and JA interpreted the data; EG wrote the first draft; EG, IG, JE, and JA critically reviewed and edited the drafts; all authors approved the final version of the manuscript.

ACKNOWLEDGMENTS

We gratefully thank Irene Madariaga for her professional assistance in exercise testing.

REFERENCES

Adami, A., Sivieri, A., Moia, C., Perini, R., and Ferretti, G. (2013). Effects of step duration in incremental ramp protocols on peak power and maximal oxygen consumption. *Eur. J. Appl. Physiol.* 113, 2647–2653. doi: 10.1007/s00421-013-2705-9

American College of Sports Medicine (2009). *ACSM's Guidelines for Exercise Testing and Prescription.* Philadelphia, PA: Lippincott Williams & Wilkins.

American Thoracic Society (1987). Standardization of spirometry: 1987 update. statement of the american thoraccic society. *Am. Rev. Respir. Dis.* 136, 1285–1298. doi: 10.1164/ajrccm/136.5.1285

Armstrong, L. E., and Costill, D. L. (1985). Variability of respiration and metabolism: responses to submaximal cycling and running. *Res. Q. Exerc. Sport* 56, 93–96. doi: 10.1080/02701367.1985.10608441

Atkinson, G., Davison, R. C., and Nevill, A. M. (2005). Performance characteristics of gas analysis systems: what we know and what we need to know. *Int. J. Sports Med.* 26(Suppl. 1), S2–S10. doi: 10.1055/s-2004-830505

Auchincloss, J. H. Jr., Gilbert, R., and Baule, G. H. (1970). Control of water vapor during rapid analysis of respiratory gases in expired air. *J. Appl. Physiol.* 28, 245–247.

Bageant, R. A. (1976). Oxygen analyzers. *Respir Care.* 21, 410–416.

Bassett, D. R. Jr., Howley, E. T., Thompson, D. L., King, G. A., Strath, S. J., McLaughlin, J. E., et al. (2001). Validity of inspiratory and expiratory methods of measuring gas exchange with a computerized system. *J. Appl Physiol. (1985).* 91, 218–224. Available online at: http://jap.physiology.org/content/91/1/218.full-text.pdf+html

Beaver, W. L., Wasserman, K., and Whipp, B. J. (1973). On-line computer analysis and breath-by-breath graphical display of exercise function tests. *J. Appl. Physiol.* 34, 128–132.

Bowen, T. S., Cannon, D. T., Begg, G., Baliga, V., Witte, K. K., and Rossiter, H. B. (2012). A novel cardiopulmonary exercise test protocol and criterion to determine maximal oxygen uptake in chronic heart failure. *J. Appl. Physiol. (1985).* 113, 451–458. doi: 10.1152/japplphysiol.01416.2011

Day, J. R., Rossiter, H. B., Coats, E. M., Skasick, A., and Whipp, B. J. (2003). The maximally attainable VO2 during exercise in humans: the peak vs. maximum issue. *J. Appl. Physiol. (1985).* 95, 1901–1907. doi: 10.1152/japplphysiol.00024.2003

Gore, C. J., Clark, R. J., Shipp, N. J., Van der Ploeg, G. E., and Withers, R. T. (2003). CPX/D underestimates VO(2) in athletes compared with an automated Douglas bag system. *Med. Sci. Sports Exerc.* 35, 1341–1347. doi: 10.1249/01.MSS.0000079045.86512.C5

Gore, C. J., Tanner, R. K., Fuller, K. L., and Stanef, F. (2013). "Determination of maximal oxygen consumption (VO2max)," in *Physiological Tests for Elite Athletes,* eds R. K. Tanner and C. J. Gore (Champaign, IL: Human Kinetics), 103–122.

Hodges, L. D., Brodie, D. A., and Bromley, P. D. (2005). Validity and reliability of selected commercially available metabolic analyzer systems. *Scand. J. Med. Sci. Sports* 15, 271–279. doi: 10.1111/j.1600-0838.2005.00477.x

Howley, E. T., Bassett, D. R. Jr., and Welch, H. G. (1995). Criteria for maximal oxygen uptake: review and commentary. *Med. Sci. Sports Exerc.* 27, 1292–1301. doi: 10.1249/00005768-199509000-00009

Jones, N. L. (1988). *Clinical Exercise Testing.* Philadelphia, PA: W.B. Saunders.

Kannagi, T., Bruce, R. A., Hossack, K. F., Chang, K., Kusumi, F., and Trimble, S. (1983). An evaluation of the Beckman Metabolic Cart for measuring ventilation and aerobic requirements during exercise. *J. Cardiac. Rehabil.* 3, 38–53.

Larsson, P. U., Wadell, K. M., Jakobsson, E. J., Burlin, L. U., and Henriksson-Larsén, K. B. (2004). Validation of the MetaMax II portable metabolic measurement system. *Int. J. Sports Med.* 25, 115–123. doi: 10.1055/s-2004-819953

Macfarlane, D. J. (2001). Automated metabolic gas analysis systems: a review. *Sports Med.* 31, 841–861. doi: 10.2165/00007256-200131120-00002

Mauritz, K. A., and Moore, R. B. (2004). State of understanding of nafion. *Chem. Rev.* 104, 4535–4585. doi: 10.1021/cr0207123

McLaughlin, J. E., King, G. A., Howley, E. T., Bassett, D. R. Jr., and Ainsworth, B. E. (2001). Validation of the COSMED K4 b2 portable metabolic system. *Int. J. Sports Med.* 22, 280–284. doi: 10.1055/s-2001-13816

Medbø, J. I., Mamen, A., Welde, B., von Heimburg, E., and Stokke, R. (2002). Examination of the Metamax I and II oxygen analysers during exercise

studies in the laboratory. *Scand. J. Clin. Lab. Invest.* 62, 585–598. doi: 10.1080/003655102764654321

Mehra, M. R., Kobashigawa, J., Starling, R., Russell, S., Uber, P. A., Parameshwar, J., et al. (2006). Listing criteria for heart transplantation: international Society for Heart and Lung Transplantation guidelines for the care of cardiac transplant candidates–2006. *J. Heart. Lung. Transplant.* 25, 1024–1042. doi: 10.1016/j.healun.2006.06.008

Myers, J., Prakash, M., Froelicher, V., Do, D., Partington, S., and Atwood, J. E. (2002). Exercise capacity and mortality among men referred for exercise testing. *N. Engl. J. Med.* 346, 793–801. doi: 10.1056/NEJMoa011858

Petot, H., Meilland, R., Le Moyec, L., Mille-Hamard, L., and Billat, V. L. (2012). A new incremental test for VO(2)max accurate measurement by increasing VO(2)max plateau duration, allowing the investigation of its limiting factors. *Eur. J. Appl. Physiol.* 112, 2267–2276. doi: 10.1007/s00421-011-2196-5

Pollock, M. L., Foster, C., Schmidt, D., Hellman, C., Linnerud, A. C., and Ward, A. (1982). Comparative analysis of physiologic responses to three different maximal graded exercise test protocols in healthy women. *Am. Heart J.* 103, 363–373. doi: 10.1016/0002-8703(82)90275-7

Prieur, F., Busso, T., Castells, J., Bonnefoy, R., Benoit, H., Geyssant, A., et al. (1998). Validity of oxygen uptake measurements during exercise under moderate hyperoxia. *Med. Sci.Sports Exerc.* 30, 958–962. doi: 10.1097/00005768-199806000-00028

Rietjens, G. J., Kuipers, H., Kester, A. D., and Keizer, H. A. (2001). Validation of a computerized metabolic measurement system (Oxycon-Pro) during low and high intensity exercise. *Int. J. Sports Med.* 22, 291–294. doi: 10.1055/s-2001-14342

Roberts, R. A., Dwyer, D., and Astorino, T. (2010). Recommendations for improved data processing from expired gas analysis indirect calorimetry. *Sports Med.* 40, 95–111. doi: 10.2165/11319670-000000000-00000

Salier Eriksson, J., Rosdahl, H., and Schantz, P. (2012). Validity of the Oxycon Mobile metabolic system under field measuring conditions. *Eur. J. Appl. Physiol.* 112, 345–355. doi: 10.1007/s00421-011-1985-1

Storer, T. W., Davis, J. A., and Caiozzo, V. J. (1990). Accurate prediction of VO2max in cycle ergometry. *Med. Sci. Sports Exerc.* 22, 704–712 doi: 10.1249/00005768-199010000-00024

Taylor, H. L., Buskirk, E., and Henschel, A. (1955). Maximal oxygen intake as an objective measure of cardio-respiratory performance. *J. Appl. Physiol.* 8, 73–80.

Versteeg, P. G., and Kippersluis, G. J. (1989). Automated systems for measurement of oxygen uptake during exercise testing. *Int. J. Sports Med.* 10, 107–112. doi: 10.1055/s-2007-1024884

Wasserman, K., Hansen, J. E., Sue, D. Y., Whipp, B. J., and Casaburi, R. (1994a). "Appendix D. Calculations, formulas, and examples," in *Principles of Exercise Testing and Interpretation,* eds K. Wasserman, J. E. Hansen, D. Y. Sue, B. J. Whipp, and R. Casaburi (Philadelphia, PA: Williams & Wilkins), 454–464.

Wasserman, K., Hansen, J. E., Sue, D. Y., Whipp, B. J., and Casaburi, R. (1994b). "Appendix F. Tables and nomogram," in *Principles of Exercise Testing and Interpretation,* eds K. Wasserman, J. E. Hansen, D. Y. Sue, B. J. Whipp, and R. Casaburi (Philadelphia, PA: Williams & Wilkins), 468–470.

Wilmore, J. H., Davis, J. A., and Norton, A. C. (1976). An automated system for assessing metabolic and respiratory function during exercise. *J. Appl. Physiol.* 40, 619–624.

Winter, E. M. (2012). Calibration and verification of instruments. *J. Sports Sci.* 30, 1197–1198. doi: 10.1080/02640414.2012.694212

Conflict of Interest Statement: The authors declare that the research was conducted in the absence of any commercial or financial relationships that could be construed as a potential conflict of interest.

3

Effect of Three Different Grip Angles on Physiological Parameters During Laboratory Handcycling Test in Able-Bodied Participants

Thomas Abel[1]*, Brendan Burkett[2], Barbara Thees[1], Stefan Schneider[1], Christopher D. Askew[2] and Heiko K. Strüder[1]

[1] Institute of Movement and Neurosciences, German Sport University Cologne, Cologne, Germany, [2] Faculty of Science, Health, Education and Engineering, School of Health and Sport Sciences, University of the Sunshine Coast, Maroochydore, QLD, Australia

Edited by:
*Pierre-Marie Leprêtre,
Université de Picardie Jules Verne,
France*

Reviewed by:
*Philip Santos Requejo,
Rancho Los Amigos National
Rehabilitation Center, USA
Arnaud Faupin,
Université de Toulon, France*

*Correspondence:
*Thomas Abel
abel@dshs-koeln.de*

Introduction: Handcycling is a relatively new wheelchair sport that has gained increased popularity for people with lower limb disabilities. The aim of this study was to examine the effect of three different grip positions on physical parameters during handcycling in a laboratory setting.

Methods: Twenty one able-bodied participants performed three maximum incremental handcycling tests until exhaustion, each with a different grip angle. The angle between the grip and the crank was randomly set at 90° (horizontal), 0° (vertical), or 10° (diagonal). The initial load was 20 W and increased by 20 W each 5 min. In addition, participants performed a 20 s maximum effort.

Results: The relative peak functional performance (W/kg), peak heart rate (bpm), associated lactate concentrations (mmol/l) and peak oxygen uptake per kilogram body weight (ml.min^{-1}.kg^{-1}) for the different grip positions during the stage test were: (a) Horizontal: 1.43 ± 0.21 W/kg, 170.14 ± 12.81 bpm, 9.54 ± 1.93 mmol/l, 30.86 ± 4.57 ml/kg; (b) Vertical: 1.38 ± 0.20 W/kg, 171.81 ± 13.87 bpm, 9.91 ± 2.29 mmol/l, 29.75 ± 5.13 ml/kg; (c) Diagonal: 1.40 ± 0.22 W/kg, 169.19 ± 13.31 bpm, 9.34 ± 2.36 mmol/l, 29.39 ± 4.70 ml/kg. Statistically significant ($p < 0.05$) differences could only be found for lactate concentration between the vertical grip position and the other grips during submaximal handcycling.

Conclusion: The orientation of three different grip angles made no difference to the peak load achieved during an incremental handcycling test and a 20 s maximum effort. At submaximal load, higher lactate concentrations were found when the vertical grip position was used, suggesting that this position may be less efficient than the alternative diagonal or horizontal grip positions.

Keywords: adapted physical activity, biomechanics, spinal cord injury

INTRODUCTION

Handcycling has opened a new world of mobilization for people who are restricted to a wheelchair, from both a health perspective (Abel et al., 2003a; Arnet et al., 2016) and for sports performance (Abel et al., 2006; Goosey-Tolfrey et al., 2006; de Groot et al., 2014). During the last 5 years, race performance has increased significantly with the adoption of elite athlete training approaches and technical developments concerning the handcycle itself. In comparison to wheelchair propulsion, handcycling has a higher mechanical efficiency (Abel et al., 2003a; Dallmeijer et al., 2004; Simmelink et al., 2015; Arnet et al., 2016), which gives the person restricted to a wheelchair the benefit of increased mobility. It has been postulated that regular engagement with handcycling will likely lead to fewer painful and debilitating overuse injuries (van der Woude et al., 2006; Arnet et al., 2014). Energy expenditure in handcycling is sufficient to offer protection against the development of secondary conditions such as cardiovascular disease (Abel et al., 2003a; van der Woude et al., 2013). As a relatively new device there have been a range of areas investigated to improve handcycle performance, such as the influence of back rest position, gear ratios (Faupin et al., 2008; Arnet et al., 2014). Whilst the efficiency of the athlete and handcycle as a complete system has been assessed, the influence of some key components within this system have not yet been quantified, such as the type or orientation of the hand grip.

As a mechanical device, the transmission of force from the athlete to the cycle plays a major role in handcycling performance. To better understand this interface between the athlete and the cycle, the influence of crank length (Goosey-Tolfrey et al., 2008; Krämer et al., 2009) and crank patterns (Verellen et al., 2004, 2008) on the transmission of forces has been investigated. In fine tuning this connection further, the configuration of cranking, either synchronous or asynchronous, has also been investigated (Hopman et al., 1995; Mossberg et al., 1999; Abel et al., 2003b; Dallmeijer et al., 2004; Goosey-Tolfrey and Sindall, 2007; van der Woude et al., 2008). To date the research on crank configurations has failed to address the critical question of hand-crank grip position. From a purely anatomical perspective, the musculoskeletal structure of the human forearm is a significant determinant of the ergonomics of the wrist, with the maximum generation of force found when the wrist is orientated near maximum flexion (Morse et al., 2006; Khan et al., 2009). Due to their disability, the users of a handcycle often have some degree of movement limitation in their forearm, therefore the optimisation of grip position for these athletes is of great importance (Bressel et al., 2001). In practice, disabled athletes commonly self-experiment with different grip angels and different grip forms. To investigate the optimal grip-crank interface, the aim of this study was to examine the effect of three different grip angles on the physiological responses to incremental and maximal handcycling in a laboratory setting. The hypothesis herby is that altering the grip orientation, and therefore altering the muscle length and specific load applied to the forearm and upper muscles, will result in changes change in power generated as well as changes in physiological reactions at submaximal and maximal load

METHODS

Participants

Twenty-one participants (15 male and six female; age 27 ± 5 years, height 178.0 ± 11.9 cm, weight 74.7 ± 13.3 kg) performed three stage tests until exhaustion with different grip angles. The participants were able-bodied and with a good training status of the upper extremity (active athletes in swimming and triathlon).

This study was carried out in accordance with the recommendations of guidelines of the International Committee of Medical Journal Editors. All subjects gave written informed consent in accordance with the Declaration of Helsinki. All investigations were approved by the German Sports University ethical advisory committee.

Experimental Overview

For all tests, participants sat in an arm-power race handcycle (Sopur Shark, Sunrisemedical Germany) connected to an ergometer (Cyclus II, Richter; Germany). The crank length was 175 mm, backrest angle approximately 45° adapted to the participants to avoid full elbow extension during crank revolutions. Crank housing position was set on a horizontal line to shoulder angle, crank configuration synchronous. The Cyclus II ergometer has been validated as an accurate measure of handcycling work load (Reiser et al., 2000). The angle between the grip and the crank was set in one of three configurations (see **Figure 1**), (a) 90° (horizontal = H), (b) 0° (vertical = V) and (c) 10°with respect to the vertical (i.e., diagonal, common way of cranking = D). Participants conducted an incremental test and a 20-s peak force test. The 20-s peak test was carried out after the incremental test und separated by 2 h. Tests were repeated three times using each of the grip configurations, in a random order, and each testing session was separated by a 3-day recovery period.

Incremental Test Protocol

After a standardized warm up period, the participants commenced hand cycling using one of the defined grip positions. Cycling cadence was freely chosen above 50 rpm. The initial load during test was 20 W and increased by 20 W every 5 min until the load where the 50 rpm cadence was not able to be maintained.

Expired air was collected continuously (ZAN 600, ZAN, Germany) during exercise for the assessment of oxygen consumption. Immediately before every test session, gas analyzers were calibrated with known reference gas mixtures (room air and a standard certified commercial gas preparation). The expiratory airflow volume was calibrated using a 1.0-l syringe. Blood samples to determine lactate concentrations were taken from the earlobe during the last 30 s of each stage (Biosen C, Eppendorf, Germany). Heart rate was monitored continuously (Polar X-Trainer, Polar, Finland).

Data Analysis

The descriptive mean and standard deviations for each of the measures of work, heart rate, blood lactate, and oxygen consumption were calculated using STATISTICA for Windows Version 7.1 F (StatSoft Inc, Tulsa, USA). An analysis of variance

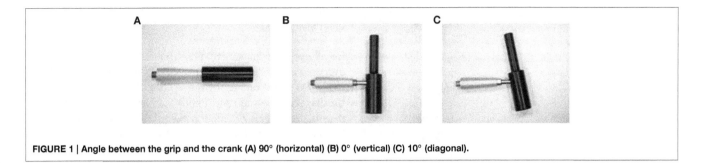

FIGURE 1 | Angle between the grip and the crank (A) 90° (horizontal) (B) 0° (vertical) (C) 10° (diagonal).

TABLE 1 | Physiological values at peak load during the stage test.

	Horizontal	Vertical	Diagonal
Relative work load (W/kg)	1.43 ± 0.21	1.38 ± 0.20	1.40 ± 0.22
Heart rate (bpm)	170.14 ± 12.81	171.81 ± 13.87	169.19 ± 13.31
Lactate (mmol/l)	9.54 ± 1.93	9.91 ± 2.29	9.34 ± 2.36
Relative oxygen uptake (ml/kg)	30.86 ± 4.57	29.75 ± 5.13	29.39 ± 4.70

with repeated measurements for submaximal and peak values was used to determine the presence of TIME and GRIP effects for heart rate, lactate and VO_{2peak}. *Post-hoc* (least significant difference Test LSD) analysis was performed where there were significant main effects and interactions to determine the precise location of differences or changes. A *P*-value less than 0.05 was considered significant.

RESULTS

The peak functional performance (W/kg), peak heart rate (bpm), the associated lactate concentrations (mmol/l), and peak oxygen uptake per kilogram body weight (ml/kg) for the three different grip positions during handcyling are shown in **Table 1**.

As shown in **Figure 2**, there were no significant differences for peak oxygen uptake between the three grip positions during the incremental test. There were also no differences between the three grip positions for the other peak variables during handcycling, including functional performance, heart rate and blood lactate. **Figure 3** shows the lactate concentrations at defined submaximal work loads of 20, 60, and 100 W during the incremental test watts. There was a statistically significant difference between the vertical grip position and the other grips at 60 and 100 W.

Peak and average data for each of the variables during the 20 s all out test are shown in **Table 2**. No significant differences were found between the three gips positions.

DISCUSSION

The aim of this study was to examine the effect of three different grip angles on functional performance and associated physiological variables during handcycling. To the authors' knowledge, this aspect of handcycling has not been previously investigated.

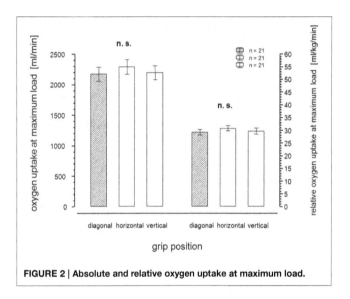

FIGURE 2 | Absolute and relative oxygen uptake at maximum load.

While absolute an relative oxygen uptake tended to be lower at submaximal and peak workloads when the diagonal grip orientation was used, this was not statistically significant. Nonetheless, small reductions in oxygen uptake during laboratory tests may translate into important and significant improvements in economy during longer endurance activities such as a handcycling road race (Fischer et al., 2015). This time dependant relationship between work load and oxygen uptake has been identified in other studies (Verellen et al., 2004).

An unexpected finding was the higher blood lactate concentration during submaximal (60 and 100 W) handcycling when the vertical grip was used compared with both the diagonal and horizontal grips. As it is unlikely that lactate clearance would be different between the three test conditions (Heck et al., 1985; Mader, 2003), this elevation in lactate with the vertical grip indicates that there is likely to be a greater reliance on anaerobic metabolism by the working muscles. As these changes are unique to the vertical grip position, a plausible hypothesis could be that the vertical position requires increased static work, throughout the entire pedal stroke, to fix the hand at the handlebar. As sweat production, and the associated grip instability, increases with exercise intensity and time, this is likely to lead to further increases in static work and a greater reliance on local anaerobic metabolism. It is likely that this explains why many athletes avoid

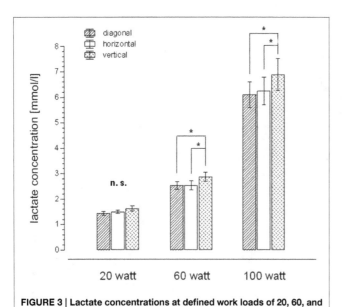

FIGURE 3 | Lactate concentrations at defined work loads of 20, 60, and 100 W for different grip angles. *Significant.

TABLE 2 | Peak and mean work load during the 20 s test.

	Horizontal	Vertical	Diagonal
Peak load (W)	589.73 ± 190.78	581.52 ± 188.24	583.67 ± 211.75
Relative peak load (W/kg)	7.74 ± 1.51	7.64 ± 1.59	7.59 ± 1.76
Mean load 20 s. (W)	350.17 ± 125.75	341.97 ± 116.18	344.02 ± 128.35
Mean relative load 20 s. (W/kg)	4.57 ± 1.08	4.48 ± 0.98	4.47 ± 1.10

using the vertical grip in practice, and instead adopt a grip with some degree of horizontal orientation.

In the present study a full 90° grip range was explored to ascertain the most appropriate orientation of the hand-crank grip. This complete range of movement was considered necessary, as previous cycling studies on crank length for example only considered small increments of change (Martin and Spirduso, 2001). Despite this maximum change in the range of motion of the grip orientation, there were no significant differences in force between the vertical, diagonal, and horizontal grip positions. The hypothesis that altering the grip orientation, and therefore altering the muscle length and specific load applied to the forearm and upper muscles, would result in a change in power generated as well as in efficiency related values was not supported. Based on the similar oxygen uptake and heart rate measures during each of the tests, the economy of the three different grip orientations showed no difference.

Training with the optimal hand-crank orientation is essential for efficiency of movement, performance and the prevention of overuse risks (Webborn and Van de Vliet, 2012; Arnet et al., 2014). As the economy of movement when handcycling with the diagonal grip was only slightly, and non-significantly, higher than the other grip orientations for the able-bodied population, it would also seem important to consider comfort when setting up the handcycle, particularly for individuals with a loss of lower limb function. Depending on the unique and individual anatomy and movement restrictions of the athlete with a disability, the optimal handcycle setup and grip orientation may alter significantly form individual to individual.

Limitations of the Study

The testing was done in a stationary laboratory situation using the Cyclus II ergometer. The absent of a need or possibility to steer the handcycling as well as the able-bodied participant with limited handcycling experience might have influenced test results. This restricts the transferability of the test results onto athletes with spinal cord injuries or other disabilities. A real competitive test setup during a handcycling race, including participants with disabilities would have simulated this more significantly, but tests like that are more or less impossible to be conducted.

Nevertheless, as all grip angles were tested under the same laboratory situation, the results allow claiming relevance for handcycling athletes.

CONCLUSION

In the present study there were no differences between three different grip positions (horizontal, vertical, and diagonal) when handcycling at maximum intensity during an incremental test and during a sprint test. There was also no difference in the economy of hand cycling during submaximal loads when each of the three grips was used. The vertical grip was associated with higher lactate concentrations during submaximal handcycling, and may be indicative of reduced efficiency caused by the static (continuous) activation of the working muscles. Further, studies should be conducted to verify these findings during prolonged exercise bouts and in athletes with a spinal cord injury or similar disabilities.

ACKNOWLEDGMENTS

The study was supported by the Federal Institute of Sport Science VF 0407/04/41.2004.

REFERENCES

Abel, T., Kröner, M., Rojas Vega, S., Peters, C., Klose, C., and Platen, P. (2003a). Energy expenditure in wheelchair racing and handbiking - a basis for prevention of cardiovascular diseases in those with disabilities. *Eur. J.*

Cardiovasc. Prev. Rehabil. 10, 371–376. doi: 10.1097/01.hjr.0000096542.305 33.59

Abel, T., Schneider, S., Platen, P., and Strüder, H. K. (2006). Performance diagnostics in handbiking during competition. *Spinal Cord* 44, 211–216. doi: 10.1038/sj.sc.3101845

Abel, T., Vega, S. R., Bleicher, I., and Platen, P. (2003b). Handbiking: physiological responses to synchronous and asynchronous crank montage. *Eur. J. Sport Sci.* 3, 1–8. doi: 10.1080/17461390300073205

Arnet, U., Hinrichs, T., Lay, V., Bertschy, S., Frei, H., and Brinkhof, M. W. G. (2016). Determinants of handbike use in persons with spinal cord injury: results of a community survey in Switzerland. *Disabil. Rehabil.* 38, 81–86. doi: 10.3109/09638288.2015.1024339

Arnet, U., van Drongelen, S., Schlüssel, M., Lay, V., van der Woude, L. H. V., and Veeger, H. E. J. (2014). The effect of crank position and backrest inclination on shoulder load and mechanical efficiency during handcycling. *Scand. J. Med. Sci. Sports* 24, 386–394. doi: 10.1111/j.1600-0838.2012.01524.x

Bressel, E., Bressel, M., Marquez, M., and Heise, G. D. (2001). The effect of handgrip position on upper extremity neuromuscular responses to arm cranking exercise. *J. Electromyogr. Kinesiol.* 11, 291–298. doi: 10.1016/S1050-6411(01)00002-5

Dallmeijer, A. J., Ottjes, L., de Waardt, E., and van der Woude, L. H. (2004). A physiological comparison of synchronous and asynchronous hand cycling. *Int. J. Sports Med.* 25, 622–626. doi: 10.1055/s-2004-817879

de Groot, S., Postma, K., van Vliet, L., Timmermans, R., and Valent, L. J. M. (2014). Mountain time trial in handcycling: exercise intensity and predictors of race time in people with spinal cord injury. *Spinal Cord* 52, 455–461. doi: 10.1038/sc.2014.58

Faupin, A., Gorce, P., Meyer, C., and Thevenon, A. (2008). Effects of backrest positioning and gear ratio on nondisabled subjects' handcycling sprinting performance and kinematics. *J. Rehabil. Res. Dev.* 45, 109–116. doi: 10.1682/JRRD.2006.10.0139

Fischer, G., Figueiredo, P., and Ardigò, L. P. (2015). Physiological performance determinants of a 22 km handbiking time trial. *Int. J. Sports Physiol. Perform.* 10, 965–971. doi: 10.1123/ijspp.2014-0429

Goosey-Tolfrey, V., Castle, P., Webborn, N., and Abel, T. (2006). Aerobic capacity and peak power output of elite quadriplegic games players. *Br. J. Sports Med.* 40, 684–687. doi: 10.1136/bjsm.2006.026815

Goosey-Tolfrey, V. L., Alfano, H., and Fowler, N. (2008). The influence of crank length and cadence on mechanical efficiency in hand cycling. *Eur. J. Appl. Physiol.* 102, 189–194. doi: 10.1007/s00421-007-0576-7

Goosey-Tolfrey, V. L., and Sindall, P. (2007). The effects of arm crank strategy on physiological responses and mechanical efficiency during submaximal exercise. *J. Sports Sci.* 25, 453–460. doi: 10.1080/02640410600702883

Heck, H., Mader, A., Hess, G., Mücke, S., Müller, R., and Hollmann, W. (1985). Justification of the 4-mmol/l lactate threshold. *Int. J. Sports Med.* 6, 117–130. doi: 10.1055/s-2008-1025824

Hopman, M. T., van Teeffelen, W. M., Brouwer, J., Houtman, S., and Binkhorst, R. A. (1995). Physiological responses to asynchronous and synchronous arm-cranking exercise. *Eur. J. Appl. Physiol. Occup. Physiol.* 72, 111–114. doi: 10.1007/BF00964124

Khan, A. A., O'Sullivan, L., and Gallwey, T. J. (2009). Effects of combined wrist deviation and forearm rotation on discomfort score. *Ergonomics* 52, 345–361. doi: 10.1080/00140130802376018

Krämer, C., Hilker, L., and Böhm, H. (2009). Influence of crank length and crank width on maximal hand cycling power and cadence. *Eur. J. Appl. Physiol.* 106, 749–757. doi: 10.1007/s00421-009-1062-1

Mader, A. (2003). Glycolysis and oxidative phosphorylation as a function of cytosolic phosphorylation state and power output of the muscle cell. *Eur. J. Appl. Physiol.* 88, 317–338. doi: 10.1007/s00421-002-0676-3

Martin, J. C., and Spirduso, W. W. (2001). Determinants of maximal cycling power: crank length, pedaling rate and pedal speed. *Eur. J. Appl. Physiol.* 84, 413–418. doi: 10.1007/s004210100400

Morse, J. L., Jung, M. C., Bashford, G. R., and Hallbeck, M. S. (2006). Maximal dynamic grip force and wrist torque: the effects of gender, exertion direction, angular velocity, and wrist angle. *Appl. Ergon.* 37, 737–742. doi: 10.1016/j.apergo.2005.11.008

Mossberg, K. C., Williams, C., Topor, M. A., Crook, H., and Patak, S. (1999). Comparison of asynchronous versus synchronous arm crank ergometry. *Spinal Cord* 37, 569–574. doi: 10.1038/sj.sc.3100875

Reiser, M., Meyer, T., Kindermann, W., and Daugs, R. (2000). Transferability of workload measurements between three different types of ergometer. *Eur. J. Appl. Physiol.* 82, 245–249. doi: 10.1007/s004210050678

Simmelink, E. K., Borgesius, E. C., Hettinga, F. J., Geertzen, J. H. B., Dekker, R., and van der Woude, L. H. V. (2015). Gross mechanical efficiency of the combined arm-leg (Cruiser) ergometer: a comparison with the bicycle ergometer and handbike. *Int. J. Rehabil. Res.* 38, 61–67. doi: 10.1097/MRR.0000000000000100

van der Woude, L. H., Horstman, A., Faas, P., Mechielsen, S., Bafghi, H. A., and de Koning, J. J. (2008). Power output and metabolic cost of synchronous and asynchronous submaximal and peak level hand cycling on a motor driven treadmill in able-bodied male subjects. *Med. Eng. Phys.* 30, 574–580. doi: 10.1016/j.medengphy.2007.06.006

van der Woude, L. H. V., de Groot, S., and Janssen, T. W. J. (2006). Manual wheelchairs: research and innovation in rehabilitation, sports, daily life and health. *Med. Eng. Phys.* 28, 905–915. doi: 10.1016/j.medengphy.2005.12.001

van der Woude, L. H. V., de Groot, S., Postema, K., Bussmann, J. B. J., Janssen, T. W. J., and Post, M. W. M. (2013). Active LifestyLe Rehabilitation interventions in aging spinal cord injury (ALLRISC): a multicentre research program. *Disabil. Rehabil.* 35, 1097–1103. doi: 10.3109/09638288.2012.718407

Verellen, J., Meyer, C., Reynders, S., Van Biesen, D., and Vanlandewijck, Y. (2008). Consistency of within-cycle torque distribution pattern in hand cycling. *J. Rehabil. Res. Dev.* 45, 1295–1302.

Verellen, J., Theisen, D., and Vanlandewijck, Y. (2004). Influence of crank rate in hand cycling. *Med. Sci. Sports Exerc.* 36, 1826–1831. doi: 10.1249/01.MSS.0000142367.04918.5A

Webborn, N., and Van de Vliet, P. (2012). Paralympic medicine. *Lancet* 380, 65–71. doi: 10.1016/S0140-6736(12)60831-9

Conflict of Interest Statement: The authors declare that the research was conducted in the absence of any commercial or financial relationships that could be construed as a potential conflict of interest.

4

Neuro-mechanical determinants of repeated treadmill sprints - Usefulness of an "hypoxic to normoxic recovery" approach

Olivier Girard[1,2]*, Franck Brocherie[1], Jean-Benoit Morin[3] and Grégoire P. Millet[1]

[1] Department of Physiology, Faculty of Biology and Medicine, Institute of Sport Sciences, University of Lausanne, Lausanne, Switzerland, [2] Athlete Health and Performance Research Center, Aspetar, Qatar Orthopaedic and Sports Medicine Hospital, Doha, Qatar, [3] Laboratory of Human Motricity, Education Sport and Health, University of Nice Sophia Antipolis, Nice, France

Edited by:
Sergej Ostojic,
University of Novi Sad, Serbia

Reviewed by:
Naoto Fujii,
University of Ottawa, Canada
Hannes Gatterer,
University of Innsbruck, Austria

*Correspondence:
Olivier Girard,
Department of Physiology,
Faculty of Biology and Medicine,
Institute of Sport Sciences, University
of Lausanne, Building Geopolis,
Campus Dorigny, CH-1015 Lausanne,
Switzerland
oliv.girard@gmail.com

To improve our understanding of the limiting factors during repeated sprinting, we manipulated hypoxia severity during an initial set and examined the effects on performance and associated neuro-mechanical alterations during a subsequent set performed in normoxia. On separate days, 13 active males performed eight 5-s sprints (recovery = 25 s) on an instrumented treadmill in either normoxia near sea-level (SL; $FiO_2 = 20.9\%$), moderate (MH; $FiO_2 = 16.8\%$) or severe normobaric hypoxia (SH; $FiO_2 = 13.3\%$) followed, 6 min later, by four 5-s sprints (recovery = 25 s) in normoxia. Throughout the first set, along with distance covered [larger sprint decrement score in SH (−8.2%) compared to SL (−5.3%) and MH (−7.2%); $P < 0.05$], changes in contact time, step frequency and root mean square activity (surface electromyography) of the quadriceps (*Rectus femoris* muscle) in SH exceeded those in SL and MH ($P < 0.05$). During first sprint of the subsequent normoxic set, the distance covered (99.6, 96.4, and 98.3% of sprint 1 in SL, MH, and SH, respectively), the main kinetic (mean vertical, horizontal, and resultant forces) and kinematic (contact time and step frequency) variables as well as surface electromyogram of quadriceps and plantar flexor muscles were fully recovered, with no significant difference between conditions. Despite differing hypoxic severity levels during sprints 1–8, performance and neuro-mechanical patterns did not differ during the four sprints of the second set performed in normoxia. In summary, under the circumstances of this study (participant background, exercise-to-rest ratio, hypoxia exposure), sprint mechanical performance and neural alterations were largely influenced by the hypoxia severity in an initial set of repeated sprints. However, hypoxia had no residual effect during a subsequent set performed in normoxia. Hence, the recovery of performance and associated neuro-mechanical alterations was complete after resting for 6 min near sea level, with a similar fatigue pattern across conditions during subsequent repeated sprints in normoxia.

Keywords: repeated-sprint ability, running mechanics, hypoxia, electromyography, recovery

Introduction

Intense physical efforts performed at or near maximal speeds are often crucial for successful participation in intermittent sports (e.g., team or racket sports). For instance, top-level soccer players complete more high-intensity running or sprinting than their lower-level counterparts (Mohr et al., 2003, 2008). However, irrespectively of competitive standard, the volume of all high-intensity actions decline over the course of a game, reflecting muscle fatigue development (Mohr et al., 2008). Although, still debated (Carling, 2013), the repeated-sprint ability (RSA) is commonly viewed as an important marker of successful physical performance in these disciplines.

While RSA has been increasingly investigated over the last decade, to date, most of the available studies focused only on the physiological features of this fitness component. Evaluation of the biomechanical aspects of running RSA have insofar been limited to either indirect measures of stride characteristics (i.e., pressure insoles) (Girard et al., 2011a; Brocherie et al., 2015) or direct sprint kinetics/kinematics assessments (i.e., force platforms), but only for a discrete number of steps at various intervals during the sprint distance (Girard et al., 2011b). Using instrumented, sprint treadmills makes now possible to deepen our knowledge about the biomechanical manifestation of fatigue during repeated sprinting (Morin et al., 2011). For instance, through direct measurement of ground reaction forces, Girard et al. (2015a) reported significant decrease in propulsive power and step frequency with fatigue while contact time and step length increased, when five maximal 5-s sprints with incomplete recoveries (25 s) were repeated.

Peripheral mechanisms, that include limitation in energy supply and the intramuscular accumulation of metabolic by-products, have been traditionally associated to fatigue development during repeated sprinting (Girard et al., 2011c). Consideration of neural factors (i.e., neural drive and muscle recruitment strategies) as significant contributors to fatigue etiology during RSA protocols stem from parallel reductions in amplitude of quadriceps surface electromyography (EMG) signals (i.e., a reasonable proxy for net motor unit activity) and in sprint performance (Mendez-Villanueva et al., 2008; Billaut et al., 2013; Bowtell et al., 2014; Brocherie et al., 2015). For instance, Brocherie et al. (2015) demonstrated a disproportionate decrease in motor unit recruitment inferred via EMG signaling [Root Mean Square (RMS) activity] of *Rectus femoris* and *Biceps femoris* muscles over sprint times when professional football players completed the repeated anaerobic sprint test on artificial turf. Although, muscle activation capacity of plantar flexors decreases from pre- to post-RSA running (Perrey et al., 2010), the question of whether this muscle group is subjected to similar neural adjustments than those seen for the quadriceps during actual sprint repetitions remains undetermined.

When attempting to evaluate RSA and its fatigue-causing factors, a single set of a fixed number of 5–15 sprints (i.e., usually of 5–10 s) with (incomplete) recovery of less than 30 s (i.e., usually passive) has most commonly been used (Girard et al., 2011c). Admittedly, while valuable knowledge on how fatigue manifests and the potential contribution of neural factors can be gained

from such RSA tests' format, derived information remains mainly descriptive. Innovative analysis methods that are based on the comparison of fatigue responses and recovery of performance during and between sets of repeated sprints, respectively, have emerged (Girard et al., 2015b). By linking the aforementioned changes to muscle metabolism and neuromuscular function, such approaches support the idea that previous repeated-sprint exercise has a negative "carry-over" impact on physiological strain, perception of effort and performance during the next bout of activity (Mendez-Villanueva et al., 2007, 2012; Billaut et al., 2013). With this in mind, it is surprising that little attention has been directed toward the usefulness of the "recovery of performance approach" to shed more light on how running mechanics and muscle activation patterns are altered during RSA run-based tests.

Extreme environments such as hypoxia [i.e., a reduction in environmental oxygen (O_2) availability] are known to lead to premature fatigue and exacerbated cardiorespiratory and perceptual responses during repeated-sprint exercise (Billaut et al., 2013; Bowtell et al., 2014; Goods et al., 2014). By majoring RSA-induced demands (and thereby recovery requirements) on the neuromuscular system during an initial set (i.e., larger changes within the central nervous system with severer hypoxic levels), it seems reasonable to speculate that performance decrement during a subsequent repeated-sprint exercise would be exacerbated. Accordingly, modifying the ensuing recovery rate of repeated-sprint performance from previous strenuous exercise highlights a context whereby neuro-mechanical determinants of RSA running performance could be explored from a new perspective (Minett and Duffield, 2014).

Our intention was therefore to manipulate hypoxia severity during an initial repeated-sprint set and examine the effect on sprinting performance, running mechanics (kinetics and kinematics) and lower-limbs neuromuscular activity (surface EMG activity) during a subsequent set performed in normoxia. We hypothesized that, with severer hypoxia levels during a first repeated-sprint set expected to major RSA-induced demands placed on the neuromuscular system, larger recovery requirements and fatigue-related residual or "carry-over" effects from the previous set would, in turn, negatively influence fatigability during the completion of a second set performed in normoxia.

Methods

Subjects

Thirteen male recreational team- (i.e., football, rugby, basketball) and racket- (i.e., tennis, squash) sport players (Mean ± SD: 31.2 ± 4.8 years; 178.4 ± 6.6 cm; 74.3 ± 8.2 kg) participated in the study. In the 6 months preceding the study, subjects trained on average 4.5 ± 2.5 h.wk^{-1}, which included activity-specific training (i.e., technical and tactical skills), aerobic and anaerobic training (i.e., on- and off-court/field exercises) and basic strength training. Although, training content of the tested athletes largely focused on accelerated runs, their sprinting skills are deemed to be "moderate" compared to "elite" (i.e., national to international level) sprinters (Rabita et al., 2015) and/or team-sport athletes (Brocherie et al., 2015). All subjects were born and raised at <1000 m and had not traveled to elevations >1000 m in the 3 months prior to investigation. They gave their informed, written consent preceding the commencement of the experiment. Experimental protocol was conducted according to the Declaration of Helsinki for use of Human Subjects and approved by the Ethics Committee of *Shafallah Medical Genetics Center*.

Experimental Procedure

About 1 week prior to testing, subjects undertook a complete preliminary session where they performed short (<5 s) "familiarization" treadmill sprints at increasing intensities while wearing a facemask for habituation (i.e., the hypoxic system was turned off at this occasion), with full recovery and until being comfortable with treadmill maximal sprint technique (which generally required 7–10 trials). Subjects then performed three maximal 5-s single sprints separated by 2 min of passive rest. All participants satisfied the criteria of having a coefficient of variation <2.2% for distance covered across three successive trials (Girard et al., 2015c). After 10 min of rest, the complete RSA test was completed. Strong verbal encouragement was given during all maximal efforts.

Subjects then came to the laboratory (well-ventilated at a constant temperature of ~25°C and 40% relative humidity) for three experimental sessions (~1 h; counterbalanced randomized crossover design in double-blind fashion), with at least 3–4 days apart, including a repeated-sprint running protocol on a treadmill sprint ergometer. They performed their trials at the same time of the day (±1 h) and wore similar sports gear (running shoes, short, and T-shirt). They were instructed to maintain their normal diet (i.e., avoiding any nutritional supplements or alcohol consumption), sleeping (i.e., ≥7 h/night) and training (i.e., avoiding vigorous exercise 24 h before every trial) habits during the 1–2 weeks period of testing to prevent any possible interference on their sprinting abilities. Subjects were instructed to drink 4–6 mL of water per kilogram of body mass every 2.5 h on the day before each experimental session to ensure euhydration at the start of exercise. They were permitted to drink *ad libitum* during the warm-up procedure.

Repeated-sprint Exercise Protocol

The exercise protocol consisted of performing first eight, 5-s "all-out" sprints interspersed with 25 s of passive rest and randomly conducted near sea level (SL; FiO_2 ~20.9%), at moderate and severe simulated altitudes (normobaric hypoxia) of 1800 m (MH; FiO_2 ~16.6%) and 3600 m (SH; FiO_2 ~13.0%), respectively. This was followed, after 6 min of passive rest (i.e., subjects breathed ambient air), by four, 5-s "all-out" sprints also interspersed by 25 s of passive rest but always performed at SL. During recovery periods, subjects stood on the treadmill. Before all tests, subjects completed a standardized warm-up (i.e., on the instrumented treadmill with subjects breathing ambient air) consisting of 10 min of running at 10 km.h^{-1}, followed by 15 min of sprint-specific muscular warm-up exercises [i.e., 3 × (high knee, high heels, butt kick, skipping for ~10 s with 30 s walking

in between), followed by 3 × (3 steps accelerations at a subjective "sense of effort" of 7, 8, and 9), then by 2 × (3-s sprints at a subjective "sense of effort" of 8 and 9] (Christian et al., 2014). Afterwards, three maximal 5-s single sprints (i.e., the best of these three trials was used as the criterion score), separated by 2 min of passive rest, were completed. Finally, after a facemask connected to a portable hypoxic generator has been attached on subjects, they were allowed 5-min of free cool down prior to the repeated-sprint protocol. Testing protocols were run in a double-blind fashion in that subjects and one investigator were blinded toward the environmental condition of the initial set. The efficacy of the subjects' blinding procedure was evaluated after each experimental session by questionnaires in which subjects were asked whether they believed to be exercising at SL, MH, or SH. We are confident that the blinding procedure was efficient, as only four athletes were able to correctly identify the order of treatment.

Altitude Simulation

Normobaric hypoxia was obtained by mixing nitrogen into ambient air under control of FiO_2 (Altitrainer, SMTec SA, Nyon, Switzerland). This gas-mixing system enriches the inspired air by adding a fixed quantity of nitrogen via a 30 L mixing chamber, with the dilution being constantly controlled by a PO_2 probe (with a precision of ± 0.82 Torr and safety set at $FiO_2 = 9.7\%$). This device allows the production of large quantities of a hypoxic gas mixture (up to 200 L.min^{-1}), with an easily adjustable O_2 fraction over a large range, and a short response time (between 15 and 45 s), expressed either by the equivalent altitude or by the O_2 partial pressure, taking into account the barometric pressure. For blinding purposes, subjects who always breathed through the same set-up (also in normoxia), inhaled the mixture contained in the buffer tank through a Hans Rudolph two-way respiratory valve. Subjects were instrumented with the facemask 5 min before the repeated-sprint exercise (i.e., after the three "reference" sprints at warm-up termination) until the end of the first set of eight sprints.

Instrumented Sprint Treadmill

The sprints were performed on an instrumented motorized treadmill (ADAL3D-WR, Medical Development—HEF Tecmachine, Andrézieux-Bouthéon, France). Briefly, it is mounted on a highly rigid metal frame fixed to the ground through four piezoelectric force transducers (KI 9077b; Kistler, Winterthur, Switzerland) and installed on a specially engineered concrete slab to ensure maximal rigidity of the supporting ground. This motorized treadmill allows subjects to sprint and produce realistic acceleration and high running velocities (Morin et al., 2010). A single-pass waist and a stiff rope (1 cm in diameter, ~2 m length) were used to tether subjects to the 0.4-m vertical rail anchored to the wall behind them. When correctly attached, subjects were required to lean forward in a typical and standardized crouched sprint-start position with their left foot forward. This starting position was used and standardized all along the sprint series. After a 5-s countdown ("5 s, 3-2-1-Go" given by both visual and audio instructions by the same investigator), the treadmill was released, and the belt began to accelerate as subjects applied a positive horizontal force.

Mechanical Variables

Data were continuously sampled at 1000 Hz over the sprints, and after appropriate filtering (Butterworth-type 30 Hz low-pass filter), instantaneous data of vertical, net horizontal and total (i.e., resultant) ground reaction forces were averaged for each support phase (vertical force above 30 N) over the 5-s sprints, and expressed in body weight (BW). These data were completed by measurements of the main step kinematic variables: contact time, aerial time, step frequency, and step length.

Electromyography

EMG signals from superficial *Rectus femoris, Vastus lateralis, Biceps femoris, Gastrocnemius medialis, Gastrocnemius lateralis,* and *Tibialis anterior* of the right lower limb were recorded using pre-amplified bi-polar surface EMG (Delsys, Trigno Wireless, Boston, Massachusetts, USA) with an inter-electrode (center-to-center) distance of 20 mm and placed according to the surface electromyography for the non-invasive assessment of muscles (SENIAM) project's recommendations. Before electrode placement, the skin was lightly abraded and washed to remove surface layers of dead skin, hair, and oil. All electrodes were secured with elastic cohesive bandage to reduce any movement of electrodes during sprinting or artifact in the signal. The position of the EMG electrodes was marked with indelible ink to ensure that they were placed in the same location during subsequent visits. The myoelectric signal was amplified (gain = 1000×) and filtered (bandwidth frequency = 20–450 Hz) to minimize extraneous noise and possible movement artifacts in the low-frequency region and to eliminate aliasing and other artifacts in the high-frequency region. Surface EMG signals were recorded continuously during each 5-s sprint with a sampling frequency of 2000 Hz using a dedicated acquisition system (CED 1401, Cambridge Electronic Design, Cambridge, UK) and analyzed offline (Spike2 v3.21; Cambridge Electronic Design, Cambridge, UK). The activity of each muscle was determined by measuring the mean value of the RMS signal between the onset and the end of the burst for each 5-s sprint. For each individual, a burst of muscle activity was identified as the amplitude of muscle activity exceeding 15% of peak activation for more than 10% of the stride (Brocherie et al., 2015). To investigate the difference in EMG frequency between the three conditions, the filtered EMG data from each sprint were further transformed into the frequency domain using a fast Fourier transformation and the median power frequency (MPF) of the resulting power spectrum density was calculated (Matsuura et al., 2006). The RMS and MPF were normalized to the first sprint value of each condition, which was assigned the value of 100% (Mendez-Villanueva et al., 2012; Brocherie et al., 2015).

Responses to Exercise

Heart rate (HR) and pulse O_2 saturation (SpO_2) were monitored and estimated, respectively, via a Polar transmitter-receiver (Wearlink T-31, Polar Electro Oy, Kempele, Finland) and non-invasive pulse oximetry using a finger probe (Palmsat 2500,

NONIN Medical Inc., Plymouth, MI, USA). The subjects were unable to view any of the HR or SpO_2 values since receivers were attached on the handrails of the treadmill facing one experimenter. Together with HR and SpO_2, ratings of perceived exertion (RPE) were recorded using the Borg 6–20 scale (i.e., 6 = no exertion at all, 20 = maximal exertion) exactly 10 s following each sprint (i.e., peak values likely to be obtained), where subjects were instructed to reflect on their perception of overall peripheral discomfort during the preceding exercise bout (Christian et al., 2014). In addition, SpO_2 was recorded between before the warm-up and 4 min into recovery between the two repeated-sprint sets. A capillary blood sample was taken from the fingertip and analyzed for blood lactate concentration with a portable analyzer (Lactate Pro LT-1710, Arkray, Japan) before the warm-up, 2 min after the first set of 8 sprints and 2 min after the second set of 4 sprints.

Data Analysis and Statistics

Subjects completed between 15 and 18 steps during each 5-s sprint. After excluding the last two ground contacts, the remaining three consecutive steps were used for final analysis of sprint kinetics/kinematics (Brocherie et al., 2015). While subjects performed a total of 12 sprints, only responses to exercise, running mechanical and surface EMG data collected for sprint number 1, 4, 8, 9, and 12 were considered for the main analysis. For the main running mechanical variables, the average of sprints number 1–4, 5–8, and 9–12 have also been compared.

Values are expressed as mean ± SD. Two-Way repeated-measures analysis of variance (ANOVAs) [Time (Sprints 1, 4, 8, 9, and 12 or Sprints number 1–4, 5–8, and 9–12) × Condition (SL, MH, and SH)] were used to compare investigated variables. To assess assumptions of variance, Mauchly's test of sphericity was performed using all ANOVA results. A Greenhouse-Geisser correction was performed to adjust the degree of freedom if an assumption was violated, while a Bonferroni *post-hoc* multiple comparison was performed if a significant main effect was observed. For each ANOVA, partial eta-squared was calculated as measures of effect size. Values of 0.01, 0.06, and above 0.14 were considered as small, medium, and large, respectively. All statistical calculations were performed using SPSS statistical software V.21.0 (IBM Corp., Armonk, NY, USA). The significance level was set at $P < 0.05$.

Results

Responses to Exercise

Responses to exercise across the three conditions are depicted in **Figure 1**. During the initial set of sprints, SpO_2 was significantly reduced for each simulated altitude ascent ($P < 0.05$). Lower SpO_2 values were recorded for both sprints 4 and 8 (no difference) vs. sprint 1 in MH and SH, while no change occurred at SL. In response to sprint 1, HR was significantly higher in MH and SH compared to SL ($P < 0.05$), while RPE values were similar. Both HR and RPE increased significantly from sprint 1–4 ($P < 0.05$), while only RPE further increased at sprint 8 in reference to sprint 4 ($P < 0.05$), yet with similar values across conditions. Compared to prior to the warm-up (96.9 ±

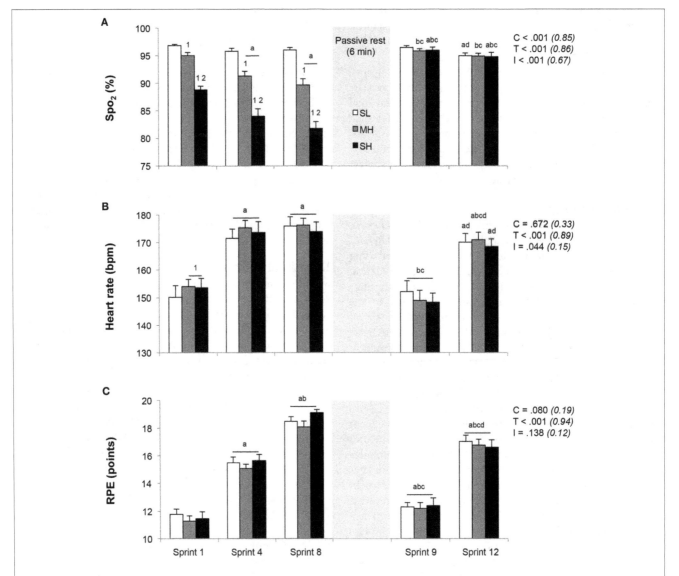

FIGURE 1 | Changes in exercise responses (A, SpO₂; B, heart rate; C, RPE). Mean ± SD ($n = 13$). The repeated-sprint exercise protocol included a first set of eight sprints performed at sea level (SL), moderate (MH), or severe hypoxia (SH), while the second set of four sprints was always performed at SL. SpO₂, arterial oxygen saturation (estimated by pulse oximetry); RPE, rating of perceived exertion. C, T, and I, respectively refer to ANOVA main effects of condition, time, and interaction between these two factors with P-value and partial eta-squared into brackets. [a], [b], [c], and [d] significantly different from sprint 1, 4, 8, and 9, respectively ($P < 0.05$). [1] and [2] significantly different from SL and MH, respectively ($P < 0.05$).

0.4%), SpO₂ were not different among conditions 4 min into recovery between the two repeated-sprint sets (96.2 ± 0.5%; all conditions compounded, $P > 0.05$). During sprint 9, after 6 min of rest, SpO₂, HR, and RPE values recovered significantly in relation to those achieved in sprint 4 and 8 ($P < 0.05$), with no difference between conditions. Whereas RPE values remained elevated compared to those measured in response to sprint 1, HR values recorded after sprint 1 and 9 were not different. At sprint 12, HR, and RPE values did not differ between conditions, while RPE was larger than in sprint 4 ($P < 0.05$).

From pre- to +2 min post-set 1, the execution of the initial set of 8 sprints resulted in similar increases in blood lactate concentration (SL: 1.4 ± 0.4 vs. 9.9 ± 1.7 mmol.L⁻¹,

MH: 1.4 ± 0.4 vs. 10.4 ± 1.8 mmol.L⁻¹, and SH: 1.4 ± 0.4 vs. 10.7 ± 2.1 mmol.L⁻¹; $P < 0.001$), irrespectively of the environmental condition. There was a further global increase of blood lactate concentration values (10.8 ± 1.9, 11.2 ± 1.7 and 10.6 ± 2.2 mmol.L⁻¹ in SL, MH, and SH, respectively; $P<0.05$) recorded +2 min post-set 2 (i.e., after the completion of 4 additional normoxic sprints) in reference to post-set 1.

Sprint Performance and Running Kinetics

Distance ran and associated running kinetics during the repeated-sprint exercise are displayed in **Figure 2**. No difference was found in distance ran during the first sprint between SL, MH and SH (24.2 ± 1.4, 24.1 ± 1.3, and 24.2 ± 2.0 m, respectively).

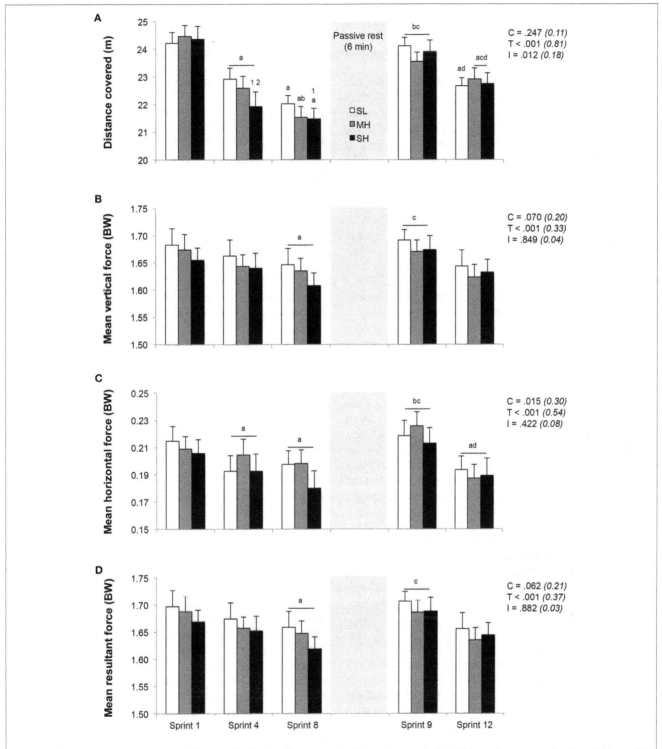

FIGURE 2 | Changes in distance covered (A) and stride kinetics (B, mean vertical force; C, mean horizontal force; D, mean resultant force). Mean ± SD (n = 13). The repeated-sprint exercise protocol included a first set of eight sprints performed at sea level (SL), moderate (MH), or severe hypoxia (SH), while the second set of four sprints was always performed at SL. C, T, and I, respectively refer to ANOVA main effects of condition, time and interaction between these two factors with P-value and partial eta-squared into brackets. [a], [b], [c], and [d] significantly different from sprint 1, 4, 8, and 9, respectively (P < 0.05). [1] and [2] significant different from SL and MH, respectively (P < 0.05).

However, sprint performance decreased to a larger extent in SH compared to SL, as evidenced by larger reductions in distance ran during sprint 4 (−8.5 ± 7.9% vs. −5.0 ± 3.0%; P < 0.05) and 8 (−11.7 ± 5.2% vs. −8.9 ± 4.1%; P < 0.05) in reference to sprint 1. Horizontal, but not vertical and total forces, significantly decreased from sprint 1 to 4 (P < 0.05). During sprint 8, values for vertical, horizontal and total forces were significantly lower (all conditions pooled; $-2.3\pm1.9\%$, $-8.6\pm6.5\%$, and $-2.4\pm1.9\%$, respectively; $P < 0.05$) in reference to sprint 1.

During sprint 9, following 6 min of rest, sprint performance and running kinetics recovered significantly, as evidenced by larger values compared to those reached during sprint 8 (distance ran and horizontal forces; $P < 0.05$). Sprint 9 values did not differ from those achieved during sprint 1 and were similar between conditions. Over the last 4 sprints (sprint 9–12), distance ran and horizontal forces decreased similarly by an average of $-4.5 \pm 2.5\%$ and $-13.1\pm9.6\%$ (all conditions pooled; $P < 0.05$), while the decrease in vertical forces ($-2.6\pm4.9\%$) and total forces ($-2.8 \pm 4.9\%$) were not significant.

Running Kinematics

Running kinematics across the repeated sprints are displayed in **Figure 3**. Whereas step length remained unchanged, both contact and aerial times lengthened and step frequency decreased from sprint 1 to 4. During sprint 4, the increase in contact time and the decrease in step frequency were significantly larger in SH compared to MH ($P < 0.05$). From sprint 1 to sprint 8, the increase in contact time ($+14.5 \pm 6.1\%$ vs. $+11.2 \pm 6.8\%$ and $+12.4 \pm 5.1\%$; $P < 0.05$) and decrease in step frequency ($-9.7 \pm 4.2\%$ vs. $-7.2 \pm 3.7\%$ and $-8.1 \pm 2.7\%$; $P < 0.05$) were larger in SH compared to SL and MH. Independently of the condition, aerial time lengthened ($+4.2 \pm 2.9\%$; $P < 0.05$) and step length decreased ($-2.5 \pm 3.0\%$; $P < 0.05$) from sprint 1 to 8. After 6 min of rest between sprints 8 and 9, sprint kinematic values during sprint 9 were not statistically different from those recorded during sprint 1, with also no significant difference between conditions. During subsequent sprints (9–12), irrespectively of the condition, contact time ($+10.2 \pm 5.2\%$) and aerial time ($+3.8 \pm 3.3\%$) lengthened ($P < 0.05$), step frequency ($-6.2 \pm 2.6\%$) decreased ($P < 0.05$) and step length ($+1.2 \pm 3.0\%$) remained unchanged.

Compared to SL and MH, contact time and step frequency values corresponding to the average of sprints 1 to 4 and sprints 5 to 8 differed under SH (**Table 1**; $P < 0.05$). The averaged values of distance covered, kinetics and kinematics for sprints 9–12 were similar across conditions and were not statistically different than the average of sprints 1–4.

Surface EMG Activity

Temporal profiles of the EMG amplitude (RMS) and frequency spectrum (MPF) for the six investigated muscles are shown in **Tables 2**, **3**. With the exception of *Rectus femoris* RMS activity displaying lower values in SH compared to SL for sprint 8 ($P < 0.05$), all other investigated muscles RMS and MPF values fell significantly over time ($P < 0.05$), independently of the condition. The decrease in RMS activity from sprint 1 to 4, expressed as a percentage of sprint 1 value, was significant for *Vastus lateralis*, *Rectus femoris*, *Gastrocnemius lateralis,* and *Tibialis anterior* muscles ($P < 0.05$), while all muscles displayed lower values in all conditions during sprint 8 (**Table 2**). After 6 min of rest, a recovery in the RMS activity of all muscles (except for *Biceps femoris*) occurred during sprint 9, which was not statistically different than that in sprint 1. During sprint 12, RMS

activities for all muscles were lower than those of sprints 4 (except for *Biceps femoris*) and 9 ($P < 0.05$). When compared to sprint 1 (100%), MPF values were reduced during sprint 8 for *Vastus lateralis* and *Rectus femoris*, during sprint 9 for *Gastrocnemius lateralis* and *Tibialis anterior* and during sprint 12 for *Biceps femoris* and *Gastrocnemius medialis* (**Table 3**; $P < 0.05$).

Discussion

Different Levels of Acute Hypoxia Alter RSA and Neuro-mechanical Adjustments

SpO_2 values were increasingly lower as O_2 availability decreased, yet cardio-vascular (HR) and perceptual (RPE) loads associated with performing repeated treadmill sprints were not incrementally higher, which may be due in part to the lower work performed at SH and the "all out" nature of the present exercise (Balsom et al., 1994). Hence, fatigue-induced decrement in sprint distance was significantly exacerbated in SH relative to SL, while sprint performance was relatively resilient to MH exposure. Single (i.e., sprint 1 in the present study) sprint performance is known to be unaffected by differing hypoxia levels (Billaut et al., 2013). For instance, treadmill sprint performance for efforts lasting 60 s or less is not adversely affected at altitude ($FiO_2 = 13\%$) (Weyand et al., 1999). This may relate to an enhanced anaerobic energy release to compensate for the reduced aerobic ATP production (Calbet et al., 2003; Ogawa et al., 2007). However, earlier and larger performance decrements usually occur when consecutive sprints are performed in O_2-deprived environments with hypoxia-related effects becoming more evident above 3000 m (Bowtell et al., 2014; Goods et al., 2014).

During set 1 of all trials, the temporal aspects of the stride cycles shifted toward an increase in contact and aerial times, along with reductions in step frequency. Collectively, it demonstrates a deteriorated ability to tolerate ground impact/stretch loads as fatigue develops with sprint repetitions. In line with these findings, similar impairments in sprint kinematics have been connected with progressively slower sprint performance during over-ground [i.e., 6×20 m – 20 s of passive recovery in U19 footballers (Girard et al., 2011a); 6×35 m – 10 s of passive recovery in elite footballers (Brocherie et al., 2015); 12×40 m – 30 s of passive recovery in team- and racquet-sports athletes (Girard et al., 2011b)] or treadmill [i.e., 5×5-s sprints–25 s of passive recovery (Girard et al., 2015a); 3 sets of 5×6-s sprints–24 s of passive recovery between sprints and 3 min between sets (Morin et al., 2011) in athletes with a team-sport background] repeated sprints. Furthermore, the larger magnitude of repeated-sprint performance alterations seen at SH compared to SL and MH was due to exacerbated increases in contact time and decreases in step frequency in the severer hypoxic condition. Slower sprints and less efficient stride characteristics in SH compared to SL or MH appear to be the result of individuals applying less forward-oriented forces. In line with previous literature (Morin et al., 2011), our primary biomechanical rationale for this conclusion is based on the fact that the magnitude of reductions for horizontal forces was three times larger than for resultant (total) forces.

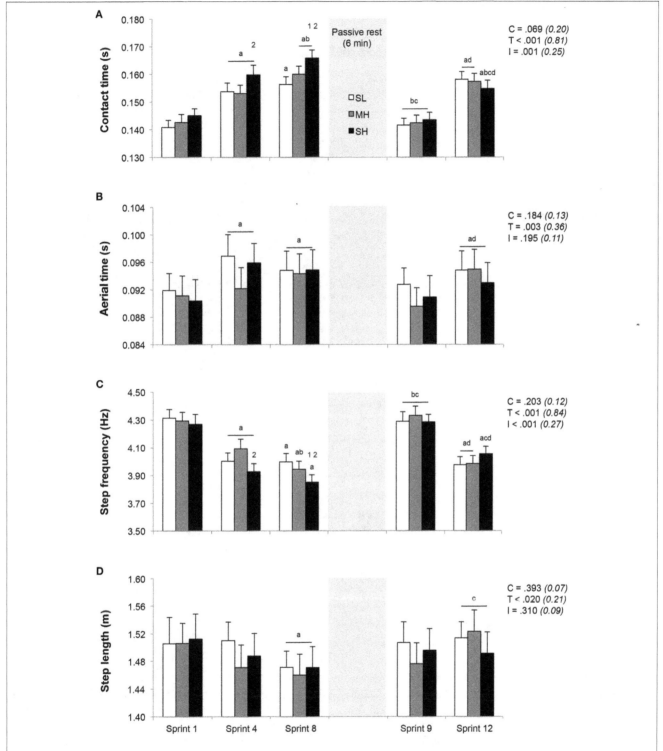

FIGURE 3 | Changes in stride kinematics (A, contact time; B, aerial time; C, step frequency; D, step length). Mean ± SD (*n* = 13). The repeated-sprint exercise protocol included a first set of eight sprints performed at sea level (SL), moderate (MH) or severe hypoxia (SH), while the second set of four sprints was always performed at SL. C, T, and I, respectively refer to ANOVA main effects of condition, time and interaction between these two factors with *P*-value and partial eta-squared into brackets. [a], [b], [c], and [d] significantly different from sprint 1, 4, 8, and 9, respectively (*P* < 0.05). [1] and [2] significant different from SL and MH, respectively (*P* < 0.05).

Remarkably, most of the alteration in performance and accompanying running mechanics was observed within the first half of the first set (sprints 1–4) with smaller changes during the second part (sprints 5–8). During the completion of ten, 10-s sprints with 180 s of recovery the rate of decline in total work was also greater during the first 5 sprints compared to the last

TABLE 1 | Sprint performance, kinetics, and kinematics averaged for sprints 1–4, 5–8, and 9–12.

Variables	Average of sprints			ANOVA p-value (partial eta-squared)		
	1–4	5–8	9–12	Condition	Time	Interaction
DISTANCE (M)						
SL	23.48 ± 1.33	22.32 ± 1.06	23.32 ± 1.53	< 0.001	0.091	0.119
MH	23.31 ± 1.36	22.04 ± 1.32	23.24 ± 1.36	(0.81)	(0.18)	(0.14)
SH	22.92 ± 1.51	21.71 ± 1.27	23.30 ± 1.29			
VERTICAL FORCE (BW)						
SL	1.67 ± 0.09	1.65 ± 0.09	1.67 ± 0.10	0.003	0.208	0.292
MH	1.67 ± 0.09	1.64 ± 0.08	1.65 ± 0.09	(0.39)	(0.12)	(0.10)
SH	1.66 ± 0.08	1.63 ± 0.09	1.66 ± 0.09			
HORIZONTAL FORCE (BW)						
SL	0.20 ± 0.04	0.20 ± 0.04	0.20 ± 0.04	0.004	0.013	0.418
MH	0.21 ± 0.04	0.20 ± 0.03	0.20 ± 0.04	(0.37)	(0.31)	(0.07)
SH	0.20 ± 0.04	0.18 ± 0.04	0.20 ± 0.04			
RESULTANT FORCES (BW)						
SL	1.69 ± 0.09	1.66 ± 0.09	1.68 ± 0.10	0.003	0.178	0.385
MH	1.68 ± 0.09	1.65 ± 0.08	1.67 ± 0.09	(0.38)	(0.13)	(0.08)
SH	1.67 ± 0.08	1.64 ± 0.09	1.68 ± 0.09			
CONTACT TIME (S)						
SL	0.148 ± 0.010	0.155 ± 0.008[a]	0.151 ± 0.011	<0.001	0.015	<0.001
MH	0.148 ± 0.010	0.158 ± 0.009[a]	0.150 ± 0.010[ab]	(0.82)	(0.30)	(0.36)
SH	0.152 ± 0.010[12]	0.163 ± 0.010[a12]	0.150 ± 0.009[ab]			
AERIAL TIME (S)						
SL	0.095 ± 0.010	0.096 ± 0.011	0.094 ± 0.010	0.026	0.583	0.886
MH	0.093 ± 0.010	0.095 ± 0.009	0.093 ± 0.010	(0.26)	(0.04)	(0.02)
SH	0.094 ± 0.010	0.096 ± 0.011	0.093 ± 0.010			
STEP FREQUENCY (HZ)						
SL	4.14 ± 0.22	4.01 ± 0.21[a]	4.11 ± 0.24[b]	<0.001	0.039	0.002
MH	4.17 ± 0.24	3.98 ± 0.22[a]	4.14 ± 0.25[b]	(0.80)	(0.24)	(0.30)
SH	4.07 ± 0.22[12]	3.88 ± 0.17[a1]	4.14 ± 0.21[b]			
STEP LENGTH (M)						
SL	1.51 ± 0.11	1.48 ± 0.09	1.51 ± 0.12	0.008	0.410	0.987
MH	1.49 ± 0.11	1.47 ± 0.10	1.50 ± 0.11	(0.33)	(0.07)	(0.01)
SH	1.49 ± 0.11	1.47 ± 0.10	1.50 ± 0.11			

Mean ± SD (n = 13). The repeated-sprint exercise protocol included a first set of eight sprints performed at sea level (SL), moderate (MH), or severe hypoxia (SH), while the second set of four sprints was always performed at SL.
[a,b] *Significant different from average of sprint 1–4 and 5–8, respectively (P < 0.05).*
[1,2] *Significant different from SL and MH, respectively (P < 0.05).*

5 sprints (−5.2% vs. −3.3%) (Pearcey et al., 2015). In this later study, neuromuscular fatigue in the first 5 sprints was mainly peripheral, whereas in the last 5 sprints it was both peripheral and central. By assessing the development of fatigability during repeated-sprint running exercise (12 × 30 m–30 s rest), it has also been reported that significant peripheral and central knee extensor fatigue becomes evident after just two maximal sprints (Goodall et al., 2015). In our study, the etiology of neuromuscular fatigability (i.e., using peripheral and/or magnetic stimulations) during or after repeated sprinting has not been specifically investigated. Using such stimulation procedure and exposure to acute moderate hypoxia (i.e., FiO_2 = 13.8%; Billaut et al.,

2013) or the induction of pre-existing locomotor muscle fatigue (i.e., following a 10-min neuromuscular electrical stimulation protocol of the quadriceps; Hureau et al., 2014) it was, however, evidenced that feedbacks from fatiguing muscles play an important role in the determination of central motor drive and force output during RSA protocols; i.e., the development of peripheral muscle fatigue would be confined to a certain level so as not to surpass a sensory tolerance limit.

During the first repeated-sprint set, RMS activity values of all investigated muscles decreased significantly over time, confirming that neural factors may have played a role in fatigue-related decrement in sprint performance (Bowtell et al., 2014;

TABLE 2 | Surface EMG root mean square (RMS) activity.

Variables (% sprint 1)	Sprints				ANOVA p-value (partial eta-squared)		
	4	8	9	12	Condition	Time	Interaction
RMS vastus lateralis							
SL	90.9 ± 9.5[a]	85.0 ± 17.0[a]	92.4 ± 16.8[c]	86.1 ± 17.2[ad]	0.987	<0.001	0.923
MH	89.2 ± 11.7[a]	86.3 ± 11.7[a]	94.3 ± 9.4[c]	84.9 ± 14.4[ad]	(0.01)	(0.52)	(0.03)
SH	88.8 ± 11.8[a]	83.0 ± 13.1[a]	96.1 ± 5.8[c]	84.8 ± 6.0[ad]			
RMS rectus femoris							
SL	88.8 ± 9.2[a]	84.8 ± 9.1[ab]	98.1 ± 11.7[c]	88.1 ± 9.9[ad]	0.166	<0.001	0.036
MH	96.8 ± 10.2[a]	85.5 ± 13.3[ab]	94.6 ± 14.2[c]	84.3 ± 17.0[ad]	(0.14)	(0.67)	(0.15)
SH	84.1 ± 10.6[a]	75.5 ± 9.9[ab1]	91.1 ± 13.7[c]	81.8 ± 12.4[ad]			
RMS biceps femoris							
SL	92.9 ± 10.4	87.1 ± 13.3[a]	94.7 ± 9.0[a]	85.1 ± 18.6[abd]	0.906	<0.001	0.535
MH	98.9 ± 9.2	91.6 ± 9.2[a]	90.2 ± 12.9[a]	85.4 ± 15.3[abd]	(0.01)	(0.53)	(0.06)
SH	93.3 ± 9.4	89.2 ± 9.5[a]	94.2 ± 11.7[a]	85.6 ± 15.5[abd]			
RMS gastrocnemius medialis							
SL	93.8 ± 5.9[a]	86.2 ± 10.2[ab]	99.6 ± 9.9[c]	91.9 ± 18.2[acd]	0.336	<0.001	0.553
MH	93.2 ± 11.2[a]	82.6 ± 13.9[ab]	92.4 ± 12.9[c]	84.5 ± 18.9[acd]	(0.09)	(0.61)	(0.06)
SH	90.3 ± 9.7[a]	81.9 ± 8.4[ab]	95.7 ± 9.5[c]	91.5 ± 11.6[acd]			
RMS gastrocnemius lateralis							
SL	94.5 ± 12.0	86.8 ± 10.4[ab]	98.0 ± 8.8[c]	88.3 ± 13.1[ad]	0.725	<0.001	0.657
MH	95.4 ± 10.3	82.5 ± 17.1[ab]	99.1 ± 14.9[c]	87.4 ± 13.6[ad]	(0.02)	(0.63)	(0.05)
SH	89.7 ± 12.1	83.0 ± 13.8[ab]	97.6 ± 8.1[c]	88.2 ± 13.4[ad]			
RMS tibialis anterior							
SL	85.6 ± 13.2[a]	72.5 ± 13.9[ab]	98.4 ± 10.8[c]	83.4 ± 16.1[ad]	0.302	<0.001	0.039
MH	87.3 ± 10.4[a]	84.4 ± 15.5[ab]	96.6 ± 10.8[c]	85.1 ± 10.8[ad]	(0.10)	(0.71)	(0.15)
SH	83.9 ± 13.3[a]	76.3 ± 13.2[ab]	90.0 ± 10.0[c]	80.5 ± 13.7[ad]			

Mean ± SD (n = 13). The repeated-sprint exercise protocol included a first set of 8 sprints performed at sea level (SL), moderate (MH), or severe hypoxia (SH), while the second set of 4 sprints was always performed at SL.
[a], [b], [c], and [d] significant different from sprint 1, 4, 8, and 9, respectively (P < 0.05).
[1] significant different from SL (P < 0.05).

Brocherie et al., 2015). This emphasis a decreased number of motor units activated and/or firing rates of the recruited motor units in exercising quadriceps and plantar flexor muscles, yet with no possible distinction between these two phenomena. Our results also feature an earlier and larger central down-regulation of skeletal muscle recruitment in SH compared to SL or MH, even though this observation is restricted to the *Rectus femoris* muscle only. Exacerbated performance decrements under severe hypoxia are likely to be explained by a reduced neural drive to the active musculature, arising secondary to a stronger reflex inhibition due to brain hypoxia (i.e., decreased brain oxygenation independently of afferent feedback and peripheral fatigue; Millet et al., 2012a) or a hypoxia-induced increased level of intramuscular metabolites known to stimulate group III-IV muscle afferents (Hogan et al., 1999). Although, hypoxia exposure would exacerbate exercise-induced demand placed upon the central nervous system to explain premature fatigue, it is important to emphasize that local metabolic factors (not measured here) may also be responsible for the greater fatigue incurred in SH vs. other conditions.

Reductions in MPF during exercise are indicative of a slowdown of muscle fiber action potential conduction velocity (Lindstrom et al., 1970). In the present study, the values of MPF from the *Vastus lateralis* and *Rectus femoris* muscles during sprint 8 were significantly lower than in sprint 1, while there was no condition effect. This result differs from that of Matsuura et al. (2006) who suggested, based on lower MPF values during repeated cycling sprints with 35-s vs. 350 s recovery periods, that a severer metabolic state (i.e., increased hypoxia severity) induces preferred recruitment of slow twitch motor units.

Restoration of Sprint Mechanical Performance between Repeated-sprint Sets

Conceivably, perceptual recovery, which is known to interact with both feed-forward/feed-back mechanisms, may well affect athlete's willingness to maintain maximal efforts during successive sprint actions. Despite distance covered and resulting HR not being different, RPE values were elevated during the second compared to the first repeated-sprint set at similar time points (sprint 9 vs. 1 and 12 vs. 4). This indicates that perception of peripheral discomfort may not be the major performance regulator during RSA running protocols. Also in line with this assumption are the well-preserved quadriceps muscle activation and associated power output that occurred during two 4-s maximal cycling bouts under hypoxic (FiO$_2$ =

TABLE 3 | Surface EMG median power frequency (MPF).

Variables (% sprint 1)	Sprints				ANOVA p-value (partial eta-squared)		
	4	8	9	12	Condition	Time	Interaction
RMS *vastus lateralis*							
SL	96.1 ± 10.0[a]	94.2 ± 13.0	97.7 ± 10.9	94.3 ± 11.9	0.977	0.024	0.923
MH	95.4 ± 13.0[a]	95.0 ± 12.6	98.0 ± 12.3	93.9 ± 16.0	(0.02)	(0.21)	(0.03)
SH	99.2 ± 8.4[a]	93.2 ± 10.0	94.4 ± 13.8	92.9 ± 14.4			
RMS *rectus femoris*							
SL	99.9 ± 5.2[a]	96.4 ± 7.6[ab]	98.8 ± 8.6[c]	99.0 ± 10.6	0.186	<0.001	0.167
MH	89.6 ± 10.9[a]	88.8 ± 8.8[ab]	97.5 ± 11.6[c]	95.1 ± 14.1	(0.14)	(0.42)	(0.13)
SH	94.1 ± 10.3[a]	87.6 ± 13.1[ab]	94.2 ± 13.2[c]	89.3 ± 16.4			
RMS *biceps femoris*							
SL	96.2 ± 7.2	95.9 ± 10.9	90.0 ± 16.4	90.1 ± 18.7	0.208	0.046	0.509
MH	99.3 ± 12.2	94.8 ± 13.0	95.1 ± 15.6	94.4 ± 11.8	(0.12)	(0.23)	(0.07)
SH	105.1 ± 6.1	101.7 ± 10.8	94.2 ± 11.2	97.1 ± 14.9			
RMS *gastrocnemius medialis*							
SL	98.7 ± 9.3	99.4 ± 9.2	92.9 ± 12.3	93.3 ± 8.8[a]	0.886	0.027	0.341
MH	94.8 ± 7.4	92.7 ± 10.6	96.0 ± 11.1	95.2 ± 11.5[a]	(0.01)	(0.20)	(0.09)
SH	97.8 ± 10.0	97.4 ± 10.9	95.0 ± 9.8	94.3 ± 10.0[a]			
RMS *gastrocnemius lateralis*							
SL	96.8 ± 5.1	99.9 ± 9.3	95.1 ± 7.7[a]	98.9 ± 12.2	0.264	0.011	0.607
MH	97.4 ± 6.3	94.4 ± 11.5	94.9 ± 12.6[a]	94.1 ± 8.3	(0.11)	(0.23)	(0.06)
SH	95.8 ± 9.4	94.6 ± 10.7	91.7 ± 12.3[a]	91.2 ± 11.2			
RMS *tibialis anterior*							
SL	97.2 ± 9.3	99.7 ± 10.8	96.3 ± 6.9	98.2 ± 11.5	0.663	0.011	0.605
MH	97.5 ± 5.9	94.5 ± 10.1	96.3 ± 15.8	93.3 ± 13.9	(0.03)	(0.23)	(0.06)
SH	97.9 ± 5.6	95.7 ± 11.0	91.8 ± 8.4	96.7 ± 6.5			

Mean ± SD (n = 13). The repeated-sprint exercise protocol included a first set of 8 sprints performed at sea level (SL), moderate (MH) or severe hypoxia (SH), while the second set of 4 sprints was always performed at SL.
[a], [b], and [c] significant different from sprint 1, 4, and 8, respectively (P < 0.05).

13%) and normoxic conditions, despite higher overall perceived peripheral discomfort and perceived difficulty breathing (Christian et al., 2014). Nevertheless, the role of effort perception during recovery should not be disregarded as, for instance, the magnitude of the core temperature decrease and the subjective perception of recovery following cold water immersion after an intense conditioning session have been related to performance enhancement in a repeated 40 m sprint protocol undertaken 24 h later (Cook and Beaven, 2013). Nonetheless, future studies should isolate perceptual responses to recovery as mitigating of improved performance.

After the 6 min of passive rest between sprint 8 and sprint 9, the temporal aspects of the stride cycle (contact and aerial times, step frequency and step length values) and force production characteristics (mean horizontal and resultant forces) during sprint 9 recovered from those recorded during sprint 8 and were not different from sprint 1. When physical education students performed four sets of five, 6-s sprints (24 s of passive recovery between sprints, 3 min of rest between sets), Morin et al. (2011) observed that the level of performance was almost systematically higher at the beginning of sets 2, 3, and 4 than at the end of sets 1, 2, and 3. Thus, to preserve RSA performance it is practically important to apply large forward-oriented total force against

the ground and minimize the decrease in step frequency (i.e., increase in contact time). Furthermore, despite differing hypoxic severity levels during sprints 1–8, distance covered as well as the main kinetic and kinematic variables measured at sprint 9 were restored near sprint 1 in all conditions. Interestingly, SpO_2 values recorded for sprint 9 were similar to those of sprint 1 in the SL condition, with also no difference between conditions for the average of the four sprint repetitions of the second normoxic set. In fact, restoration of SpO_2 levels near baseline SL values is virtually complete after 6 min of normoxic exposure. Collectively, it shows that hypoxia level of an initial sprint bout may not blunt the post-exercise recovery of single and repeated-sprint performance and its mechanical basis.

Restoration of EMG indices (RMS and MPF values) appear to align with sprint mechanical performance recovery between sprints 8 and 9, with no difference when comparing initial efforts of the two repeated-sprint sets (sprints 1 vs. 9). This reinforces that the ability to fully activate the contracting musculature and/or optimal inter-muscle recruitment strategies are important regulators of RSA. These results, however, are in disagreement with those reporting that EMG amplitude remained depressed (≈ 13%), after 6 min of rest, during the initial repetition of the second exercise set, despite mechanical performance being matched for first sprint of the two repeated-sprint series (Mendez-Villanueva et al., 2007). Compared to normoxia, cycling performance and quadriceps muscle activation during a multiple sets RSA protocol (three sets of five 5-s cycling sprints with 25 s of passive recovery between sprints and 120 s of rest between sets) was lower in moderate hypoxia (FiO_2 ~0.14), with also incomplete apparent recoveries of performance between the last repetition of sets 1 and 2 (i.e., sprints 5 and 10) and the initial repetition of sets 2 and 3 (i.e., sprints 6 and 11) (Billaut et al., 2013). Accordingly, it is difficult to directly compare our results with other experimental/environmental conditions. In the present study, restoration of sprint mechanical performance following prior repeated sprints at differing hypoxia severity resulted from the recovery of muscle recruitment patterns, which implicates a role for central mechanisms in the regulation of post-exercise recovery. However, the role of peripheral recovery should not be overlooked since it was demonstrated, using a similar exercise protocol, that phosphocreatine re-synthesis was associated with total work done during the first sprint of the second set ($r = 0.79$, $P < 0.05$) and total work done during the five sprints of the second set ($r = 0.67$, $P < 0.05$) (Mendez-Villanueva et al., 2012).

Hypoxia has no Residual Effect during a Subsequent Normoxic Repeated-sprint Performance

An important determinant of fatigue during repeated sprinting is the initial (i.e., first sprint) mechanical output, which has consistently been positively correlated with performance decrement over subsequent sprints (Girard et al., 2011c). In this study, similar performance was observed during initial sprints of both sets with no difference between conditions. Furthermore, the averaged values of distance covered, kinetics and kinematics for the four sprints of the second set (i.e., sprints 9–12; fatigued muscles) were similar across conditions and were not statistically different in reference to the average of the first four sprints of the initial set (i.e., sprints 1–4; non-fatigued muscles). With this in mind, our results indicate that recent muscle activation (completion of the first set) does not alter the muscle recruitment pattern and fatigability during a second set of repeated sprints completed near sea level after a 6 min (normoxic) resting period. These results contrast with those of Mendez-Villanueva et al. (2007) who indicated that after 6 min of rest following 10, 6-s cycling sprints, participants were able to reproduce during sprint 11 the mechanical performance achieved during sprint 4, but not RSA. In the above study, greater fatigability was evident in the five repetitions of the second (i.e., sprints 11–15) vs. the first set (i.e., sprints 4–8), suggesting different recovery time courses after single sprint and RSA performances. Despite severer hypoxia levels during a first repeated-sprint exercise bout, majoring exercise-induced demands placed on the neuromuscular system (i.e., contact times and step frequencies for sprints 5–8 differed from sprints 1 to 4 and 9 to 12), there was no apparent fatigue-related residual or "carry-over" effects from this previous set. Hence, RSA was similar across conditions during the completion of a second set of normoxic repeated sprints.

With different exercise-to-rest ratios influencing, to a large extent, the oxidative vs. glycolytic component (Tabata et al., 1997), RSA may not be similarly affected by hypoxia exposure, which complicates comparison of our results with those of previous studies. Although, evidence is currently lacking, it is anticipated that narrower exercise-to-rest ratios (1:2–1:4 vs. 1:5 as used here) and severer hypoxic conditions, inducing a decreased O_2 availability and an increased reliance on O_2-independent glycolysis for ATP resynthesis together with a larger recruitment of fast-twitch fibers, may exacerbate sprint performance decrements. While similar blood lactate concentration levels observed here may suggest otherwise, whether glycolytic vs. aerobic contributions actually differed between our three conditions would need to be confirmed from muscle oxygenation, phosphocreatine metabolism and/or pH recordings. RSA protocols using different exercise-to-rest ratios and hypoxia levels in the same group of participants would also be helpful in this instance. The resting period duration between the two sets is obviously a key parameter for any type of multiple repeated-sprint sets. In the "hypoxia-to-normoxia recovery" protocols, this duration is paramount as it determines SpO_2 levels at the start of the second set. In this study, SpO_2 values measured 4 min into recovery between the two repeated-sprint sets returned near baseline and did not differ between conditions. It is, however, likely that SpO_2 recovery to initial values was even shorter. Hence, Krivoshchekov et al. (2014) reported that the SpO_2 recovery response after an acute exposure to normobaric hypoxia ($FiO_2 = 0.10$) decreasing SpO_2 to 85% was ~120 s.

Limitations

Before concluding, we must acknowledge several limitations that may affect generalization of our findings. Firstly, although the data were collected continuously (step-by-step), our analysis was concentrated on 3 steps at top speed (i.e., usually corresponding to the 20 m mark of the sprints). It is noteworthy, however, that considering all steps or only a few steps during early, middle or late phases of 5-s sprints provides similar mechanical outcomes during repeated treadmill sprinting, although acceleration induces noticeable differences between the sections studied (Girard et al., 2015a). It must also be appreciated that running speed reached on our treadmill is 15–20% slower than over-ground, even though changes in running mechanics are relatively similar (Rabita et al., 2015) and overall sprint performance is highly correlated between these two sprinting modes (Morin and Sève, 2011). Although, an effect on performance induced by EMG electrodes or mask breathing cannot be completely ruled out, the use of wireless technology and the fact that resistance and increase in dead space are negligible (Sheel, 2002) suggests that their influence did not modify the main findings of the present study.

Secondly, several concerns may affect EMG analysis and include: (1) surface EMG amplitude cancellation; (2) the stability of neuromuscular propagation and sarcolemmal excitability (i.e., absence of supra-maximal stimulation to evoke a M-wave for normalization of the EMG signal); (3)

fatigue-related reflex inhibition (i.e., reflex effects in the spinal cord). With differences <5%, the surface EMG signal may not be sufficiently sensitive to measure meaningful (i.e., clinically relevant) difference in muscle activation between conditions. Therefore, declines in the magnitude of efferent descending motor outflow, as a key factor in neuromuscular recovery following repeated sprints, would need to be confirmed through the use of multiple neurophysiological measures (TMS, EEG) during resting intervals. The kinetics of muscle oxygenation (NIRS) would also be valuable for better comparing the metabolic differences between hypoxic conditions.

Thirdly, we have used three known values of FiO_2 as hypoxic stimulus. For exposure to the same simulated altitude ($FiO_2 = 10\%$), however, it is conceded that there is a larger inter-individual variability in the degree of arterial hypoxemia compared to clamped values of SpO_2 (at 75%) (Hamlin et al., 2010). While clamping of SpO_2 would likely cause a more consistent hypoxic stimulus across individuals, it remains to be demonstrated that it will also induce a better heterogeneity in neuro-mechanical responses to repeated sprinting. Furthermore, hypobaric hypoxia has been shown to induce severer physiological responses (SpO_2 and HR) than normobaric hypoxia (Millet et al., 2012b). One may therefore speculate that the performance and mechanical alterations would be larger at natural altitude than in the present laboratory study. Direct comparisons of repeated sprint exercises between normobaric and hypobaric hypoxia are required.

Finally, in our study, we implemented 6 min of rest between the two sets of repeated treadmill sprints, so as to compare our results with previous findings (Mendez-Villanueva et al., 2007, 2012). However, not only are the acute neuro-mechanical adjustments and the ensuing recovery of SpO_2 and performance influenced by the duration/nature of the between-sets normoxic rest period but also the details of the RSA protocols (e.g., exercise-to-rest ratio, exercise mode, environment encountered; Girard et al., 2011c) and participants' background (e.g., training status, "aerobic" vs. "anaerobic" profile, gender; Calbet et al., 2003). Given the task-dependency of the effects of fatigue, our conclusions must remain specific to the circumstances of this study and would need to be confirmed using other RSA protocols and participants.

Conclusion

To improve our understanding of neuro-mechanical determinants of RSA, we manipulated the hypoxia severity during an initial set of repeated sprints and examined the effect on alterations in performance, running mechanics and lower-limbs neuromuscular activity during a subsequent set completed in normoxia. Under the circumstances of this study (participants' background, exercise-to-rest ratio, hypoxia exposure), the magnitude of performance and neuro-mechanical alterations (kinetics, kinematics, EMG indices) and the severity of physiological and perceptual responses were larger in SH compared to SL and MH. The novel findings from our "recovery of performance" approach are that recoveries of performance and neuro-mechanical alterations are almost complete after resting for 6 min near sea level, with also a similar fatigue pattern across conditions during subsequent repeated sprints in normoxia. To preserve RSA performance, it is therefore important to apply large forward-oriented ground reaction force and minimize the decrease in step frequency (i.e., increase in contact time), which at least in part result from more optimal neural drive strategies. However, no singular factor may represent a direct causative mechanism determining RSA so that studying the potential for other drivers of recovery (e.g., muscle damage or metabolic factors) may also be relevant.

Author Contributions

Conceived and designed the experiments: OG and FB. Performed experiments: OG and FB. Analyzed data: OG, FB, and JM. Interpreted results of research: OG, FB, JM, and GM. Drafted manuscript and prepared tables/figures: OG. Edited critically revised paper and approved final version of manuscript: OG, FB, JM, and GM.

Funding

This work is based on research funded by QNRF (NPRP 4 – 760 – 3 – 217).

Acknowledgments

The authors thank the participants for their maximal efforts and cooperation.

References

Balsom, P. D., Gaitanos, G. C., Ekblom, B., and Sjödin, B. (1994). Reduced oxygen availability during high intensity intermittent exercise impairs performance. *Acta Physiol. Scand.* 152, 279–285. doi: 10.1111/j.1748-1716.1994.tb09807.x

Billaut, F., Kerris, J. P., Rodriguez, R. F., Martin, D. T., Gore, C. J., and Bishop, D. J. (2013). Interactions of central and peripheral factors using repeated sprints at different levels of arterial O_2 saturation. *PLoS ONE* 8:e77297. doi: 10.1371/journal.pone.0077297

Bowtell, J. L., Cooke, K., Turner, R., Mileva, K. N., and Sumners, D. P. (2014). Acute physiological and performance responses to repeated sprints in varying degrees of hypoxia. *J. Sci. Med. Sport.* 17, 399–403. doi: 10.1016/j.jsams.2013.05.016

Brocherie, F., Millet, G. P., and Girard, O. (2015). Neuro-mechanical and metabolic adjustments to the repeated anaerobic sprint test in professional football players. *Eur. J. Appl. Physiol.* 115, 891–903. doi: 10.1007/s00421-014-3070-z

Calbet, J. A., De Paz, J. A., Garatechea, N., Cabeza de Veca, S., and Chavarren, J. (2003). Anaerobic energy provision does not limit Wingate exercise performance in endurance-trained cyclists. *J. Appl. Physiol.* 94, 668–676. doi: 10.1152/japplphysiol.00128.2002

Carling, C. (2013). Interpreting physical performance in professional soccer match-play: should we be more pragmatic in our approach? *Sports Med.* 43, 655–663. doi: 10.1007/s40279-013-0055-8

Christian, R. J., Bishop, D. J., Billaut, F., and Girard, O. (2014). The role of sense of effort on self-selected cycling power output. *Front Physiol.* 5:115. doi: 10.3389/fphys.2014.00115

Cook, C. J., and Beaven, C. M. (2013). Individual perception of recovery is related to subsequent sprint performance. *Br. J. Sports Med.* 47, 705–709. doi: 10.1136/bjsports-2012-091647

Girard, O., Brocherie, F., and Millet, G. P. (2015b). Can analysis of performance and neuromuscular recoveries from repeated sprints shed more light on its fatigue-causing mechanisms? *Front. Physiol.* 6:5. doi: 10.3389/fphys.2015.00005

Girard, O., Brocherie, F., Morin, J.-B., Degache, F., and Millet, G. P. (2015a). Comparison of four sections for analysing running mechanics alterations during repeated treadmill sprints. *J. Appl. Biomech.* doi: 10.1123/jab.2015-0049. [Epub ahead of print].

Girard, O., Brocherie, F., Morin, J.-B., and Millet, G. P. (2015c). Intra- and inter-session reliability of running mechanics during treadmill sprints. *Int. J. Sports Physiol. Perf.* doi: 10.1123/ijspp.2015-0145. [Epub ahead of print].

Girard, O., Mendez-Villanueva, A., and Bishop, D. J. (2011c). Repeated-sprint ability—Part I. *Sports Med.* 41, 673–694. doi: 10.2165/11590550-000000000-00000

Girard, O., Micallef, J. P., and Millet, G. P. (2011b). Changes in spring-mass model characteristics during repeated running sprints. *Eur. J. Appl. Physiol.* 111, 125–134. doi: 10.1007/s00421-010-1638-9

Girard, O., Racinais, S., Kelly, L., Millet, G. P., and Brocherie, F. (2011a). Repeated sprinting on natural grass impairs vertical stiffness but does not alter plantar loading in soccer players. *Eur. J. Appl. Physiol.* 111, 2547–2555. doi: 10.1007/s00421-011-1884-5

Goodall, S., Charlton, K., Howatson, G., and Thomas, K. (2015). Neuromuscular fatigability during repeated-sprint exercise in male athletes. *Med. Sci. Sports Exerc.* 47, 528–536. doi: 10.1249/MSS.0000000000000443

Goods, P. S. R., Dawson, B. T., Landers, G. J., Gore, C. J., and Peeling, P. (2014). Effect of different simulated altitudes on repeat-sprint performance in team-sport athletes. *Int. J. Sports Physiol. Perform.* 9, 857–862. doi: 10.1123/ijspp.2013-0423

Hamlin, M. J., Marshall, H. C., Hellemans, J., and Ainslie, P. N. (2010). Effect of intermittent hypoxia on muscle and cerebral oxygenation during a 20-km time trial in elite athletes: a preliminary report. *Appl. Physiol. Nutr. Metab.* 35, 548–559. doi: 10.1139/H10-044

Hogan, M. C., Richardson, R. S., and Haseler, L. J. (1999). Human muscle performance and PCr hydrolysis with varied inspired oxygen fractions: a 31P-MRS study. *J. Appl. Physiol.* 86, 1367–1373.

Hureau, T. J., Olivier, N., Millet, G. Y., Meste, O., and Blain, G. M. (2014). Exercise performance is regulated during repeated sprints to limit the development of peripheral fatigue beyond a critical threshold. *Exp. Physiol.* 99, 951–963. doi: 10.1113/expphysiol.2014.077974

Krivoshchekov, S. G., Balioz, N. V., Nekipelova, N. V., and Kapilevich, L. V. (2014). Age, gender, and individually-typological features of reaction to sharp hypoxic influence. *Hum. Physiol.* 40, 34–45. doi: 10.1134/S0362119714060061

Lindstrom, L., Magnusson, R., and Petersén, I. (1970). Muscular fatigue and action potential conduction velocity changes studied with frequency of EMG signals. *Electromyography* 10, 341–356.

Matsuura, R., Ogata, H., Yunoki, T., Arimitsu, T., and Yano, T. (2006). Effect of blood lactate concentration and the level of oxygen uptake immediately before a cycling sprint on neuromuscular activation during repeated cycling sprints. *J. Physiol. Anthropol.* 25, 267–273. doi: 10.2114/jpa2.25.267

Mendez-Villanueva, A., Edge, J., Suriano, R., Hamer, P., and Bishop, D. J. (2012). The recovery of repeated-sprint exercise is associated with PCr resynthesis, while muscle pH and EMG amplitude remain depressed. *PLoS ONE* 7:e51977. doi: 10.1371/journal.pone.0051977

Mendez-Villanueva, A., Hamer, P., and Bishop, D. J. (2007). Fatigue responses during repeated sprints matched for initial mechanical output. *Med. Sci. Sports Exerc.* 39, 2219–2225. doi: 10.1249/mss.0b013e31815669dc

Mendez-Villanueva, A., Hamer, P., and Bishop, D. J. (2008). Fatigue in repeated-sprint exer- cise is related to muscle power factors and reduced neuromuscular activity. *Eur. J. Appl. Physiol.* 103, 411–419. doi: 10.1007/s00421-008-0723-9

Millet, G. P., Faiss, R., and Pialoux, V. (2012b). Point: hypobaric hypoxia induces different physiological responses from normobaric hypoxia. *J. Appl. Physiol*, 112, 1783–1784. doi: 10.1152/japplphysiol.00067.2012

Millet, G. Y., Muthalib, M., Jubeau, M., Laursen, P. B., and Nosaka, K. (2012a). Severe hypoxia affects exercise performance independently of afferent feedback and peripheral fatigue. *J. Appl. Physiol.* 112, 1335–1344. doi: 10.1152/japplphysiol.00804.2011

Minett, G. M., and Duffield, R. (2014). Is recovery driven by central or peripheral factors? A role for the brain in recovery following intermittent-sprint exercise. *Front. Physiol.* 5:24. doi: 10.3389/fphys.2014.00024

Mohr, M., Krustrup, P., Andersson, H., Kirkendal, D., and Bangsbo, J. (2008). Match activities of elite women soccer players at different performance levels. *J. Strength Cond. Res.* 22, 341–349. doi: 10.1519/JSC.0b013e318165fef6

Mohr, M., Krustrup, P., and Bangsbo, J. (2003). Match performance of high-standard soccer players with special reference to development of fatigue. *J. Sports Sci*, 21, 519–528. doi: 10.1080/0264041031000071182

Morin, J. B., Samozino, P., Bonnefoy, R., Edouard, P., and Belli, A. (2010). Direct measurement of power during one single sprint on treadmill. *J. Biomech.* 43, 1970–1975. doi: 10.1016/j.jbiomech.2010.03.012

Morin, J.-B., Samozino, P., Edouard, P., and Tomazin, K. (2011). Effect of fatigue on force production and force application technique during repeated sprints. *J. Biomech.* 44, 2719–2723. doi: 10.1016/j.jbiomech.2011.07.020

Morin, J.-B., and Sève, P. (2011). Sprint running performance: comparison between treadmill and field conditions. *Eur. J. Appl. Physiol.* 111, 1695–1703. doi: 10.1007/s00421-010-1804-0

Ogawa, T., Hayashi, K., Ichinose, M., Wada, H., and Nishiyasu, T. (2007). Metabolic response during intermittent graded sprint running in moderate hypobaric hypoxia in competitive middle-distance runners. *Eur. J. Appl. Physiol.* 99, 39–46. doi: 10.1007/s00421-006-0315-5

Pearcey, G. E., Murphy, J. R., Behm, D. G., Hay, D. C., Power, K. E., and Button, D. C. (2015). Neuromuscular fatigue of the knee extensors during repeated maximal intensity intermittent-sprints on a cycle ergometer. *Muscle Nerve* 51, 569–579. doi: 10.1002/mus.24342

Perrey, S., Racinais, S., Saimouaa, K., and Girard, O. (2010). Neural and muscular adjustments following repeated running sprints. *Eur. J. Appl. Physiol.* 109, 1027–1036. doi: 10.1007/s00421-010-1445-3

Rabita, G., Dorel, S., Slawinski, J., Sàez-de-Villarreal, E., Couturier, A., Samozino, P., et al. (2015). Sprint mechanics in world-class athletes: a new insight into the limits of human locomotion. *Scand. J. Med. Sci. Sports* 25, 583–594. doi: 10.1111/sms.12389

Sheel, A. W. (2002). Respiratory muscle training in healthy individuals: physiological rationale and implications for exercise performance. *Sports Med.* 32, 567–581. doi: 10.2165/00007256-200232090-00003

Tabata, I., Irisawa, K., Kouzaki, M., Ishimura, K., Ogita, F., and Miyachi, M. (1997). Metabolic profile of high intensity intermittent exercises. *Med. Sci. Sports Exerc.* 29, 390–395. doi: 10.1097/00005768-199703000-00015

Weyand, P. G., Lee, C. S., Martinez-Ruiz, R., Bundle, M. W., Bellizzi, M. J., and Wright, S. (1999). High-speed running performance is largely unaffected by hypoxic reductions in aerobic power. *J. Appl. Physiol.* 86, 2059–2064.

Conflict of Interest Statement: The authors declare that the research was conducted in the absence of any commercial or financial relationships that could be construed as a potential conflict of interest.

5

Salivary Hormones Response to Preparation and Pre-competitive Training of World-class Level Athletes

Gaël Guilhem[1]*, Christine Hanon[1], Nicolas Gendreau[1], Dominique Bonneau[1,2], Arnaud Guével[3] and Mounir Chennaoui[2]

[1] Laboratory Sport, Expertise and Performance (EA 7370), Research Department, French National Institute of Sport (INSEP), Paris, France, [2] Fatigue and Vigilance Unit (EA 7330), Neurosciences and Operational Constraints Department, French Armed Forces Biomedical Research Institute (IRBA), Paris Descartes University, Brétigny-sur-Orge, France, [3] Laboratory "Movement, Interactions, Performance" (EA 4334), University of Nantes, Nantes, France

This study aimed to compare the response of salivary hormones of track and field athletes induced by preparation and pre-competitive training periods in an attempt to comment on the physiological effects consistent with the responses of each of the proteins measured. Salivary testosterone, cortisol, alpha-amylase, immunoglobulin A (IgA), chromogranin A, blood creatine kinase activity, and profile of mood state were assessed at rest in 24 world-class level athletes during preparation (3 times in 3 months) and pre-competitive (5 times in 5 weeks) training periods. Total mood disturbance and fatigue perception were reduced, while IgA (+61%) and creatine kinase activity (+43%) increased, and chromogranin A decreased (−27%) during pre-competitive compared to preparation period. A significant increase in salivary testosterone (+9 to +15%) and a decrease in testosterone/cortisol ratio were associated with a progressive reduction in training load during pre-competitive period ($P < 0.05$). None of the psycho-physiological parameters were significantly correlated to training load during the pre-competitive period. Results showed a lower adrenocortical response and autonomic activity, and an improvement of immunity status, in response to the reduction in training load and fatigue, without significant correlations of salivary hormones with training load. Our findings suggest that saliva composition is sensitive to training contents (season period) but could not be related to workload resulting from track and field athletics training.

Keywords: alpha-amylase, immunoglobulin A, chromogranin A, creatine kinase, athletics training

Edited by:
Vincent Pialoux,
Université Claude Bernard Lyon 1,
France

Reviewed by:
Robert Hester,
The University of Mississippi, USA
Tadej Debevec,
Jozef Stefan Institute, Slovenia

***Correspondence:**
Gaël Guilhem
gael.guilhem@insep.fr

INTRODUCTION

During the last few decades, the exponential increase in international competition has progressively led the top-level athletes to extend the time spent to train in order to enhance their performance. Although successful training must involve such high training load phases (i.e., increased volume and intensity), it must also avoid the combination of excessive overload and inadequate recovery (Meeusen et al., 2006). Indeed, a disrupted balance between training stress and rest period following exercise can increase fatigue associated with short-term withdrawal of performance capacity, defined as functional "overreaching" syndrome (Meeusen et al., 2006). When intensive training is maintained, overreaching might evolve to a non-functional overreaching state determined by "qualitative" changes (i.e., symptoms of psychological and/or endocrine distress), which necessitate several weeks or months to restore initial performance (Meeusen et al., 2006). In a monitoring training study, Foster (1998) noted a correspondence between excessive training load and injury and illness occurrence, thereby highlighting the interest of methods for the identification of non-functional overreaching development in elite athletes. Although a very large panel of variables exist to detect non-functional overreaching, on the one hand, there is a lack of consensus regarding their significance when considered independently (Meeusen et al., 2006). On the other hand, multivariate approaches have shown promising results (Le Meur et al., 2013), but have to be validated in the natural context of training and may consequently have limited practicality when used in field conditions of high-level training.

Physical activity is an external stimulus able to trigger an adaptive response coordinated by the stress system (Chennaoui et al., 2004). The main components of the stress system include the autonomic nervous system (ANS) and the hypothalamic-pituitary adreno-cortical (HPA) axis, whose function is sensitive to psychological and physiological stressors (Tsigos and Chrousos, 2002). The ANS mediates the stress response via parasympathetic and sympathetic nerves to the adrenal medulla to produce catecholamines, while steroid hormones are the final effectors of HPA. Thereby, the plasma concentrations of catecholamines, or corticosteroids, testosterone (T) and cortisol (C), have been used as an indicator of autonomic activity (Urhausen et al., 1995). However, the quantification of these proteins also require invasive, stressful procedures (sting venipuncture) and qualified personnel to collect blood samples. Released in blood circulation, steroid hormones may also reach saliva by passive diffusion or active transport.

Scientific evidence also suggests that autonomic activity can indirectly be assessed by hormones released in saliva under the control of ANS (Nater and Rohleder, 2009). Several studies reported fatigue-induced variations in salivary testosterone, signaling a catabolic state, in relation to the intensity and duration of a preceding physical load (Gatti and De Palo, 2011), with an effect of age and gender on basal values (250–600 for males vs. 200 pmol.L^{-1} for females) (Wood, 2009). Similarly, salivary cortisol can be used to determine psychophysiological stress during single and repeated exercise sessions even if a non-univocal relationship has been found between stress and cortisol concentration (Gatti and De Palo, 2011). In addition, during physiological stress experience, similar mechanisms underlie the secretion of alpha-amylase (AA), and catecholamines (norepinephrine and epinephrine), which are co-stored and co-released in saliva with chromogranin A (Montero-Hadjadje et al., 2008). Similarly, subjects exposed to excessive stress could experience immunodepression, which is manifested by decreased levels of immunoglobulin A (IgA), secreted in saliva under autonomic control (Papacosta and Nassis, 2011). Interestingly, repeated training sessions have been shown to increase the levels of salivary IgA and AA activity (Born et al., 2015) or decrease the salivary CgA concentration (Díaz Gómez et al., 2013). Taking together, these elements make saliva a useful, non-invasive, rapid and stress-free alternative to the collection of serum and plasma, allowing for frequent and easy appraisal of stress response.

In this context, the impact of training on salivary markers is currently receiving growing attention. Indeed, the response of aforementioned proteins (e.g., T, C, AA, CgA, IgA) has been applied to predict exercise intensity in well-trained athletes with variable outcomes (Gatti and De Palo, 2011). These different findings have been notably attributed to the high inter-individual variability of the salivary biomarkers, suggesting that repeated sampling can provide more accurate results than unique measure (Papacosta and Nassis, 2011). Whereas most of the studies measured response to acute exercise, those reporting association with chronic exercise (long-term training) in humans are scarce (Nater and Rohleder, 2009). Recently, Diaz et al. (2013) showed that salivary AA response was proportional to training load and intensity in swimmers. However, little is known about the potential usefulness of salivary markers in the identification of non-functional OR over prolonged periods, notably in sport activities with high incidence of injury (e.g., team sports, running, jumping).

Thus, the aim of the present study was to determine the long-term changes in endocrine, psychological, and muscle damage response of training stimulus during an injurious period of elite track and field athletics season, in comparison to a normal preparation phase. Preliminary data and previous studies showed that injury incidence increased during the pre-competitive period, where training volume progressively decreases to increase session intensity and focus on technical contents (D'Souza, 1994). We hypothesized that such modifications in the training stress influence salivary proteins throughout training. Such quantified changes could help to reduce the risk of injury, adjust volume and intensity of training, and in turn lead to enhance functional gains.

METHODS

Participants
Twenty-four high-level track and field athletes (9 men, 15 female, 25 ± 4 years; 177 ± 12 cm; 67 ± 12 kg), including short and long distance sprinters (100–400 m), long jumpers, middle distance runners (800–1500) and combined events athletes, all members of the French national team and competing at the international level during the year of the experiment, participated in this study. The sample included two World champions and one Olympic champion, and several medallists at the European championships, all ranked between the 70th and the 1st place at the International Association of Athletics Federations at the moment of the study. All participants were informed regarding the nature, aims, and risks associated with the experimental procedures before they gave their written consent to participate. None of them smoked, had significant medical or oral health history, or were taking regular or incidental medication during the study. The study was approved by the ethics committee of Paris XI and the French health and safety agency. All experiments were conducted in accordance with the Declaration of Helsinki.

Experimental Design
All participating athletes were followed throughout a 20 week (i.e., 4.5 months) period prior to the major international

competitions (**Figure 1**). The follow-up was spread over two main periods: a preparation period of 3 months (PREP), characterized by a high training volume, and a pre-competitive period (COMP) of 1.5 month including high-intensity and specific training, with a reduced training volume (Issurin, 2010). This part of the season was previously identified as the period where injury incidence was the highest for the athletes (personal data; D'Souza, 1994). During the preparation period, aimed at determining basal hormonal profile, participants attended a test session every first Monday of each month. During pre-competitive period, tests were performed every Monday during 5 consecutive weeks to provide more accurate salivary hormones quantification throughout this phase where injury incidence increases (Papacosta and Nassis, 2011). Each test session consisted of psychological questionnaires filling, and collection of saliva and blood samples. The participants refrained from intense exercise at least 24 h prior to the each collection of samples.

Data Collection
Psychometric Measurements
The participants completed the Profile Of Mood States (POMS) immediately before saliva collection (Cayrou et al., 2003). The participants were asked to state how they felt over the week. The POMS is a 65-item questionnaire measuring tension, depression, anger, confusion, vigor, and fatigue on a 5-point Likert scale. The internal consistency for the POMS (Cronbach's alpha coefficient) was 0.96.

Samples
Whole saliva and blood samples were performed after at least 24 h of rest, the same day of the week, at the same time of

the day (4 p.m.) for all athletes to control for diurnal variation (Gatti and De Palo, 2011). T, C, AA, IgA, and CgA were measured from saliva samples, while CK activity was determined from blood sample. According to standard recommendations, the participants were asked to refrain from drinking or eating during the 2 h prior to the collection of the samples. They were instructed not to perform any physical exercise 2 h and not to brush their teeth 45 min prior to sampling to avoid micro-injuries or abrasion that could induce blood contamination of saliva. Athletes washed their mouth with water 10 min before collection and swallowed the first amount of saliva. Whole saliva was collected by passive drool with no exogenous stimulation, recognized as the most reliable option (Granger et al., 1994). The saliva was allowed to pool in the mouth and then drooled into pre-weighted collection vials after 2 min. Immediately after collecting saliva, 5-mL blood samples were collected in vacutainer EDTA-coated tubes via antecubital venipuncture on the resting arm. Tubes were then mixed and placed on ice before centrifugation (10 min at 2000 bpm at 4°C) and plasma was transferred using a pipette into Eppendorf tubes. Tubes containing plasma and saliva were stored at −80°C for further analysis.

Training Load
During PREP, the training sessions focused on strength and aerobic development with the objective of maintaining the qualities of velocity and the technical abilities. The COMP period consisted of improvement of the anaerobic qualities (velocity and speed endurance) while preserving the retention of the aerobic level. Over this period, the technical exercises were performed at a maximal velocity. Training load was quantified for each week of COMP, in order to relate psychometrical and biological

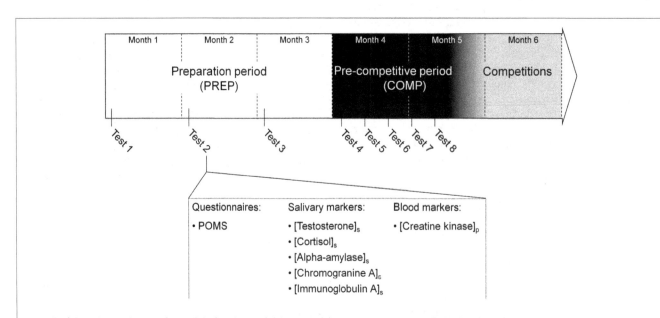

FIGURE 1 | Overview of the experimental design. A total of eight tests sessions were spread over the 5 months prior to the international competition period. The first three tests were performed during the first week of 3 month of the preparation period (PREP) consisted of high volume and low intensity contents. During the pre-competitive period (COMP) characterized by low volume and high intensity training, identical tests sessions were performed every Monday during 5 weeks. Each test session included a Profile Of Mood State (POMS) questionnaire, salivary and blood samples to assess total mood disturbance, salivary concentration of testosterone, cortisol, alpha-amylase, immunoglobulin A and chromogranin A and plasma creatine kinase activity.

changes to training stimulus throughout the injurious period (i.e., COMP). According to the Foster model, the training load of each athlete was determined for each session by integrating the exercise session rating of perceived exertion (RPE) and the duration of the training session (Foster, 1998).

Data Analyses

Salivary concentrations of testosterone, cortisol, and IgA and AA activity were determined using a spectrophotometer Dynex MRXe (Magellan Biosciences, Chelmsford, USA) and standard assay kits (Salimetrics, State College, PA, USA). Chromogranin A was assayed using a kit from Yanaihara Institute (YK070 Human CgA EIA, Yanaihara Institute, Shizuoka, Japan). Salivary concentrations were determined from duplicates of the samples obtained during the preparation, resulting in an intra-assay coefficient of variation below 5% for all salivary markers (4.5 ± 2.1% on average). Subsequent analyses (pre-competitive phase) were thus performed in simple measurement. Measurements performed during both periods were averaged to obtain a representative value for each period (3 values for preparation period, 6 values for pre-competitive period).

Testosterone (T)

The concentration of salivary testosterone in the sample is inversely proportional to the testosterone peroxidase, which was measured by the reaction of the peroxidase enzyme on the substrate tetramethylbenzidine. The optical density resulting from this reaction was measured at 450 nm.

Cortisol (C)

The amount of cortisol peroxidase, measured by the intensity of color originate from the reaction of the peroxidase enzyme on the substrate tetramethylbenzidine, is inversely proportional to the amount of cortisol present. The optical density was measured at 450 nm. The ratio between testosterone and cortisol salivary concentration was expressed as the T/C ratio (Adlercreutz et al., 1986).

Alpha-amylase (AA)

The reagents in the kit contain a chromagenic substrate, 2-chloro-p-nitrophenol linked with maltotriose. The amount of AA activity present in the sample is directly proportional to the increase in absorbance resulting from the enzymatic action of AA on this substrate yields 2-chloro-p-nitrophenol, which was spectrophotometrically measured at 405 nm. Inter- and intra-assay variance was below 1%.

Immunoglobulin A (IgA)

The salivary concentration of IgA was determined by measuring the optical density of the reaction of the peroxidase enzyme on the substrate tetramethylbenzidine, at 450 nm. The amount of peroxidase is inversely proportional to the amount of IgA present in the sample.

Chromogranin A (CgA)

The salivary concentration of CgA was determined by competitive enzyme immunoassay using combination of highly specific antibody to human CgA (344–374) and biotin-avidin affinity system. The 96-wells plate was coated with goat anti rabbit IgG. Human CgA standard or samples, labeled antigen and specific antibody, were added to the wells for competitive immunoreaction. After incubation and plate washing, HRP labeled streptoavidin (SA-HRP) were added to form HRP labeled streptoavidin-labeled antigen-specific antibody complex on the surface of the wells. Finally, HRP enzyme activity was determined by o-Phenylenediamine dihydrochloride (OPD) and the concentration of human CgA is calculated by measuring the absorbance at 490 nm.

Plasma CK Activity

As a marker of sarcolemma disruption, plasma CK activity was measured spectrophotometrically by using commercially available reagents (Roche/Hitachi, Meylan, France) with an inter-assay precision (CV) of 2.7 ± 1.3%.

Statistical Analysis

All analyses were performed with Statistica Version 7.1 (StatSoft, Tulsa, Oklahoma, USA). Data distributions consistently passed the Shapiro-Wilk normality test. All data being normally distributed, Two-way ANOVAs with repeated measures (gender × training period) were performed to determine potential differences in average values of psychometric measurements (POMS scores), salivary concentrations of T, C, AA, IgA, CgA, and blood CK activity between preparation and pre-competitive periods. One-way ANOVAs (time effect) with repeated measures were applied to determine changes in POMS scores, [T], [C], AA activity, [IgA], [CgA], CK activity, and training load throughout the pre-competitive period. A Geisser-Greenhouse correction was used when the sphericity assumption in repeated measures ANOVAs was violated (Mauchly's test). *Post-hoc* tests were performed by means of Newman-Keuls procedures. Separate linear Pearson correlations (r) were performed between each indicators and training load. The significance level was set at $P < 0.05$ for all tests. The data are presented as mean ± SD.

RESULTS

Mood Disturbance

Tension—anxiety, depression, anger and confusion—bewilderment scores significantly decreased from PREP to COMP ($P < 0.05$), whereas vigor—activity ($P = 0.4$) and fatigue ($P = 0.07$) were not affected between both training periods As a result, total mood disturbance was significantly decreased when competitions approached, in comparison to the PREP (**Table 1**). All POMS subscale scores and total mood disturbance did not change significantly throughout COMP ($P = 0.15–0.68$; **Table 2**).

Salivary Hormones
Testosterone

Salivary testosterone concentration during PREP was 405.5 ± 112.7 and 164.7 ± 60.9 pmol.L^{-1} for male and female athletes, respectively vs. 409.6 ± 76.9 and 205.9 ± 83.2 pmol.L^{-1} during COMP. We observed a main effect of gender ($P <$

TABLE 1 | Mood disturbance scores of track and field athletes during the preparation (PREP) and pre-competitive (COMP) period of the sport season.

POMS subscale scores	PREP	COMP
Tension—anxiety	8.6 (4.5)	6.8 (4.0)*
Depression	7.6 (9.1)	4.6 (6.2)*
Anger—hostility	10.4 (8.2)	7.0 (7.7)*
Vigor—activity	16.5 (4.2)	15.8 (4.8)
Fatigue	7.0 (4.2)	5.5 (3.2)
Confusion—bewilderment	7.1 (4.3)	5.1 (3.2)*
Total mood disturbance	43.1 (20.4)	33.7 (17.6)*

The results are means (SD).
*Significant difference (P > 0.05).

TABLE 2 | Training load and mood disturbance of track and field athletes throughout the 5 weeks of the pre-competitive (COMP) period of the sport season.

POMS subscale scores	Training week of the pre-competitive period (COMP)				
	1	2	3	4	5
Training load	3746.4 (4353.3)	2479.1 (3044.2)	2953.2 (2556.3)	1230.8 (1694.2)	1072.7 (1428.2)*
Tension—anxiety	7.7 (4.8)	7.4 (4.4)	7.0 (5.3)	6.6 (5.0)	5.5 (4.8)
Depression	5.1 (6.8)	5.5 (7.9)	4.3 (8.7)	7.5 (10.2)	3.6 (6.0)
Anger—hostility	8.1 (9.0)	6.8 (7.5)	6.6 (9.8)	9.7 (11.0)	6.7 (6.9)
Vigor—activity	16.2 (5.3)	15.2 (5.6)	16.1 (6.5)	16.0 (6.2)	15.0 (6.0)
Fatigue	6.0 (4.7)	6.6 (4.9)	5.0 (4.5)	5.6 (4.3)	4.8 (4.0)
Confusion—bewilderment	6.0 (3.9)	5.8 (4.6)	4.9 (4.3)	4.4 (4.2)	4.3 (4.0)
Total mood disturbance	37.0 (19.9)	35.5 (16.9)	32.6 (24.7)	33.4 (25.4)	31.3 (17.0)

The results are means (SD).
*Significant effect of time (P > 0.05).

0.0001), while no main effect of training period ($P = 0.29$) or gender × training period interaction ($P = 0.38$) were found for testosterone concentration (**Figure 2A**). However, the variations of testosterone during COMP showed a significant effect of time ($P = 0.03$), with a significant increase of salivary testosterone at week 5 in comparison to week 2 ($+14.5 \pm 44.7\%$), week 3 ($+9.2 \pm 51.4\%$), and week 4 ($+8.9 \pm 50.5\%$; $P < 0.05$; **Table 3**).

Cortisol

Salivary cortisol concentration during PREP was 6.8 ± 4.4 and 4.6 ± 2.3 nmol.L^{-1} for male and female athletes, respectively vs. 4.1 ± 1.8 and 5.6 ± 3.7 nmol.L^{-1} during COMP. No main effect of gender ($P = 0.76$) or time ($P = 0.15$) were found for salivary cortisol. A gender × training period interaction was obtained on cortisol concentration ($P < 0.007$), whereas *post-hoc* did not show significant differences between the different time points ($P > 0.05$; **Figure 2B**). Detailed analysis of the amount of cortisol in saliva did not reveal any significant variation throughout COMP ($P =$

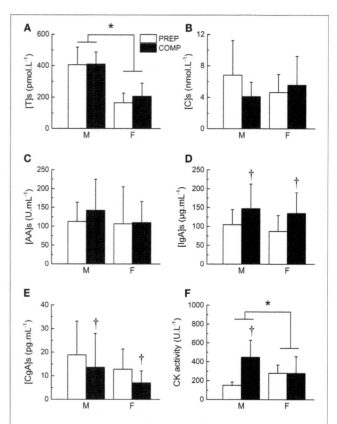

FIGURE 2 | Changes in biological markers between preparation and competitive training periods. Mean salivary concentration of testosterone ([T]s, **A**), cortisol ([C]s, **B**), alpha-amylase ([AA]s, **C**) immunoglobulin A ([IgA]s, **D**) and chromogranin A ([CgA]s, **E**), and plasma creatine kinase (CK) activity (**F**) during preparation (PREP) and pre-competitive (COMP) periods for male (M) and female (F) athletes. *Significant effect of gender (P < 0.05). †Significant difference between PREP and COMP (P < 0.05). Values are presented as mean ± SD.

TABLE 3 | Salivary markers and plasma CK activity of track and field athletes throughout the 5 weeks of the pre-competitive (COMP) period of the sport season.

POMS subscale scores	Training week of the pre-competitive period (COMP)				
	1	2	3	4	5
[Testosterone]s	287.2 (150.2)	262.5 (124.9)	282.4 (128.7)	265.6 (119.1)	328.9 (175.9)*
[Cortisol]s	5.1 (3.2)	4.6 (3.0)	4.6 (2.6)	4.9 (4.6)	6.1 (4.3)
[Alpha-amylase]s	109.0 (72.5)	116.6 (69.8)	139.2 (89.0)	112.4 (70.2)	125.2 (77.9)
[Immunoglobulin A]s	139.2 (46.3)	111.5 (57.2)	143.1 (71.6)	151.3 (97.0)	141.6 (68.7)
[Chromogranin A]s	9.4 (15.4)	4.4 (1.8)	8.5 (9.7)	7.9 (11.7)	9.7 (9.8)
Creatine kinase activity	386.8 (243.4)	310.1 (186.9)	381.1 (240.6)	297.1 (230.8)	279.1 (168.4)

The results are means (SD).
*Significant effect of time (P > 0.05).

0.64; **Table 3**). The T/C ratio ($\times 10^{-3}$) was higher in COMP compared to PREP (58.5 ± 39.9 vs. 80.9 ± 44.3; $P = 0.01$).

AA

Salivary AA concentration during PREP was 112.6 ± 50.7 and $106.7 \pm 98.3 \, \text{nmol.L}^{-1}$ for male and female athletes, respectively vs. 142.2 ± 82.7 and $109.8 \pm 55.6 \, \text{nmol.L}^{-1}$ during COMP. No effect of gender ($P = 0.58$), training period ($P = 0.30$) or gender × training period ($P = 0.40$) were observed (**Figure 2C**). No significant difference was observed between the 5 consecutive weeks of COMP ($P = 0.23$; **Table 3**) in salivary AA activity.

IgA

Salivary IgA concentration during PREP was 104.5 ± 39.9 and $87.2 \pm 42.0 \, \text{nmol.L}^{-1}$ for male and female athletes, respectively vs. 146.9 ± 65.7 and $134.8 \pm 55.1 \, \text{nmol.L}^{-1}$ during COMP. No main effect of gender ($P = 0.43$) was observed, whereas a significant effect of training period ($P = 0.006$) was obtained on salivary IgA, with no gender × training period interaction ($P = 0.86$). On average, salivary IgA levels measured in saliva of the elite athletes showed a significant increase between PREP and COMP ($+60.5 \pm 80.3\%$; $P = 0.003$; **Figure 2D**). No significant variation of salivary IgA was observed throughout COMP ($P = 0.22$; **Table 3**).

CgA

Salivary CgA concentration during PREP was 18.8 ± 14.4 and $13.6 \pm 14.3 \, \text{nmol.L}^{-1}$ for male and female athletes, respectively vs. 13.6 ± 14.3 and $7.1 \pm 5.0 \, \text{nmol.L}^{-1}$ during COMP. No main effect of gender was observed on salivary CgA ($P = 0.37$). A significant main effect of training period was obtained ($P = 0.04$), with no gender × training period interaction ($P = 0.93$). On average, CgA concentration decreased by $27.0 \pm 82.8\%$ from PREP to COMP ($P = 0.005$; **Figure 2E**). Week-by-week results did not show any main effect of time during the COMP period ($P = 0.69$; **Table 3**).

CK Activity

We observed a main effect of gender ($P < 0.0001$), training period ($P < 0.0001$) and a gender × training period interaction for plasma CK activity ($P = 0.006$). On average, CK activity significantly increased from 151.4 ± 35.9 to $448.4 \pm 179.6 \, \text{U.L}^{-1}$ between PREP and COMP for male ($P = 0.001$) with no significant changes for female athletes ($P = 0.48$; **Figure 2F**). No effect of time was observed throughout COMP for CK activity ($P = 0.09$; **Table 3**).

Correlation with Training Load

None of the psychological or physiological parameters were significantly correlated to the amount of training load during COMP ($P > 0.05$).

DISCUSSION

The present study aimed to compare the endocrine, psychological, and muscle damage response of world-class level athletes in preparation and pre-competitive period, where the injury incidence has been shown to increase. On the one hand, according to our hypothesis we observed changes in stress response manifested by a decrease in salivary chromogranin

A concentration, and an immunological status improvement as shown by the increase in salivary IgA. On the other hand, the diminution of the psychological component of fatigue and training load during the pre-competitive period was not accompanied by significant variations in testosterone and cortisol responses. However, elite athletes exhibited higher CK activity during the pre-competitive period compared to the preparation period. This interesting result could potentially mirror the effect of high-intensity and specialized training, which could exacerbate the exercise-induced muscle damage resulting from this training cycle.

Due to the characteristics of the sample (international level track and field athletes), conditioning and training programs were determined entirely by the coaches. Although we were not allowed to define the training stimulus in this context, this study is the first to present the psycho-physiological response to long-term elite athletic training (4.5 months), under real conditions. According to the well-known classical models of training periodization, preparatory period programs contain extensive, high volume, and diversified exercises, whereas the competitive period is focused mainly on more intensified, specialized exercises of reduced volume (Issurin, 2010). Such a training design aims to lead the athletes to their seasonal peak performance at the moment of competition. Track and field athletics encompassed a wide variety of athletes with different training contents to reach the targeted performance level. The quantification of the workload resulting from such various training is noticeably complex. For this reason, the training load was measured using the calculation method proposed by Foster (1998), which provides a global evaluation of the exercise stimulus, applicable to the various activities. Based on this methodological approach, as expected, the training load progressively decreased as competition was approaching (**Table 2**). It must be kept in mind that varied training regimes are employed to prepare sprinters, middle distance runners, and combined events. Therefore, further investigations are required to specifically address the hormonal response to these respective physical loads.

This well-known reduction in training volume that precedes the competition was associated with a reduced fatigue perception as shown by the lower level of tension, depression, anger, confusion, and total mood disturbance in pre-competitive in comparison with the PREP (**Table 1**). Our findings are in accordance with previous studies that show a lower mood disturbance in low-load periods (e.g., recovery, taper) than in high-load periods (e.g., high-volume training) (Faude et al., 2008). Conversely, psychological alterations have been reported in athletes submitted to a training stress leading to an overreached state (Coutts et al., 2007). If the athletes' mood states were close to high-volume training in our study (Rietjens et al., 2005), they did not reach values observed in overreached subjects. This suggests that training contents are properly adjusted by the coaches to avoid chronic fatigue or overreaching at international competitive level, even during high-load programs, which are recognized as a potential cause of psychological disturbance.

The pre-competitive phase was identified as a season period conducive to an increased injury incidence in track and field athletes (D'Souza, 1994). Such interruption in the training process before competition could be related to an imbalance between training stimulus and subsequent recovery (Foster, 1998). Overreached athletes have been shown to exhibit an exhaustion of the HPA axis (Meeusen et al., 2006). Although such influence on the higher brain centers can be inferred from changes in blood catecholamines, stress response was appraised based on hormonal variations in saliva. This easy-to-sample fluid allowed for non-invasive and stress-free determination of the physiological status of elite athletes with important time constraints. In addition, studies have shown that hormonal changes in response to exercise are more pronounced in saliva compared to blood (Gozansky et al., 2005). Given that steroids concentration may exhibit large fluctuations (Gatti and De Palo, 2011), we collected multiple samples to obtain relevant data. Saliva was collected in the middle of the afternoon when hormones concentrations exhibit reduced fluctuations in comparison with morning measurements, which could be influenced by the awakening response.

The present group of world-class level athletes presented slightly higher rates of salivary testosterone when compared to elite male ($286.5\,pg.mL^{-1}$; Kivlighan and Granger, 2006) and female athletes ($87\,pg.mL^{-1}$; Cook et al., 2012). As salivary testosterone has been reported to be related to the training level (Cook et al., 2012), our values could thus reflect the very high training level of the present group of athletes. Such higher testosterone baseline could indicate a greater capacity for performance at higher work rates. Hormones with anabolic or catabolic properties like testosterone show quantitative changes, reflective of a catabolic state, in relation to the intensity and duration of training load (Gatti and De Palo, 2011). Indeed, a negative relationship between training load and resting testosterone has been reported (Elloumi et al., 2008). Although training load and psychological perception of fatigue were lower in the pre-competitive period than in the preparation period in our study, testosterone concentration was similar in both phases (**Figure 2A**). This lack of variation between preparation and pre-competitive periods could be interpreted as a compensatory process between the load diminution (which potentially increases [T]s) associated with the reduction in strength training contents (which potentially decreases [T]s) (Gatti and De Palo, 2011).

Salivary cortisol is also recommended and extensively used as an index of training stress (Gatti and De Palo, 2011). The present cortisol values are in the range obtained for athletes ($1.8\text{–}19.9\,nmol.L^{-1}$; Cook et al., 2013), and close to the lowest concentrations commonly reported in the literature. This could be explained by the fact that measurements were performed in the middle of the afternoon (3–4 p.m.) when cortisol reaches a low-level plateau (Strahler et al., 2010). Moreover, the rise in cortisol induced by a psychobiological stress (i.e., training) has been demonstrated to be lower in trained than in untrained subjects (Rimmele et al., 2007), which is confirmed by our results obtained on highly trained athletes. A robust rise in resting cortisol has been reported as a complementary approach to assess excessive fatigue at the onset of overreaching (Urhausen et al., 1998). However, as for testosterone, we did not observe

significant changes in cortisol concentration between preparation and pre-competitive periods. Only the T/C ratio was increased in pre-competitive period, which could reflect the lower amount of training load during this training cycle. Our findings thus suggest a similar response of HPA axis to high-load or high-intensity training in track and field elite athletes. Such a result could also originate from the expertise of the coaches and the athletes themselves in their aptitude to properly regulate the training load according to the athletes' capacities, as reported for elite subjects (Cook and Beaven, 2013).

However, stress is a multi-faceted phenomenon that requires a multidimensional measurements approach (Nater et al., 2006). Indeed, except HPA axis, exercise-induced stress is also mediated by the ANS, which stimulates the adrenal medulla to produce catecholamines. Intense training (e.g., pre-competitive period) can deplete the amount of catecholamines in the blood. As AA and CgA are co-released with catecholamines in saliva, and these hormones have been proposed as non-invasive markers of autonomic activity. Although previous data on elite athletes are scarce, our study showed similar AA concentrations as those obtained by Filaire et al. (2013) on tennis players ($125\,U.mL^{-1}$). CgA values also showed salivary concentrations close to active subjects ($8.9\,pg.mL^{-1}$; Gallina et al., 2011). Competition involves social comparison and evaluation, which represents a potential source of pressure for athletes. Competitive periods are thus recognized for increasing sympathetic activity both in the anticipation and in the response to the event, which results in significant increase in salivary AA and CgA (Kraemer et al., 2001). While salivary AA increases might reflect the interaction of stress-dependent sympathetic and parasympathetic stimulation via central noradrenergic input, AA response depends on the nature of the stressor (Nater and Rohleder, 2009). Consequently, the changes in training contents between preparation and pre-competitive phases could have different effects on the AA response in the present group of elite athletes. This hypothesis was not verified, because similar concentrations were measured in both periods (**Figure 2C**). Inversely, CgA concentration was significantly decreased during the pre-competitive phase. Even though the mechanisms underlying its salivary secretion are complex, it is suggested that CgA is involved in the secretory responses to α-adrenergic agonists and is therefore considered a reliable index of autonomic activity (Gallina et al., 2011). Most of the studies based on salivary CgA were interested in the acute response to exercise, whereas long-term studies are scarce. Our findings suggest that a reduced training load decreases the salivary release of CgA at rest, and this could potentially indicate a lower autonomic activity in pre-competitive phases for elite athletes (Montero-Hadjadje et al., 2008).

As immunoglobulins A act as the first line of defense via mucosal surface, the assessment of IgA represents the effects of exercise on mucosal immunity. While variable effects of acute exercise on IgA have been reported in the literature, chronic exercise (training) can decrease the salivary concentration of IgA (Libicz et al., 2006). Such a decline in IgA appears to contribute to increase the athletes' susceptibility for upper respiratory tract infection (Neville et al., 2008; Papacosta and Nassis, 2011). The present IgA concentrations existed in the variations reported of a training season of athletes (35–314 μg.mL^{-1}; Neville et al., 2008), with significant higher values in pre-competitive compared to preparation period (**Figure 2D**). The reduction in training load as competitive events approach seemed to positively affect the mucosal immunity of elite athletes. Together with the reduced autonomic activity inferred from CgA results, these findings suggest that the rise in injury incidence during pre-competitive periods could not be attributed to an excessive general fatigue that could have triggered ANS disturbance or immunodepression.

Blood CK activity increased in pre-competitive period when compared with preparation period. Such increase in CK content is observed in the case of degeneration and regeneration of skeletal muscle damage (Guilhem et al., 2010). Although our CK values are comprised in the ranges reported throughout an athletic season (Meyer and Meister, 2011), the significant increase observed in pre-competitive period could be reflective of higher levels of muscle damage induced by intensified and specialized exercises, which increase the mechanical strain and the risk of injury in muscular tissues (Fiorentino et al., 2014). However, CK is recognized for being influenced by factors other than the level of muscle damage (e.g., soft tissue trauma, exercise-induced hemoconcentration and/or hemodilution, alterations of tissue clearance). Hence, the measurement of muscle injury cannot be solely based on the changes of CK activity (Guilhem et al., 2013). Furthermore, week-to-week analysis of salivary contents did not reveal significant changes in any of the assessed hormones (**Table 3**). Although ANS and HPA response could serve to identify overstressed athletes (i.e., functional or non-functional overreaching; Papacosta and Nassis, 2011), these data also illustrate the high inter- and intra-individual variability of hormonal response to exercise. Consequently, taken together with the lack of acute changes during pre-competitive period when injury incidence increases, our study suggests that potential increase in risk of injury from an increase in training load is less likely than from an increase in musculo-articular load. Innovative markers (e.g., micro-ARN; Banzet et al., 2013), more specific to tissue lesions resulting from high-intensity workouts, should be thus considered in power-oriented activities with repeated breaking (eccentric) actions, such as track and field athletics. Such indicators would benefit from optimization in the quantification procedure and increase in the capacity to perform large number of simultaneous measurements to allow for their implementation in high-level training conditions.

The present study aimed to determine the psychological, endocrinological, immunological, and muscle damage status throughout the season of world-class level track and field athletes,

based on the concentration of hormones contained in saliva and plasma CK activity. The reduction in training load during pre-competitive period compared to preparation period was associated with a decrease in psychological fatigue. Although T/C ratio and IgA were increased, and CgA decreased in response to the reduction in training load and fatigue perception, these parameters were not correlated to the training load. These findings suggest that saliva composition is sensitive to the type of training workouts performed by track and field athletes during the various season periods. Nonetheless, salivary hormones could not be related to the amount of workload resulting from athletics training, particularly during pre-competitive training period where injury incidence has been reported to increase. Our findings suggest that innovative markers, more specific to muscle tissue lesions, should be considered in the future to diagnose muscular overuse. The implementation of such indicators would help coaches and athletes to optimize the regulation of training contents throughout the season, particularly when high-intensity specialized workouts are used to increase technical performance as competition approaches.

AUTHOR CONTRIBUTIONS

Conception or design of the work: GG, CH, AG, MC. Acquisition, analysis, or interpretation of data for the work: GG, CH, NG, DB, AG, MC. Drafting the work or revising it critically for important intellectual content: GG, CH, NG, DB, AG, MC. Final approval of the version to be published: GG, CH, NG, DB, AG, MC. Agreement to be accountable for all aspects of the work in ensuring that questions related to the accuracy or integrity of any part of the work are appropriately investigated and resolved: GG, CH, NG, DB, AG, MC.

FUNDING

The study was funded by the French Ministry of Sports (contract no. 10-i-008) and received grants from the French Athletics Federation.

ACKNOWLEDGMENTS

We are grateful to the nurses, Mrs Pascale Raboisson and Mrs Christine Morlet, who performed the samples throughout the study. We are also indebted to the athletes and the coaches of the French national team for their participation and exceptional effort.

REFERENCES

Adlercreutz, H., Härkönen, M., Kuoppasalmi, K., Näveri, H., Huhtaniemi, I., Tikkanen, H., et al. (1986). Effect of training on plasma anabolic and catabolic steroid hormones and their response during physical exercise. *Int. J. Sports Med.* 7(Suppl. 1), 27–28. doi: 10.1055/s-2008-1025798

Banzet, S., Chennaoui, M., Girard, O., Racinais, S., Drogou, C., Chalabi, H., et al. (2013). Changes in circulating microRNAs levels with exercise modality. *J. Appl. Physiol.* 115, 1237–1244. doi: 10.1152/japplphysiol.00075.2013

Born, D. P., Faiss, R., Willis, S. J., Strahler, J., Millet, G. P., Holmberg, H. C., et al. (2015). Circadian variation of salivary immunoglobin A, alpha-amylase activity

and mood in response to repeated double-poling sprints in hypoxia. *Eur. J. Appl. Physiol.* doi: 10.1007/s00421-015-3236-3. [Epub ahead of print].

Cayrou, S., Dickès, P., and Dolbeault, S. (2003). [French version of the Profile of Mood State (POMS-f)]. *Sci. Sport* 13, 83–88.

Chennaoui, M., Gomez-Marino, D., Drogou, C., Bourrilhon, C., Sautivet, S., and Guezennec, C. Y. (2004). Hormonal and metabolic adaptation in professional cyclists during training. *Can. J. Appl. Physiol.* 29, 714–730. doi: 10.1139/h04-046

Cook, C. J., and Beaven, C. M. (2013). Salivary testosterone is related to self-selected training load in elite female athletes. *Physiol. Behav.* 116–117, 8–12. doi: 10.1016/j.physbeh.2013.03.013

Cook, C. J., Crewther, B. T., and Kilduff, L. P. (2013). Are free testosterone and cortisol concentrations associated with training motivation in elite male athletes? *Psychol. Sport Exerc.* 14, 882–885. doi: 10.1016/j.psychsport.2013.08.001

Cook, C. J., Crewther, B. T., and Smith, A. A. (2012). Comparison of baseline free testosterone and cortisol concentrations between elite and non-elite female athletes. *Am. J. Hum. Biol.* 24, 856–858. doi: 10.1002/ajhb.22302

Coutts, A. J., Wallace, L. K., and Slattery, K. M. (2007). Monitoring changes in performance, physiology, biochemistry, and psychology during overreaching and recovery in triathletes. *Int. J. Sports Med.* 28, 125–134. doi: 10.1055/s-2006-924146

Díaz Gómez, M. M., Bocanegra Jaramillo, O. L., Teixeira, R. R., and Espindola, F. S. (2013). Salivary surrogates of plasma nitrite and catecholamines during a 21-week training season in swimmers. *PLoS ONE* 8:e64043. doi: 10.1371/journal.pone.0064043

Diaz, M. M., Bocanegra, O. L., Teixeira, R. R., Soares, S. S., and Espindola, F. S. (2013). Salivary nitric oxide and alpha-amylase as indexes of training intensity and load. *Int. J. Sports Med.* 34, 8–13. doi: 10.1055/s-0032-1316318

D'Souza, D. (1994). Track and field athletics injuries—a one-year survey. *Br. J. Sports Med.* 28, 197–202. doi: 10.1136/bjsm.28.3.197

Elloumi, M., Ben Ounis, O., Tabka, Z., Van Praagh, E., Michaux, O., and Lac, G. (2008). Psychoendocrine and physical performance responses in male Tunisian rugby players during an international competitive season. *Aggress. Behav.* 34, 623–632. doi: 10.1002/ab.20276

Faude, O., Meyer, T., Scharhag, J., Weins, F., Urhausen, A., and Kindermann, W. (2008). Volume vs. intensity in the training of competitive swimmers. *Int. J. Sports Med.* 29, 906–912. doi: 10.1055/s-2008-1038377

Filaire, E., Ferreira, J. P., Oliveira, M., and Massart, A. (2013). Diurnal patterns of salivary alpha-amylase and cortisol secretion in female adolescent tennis players after 16 weeks of training. *Psychoneuroendocrinology* 38, 1122–1132. doi: 10.1016/j.psyneuen.2012.11.001

Fiorentino, N. M., Rehorn, M. R., Chumanov, E. S., Thelen, D. G., and Blemker, S. S. (2014). Computational models predict larger muscle tissue strains at faster sprinting speeds. *Med. Sci. Sports Exerc.* 46, 776–786. doi: 10.1249/MSS.0000000000000172

Foster, C. (1998). Monitoring training in athletes with reference to overtraining syndrome. *Med. Sci. Sports Exerc.* 30, 1164–1168. doi: 10.1097/00005768-199807000-00023

Gallina, S., Di Mauro, M., D'Amico, M. A., D'Angelo, E., Sablone, A., Di Fonso, A., et al. (2011). Salivary chromogranin A, but not alpha-amylase, correlates with cardiovascular parameters during high-intensity exercise. *Clin. Endocrinol. (Oxf.)* 75, 747–752. doi: 10.1111/j.1365-2265.2011.04143.x

Gatti, R., and De Palo, E. F. (2011). An update: salivary hormones and physical exercise. *Scand. J. Med. Sci. Sports* 21, 157–169. doi: 10.1111/j.1600-0838.2010.01252.x

Gozansky, W. S., Lynn, J. S., Laudenslager, M. L., and Kohrt, W. M. (2005). Salivary cortisol determined by enzyme immunoassay is preferable to serum total cortisol for assessment of dynamic hypothalamic—pituitary—adrenal axis activity. *Clin. Endocrinol. (Oxf.)* 63, 336–341. doi: 10.1111/j.1365-2265.2005.02349.x

Granger, D. A., Weisz, J. R., McCracken, J. T., Kauneckis, D., and Ikeda, S. (1994). Testosterone and conduct problems. *J. Am. Acad. Child Adolesc. Psychiatry* 33, 908. doi: 10.1097/00004583-199407000-00020

Guilhem, G., Cornu, C., and Guével, A. (2010). Neuromuscular and muscle-tendon system adaptations to isotonic and isokinetic eccentric exercise. *Ann. Phys. Rehabil. Med.* 53, 319–341. doi: 10.1016/j.rehab.2010.04.003

Guilhem, G., Hug, F., Couturier, A., Regnault, S., Bournat, L., Filliard, J. R., et al. (2013). Effects of air-pulsed cryotherapy on neuromuscular recovery subsequent to exercise-induced muscle damage. *Am. J. Sports Med.* 41, 1942–1951. doi: 10.1177/0363546513490648

Issurin, V. B. (2010). New horizons for the methodology and physiology of training periodization. *Sports Med.* 40, 189–206. doi: 10.2165/11319770-000000000-00000

Kivlighan, K. T., and Granger, D. A. (2006). Salivary alpha-amylase response to competition: relation to gender, previous experience, and attitudes. *Psychoneuroendocrinology* 31, 703–714. doi: 10.1016/j.psyneuen.2006.01.007

Kraemer, W. J., Fry, A. C., Rubin, M. R., Triplett-McBride, T., Gordon, S. E., Koziris, L. P., et al. (2001). Physiological and performance responses

to tournament wrestling. *Med. Sci. Sports Exerc.* 33, 1367–1378. doi: 10.1097/00005768-200108000-00019

Le Meur, Y., Hausswirth, C., Natta, F., Couturier, A., Bignet, F., and Vidal, P. P. (2013). A multidisciplinary approach to overreaching detection in endurance trained athletes. *J. Appl. Physiol.* 114, 411–420. doi: 10.1152/japplphysiol.01254.2012

Libicz, S., Mercier, B., Bigou, N., Le Gallais, D., and Castex, F. (2006). Salivary IgA response of triathletes participating in the French Iron Tour. *Int. J. Sports Med.* 27, 389–394. doi: 10.1055/s-2005-865747

Meeusen, R., Duclos, M., Gleeson, M., Rietjens, G., Steinacker, J., and Urhausen, A. (2006). Prevention, diagnosis and treatment of the Overtraining Syndrome. *Eur. J. Sport Sci.* 6, 1–14. doi: 10.1080/17461390600617717

Meyer, T., and Meister, S. (2011). Routine blood parameters in elite soccer players. *Int. J. Sports Med.* 32, 875–881. doi: 10.1055/s-0031-1280776

Montero-Hadjadje, M., Vaingankar, S., Elias, S., Tostivint, H., Mahata, S. K., and Anouar, Y. (2008). Chromogranins A and B and secretogranin II: evolutionary and functional aspects. *Acta Physiol.* 192, 309–324. doi: 10.1111/j.1748-1716.2007.01806.x

Nater, U. M., La Marca, R., Florin, L., Moses, A., Langhans, W., Koller, M. M., et al. (2006). Stress-induced changes in human salivary alpha-amylase activity—associations with adrenergic activity. *Psychoneuroendocrinology* 31, 49–58. doi: 10.1016/j.psyneuen.2005.05.010

Nater, U. M., and Rohleder, N. (2009). Salivary alpha-amylase as a non-invasive biomarker for the sympathetic nervous system: current state of research. *Psychoneuroendocrinology* 34, 486–496. doi: 10.1016/j.psyneuen.2009.01.014

Neville, V., Gleeson, M., and Folland, J. P. (2008). Salivary IgA as a risk factor for upper respiratory infections in elite professional athletes. *Med. Sci. Sports Exerc.* 40, 1228–1236. doi: 10.1249/MSS.0b013e31816be9c3

Papacosta, E., and Nassis, G. P. (2011). Saliva as a tool for monitoring steroid, peptide and immune markers in sport and exercise science. *J. Sci. Med. Sport* 14, 424–434. doi: 10.1016/j.jsams.2011.03.004

Rietjens, G. J., Kuipers, H., Adam, J. J., Saris, W. H., van Breda, E., van Hamont, D., et al. (2005). Physiological, biochemical and psychological markers of strenuous training-induced fatigue. *Int. J. Sports Med.* 26, 16–26. doi: 10.1055/s-2004-817914

Rimmele, U., Zellweger, B. C., Marti, B., Seiler, R., Mohiyeddini, C., Ehlert, U., et al. (2007). Trained men show lower cortisol, heart rate and psychological responses to psychosocial stress compared with untrained men. *Psychoneuroendocrinology* 32, 627–635. doi: 10.1016/j.psyneuen.2007.04.005

Strahler, J., Berndt, C., Kirschbaum, C., and Rohleder, N. (2010). Aging diurnal rhythms and chronic stress: distinct alteration of diurnal rhythmicity of salivary alpha-amylase and cortisol. *Biol. Psychol.* 84, 248–256. doi: 10.1016/j.biopsycho.2010.01.019

Tsigos, C., and Chrousos, G. P. (2002). Hypothalamic-pituitary-adrenal axis, neuroendocrine factors and stress. *J. Psychosom. Res.* 53, 865–871. doi: 10.1016/S0022-3999(02)00429-4

Urhausen, A., Gabriel, H., and Kindermann, W. (1995). Blood hormones as markers of training stress and overtraining. *Sports Med.* 20, 251–276. doi: 10.2165/00007256-199520040-00004

Urhausen, A., Gabriel, H. H., and Kindermann, W. (1998). Impaired pituitary hormonal response to exhaustive exercise in overtrained endurance athletes. *Med. Sci. Sports Exerc.* 30, 407–414. doi: 10.1097/00005768-199803000-00011

Wood, P. (2009). Salivary steroid assays - research or routine? *Ann. Clin. Biochem.* 46, 183–196. doi: 10.1258/acb.2008.008208

Conflict of Interest Statement: The authors declare that the research was conducted in the absence of any commercial or financial relationships that could be construed as a potential conflict of interest.

6

Monitoring Fatigue Status with HRV Measures in Elite Athletes: An Avenue Beyond RMSSD?

Laurent Schmitt[1,2], Jacques Regnard[3] and Grégoire P. Millet[2]*

[1] Centre National de Ski Nordique et de Moyenne Montagne, Ecole Nationale des Sports de Montagne, Prémanon, France, [2] Faculty of Biology and Medicine, Institute of Sport Sciences, University of Lausanne, Lausanne, Switzerland, [3] Unité de Recherche EA3920, Marqueurs Pronostiques et Facteurs de Régulations des Pathologies Cardiaques et Vasculaires, Hôpital Universitaire de Besançon, Université de Franche-Comté, Besançon, France

Among the tools proposed to assess the athlete's "fatigue," the analysis of heart rate variability (HRV) provides an indirect evaluation of the settings of autonomic control of heart activity. HRV analysis is performed through assessment of time-domain indices, the square root of the mean of the sum of the squares of differences between adjacent normal R-R intervals (RMSSD) measured during short (5 min) recordings in supine position upon awakening in the morning and particularly the logarithm of RMSSD (LnRMSSD) has been proposed as the most useful resting HRV indicator. However, if RMSSD can help the practitioner to identify a global "fatigue" level, it does not allow discriminating different types of fatigue. Recent results using spectral HRV analysis highlighted firstly that HRV profiles assessed in supine and standing positions are independent and complementary; and secondly that using these postural profiles allows the clustering of distinct sub-categories of "fatigue." Since, cardiovascular control settings are different in standing and lying posture, using the HRV figures of both postures to cluster fatigue state embeds information on the dynamics of control responses. Such, HRV spectral analysis appears more sensitive and enlightening than time-domain HRV indices. The wealthier information provided by this spectral analysis should improve the monitoring of the adaptive training-recovery process in athletes.

Keywords: heart rate variability, RMSSD, overreaching, fatigue, monitoring, physiologic

Edited by:
Niels H. Secher,
University of Copenhagen, Denmark

Reviewed by:
Stefanos Volianitis,
Aalborg University, Denmark
Stuart Goodall,
Northumbria University, UK

*Correspondence:
Grégoire P. Millet
gregoire.millet@unil.ch

The optimization of the training process in elite athletes requires the quantification of the training loads (Borresen and Lambert, 2009) and a thorough analysis of the training program (Tønnessen et al., 2014). Adjusting the training content aims at allowing optimal improvement in fitness. Therefore training has to be customized according to environmental conditions (e.g., altitude Schmitt et al., 2008; ambient temperature Brocherie et al., 2014), cross-transfer between training components (Millet et al., 2002), training phases (Issurin, 2010). It is also crucial to take into account any athlete's fatigue state and/or performance responses to the training load. Among the methods available for diagnosing a particular kind of "fatigue" (e.g., non-functional overreaching NFOR or overtraining, Meeusen et al., 2013), the heart rate variability (HRV) is widely used as its alterations depend largely on changes in cardiac autonomic control which continuously attempts to adapting cardiovascular function. HRV has been assessed either at rest, awake (Schmitt et al., 2006; Plews et al., 2013a), or sleeping (Pichot et al., 2000; Garet et al., 2004), during exercise

(Sandercock and Brodie, 2006) or during the post-exercise recovery phase (Buchheit et al., 2007; Seiler et al., 2007; Hug et al., 2014).

In a recent review (Buchheit, 2014), the pros and cons of these different measures have been elegantly presented. The suggested outcome was that the most useful resting HRV indicator would be the time domain index RMSSD (square root of the mean of the sum of the squares of differences between adjacent normal R-R intervals) measured during short (5 min) recordings in supine position upon awakening in the morning. The method gathers several advantages as an easy and quick accessibility, a short recording time not disturbing the athlete's recovery and a lower sensitivity to breathing pattern than spectral variables (Saboul et al., 2013). For all these reasons, the logarithm of RMSSD (LnRMSSD) is described as the *"most reliable and practically applicable measure for day-to-day monitoring"* (Plews et al., 2013b) and different recommendations have been proposed to improve the quality of the "fatigue" diagnosis: the use of weekly average (Plews et al., 2013a) of a minimum of three (ideally, randomly selected) measures of Ln RMSSD per week (Plews et al., 2014); a 7-day running average of LnRMSSD (Plews et al., 2012) instead of daily measures; the use of LnRMSSD/RR ratio (Plews et al., 2012, 2013b; Buchheit, 2014) for identifying any vagal-related saturation phenomena; the interpretation that coefficient of variation (CV) of LnRMSSD is linearly decreased toward NFOR (Plews et al., 2013a; Buchheit, 2014). All these information are useful and relevant, increase the signal-to-noise ratio, the reproducibility of these measures and therefore improve the quality/robustness of the monitoring of the "fatigue" status.

However, despite its accessibility/simplicity, even with all the above-mentioned methodological improvements (see Plews et al., 2013a; Buchheit, 2014, for further details), in our view, using only time-domain HRV indices for monitoring the training status in elite athletes has limitations, and might even lead to a dead-end (Schmitt et al., 2013, 2015). RMSSD and its proposed derivatives are taken as a vagal index (Berntson et al., 2005). Indeed, an increase in vagal heart control reflects often a fitness improvement, while athete's fatigue and performance impairment are often concomitant with a decreased vagal HRV (Pichot et al., 2000; Iellamo et al., 2002; Gratze et al., 2005). However, vagal heart control is influenced by sympathetic activity that can either impede or bolster it (Task-Force, 1996). In addition, the interplay between sympathetic and parasympathetic influences changes along the resting—exercising scale, to adapt the distribution of muscle blood flow and heart work (Harms et al., 1998). Thus, autonomic patterns differ according to different functional requirements in different training phases and in different types of sport activity. As from lying supine to standing (Stewart, 2012), from rest to various exercising levels the fine tuning of autonomic adjustments relies on fine resetting of baroreflex activity (Ogoh et al., 2007) with a complex interplay, as e.g., modulation of carotid-aortic baroreflex activity by low pressure cardiopulmonary receptors (Halliwill et al., 2014). Indeed, performing at high level requires an optimal interplay of parasympathetic and sympathetic controls (Hedelin et al., 2001; Pagani and Lucini, 2009; Hug et al., 2014). RMSSD does not provide any information on the sympathetic-related

modulation. A decrease in RMSSD may have also a biased interpretation due to vagal saturation (Kiviniemi et al., 2004), as it could result of a sympathetic overactivity combined with a vagal-related saturation. By measuring RMSSD alone in the sole supine position, the use of LnRMSSD/RR ratio is not unambiguous since an increase in this ratio may be taken in both opposite ways (either reflecting a fitness improvement or an increased fatigue). Lastly, the values obtained from the sole lying data recording do not provide any clue about the preserved or altered ability to dynamic control adjustment.

In our view, recording HRV clues in both supine and standing positions is also convenient and provides more information about the actual autonomic settings, their interplay and how they are resorted (Schmitt et al., 2013, 2015). We believe that the analysis of changes in HRV between supine and standing provides information about the ability of autonomic control to assume resetting for functional adaptation. In orthostatic tolerance assessment, HRV patterns in both supine and standing positions are affected by different involvement of cardiopulmonary receptors, i.e., cardiac preload and hence tuned changes in plasma volume and/or peripheral vasomotor tone (Iwasaki et al., 2000; Stewart, 2012). Among other factors, these latter parameters likely support changes in autonomic patterns and HRV also during exercising settings, upon different training loads and phases, as in day to day changes in sleep quality or appetite.

A recently published study accurately displayed how individual patterns of spectral analysis of HRV divert in "fatigue" states from "no fatigue" condition (Schmitt et al., 2013), and the data analysis describes the clustering of different types of fatigue through mathematical proximity of heart rate and main variables of spectral analysis (Schmitt et al., 2015). These distinct patterns encompass increases and/or decreases in HR as well as in spectral low frequency (LF) and high frequency (HF) components, and these changes are differently sized in supine and standing positions, and also sometimes contrariwise directed in each position. A main outcome of the analysis was that supine and standing HRV variables were fully independent, and non-commutable in the clustering of alterations from the individual normal "no fatigue" patterns. Indeed, low pressure baroreceptors are not activated similarly in supine and standing positions, and other inputs of autonomic control are likely differently active in each position. This study highlights the importance to combine HRV analysis in supine and standing positions. The new HRV-based sub-categories of "fatigue" may open doors for a more precise monitoring of athlete status and for different specific recovery strategies (that remain to be validated). We believe it represents an interesting step forward in using HRV for diagnosing NFOR and overtraining in athletes.

In summary, RMSSD measures and their derived variables have an effective practical usefulness, which can help the practitioner to identify a global "fatigue" level. However these variables do not allow the clustering of different sub-categories of "fatigue," at variance with the spectral HRV analysis in both supine and standing positions, which likely consider the current ability to control in a dynamic setting.

REFERENCES

Berntson, G. G., Lozano, D. L., and Chen, Y. J. (2005). Filter properties of root mean square successive difference (RMSSD) for heart rate. *Psychophysiology* 42, 246–252. doi: 10.1111/j.1469-8986.2005.00277.x

Borresen, J., and Lambert, M. I. (2009). The quantification of training load, the training response and the effect on performance. *Sports Med.* 39, 779–795. doi: 10.2165/11317780-000000000-00000

Brocherie, F., Girard, O., Pezzoli, A., and Millet, G. P. (2014). Outdoor exercise performance in ambient heat: time to overcome challenging factors? *Int. J. Hyperthermia* 30, 547–549. doi: 10.3109/02656736.2014.979257

Buchheit, M., Papelier, Y., Laursen, P. B., and Ahmaidi, S. (2007). Noninvasive assessment of cardiac parasympathetic function: postexercise heart rate recovery or heart rate variability? *Am. J. Physiol. Heart Circ. Physiol.* 293, H8–H10. doi: 10.1152/ajpheart.00335.2007

Buchheit, M. (2014). Monitoring training status with HR measures: do all roads lead to Rome? *Front. Physiol.* 5:73. doi: 10.3389/fphys.2014.00073

Garet, M., Tournaire, N., Roche, F., Laurent, R., Lacour, J. R., Barthélémy, J. C., et al. (2004). Individual Interdependence between nocturnal ANS activity and performance in swimmers. *Med. Sci. Sports Exerc.* 36, 2112–2118. doi: 10.1249/01.MSS.0000147588.28955.48

Gratze, G., Rudnicki, R., Urban, W., Mayer, H., Schlogl, A., and Skrabal, F. (2005). Hemodynamic and autonomic changes induced by Ironman: prediction of competition time by blood pressure variability. *J. Appl. Physiol.* 99, 1728–1735. doi: 10.1152/japplphysiol.00487.2005

Halliwill, J. R., Sieck, D. C., Romero, S. A., Buck, T. M., and Ely, M. R. (2014). Blood pressure regulation X: what happens when the muscle pump is lost? Post-exercise hypotension and syncope. *Eur. J. Appl. Physiol.* 114, 561–578. doi: 10.1007/s00421-013-2761-1

Harms, C. A., Wetter, T. J., McClaran, S. R., Pegelow, D. F., Nickele, G. A., Nelson, W. B., et al. (1998). Effects of respiratory muscle work on cardiac output and its distribution during maximal exercise. *J. Appl. Physiol. (1985)* 85, 609–618.

Hedelin, R., Bjerle, P., and Henriksson-Larsén, K. (2001). Heart rate variability in athletes: relationship with central and peripheral performance. *Med. Sci. Sports Exerc.* 33, 1394–1398. doi: 10.1097/00005768-200108000-00023

Hug, B., Heyer, L., Naef, N., Buchheit, M., Wehrlin, J. P., and Millet, G. P. (2014). Tapering for marathon and cardiac autonomic function. *Int. J. Sports Med.* 35, 676–683. doi: 10.1055/s-0033-1361184

Iellamo, F., Legramante, J. M., Pigozzi, F., Spataro, A., Norbiato, G., Lucini, D., et al. (2002). Conversion from vagal to sympathetic predominance with strenuous training in high-performance world class athletes. *Circulation* 105, 2719–2724. doi: 10.1161/01.CIR.0000018124.01299.AE

Issurin, V. B. (2010). New horizons for the methodology and physiology of training periodization. *Sports Med.* 40, 189–206. doi: 10.2165/11319770-000000000-00000

Iwasaki, K. I., Zhang, R., Zuckerman, J. H., Pawelczyk, J. A., and Levine, B. D. (2000). Effect of head-down-tilt bed rest and hypovolemia on dynamic regulation of heart rate and blood pressure. *Am. J. Physiol. Regul. Integr. Comp. Physiol.* 279, R2189–R2199.

Kiviniemi, A. M., Hautala, A. J., Seppänen, T., Makikällio, T. H., Huikuri, H. V., and Tulppo, M. P. (2004). Saturation of high-frequency oscillations of R-R intervals in healthy subjects and patients after acute myocardial infarction during ambulatory conditions. *Am. J. Physiol. Heart Circ. Physiol.* 287, H1921–H1927. doi: 10.1152/ajpheart.00433.2004

Meeusen, R., Duclos, M., Foster, C., Fry, A., Gleeson, M., Nieman, D., et al. (2013). Prevention, diagnosis, and treatment of the overtraining syndrome: joint consensus statement of the European College of Sport Science and the American College of Sports Medicine. *Med. Sci. Sports Exerc.* 45, 186–205. doi: 10.1249/MSS.0b013e318279a10a

Millet, G. P., Candau, R. B., Barbier, B., Busso, T., Rouillon, J. D., and Chatard, J. C. (2002). Modelling the transfers of training effects on performance in elite triathletes. *Int. J. Sports Med.* 23, 55–63. doi: 10.1055/s-2002-19276

Ogoh, S., Fisher, J. P., Raven, P. B., and Fadel, P. J. (2007). Arterial baroreflex control of muscle sympathetic nerve activity in the transition from rest to steady-state dynamic exercise in humans. *Am. J. Physiol. Heart Circ. Physiol.* 293, H2202–H2209. doi: 10.1152/ajpheart.00708.2007

Pagani, M., and Lucini, D. (2009). Can autonomic monitoring predict results in distance runners? *Am. J. Physiol. Heart Circ. Physiol.* 296, 1721–1722. doi: 10.1152/ajpheart.00337.2009

Pichot, V., Roche, F., Gaspoz, J. M., Enjolras, F., Antoniadis, A., Minini, P., et al. (2000). Relation between heart rate variability and training load in middle-distance runners. *Med. Sci. Sports Exerc.* 32, 1729–1736. doi: 10.1097/00005768-200010000-00011

Plews, D. J., Laursen, P. B., Kilding, A. E., and Buchheit, M. (2012). Heart rate variability in elite triathletes, is variation in variability the key to effective training? A case comparison. *Eur. J. Appl. Physiol.* 112, 3729–3741. doi: 10.1007/s00421-012-2354-4

Plews, D. J., Laursen, P. B., Kilding, A. E., and Buchheit, M. (2013a). Evaluating training adaptation with heart-rate measures: a methodological comparison. *Int. J. Sports Physiol. Perform.* 8, 688–691.

Plews, D. J., Laursen, P. B., Le Meur, Y., Hausswirth, C., Kilding, A. E., and Buchheit, M. (2014). Monitoring training with heart rate-variability: how much compliance is needed for valid assessment? *Int. J. Sports Physiol. Perform.* 9, 783–790. doi: 10.1123/IJSPP.2013-0455

Plews, D. J., Laursen, P. B., Stanley, J., Kilding, A. E., and Buchheit, M. (2013b). Training adaptation and heart rate variability in elite endurance athletes: opening the door to effective monitoring. *Sports Med.* 43, 773–781. doi: 10.1007/s40279-013-0071-8

Saboul, D., Pialoux, V., and Hautier, C. (2013). The impact of breathing on HRV measurements: implications for the longitudinal follow-up of athletes. *Eur. J. Sport Sci.* 13, 534–542. doi: 10.1080/17461391.2013.767947

Sandercock, G. R., and Brodie, D. A. (2006). The use of heart rate variability measures to assess autonomic control during exercise. *Scand. J. Med. Sci. Sports* 16, 302–313. doi: 10.1111/j.1600-0838.2006.00556.x

Schmitt, L., Fouillot, J. P., Millet, G. P., Robach, P., Nicolet, G., Brugniaux, J., et al. (2008). Altitude, heart rate variability and aerobic capacities. *Int. J. Sports Med.* 29, 300–306. doi: 10.1055/s-2007-965355

Schmitt, L., Hellard, P., Millet, G. P., Roels, B., Richalet, J. P., and Fouillot, J. P. (2006). Heart rate variability and performance at two different altitudes in well-trained swimmers. *Int. J. Sports Med.* 27, 226–231. doi: 10.1055/s-2005-865647

Schmitt, L., Regnard, J., Desmarets, M., Mauny, F., Mourot, L., Fouillot, J. P., et al. (2013). Fatigue shifts and scatters heart rate variability in elite endurance athletes. *PLoS ONE* 8:e71588. doi: 10.1371/journal.pone.0071588

Schmitt, L., Regnard, J., Parmentier, A. L., Mauny, F., Mourot, L., Coulmy, N., et al. (2015). Typology of "Fatigue" by heart rate variability analysis in Elite Nordic-skiers. *Int. J. Sports Med.* 36, 999–1007. doi: 10.1055/s-0035-1548885

Seiler, S., Haugen, O., and Kuffel, E. (2007). Autonomic recovery after exercise in trained athletes: intensity and duration effects. *Med. Sci. Sports Exerc.* 39, 1366–1373. doi: 10.1249/mss.0b013e318060f17d

Stewart, J. M. (2012). Mechanisms of sympathetic regulation in orthostatic intolerance. *J. Appl. Physiol. (1985)* 113, 1659–1668. doi: 10.1152/japplphysiol.00266.2012

Task-Force (1996). Task Force of the european society of cardiology and the North American Society of pacing and electrophysiology. Heart rate variability. standards of measurement, physiological interpretation, and clinical use. *Eur. Heart J.* 17, 354–381. doi: 10.1093/oxfordjournals.eurheartj.a014868

Tønnessen, E., Sylta, Ø., Haugen, T. A., Hem, E., Svendsen, I. S., and Seiler, S. (2014). The road to gold: training and peaking characteristics in the year prior to a gold medal endurance performance. *PLoS ONE* 9:e101796. doi: 10.1371/journal.pone.0101796

Conflict of Interest Statement: The authors declare that the research was conducted in the absence of any commercial or financial relationships that could be construed as a potential conflict of interest.

7

The Averaged EMGs Recorded from the Arm Muscles During Bimanual "Rowing" Movements

Tomasz Tomiak[1], Andriy V. Gorkovenko[2], Arkadii N. Tal'nov[2], Tetyana I. Abramovych[2], Viktor S. Mishchenko[1], Inna V. Vereshchaka[2] and Alexander I. Kostyukov[2]*

[1] Unit of the Theory of Sport and Motorics, Chair of Individual Sports, Gdansk University of Physical Education and Sport, Gdańsk, Poland, [2] Department of Movement Physiology, Bogomoletz Institute of Physiology, National Academy of Sciences, Kiev, Ukraine

The main purpose was to analyze quantitatively the the average surface EMGs of the muscles that function around the elbow and shoulder joints of both arms in bimanual "rowing" movements, which were produced under identical elastic loads applied to the levers ("oars"). The muscles of PM group (*"pulling" muscles*: elbow flexors, shoulder extensors) generated noticeable velocity-dependent dynamic EMG components during the pulling and returning phases of movement and supported a steady-state activity during the hold phase. The muscles of RM group (*"returning" muscles*: elbow extensors, shoulder flexors) co-contracted with PM group during the movement phases and decreased activity during the hold phase. The dynamic components of the EMGs strongly depended on the velocity factor in both muscle groups, whereas the side and load factors and combinations of various factors acted only in PM group. Various subjects demonstrated diverse patterns of activity redistribution among muscles. We assume that central commands to the same muscles in two arms may be essentially different during execution of similar movement programs. Extent of the diversity in the EMG patterns of such muscles may reflect the subject's skilling in motor performance; on the other hand, the diversity can be connected with redistribution of activity between synergic muscles, thus providing a mechanism directed against development of the muscle fatigue.

Keywords: bimanual movements, two-joint movements, motor control, muscle synergy, electromyogram

Edited by:
Ronaldo M. Ichiyama,
University of Leeds, UK

Reviewed by:
Andrea Utley,
University of Leeds, UK
Thomas J. Burkholder,
Georgia Institute of Technology, USA

*Correspondence:
Alexander I. Kostyukov
kostyuko@biph.kiev.ua

INTRODUCTION

Simplified, constrained movements are often used to study the control of complex movement. (Gomi and Osu, 1998; Gribble and Ostry, 1998; Gribble et al., 2003; Tal'nov et al., 2014). To obtain the maximal extent of reproduction of the same movement paradigm, one of the most suitable procedures consists of the visual tracking of a basic movement parameter in accordance with a given command signal, which presents a desirable movement trajectory (Tal'nov et al., 1997, 1999, 2014; Gribble et al., 2003) or generated muscle force (Nijhof and Gabriel, 2006). The central commands directed to the muscles have typically been evaluated in experiments with many-fold repetitions of identical movement programs that were followed by an off-line averaging procedure applied to both the surface EMG activities recorded from the muscles that provide the movement

---

Abbreviations: bic.b., m. biceps brachii caput breve; bic.l., m. biceps brachii caput longum; br., m. brachioradialis; delt., m. deltoideus pars scapularis; EMG, electromyogram; MVC, maximal voluntary contraction; pect., m. pectoralis pars major; tric., m. triceps brachii caput longum; PM, "pulling" muscles; RM, "returning" muscles.

and the basic mechanical parameters. Some motor control theories, such as the equilibrium state hypotheses (Feldman, 1966; Hogan, 1985; Feldman and Levin, 2009), are typically considered to be a single-valued correspondence between efferent activities directed to the joint muscles and its mechanical parameters. The analysis of the EMG patterns in the stereotyped isotorque single-joint movements simultaneously demonstrated evident movement-dependent uncertainties in the relationships between EMGs and the positioning parameters (Tal'nov and Kostyukov, 1994). The dynamics of the skeletal muscle behavior in the stretch reflex system are also essentially non-linear because they depend not only on the instantaneous values of neural activation and external load but also on the direction of previous movement and activation prehistory (Kostyukov, 1986, 1998; Herzog et al., 2006). Contractions of agonist and antagonist muscle groups evoke movements around a limb joint, whereas the muscle antagonists change their lengths in opposite directions during a movement. Because the dynamic muscle properties crucially depend on the direction of length change, the joint dynamics will reflect the complex interactions of the direction-dependent asymmetries in the behavior of the muscle antagonists.

The activation patterns of the antagonistic muscle groups are changed not only in different motor tasks but can markedly vary even in identical movements, depending on the balance between the activation intensities of the antagonists. It is quite clear that for a given movement amplitude, the required level of agonist activation will depend on the antagonist activity. Real movements quite often contain elements of co-activation; it is commonly accepted that the co-activation of antagonists increases the mechanical stiffness of the joint, which is especially important for the most proximal joints in multi-joint movements (Dounskaia et al., 2002). Increased stiffness is also important to overcome joint instability under different external loads; co-activation of antagonistic muscles is one of the main factors that improve movement precision (Gribble and Ostry, 1998; Gribble et al., 2003). The muscles from different joints can form different temporary groups that act in a synergic mode; some muscles participate in producing a given movement, whereas other muscles function in an opposing mode at various phases of the movement. It can be hypothesized that the patterns of the central commands that arrive at different muscles in the same synergic group will have both similarities and diversities. Two-joint movements present the simplest form of multi-joint movements that enable the comparison of dynamic and static EMG components in muscles that belong to different joints. Despite numerous studies devoted to the investigation of bimanual movements (Swinnen et al., 1996; Dounskaia et al., 1998, 2002; Soteropoulos and Perez, 2011; Gueugnon et al., 2014), we did not identify papers devoted to the quantitative comparative analysis of EMGs in identical muscles in both arms. The various problems regarding the hierarchical control of different coordination patterns in multi-joint movements are discussed in details elsewhere (Kelso, 1994; Dounskaia et al., 1998, 2002; Diedrichsen and Dowling, 2009).

The main aims of the current study include a detailed analysis of the EMG intensities of the muscles in the elbow and shoulder joints in both arms during the execution of identical bimanual pulling and returning movements of ramp-and-hold profile. We compared the EMG reactions in different muscles participating in these movements for two levels of external loading and three movement velocities. It was assumed that the extent of variability in EMG intensities would be different in different subjects even during the fulfillment of identical movements. Potential differences in the reactions of similar muscles in both arms during fulfillment of identical bimanual movements are considered.

METHODS

Experimental Setup

Experiments were conducted with nine adult right-handed men, 19–39 years old (24.8 ± 5.5). An informed consent was signed by each subject before the experiments. All study procedures were in accordance with the ethical standards of the institutional and/or national research committee of A. A. Bogomoletz Institute of Physiology, National Academy of Sciences, Kiev, Ukraine, and with the 1964 Helsinki declaration and its subsequent amendments or comparable ethical standards. Informed consent was obtained from all individual participants included in the study. The experimental procedure lasted ~1 h. The mechanical part of the experimental setup is schematically presented in **Figure 1**. The subject sat near a special table in a chair with a regulated position of the chair-bottom; his position was adjusted via the elevation of his armpits 10–15 cm over the table plate. The chair was rigidly fixed to the floor, and the subject's trunk was fixed to the chair back by special belts. The subject held two rotating wood levers that imitated boat oars; the levers could move around vertical axes ("oarlocks") only in horizontal plane due to a special ball-bearing fixation to the axes. The plane of the levers' axes movement approximately coincided with positioning of the shoulder joints; therefore, it was most convenient for subjects to move the arms' segments in this plane without any additional suspension supports of his arms. Rubber bands (4 m length in the non-stretched state) connected the levers as shown in **Figure 1A** and created identical loads on the subject's arms; the loads could be increased by the connection of additional bands. In the initial positions of the levers prior to the beginning of movement (point s in **Figure 1A**), the subject's arms were fully extended; the initial forces that acted on the subject's hands (points H_L, H_R) were approximately 32 and 64 N for the single and double bands of loading properly. When the levers were pulled, the loads were raised linearly, which achieved the final positions (point f in **Figure 1A**) of 44 and 88 N. Precision potentiometers were used to measure the rotating angles of the levers (θ_L; θ_R); zero values of the signals were installed at the middle levers' positions as shown in **Figure 1**. The positive deflection corresponded to the pulling movement direction, which coincided with the clockwise turning of the left lever and the anti-clockwise turning of the right lever. The subjects executed the symmetrical bimanual pulling and returning movements through a combination on the monitor screen of the beam that reflected the angle position of the left

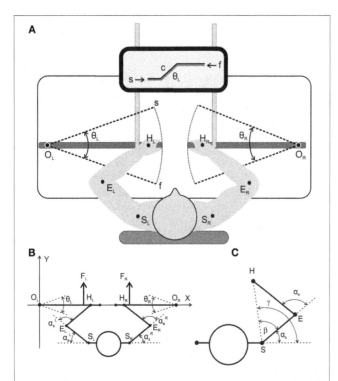

FIGURE 1 | (A) general scheme of the experimental setup from a top view **(A)** and a detailed geometry description regarding the relative arrangement of the moving arm segments and levers **(B,C)**. **(A)** The subjects produced symmetrical bimanual movements using a visual tracking procedure. The target movements were executed via the combination of two beams on the monitor screen: the command signal (c) evolving with time as a trapezoid and the signal from the joint angle sensor of the left lever (θ_L). **(B)** General scheme of the experimental setup from a top view with a detailed geometry description regarding the relative arrangement of the moving arm segments and levers. Real parameters of the arm's segments (*EH, ES*) and the distance between the rotation centers at the shoulders ($S_L S_R$) were defined for each subject prior to the experiment. **(C)** Geometrical drawing used to define the precise joint angle changes in the shoulder and elbow joints (α_s, α_e) based on real records of the levers' turning angles (θ_L, θ_R); a detailed description is provided in the text.

lever (θ_L) with the command signal (*c*) unwrapping over the screen as a trapezoid with a duration of the ramp phases 0.4, 1.0, or 2.0 s.

Off-line Computation of the Joint Angles

Figures 1B,C show definition of the movement parameters. A rigid mechanical coupling of the subject's arm segments with levers during movement enables a precise computation of the joint angle traces [$\alpha_e(t),, \alpha_s(t)$] based on the change in position of the corresponding lever [turning angle, $\theta(t)$]. In this scheme, the abscissa of the drawing passes through the centers of the levers' rotation O_L and O_R, and the origin of the coordinates coincides with the left center (O_L). The coordinates of the shoulder joints (points S_L, S_R) and the length of the shoulder and forearm segments ($SE = L_s$; $EH = L_e$) were defined prior to the initiation of the experiments; the positions of the hands at the levers were standard for all subjects ($R = OH = 66\ cm$). Zero value of the turning angle ($\theta = 0$) coincides with abscissa axis and positive values assumed for anti-clockwise rotation of the right lever and

clockwise of the left one in a pulling direction. The coordinates of the hand positions (H_L, H_R) for the different turning angles of the levers are defined by the following trigonometry expressions:

$$H_R = O_R + R \cdot \begin{bmatrix} -\cos(-\theta_R) \\ \sin(-\theta_R) \end{bmatrix}; H_L = O_L + R \cdot \begin{bmatrix} \cos(-\theta_L) \\ \sin(-\theta_L) \end{bmatrix} \quad (1)$$

The formulae for the calculations of the angles at the shoulder (α_s) and elbow (α_e) joints are subsequently presented for the right arm; similar expressions are used for left arm. First, there are defined polar coordinates for the changing position of the hand at the plain:

$$L = \sqrt{(H_x - S_x)^2 + (H_y - S_y)^2}; \gamma = arctg\left(\frac{H_y - S_y}{H_x - S_x}\right), \quad (2)$$

where H_x, H_y, S_x, S_y are the corresponding Cartesian coordinates of the hand and shoulder joints, respectively.

Finally, the joint angles α_s and α_e are defined by the expressions (3) and (4):

$$\beta = arccos\left(\frac{L^2 + L_s^2 - L_e^2}{2 \cdot L_e \cdot L_s}\right); \alpha_s = \gamma - \beta; \quad (3)$$

$$\alpha_e = \pi - arccos\left(\frac{L_e^2 + L_s^2 - L^2}{2 \cdot L_e \cdot L_s}\right) \quad (4)$$

EMG Recording and Off-line Handling

Surface EMGs were recorded using surface electrode pairs (Biopac System EL 503, USA; center to center distance 25 mm), which were fixed at both arms on the subject's skin over the muscles' bellies. The activity was registered from the following muscles: *pectoralis major, deltoideus scapularis, biceps brachii caput longum et breve, brachioradialis*, and *triceps brachii caput longum*. The recorded muscle activity was amplified via a multichannel amplifier (16-channel Bioamplifier, CWE, Inc., PA 19003 USA) using a bandpass filter in the range of 10–5000 Hz (**Figure 2A**). All raw EMG records were inspected visually, and possible mechanical artifacts (De Luca et al., 2010) were identified and removed. The EMGs together with the two position signals (θ_L, θ_R) were collected via a CED Power 1401 data acquisition system, using the program Spike 2 (Cambridge Electronic Design, UK). The EMGs and position signals were digitized at 10.0 and 2.0 kHz, respectively. Origin 8.0 (OriginLab Corporation, USA) and SPSS 17.0 (IBM Business Analytics software) were used for the off-line data analysis. Procedure of EMG recording and data handling is presented in **Figure 2**. The EMG records were full-wave rectified and additionally filtered (Batterworth filter of fourth order, bandwidth 0–10 Hz) in an off-line regimen; this procedure introduced a phase lag with respect to the real changes in the EMG intensity near 130–150 ms (Tal'nov et al., 2014). All tests were repeated 10 times to average the corresponding records. When necessary, the averaged trajectories of movement also underwent numerical differentiation to obtain the velocity and acceleration of the movement. Prior to each experiment, the maximal voluntary

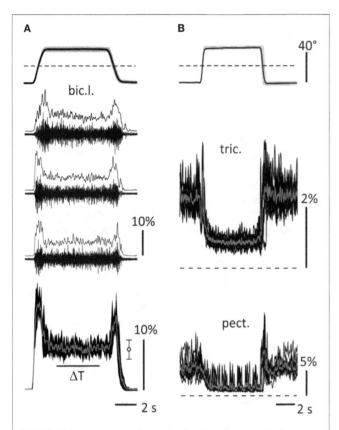

FIGURE 2 | General description of the data handling used in the study.
(A) A part of standard movement tests (subject 23A, left *bic.l.*); upper panel
shows averaging of 10 records of the turning angle of the left lever (black) and
their trial-to-trial variability (± *SD,* gray area), dash line marks zero angle
corresponding to the middle lever' positions in **Figures 1A,B**; middle panels
(2–4)—single raw EMGs recorded in 10–5000 Hz range and results of the full
wave rectification and smoothing by 4th order Batherworth low-pass filter with
10 Hz cut-off frequency; bottom panel—averaging of 10 smoothed records
(red), three of which are shown in panels 2–4, and their trial-to-trial variability
(± *SD,* black area); statistical parameters of the averaging within ΔT interval
are presented at the right (*m* ± *SD*). **(B)** Examples of activity of the right *tric.*
and *pect.* (subject 25B); upper panel show superposition of 10 turning angle
records (gray) and their averaging (black); middle and bottom panels show
superpositions of 10 smoothed rectified EMG records (black) and their
averaging (red). The EMG calibration is given in % of MVC.

contractions (MVC) of all muscles were registered to normalize
the averaged EMG records in the percentage of MVC. During the
procedure, the maximal EMG intensities of the corresponding
muscles were registered in either pulling or returning bimanual
isometric contractions produced when a participant sat in a
standard experimental position, and the elbow and shoulder
joint angles constituted ∼90° and 40°, respectively. Examples
of the raw EMGs and various stages of the signals handling are
presented in **Figure 2** for *bic.l, tric.,* and *pect.* muscles. Recording
of the raw EMG in a single movement test and result of the low-
pass filtering of the full-wave rectified records are shown for *bic.l.,*
rest of the EMGs include superpositions of 10 records and their
averaging. The elbow flexors and shoulder extensors were almost
inactive before and after test movements, therefore these parts
of the records can be used to determine the zero activation levels.

On the contrary, the elbow extensors and shoulder flexors usually
demonstrated some activity before and after tests, the dashed
lines in this and other Figures show additionally the zero levels of
activity. The EMGs in *pect.* muscles in many cases are distorted
by the ECG waves, and their averaged records contain clearly seen
oscillations (**Figure 2B**, bottom panel). In the framework of the
present experimental approach, we cannot completely exclude
contamination of the EMG records by mechanical artifacts,
which may be likely added during fast movements. The frequency
range of these artifacts is not significantly different from that
of the raw EMGs, therefore this noise cannot be removed by a
simple filtering, and more sophisticated computation procedures
must be applied.

Estimation of the Static and Dynamic Components in the Averaged EMG Records

The following method was proposed to quantitatively compare
the activation intensities of different muscles (**Figure 3**). This
approach enables an evaluation of weights of the dynamic
and static components in the averaged EMG records. First,
within 2 s intervals ΔT_0 and ΔT_1, two static levels were
defined in the averaged EMG records: E_0—the background
EMG intensity, and E_1—the stationary activation intensity prior
to the start of the returning phase in the test movement
(**Figure 3A**). E_0 was primarily close to zero in the elbow flexors
and shoulder extensors, and typically achieved small positive
values in the elbow extensors and shoulder flexors. During the
hold phase, the E_1 increased compared with the E_0 in the
elbow flexors and shoulder extensors and primarily decreased
in in the elbow extensors and shoulder flexors (**Figure 3B**).
The static components E_{st} in the averaged EMG reactions were
approximated using the following expressions:

$$E_{st}(t) = E_0 + \frac{\alpha(t) - \alpha_0}{\alpha_1 - \alpha_0}(E_1 - E_0), \qquad (5)$$

where the parameters α_0, E_0, and α_1, E_1 represent the averaged
values of the joint angle and EMG intensity computed within the
2 s intervals ΔT_0 and ΔT_1 prior to the movement phases.

The dynamic part of reaction was determined by subtraction
from the initial EMG record the previously defined static
component:

$$E_{dyn} = E - E_{st} \qquad (6)$$

The integral dynamic components (I_{dc}), which describe the EMG
activity changes during the movement phases, were defined by
the integration of E_{dyn} within the correspondent time intervals
Δt_1 and Δt_2. These intervals were evaluated using the first
derivative of the correspondent joint angle changes (lowest rows
in **Figures 3A,B**). Because the dynamic changes of the activity
ordinarily exceeded the durations of the movement phases, the
integration times Δt_1 and Δt_2 were subsequently obtained by
elongation of the durations of the derivative waves 1.5 times.
Finally, the integral dynamic components during the pulling (1)

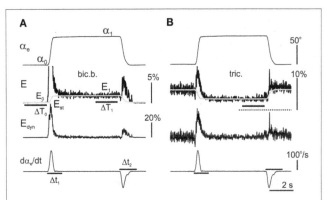

FIGURE 3 | Extraction of the dynamic components within the averaged EMG records (see detailed description in the text). The same procedure was applied to analyse the reactions in both the flexor **(A)** and extensor **(B)** muscles. First, the amplitude of the static component E_{st} was determined by averaging the EMG activities over 2 s periods ΔT_1 prior to the end of the hold phases in the test movements. Finally, the time course of the static components in the EMGs was assumed to repeat the time course of the angle changes in the corresponding joint; Equation (5) had been proposed for its description (shown by the gray lines in the second row from top). The dynamic EMG components were determined using the difference between the initial EMG record and the static component evaluation E_{st}. In flexors, the resulting dynamic components $E_{dyn} = E - E_{st}$ predominantly include two different waves of activity connected directly with the phases of active muscle shortening (D_P) or lengthening (D_R). If the E_{dyn} traces are compared with the first derivative of the movement records ($d\alpha_e/dt$), one can conclude that the durations of D_P and D_R waves exceed the durations of the movement phases. Therefore, for the correct assessment of the areas of the components, the integration times were elongated 1.5 times with respect to the duration of the derivative waves (lines Δt_1 and Δt_2 in the bottom panels, $d\alpha_e/dt$ graphs). The EMG calibration is given in % of MVC.

and returning (2) phases of the test movements were defined by the following expression:

$$D_{P,\ R} = \frac{\int_{\Delta t_{1,2}} E_{dyn}(t)dt}{\Delta R}, \tag{7}$$

where E_{dyn} is defined according to Equations (5) and (6); Δt_1 and Δt_2 represent the integration times during the pulling and returning phases, respectively; and ΔR represents the duration of the ramp phases in the command signal, i.e., 2.0, 1.0, or 0.4 s.

RESULTS

The Averaged EMGs Recorded from the Muscles of Both Arm

An example of the averaged EMGs recorded from the same muscles in both arms is shown in **Figure 4**. The angle trajectory changes in the elbow (α_e) and shoulder (α_s) joints in both arms (*left*–L; *right*–R) were calculated based on θ_L, θ_R, which represent the turning angle records of the proper levers in conformity with the procedure described in Section Off-line Computation of the Joint Angles (**Figure 1C**). The dynamic components of the EMG reactions recorded during the pulling and returning phases of movement were quite different in various muscles and were dependent on the direction and velocity of

the movement. In contrast, the steady-state activities during the hold phases were not noticeably different in their dependence on the velocity; however, these components occasionally varied, with a predominant tendency to increase at higher velocities of movement (see the EMG records from the right *bic.b.* and right *delt.* in **Figure 4**). In the test movements, the elbow flexor muscles (*bic.b.*, *bic.l.*, and *br.*) act in a similar way with the shoulder extensors (*delt.*); a certain similarity is also present in the reactions of the elbow extensors (*tric.*) and the shoulder flexors (*pect.*). The functional associations of the elbow flexors with the shoulder extensors and the elbow extensors with the shoulder flexors enable the selection of two groups of the synergist muscles that belong to different joints in antagonistic relationships with one another. The muscles of *PM group* (elbow flexors and shoulder extensors) generated powerful bursts of activity during the pulling movements; in contrast, their activities predominately decreased during the returning phases of the movement, when they contracted in the "yielding" regimen. In contrast to the muscles of *PM group*, *RM group* muscles (elbow extensors and shoulder flexors) typically exhibited a weak background activity in the initial position. The pulling movements in these muscles were associated with complex velocity-dependent oscillations of activity with a tendency to decrease; during the hold phases, the EMG intensities predominantly decreased until full disappearance. In the following returning phases of the movement, the EMG intensity in these muscles often recovered to a background level; thus, following an increase in the movement velocity, clear, dynamic oscillations of activity appeared.

When the EMG reactions in the same muscles that belong to different arms are compared, their similarities may often be noted, such as in the experiment presented in **Figure 4**. The subject who participated in this experiment demonstrated stable and similar EMG reactions in the same muscles in both arms. However, several differences exist, which consist, in particular, of velocity-dependent shifts in the stationary EMG levels in the *bic.b.* and *delt.* muscles in the right arm, whereas these shifts are absent in the left arm. These differences may be explained, at least in part, by the increased movement amplitudes produced by the right arm (compare the joint angle traces in **Figure 4**). The larger movement amplitudes of the right arm are likely connected with the absence of the direct visual control of its movement (see Methods). In contrast, the observed inconstancy of the EMG activities may also reflect the redistribution of activity among muscles of *PM group*, as well as a corresponding change in the opposing forces generated by *RM group*. In addition, it should be noted that the present experimental approach could not provide control of all muscles in the movement tests.

An example of the unstable EMG reactions with non-uniform distribution of activity among different muscles in both arms is presented in **Figure 5**. This subject exhibited quite good movement tracking and precise fixation of the hold positions by both arms; at the same time, in contrast with the experiment presented in **Figure 4**, the averaged EMG records were mainly different for the identical muscles that belonged to these arms. Within *PM group*, a similarity of reactions was registered only in the *delt.*, whereas in all muscles of the elbow joint, the EMG

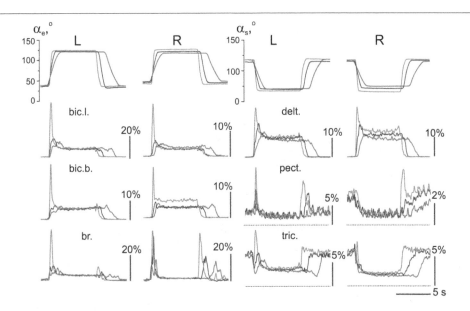

FIGURE 4 | The averaged joint angle trajectories and EMGs recorded from identical muscles in the *left* (L) and *right* (R) arms during test movements (*subject 25B*). Responses to the command signals with three durations of ramp phases 2.0, 1.0, and 0.4 s are compared; the corresponding reactions are marked by different colors. Two rubber bands were used at each side for loading the test movements; at the middle positions of the levers (as shown in **Figure 1**), the loads that acted in area of the subject's hands constituted approximately 76 N. EMG records are mainly placed below the angle traces of the corresponding joint, including the elbow (α_e, left half of Figure) or shoulder (α_s, right half); the triceps EMGs are shifted into the right half of the Figure to obtain a better picture format. Other abbreviations used in this and the following Figures: *bic.l., m. biceps brachia cap. longum; bic.b., m. biceps brachia cap. breve; br., m. brachioradialis*; delt., *m. deltoideus pars scapularis*; pect., *m. pectoralis pars major*; and tric., *m. triceps brachii caput longum*. Note that the *pect.* and *tric.* largely exhibited background activation at the initial position preceding the test movements; the dashed lines note zero levels of activity in the EMGs recorded from these muscles. Rest muscles were inactive before and after movement test, therefore the zero levels are presented by straight lines at the EMG records before and after movements. The EMG calibration is given in % of MVC.

reactions were remarkably different. A common peculiarity in the muscle reactions of *PM group* was evident dependent on the hold EMG levels on the movement velocity; an increase in the velocity typically led to an increase in the static EMG intensity. Another apparent property of these reactions was the presence of well-expressed dynamic components during the returning phases of the movements; moreover, in some muscles (left *bic.l.*, left and right *delt.*), these components even exceeded the components recorded during slower movements. During fast movements, quite similar strong dynamic reactions appeared almost synchronously in *RM group* of muscles; therefore, the antagonist muscles that act at both joints were co-contracted in these cases. It should also be emphasized that these mainly unpredictable features of the central commands in this subject were not associated with a worse movement quality compared with the other subjects.

Velocity of movement is essential factor defining reactions of the elbow extensors and shoulder flexors, what is well seen in **Figures 4, 5**. At minimal velocity, subjects provide the necessary movement predominantly by lowering intensity of activation in these muscles. It seems that the drop of activity in these muscles become insufficient with velocity rise, what may be compensated for by the dynamic components of EMG in the elbow flexors and shoulder extensors, thus switching on a process of redistribution of the central commands between muscles-antagonists.

Statistical Analysis of the Integral Dynamic Components of EMGs

The integral dynamic components D_P and D_R (in accordance with the quantitative method described in Section Estimation of the Static and Dynamic Components in the Averaged EMG Records) are summarized in **Figure 6** for the group of nine subjects; these parameters have been defined at three durations of the test movements and two levels of loading. A Four-way ANOVA for repeated measurements was applied to estimate the potential dependences of the dynamic components on the used experimental conditions for each particular muscle (**Table 1**). The following independent factors are taken into account: **D**—the movement direction factor: pulling (D_P) or returning (D_R); **S**—the side factor: the *left* (L) or *right* (R) arm; **P**—the load factor: one or two rubber bands; and **V**—the movement velocity factor (ramp duration: 0.4, 1.0, or 2.0 s). In *PM group* of synergic muscles (*bic.b., bic.l., br., delt.*), in most cases, the D_P components were significantly increased compared with the D_R components; however, at lower movement velocities (1.0, 2.0 s), these differences were less expressed. Moreover, in some cases, a reverse ratio between the component values was identified. Nevertheless, while considering the influence of the velocity factor on the dynamic components of EMG, significant effects were identified in all studied muscles (**Table 1**). The action of the load factor was significant in all muscles of *PM group*, whereas

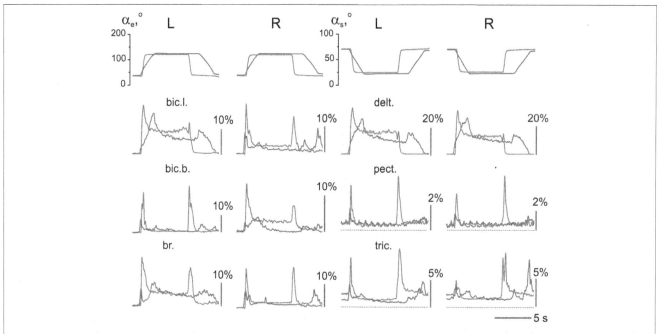

FIGURE 5 | Example of unstable patterns in the averaged EMG records; the test movements with 2.0 and 0.4 s ramp phases in the command signals are shown (subject 25A). The EMG calibration is given in % of MVC; the same designations as in **Figure 4**.

the muscles of *RM group* did not react in this way, which could, at least in part, be connected with the low intensity and instability of their reactions (*P* column in **Table 1**). A significant action of the side factor was fixed only in the *bic.b.* reactions (*S* column in **Table 1**). Significant differences in the D_P component at different sides were identified for the double loading and all durations of movement (0.4, 1.0, and 2.0 s); the D_R component exhibited similar differences for the single band loading and 0.4 s of movement duration (Bonferroni *post-hoc* analysis $p < 0.05$).

The combined actions of various factors (**DP, SP, DV, PV, DPV**) may provide additional information regarding the central programs in the bimanual movements (**Table 1**). Weakness and frequent instability in the reactions of *the RM group* muscles are accompanied by the absence of a significant interaction of the factors (see *tric.* and *pect.* rows in **Table 1**). In contrast, this type of interaction was identified in the *delt.* muscle, which demonstrated highly repeatable, powerful and stable reactions in all experiments. Most likely, because of this stability, all combinations of the factors exerted a significant influence on the dynamic components of the EMGs in this muscle; however, these combinations were only partly effective in the biceps and completely ineffective in the *br.* During the movement phases, the central commands to the elbow flexors were more flexible and variable compared with the *delt.*; however, the *br.* could be identified in this muscle group because of a relative weakness of the steady-state reactions and, in many cases, the somewhat higher amplitudes of the D_R components (**Figure 4**). Peculiarities in the EMG reactions in the *br.* were also characterized by a significant combined action of three factors (**DPV**); however, the same combination of the factors was significant in both the *delt.* and *bic.l.* (**Table 1**).

Statistical Analysis of Relative Differences between the Integral Dynamic Components at the Pulling and Returning Movement Phases

Based on the pattern of the integral dynamic components in *PM group* of synergic muscles (two upper rows in **Figure 6**), one can assume that D_R components are likely less expressed in the *delt.* muscle compared with the elbow flexors. To further confirm this assumption, we introduced the difference coefficients that define the relative differences between the integral dynamic components that belong to the pulling and returning movement phases:

$$k = \frac{(\overline{D}_P - \overline{D}_R)}{(\overline{D}_P + \overline{D}_R)/2}, \tag{8}$$

where $\overline{D}_P$ and $\overline{D}_R$ indicate the mean values of *PM* and *RM* integral dynamic components in the group of nine subjects (i.e., the bar amplitudes in **Figure 6**).

In accordance with this previous definition of the difference coefficients, maximum or minimum values (+2 or −2, respectively) will be achieved in the following conditions: 1) $\overline{D}_P \neq 0$; $\overline{D}_R = 0$ and 2) $\overline{D}_P = 0$; $\overline{D}_R \neq 0$; zero values of the coefficient will correspond to the condition: $\overline{D}_P = \overline{D}_R \neq 0$; its positivity (negativity) would signify that $\overline{D}_P$ ($\overline{D}_R$) prevails. When various muscles of the group (*bic.b., bic.b., br.,* and *delt.*) were compared with respect to the difference coefficients, the distinctions between the arms, movement velocities, and loading levels were not taken into account; therefore, the coefficient sets included 12 quantities for each muscle. The sets of the difference coefficients were analyzed using One-way ANOVA with repeated

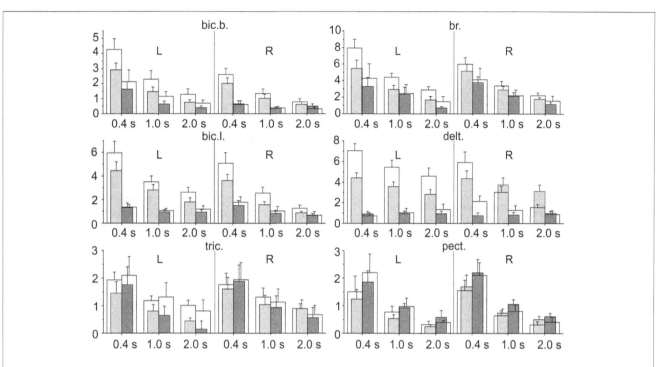

FIGURE 6 | Statistical analysis of the integral dynamic components of the EMGs during the pulling (D_P) and returning (D_R) phases of the test movements produced with three different movement durations and two values of external load ($m \pm SE$, group of nine subjects). For each EMG recording at a given ramp duration, four parameters are shown: the gray (white) bars correspond to the tests for one (two) rubber band loading; the left pairs of bars (light gray and white) describe D_P, and the right pairs (dark gray and white) describe the D_R components. The numbers under the separate bar groups (abscissa axes) signify the duration of the ramp phases; L, R indicate left and right arms, respectively; ordinates are given as the percentage of MVC.

TABLE 1 | Four-way ANOVA with repeated measurements for the dynamic EMG components.

	D	S	P	V	DS	DP	SP	DSP	DV	SV	DSV	PV	DPV	SPV	DSPV
bic. b.	0.019	0.037	0.000	0.001	0.720	0.071	0.034	0.882	0.023	0.083	0.874	0.048	0.273	0.753	0.679
bic. l.	0.000	0.129	0.001	0.000	0.183	0.005	0.938	0.871	0.003	0.704	0.375	0.413	0.034	0.074	0.055
br.	0.015	0.685	0.034	0.016	0.517	0.227	0.211	0.226	0.089	0.727	0.299	0.164	0.010	0.392	0.153
tric.	0.882	0.789	0.746	0.003	0.760	0.923	0.178	0.685	0.209	0.740	0.197	0.500	0.775	0.316	0.164
delt.	0.000	0.330	0.002	0.007	0.897	0.000	0.024	0.152	0.000	0.862	0.376	0.004	0.000	0.101	0.915
pect.	0.008	0.788	0.930	0.012	0.582	0.645	0.392	0.567	0.166	0.516	0.878	0.712	0.422	0.669	0.360

The following parameters are considered: **D**—direction factor (D_P–pulling/D_R–returning); **S**—side factor (left/right arm); **P**—load factor (one/two rubber bands); **V**—factor of the movement velocity (ramp duration: 0.4, 1.0, or 2.0 s). The header of table consists of marks of factors and their interactions. Combination of letters in header marks the interaction of respective factors. The cells with $p < 0.05$ are marked by gray color.

measurements for each specific muscle; significant differences in a parameter were identified within PM group ($F = 309.788$, $p < 0.001$). The statistical characteristics of the difference coefficients are shown in **Figure 7**; the results of the Bonferroni post-hoc analysis of the pairwise comparisons for specific muscles are schematically presented by the corresponding arrowed lines. The positivity of the coefficients for all muscles of the group signifies that the first dynamic coefficient is higher compared with the second value. Therefore, it could be concluded that weights of the second dynamic components were smaller in the shoulder extensor muscle (delt.) compared with the elbow flexors.

Statistical Analysis of the Static Components of the EMGs in the Test Movements

A Three-way ANOVA for repeated measurements for all muscles was used to estimate the dependence of the static component E_{st} (Equation 5) on the **S**, **P**, and **V** factors. The muscles of RM group did not exhibit dependency on any of these factors, whereas all muscles of PM group depended on **P** factor; the static component increased with an increase in the external load (**Figure 8**). In addition, it was observed that the static component of the bic.b. significantly increased in the left arm compared with the right arm for the higher loads (two rubber

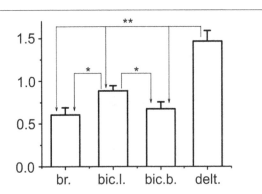

FIGURE 7 | Statistical analysis of the difference coefficients determined by Equation 8. The difference coefficients were defined for the mean values D_P and D_R presented as the bar amplitudes in **Figure 6**. Shared populations of the coefficients for each of the four muscles, *bic.b.*, *bic.b. br.*, and *delt.*, included the results obtained for all movement velocities at both arms, which thus consisted of 12 values for each muscle under study. The potential differences in the coefficients were analyzed by One-way ANOVA with repeated measurements, which indicated their significant dependence within a given group of synergist muscles ($F = 309.788$, $p < 0.001$). The results of the Bonferroni *post-hoc* analysis of pairwise comparisons for particular muscles are schematically indicated by the arrowed lines; one and two asterisks above the lines signify $p < 0.05$ and $p < 0.005$, respectively. The EMG calibration is given in % of MVC.

bands) and slower movements (1.0 and 2.0 s ramp durations). An ANOVA analysis indicated a significant action of the interaction between the **S** and **P** factors in the reactions of the *bic.b.* and *br.*; a *post-hoc* Bonferroni analysis supported the existence of significant differences in these cases ($p < 0.05$). Noticeable dynamic components in the reactions of the *br.* muscle were associated with a relative weakness and instability of the stationary components, especially with a small loading. For the one band load, the mean values of the parameter in the left arm registered quite low; higher stationary values of the EMG activities in the right *br.* were simultaneously present with the high dispersion levels (**Figure 8**).

DISCUSSION

The present study was devoted to the analysis of simple, visually tracked, bimanual, symmetrical, ramp-and-hold movements executed against similar elastic loads. The focus of the investigation was to identify the patterns of the averaged EMGs in different muscles that act at the elbow and shoulder joints and to compare the reactions of similar muscles in the left and right arms. We did not take into account the hand muscle activity, which evidently plays an important role in the test movements; for a sake of simplicity, a complex multi-joint movement was reduced to the two-joint movement. The bimanual two-joint movements were fulfiled in the horizontal plane; these movements included symmetrical pulling and returning phases separated by the position fixation. Despite the simplicity, these movements are provided by the concerted action of many muscles; therefore, recording surface EMGs only in part of the muscles can present rather restricted information regarding the

central commands that provide these movements. Moreover, the reliability of the EMG measures in the characterisation of activity patterns is known to be dependent on the variability that can occur in electrode placements. The proximity of the EMG electrodes to a muscle's innervation zone can affect the EMG signal (De Luca and Contessa, 2012), and the innervation zone may exhibit considerable variability in its location for certain muscles (Rainoldi et al., 2004). We understand that the influence of these problems become more essential if the EMG activities in similar muscles of different limbs are compared, which was accomplished in the present study.

Velocity of movement is essential factor defining reactions of the elbow extensors and shoulder flexors, what is can be seen in **Figures 6**, 7. At minimal velocity, subjects provide the necessary movement predominantly by lowering intensity of activation in these muscles. On the other hand, the drop of activity in these muscles become insufficient with velocity rise, what may be compensated for by the dynamic components of EMG in the elbow flexors and shoulder extensors. The simultaneous appearance of intensive dynamic EMG components in muscles-antagonists may reflect a tuning process of redistribution of activity between these muscles during fulfillment of fast movements.

PM group of synergy consists of the muscles that flex the elbow joint and extend the shoulder joint; these muscles provide an active pulling movement at the beginning of the test, support steady-state positions during the hold phase, and work in the yielding regimen during the returning phase. The general forms of the EMG intensity changes in actively contracting muscles and their rearrangement with an increase in the movement velocity are well corresponded with the reactions of the elbow flexors in single-joint isotorque movements (Kostyukov and Tal'nov, 1991). The central commands to the muscles during ramp-and-hold flexing movements also include the dynamic and static components, which are crucially dependent on the muscle hysteresis (Kostyukov and Korchak, 1998); it has been assumed that hysteresis effects allow the intensity of the coming efferent activity to be diminished for clamping the muscle length after shortening (Kostyukov, 1998). During the returning phase of the test movements, when the muscles lengthen in the regimen of the yielding work, more complex reactions are registered (**Figures 4**, **5**). Fundamental difficulties in the explanation of muscle behavior during lengthening exist even for experiments on nerve-muscle preparations in which the intensity in the incoming efferent activity can be completely controlled (Kostyukov, 1987, 1998). For the analysis of a real multi-joint movement, these difficulties are raised because of the restricted quantity of the muscles that produce the EMG records; another problem consists of the potential redistribution of activity among muscles, which is likely needed in the development of additional methodical approaches with a higher time resolution compared with the averaging technique.

RM group of synergy includes the muscles that are in antagonistic relationships with the muscles of *PM group*. During both movement phases, these muscles predominantly increase their activities, which thus opposes the forces generated by the actively contracting muscles of *PM group*. At the same

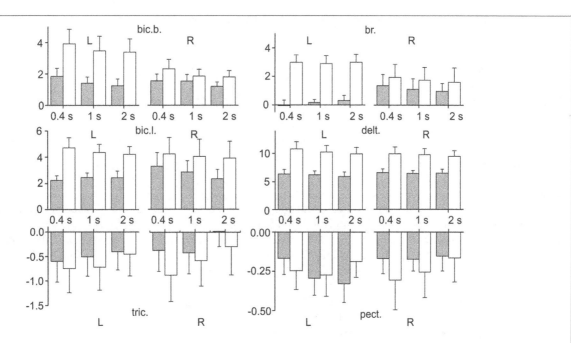

FIGURE 8 | Statistical analysis of the static components of the EMGs in the test movements produced with three different movement durations and two values of external load (m ± SE, N = 9). Tests with loading by one and two rubber bands are shown as *gray* and *white bars, respectively*; the other designations are similar to **Figure 6**. Note that the negativity in the reactions of the *mm. triceps, pectoralis* indicate that the levels of their stationary activity decrease with respect to their initial states. The EMG calibration is given in % of MVC.

time, during the hold phases of the test movements, they largely decrease activity, which therefore assists the actions of these muscles. The relatively low amplitudes of the dynamic components and frequently observed variability in the activity during the hold phases in these muscles are likely connected with their predominately subsidiary role in the given movements. It should be noted that the division of the muscles under study in accordance with their attitude to a definite joint is oversimplified. The places of the force applications are single-valued only for mono-articular muscles, such as the *bic.l., br.,* and *delt. pect.,* whereas the *bic.b. (m. biceps brachii breve)* and *tric. (m. triceps brachii caput longum)* are bi-articular muscles; however, these bi-articular muscles primarily provide movements around the elbow joint (van Bolhuis et al., 1998).

A common feature of *PM* and *RM groups* of synergic muscles consists of the strong dependency of the dynamic components on movement velocity, whereas the actions of the other factors, as well as the combinations of different factors are significant only in the muscles of *PM group* (**Tables 1, 2**). Side-dependent differences are identified only for the dynamic components of the EMG reactions in the *bic. b.*; in the other muscles, these differences are not significant. In all muscles of *PM group,* the load factor influences the steady-state EMG reactions, whereas the side and velocity factors do not evoke effects (**Table 2**). The strong action of the load factor is likely the main reason that the combination of the load and side factors is also effective in the *br.* and *bic. b.*

A set of the efferent activities that control the two-joint test movements can be localized within separate time zones, in which the programs of co-contraction (co-activation) or reciprocal activation predominate. The movement phases are primarily

accompanied by antagonist co-contractions, whereas the steady-states are connected with a preferential use of reciprocal activation. Recently, the movement dynamic under these basic patterns of the antagonist activations was studied via the experimental model of two antagonistic muscles (Gorkovenko et al., 2012). It has been demonstrated that a reciprocal activation pattern can essentially linearise the movements after a change in their direction, providing they also exhibit a fast beginning; the co-contraction patterns can distinctly reduce the undesirable hysteresis after-effects, such as the ongoing residual movements at the apexes of activity. Thus, the co-activation of the antagonistic muscles could reduce the uncertainty effects in the motor control system connected, in particular, with muscle hysteresis (Kostyukov, 1998; Gorkovenko et al., 2012). Behavioral studies of postural tasks have demonstrated that subjects use muscle co-contraction as a strategy to stabilize limb joints in the presence of external loads (Kearney and Hunter, 1990; De Serres and Milner, 1991; Milner and Cloutier, 1998); these subjects are also able to independently modulate the relative balance of the co-contraction and limb stiffness in different spatial directions (Gomi and Osu, 1998; Burdet et al., 2001) and at different joints (Gribble and Ostry, 1998). It has been suggested that the CNS may use co-contraction as a strategy to facilitate the accuracy of the limb movement (Gribble and Ostry, 1998; Gribble et al., 2003).

Despite a sufficiently good quantity of execution of the test movements by all subjects in the present study, the patterns of the EMG reactions are essentially diverse. In some subjects, the reactions of the identical muscles that belonged to the left and right arms were quite similar. Simultaneously, the activities recorded during the hold phases in these subjects did

TABLE 2 | Result of the Three-way ANOVA with repeated measurements for static components.

	S	P	V	SP	SV	PV	SPV
bic. b.	0.081	0.005	0.151	0.010	0.378	0.451	0.529
bic. l.	0.977	0.000	0.125	0.266	0.500	0.465	0.187
br.	0.912	0.002	0.695	0.004	0.260	0.765	0.149
tric.	0.544	0.386	0.053	0.405	0.092	0.613	0.127
delt.	0.756	0.000	0.290	0.093	0.515	0.870	0.163
pect.	0.446	0.844	0.057	0.423	0.054	0.053	0.530

Similar symbols as in **Table 1**.

not contain noticeable oscillations or substantial trends; thus, the mean EMG intensities in these phases were close to one another for the different velocities of movements executed at the same levels of loading (**Figure 4**). In contrast, in other subjects, essential and often unpredictable side- or velocity dependent changes in the basic EMG components were identified (**Figure 5**). Our data indicate that the EMG variability during the hold sections of movements can differ in the muscles of *PM group*. The quality of the test executions was almost identical in all subjects; therefore, the variability of the EMG reactions may signify the presence of the activation redistribution among different muscles or motor units within the same muscles. One can speculate that the activity redistribution processes could decrease the development of fatigue in the actively contracting muscle groups, which has been demonstrated for the natural labor movements of professional butchers (Madeleine et al., 2003). However, muscle fatigue itself can essentially modify the central programs of movement execution (Lacquaniti, 1992; Haruno and Wolpert, 2005; Huffenus et al., 2006; Prilutsky et al., 2009; Fuller et al., 2013; Lampropoulou and Nowicky, 2014; Rampichini et al., 2014); thus, the observed EMG rearrangements might be, at least in part, secondary with respect to the fatigue effects. Nevertheless, we can assume that different subjects use different motor strategies, which differ to various extents, of the activity rearrangement among different muscles or within these muscles. In our opinion, the analysis of these processes might be expanded by the simultaneous recording of activities from different motor units; however, there are known methodological difficulties in using this approach during large-scaled movements under noticeable loads (Tal'nov et al., 2014). Thus, indirect methods of recording appear to be more valid for these purposes (Akazawa and Okuno, 2000). The identification of potential side-dependent asymmetries in the central motor programs cannot likely be effective using standard EMG methods, such as in the present study; however, some prerequisites for the existence of this asymmetry in spinal cord circuitries have recently been demonstrated in animal experiments (Pilyavskii et al., 2013). In the present study, the right-handed subjects participated, and experiments were not directed on searching possible asymmetries in the EMG patterns related to the handedness. Nevertheless, we

suppose that application of the present experimental approach to more complex movement paradigms, which are traditionally elaborated in classical studies of bimanual coordination (Walter and Swinnen, 1992; Swinnen et al., 1995), might be suitable for analysis of more intimate processes within the motor control system.

CONCLUSIONS

The muscles of *PM group* (which flex the elbow joint and extend the shoulder joint) generated noticeable, velocity-dependent, dynamic EMG components during the pulling and returning phases of the trapezoidal test movements, which supports a steady-state activity during their hold phases. The muscles of *RM group* (which extend the elbow joint and flex the shoulder joint) co-contracted with *PM group* during the movement phases and decreased activity during the hold phase. A Multi-way ANOVA analysis for particular muscles demonstrated that in both muscle groups, the dynamic components of the EMGs strongly depended on the velocity factor, whereas the side and load factors, as well as the combinations of various factors, were significant only in the muscles of *PM group*. The extent of the EMG variability changed in various subjects, which could signify that the same movements may be realized by central commands with different extents of activity redistribution among muscles. It has been assumed that the activity redistributions may decrease the development of fatigue effects in actively contracted muscles.

AUTHOR CONTRIBUTIONS

TT, data analysis and discussion; AG, statistical analysis and data discussion; AT, data analysis and discussion; TA, data analysis and discussion; VM, data discussion; IV, data analysis and discussion; AK, data analysis and discussion.

ACKNOWLEDGMENTS

This work was supported by Fund "Academic Sports Development" of Ministry High Education and Science of Poland.

REFERENCES

Akazawa, K., and Okuno, R. (2000). "Firing behaviors of single motor units in m. biceps brachii during isovelocity elbow flexion," in *Proceedings of the 10th International Conference on Biomedical Engineering* (Singapore), 249–250.

Burdet, E., Osu, R., Franklin, D. W., Milner, T. E., and Kawato, M. (2001). The central nervous system stabilizes unstable dynamics by learning optimal impedance. *Nature* 414, 446–449. doi: 10.1038/35106566

De Luca, C. J., and Contessa, P. (2012). Hierarchical control of motor units in voluntary contractions. *J. Neurophysiol.* 107, 178–195. doi: 10.1152/jn.00961.2010

De Luca, C. J., Gilmore, L. D., Kuznetsov, M., and Roy, S. H. (2010). Filtering the surface EMG signal: movement artifact and baseline noise contamination. *J. Biomech.* 43, 1573–1579. doi: 10.1016/j.jbiomech.2010.01.027

De Serres, S. J., and Milner, T. E. (1991). Wrist muscle activation patterns and stiffness associated with stable and unstable mechanical loads. *Exp. Brain Res.* 86, 451–458. doi: 10.1007/BF00228972

Diedrichsen, J., and Dowling, N. (2009). Bimanual coordination as task-dependent linear control policies. *Hum. Mov. Sci.* 28, 334–347. doi: 10.1016/j.humov.2008.10.003

Dounskaia, N. V., Ketcham, C., and Stelmach, G. E. (2002). Influence of biomechanical constraints on horizontal arm movements. *Motor Control* 6, 366–387.

Dounskaia, N. V., Swinnen, S. P., Walter, C. B., Spaepen, A. J., and Verschueren, S. M. P. (1998). Hierarchical control of different elbow-wrist coordination patterns. *Exp. Brain. Res.* 121, 239–254. doi: 10.1007/s002210050457

Feldman, A. G. (1966). Functional tuning of nervous system with control of movement or maintenance of a steady posture: 2. Controllable parameters of the muscle. *Biophysics* 11, 565–578.

Feldman, A. G., and Levin, M. F. (2009). The equilibrium-point hypothesis-past, present and future. *Adv. Exp. Med. Biol.* 629, 699–726. doi: 10.1007/978-0-387-77064-2_38

Fuller, J. R., Fung, J., and Côté, J. N. (2013). Posture-movement responses to stance perturbations and upper limb fatigue during a repetitive pointing task. *Hum. Mov. Sci.* 32, 618–632. doi: 10.1016/j.humov.2013.03.002

Gomi, H., and Osu, R. (1998). Task dependent viscoelasticity of human multijoint arm and spatial characteristic for interaction with environment. *J. Neurosci.* 18, 8965–8978.

Gorkovenko, A. V., Sawczyn, S., Bulgakova, N. V., Jasczur-Nowicki, J., Mishchenko, V. S., and Kostyukov, A. I. (2012). Muscle agonist-antagonist interactions in an experimental joint model. *Exp. Brain Res.* 222, 399–414. doi: 10.1007/s00221-012-3227-0

Gribble, P. L., Mullin, L. I., and Mattar, A. (2003). Role of contraction in arm movement accuracy. *J. Neurophysiol.* 89, 2396–2405. doi: 10.1152/jn.01020.2002

Gribble, P. L., and Ostry, D. J. (1998). Independent coactivation of shoulder and elbow muscles. *Exp. Brain Res.* 123, 335–360. doi: 10.1007/s002210050580

Gueugnon, M., Torre, K., Mottet, D., and Bonnetblanc, F. (2014). Asymmetries of bilateral isometric force matching with movement intention and unilateral fatigue. *Exp. Brain Res.* 232, 1699–1706. doi: 10.1007/s00221-014-3862-8

Haruno, M., and Wolpert, D. M. (2005). Optimal control of redundant muscles in step tracing wrist movements. *J. Neurophysiol.* 94, 4244–4255. doi: 10.1152/jn.00404.2005

Herzog, W., Lee, E. J., and Rassier, D. E. (2006). Residual force enhancement in skeletal muscle. *J. Physiol.* 574, 635–642. doi: 10.1113/jphysiol.2006.107748

Hogan, N. (1985). The mechanics of multi-joint posture and movement control. *Biol. Cybern.* 52, 315–331. doi: 10.1007/BF00355754

Huffenus, A. F., Amarantini, D., and Forestier, N. (2006). Effects of distal and proximal arm muscles fatigue on multijoint movement organization. *Exp. Brain Res.* 170, 438–447. doi: 10.1007/s00221-005-0227-3

Kearney, R. E., and Hunter, I. W. (1990). System identification of human joint dynamics. *Crit. Rev. Biomed. Eng.* 18, 55–87.

Kelso, J. A. S. (1994). The informational character of self-organized coordination dynamics. *Hum. Mov. Sci.* 13, 393–413. doi: 10.1016/0167-9457(94)90047-7

Kostyukov, A. I. (1986). Muscle dynamic: dependence of muscle length on changes in external load. *Biol. Cybern.* 56, 375–387. doi: 10.1007/BF00319517

Kostyukov, A. I. (1987). Muscle dynamic: dependence of muscle length on changes in external load. *Biol. Cybern.* 56, 375–387. doi: 10.1007/bf00319517

Kostyukov, A. I. (1998). Muscle hysteresis and movement control: a theoretical study. *Neuroscience* 83, 303–320. doi: 10.1016/S0306-4522(97)00379-5

Kostyukov, A. I., and Korchak, O. E. (1998). Length changes of the cat soleus muscle under frequency-modulated distributed stimulation of efferents in isotony. *Neuroscience* 82, 943–955. doi: 10.1016/S0306-4522(97)00105-X

Kostyukov, A. I., and Tal'nov, A. N. (1991). Effects of torque disturbances on elbow joint movements evoked in unanesthetized cats by microstimulation of the motor cortex. *Exp. Brain Res.* 84, 374–382.

Lacquaniti, F. (1992). Automatic control of limb movement and posture. *Curr. Neurobiol.* 2, 807–814. doi: 10.1016/0959-4388(92)90138-B

Lampropoulou, S. I., and Nowicky, A. V. (2014). Perception of effort changes following an isometric fatiguing exercise of elbow flexors. *Motor Control* 18, 146–164. doi: 10.1123/mc.2013-0010

Madeleine, P., Lundager, B., Voigt, M., and Arendt-Nielsen, L. (2003). Standardized low-load repetitive work: evidence of different motor control strategies between experienced workers and a reference group. *Appl. Ergon.* 34, 533–542. doi: 10.1016/S0003-6870(03)00083-8

Milner, T. E., and Cloutier, C. (1998). Damping of the wrist joint during voluntary movement. *Exp. Brain Res.* 122, 309–317. doi: 10.1007/s002210050519

Nijhof, E. J., and Gabriel, D. A. (2006). Maximum isometric arm forces in the horizontal plane. *J. Biomech.* 39, 708–716. doi: 10.1016/j.jbiomech.2005.01.004

Pilyavskii, A. I., Moska, W., Kochanowicz, K., Bulgakova, N. V., Maznychenko, A. V., Vereshchaka, I. V., et.al. (2013). Dynorphin B induces lateral asymmetric changes in feline spinal cord reflexes. *Front. Neurosci.* 7:244. doi: 10.3389/fnins.2013.00244

Prilutsky, B. I., Klishko, A. N., Farrell, B., Harley, L., Phillips, G., and Bottasso, C. L. (2009). "Movement coordination in skilled tasks: insights from optimization," in *Advances in Neuromuscular Physiology of Motor Skills and Muscle Fatigue*, ed M. Shinohara (Trivandrum: Research Signpost), 139–171.

Rainoldi, A., Melchiorri, G., and Caruso, I. (2004). A method for positioning electrodes during surface EMG recordings in lower limb muscles. *J. Neurosci. Methods* 134, 37–43. doi: 10.1016/j.jneumeth.2003.10.014

Rampichini, S., Cè, E., Limonta, E., and Esposito, F. (2014). Effects of fatigue on the electromechanical delay components in gastrocnemius medialis muscle. *Eur. J. Appl. Physiol.* 114, 639–651. doi: 10.1007/s00421-013-2790-9

Soteropoulos, D. S., and Perez, M. A. (2011). Physiological changes underlying bilateral isometric arm voluntary contractions in healthy humans. *J. Neurophysiol.* 105, 1594–1602. doi: 10.1152/jn.00678.2010

Swinnen, S. P., Jardin, K., and Meulenbroek, R. (1996). Between-limb asynchronies during bimanual coordination: effects of manual dominance and attentional cueing. *Neuropsychologia* 34, 1203–1213. doi: 10.1016/0028-3932(96)00047-4

Swinnen, S. P., Serrien, D. J., Walter, C. B., and Philippaerts, R. (1995). The organization of patterns of multilimb coordination as revealed through reaction time measures. *Exp. Brain. Res.* 104, 153–162. doi: 10.1007/BF00229865

Tal'nov, A. N., Cherkassky, V. L., and Kostyukov, A. I. (1997). Movement-related and steady-state electromyographic activity of human elbow flexors in slow transition movements between two equilibrium states. *Neuroscience* 79, 923–933.

Tal'nov, A. N., and Kostyukov, A. I. (1994). Hysteresis aftereffects in human single-joint voluntary movements. *Neurophysiology* 26, 65–71.

Tal'nov, A. N., Serenko, S. G., Strafun, S. S., and Kostyukov, A. I. (1999). Analysis of the electromyographic activity of human elbow joint muscles during slow linear flexion movements in isotorque conditions. *Neuroscience* 90, 1123–1136.

Tal'nov, A. N., Tomiak, T., Maznychenko, A. V., Dovgalets, G. V., and Kostyukov, A. I. (2014). Firing patterns of human biceps brachii motor units during isotorque ramp-and-hold movements in the elbow joint. *Neurophysiology* 46, 212–220. doi: 10.1007/s11062-014-9431-8

van Bolhuis, B. M., Gielen, C. C., and van Ingen Schenau, G. J. (1998). Activation patterns of mono- and bi-articular arm muscles as a function of force and movement direction of the wrist in humans. *J. Physiol.* 508, 313–324. doi: 10.1111/j.1469-7793.1998.313br.x

Walter, C. B., and Swinnen, S. P. (1992). Adaptive tuning of interlimb attraction to facilitate bimanual decoupling. *J. Mot. Behav.* 24, 95–104. doi: 10.1080/00222895.1992.9941605

Conflict of Interest Statement: The authors declare that the research was conducted in the absence of any commercial or financial relationships that could be construed as a potential conflict of interest.

8

An Ultra-High Field Magnetic Resonance Spectroscopy Study of Post Exercise Lactate, Glutamate and Glutamine Change in the Human Brain

Andrea Dennis[1][*][†], Adam G. Thomas[1,2][†], Nancy B. Rawlings[1], Jamie Near[1,3],
Thomas E. Nichols[1,4], Stuart Clare[1], Heidi Johansen-Berg[1] and Charlotte J. Stagg[1,5]

[1] Oxford Centre for Functional MRI of the Brain (FMRIB), Nuffield Department of Clinical Neurosciences, University of Oxford, Oxford, UK, [2] Section on Functional Imaging Methods, National Institute of Mental Health, National Institutes of Health, Department of Health and Human Services, Bethesda, MD, USA, [3] Douglas Mental Health University Institute and Department of Psychiatry, McGill University, Montreal, QC, Canada, [4] Department of Statistics and Warwick Manufacturing Group, University of Warwick, Coventry, UK, [5] Physiological Neuroimaging Group, Oxford Centre for Human Brain Activity (OHBA), University of Oxford, Oxford, UK

Edited by:
J. A. Taylor,
Harvard University, USA

Reviewed by:
Can Ozan Tan,
Harvard Medical School, USA
Alexander Peter Lin,
Brigham and Women's Hospital, USA

*Correspondence:
Andrea Dennis
andrea.dennis@ndcn.ox.ac.uk

[†] These authors have contributed equally to this work.

During strenuous exercise there is a progressive increase in lactate uptake and metabolism into the brain as workload and plasma lactate levels increase. Although it is now widely accepted that the brain can metabolize lactate, few studies have directly measured brain lactate following vigorous exercise. Here, we used ultra-high field magnetic resonance spectroscopy of the brain to obtain static measures of brain lactate, as well as brain glutamate and glutamine after vigorous exercise. The aims of our experiment were to (a) track the changes in brain lactate following recovery from exercise, and (b) to simultaneously measure the signals from brain glutamate and glutamine. The results of our experiment showed that vigorous exercise resulted in a significant increase in brain lactate. Furthermore, both glutamate and glutamine were successfully resolved, and as expected, although contrary to some previous reports, we did not observe any significant change in either amino acid after exercise. We did however observe a negative correlation between glutamate and a measure of fitness. These results support the hypothesis that peripherally derived lactate is taken up by the brain when available. Our data additionally highlight the potential of ultra-high field MRS as a non-invasive way of measuring multiple brain metabolite changes with exercise.

Keywords: brain, lactate, glutamate, magnetic resonance spectroscopy, exercise

INTRODUCTION

In the non-activated state, the brain's energy needs are met primarily by glucose. However, the brain has been shown to be capable of using substrates other than glucose when they are available to support activity, including lactate (Schurr et al., 1997; Bouzier-Sore et al., 2003; Overgaard et al., 2012; Schurr, 2014), pyruvate (Cruz et al., 2001; Sharma et al., 2003), and ketone bodies (Nybo et al., 2003; Chowdhury et al., 2014). During recovery from exercise, lactate is perhaps the most important of these additional substrates (Dalsgaard et al., 2002) as during high intensity exercise there is an increase in blood and brain lactate (Quistorff et al., 2008; van Hall et al., 2009). It has even been suggested that lactate may be preferred to glucose, possibly 'sparing' brain glucose metabolism during exercise (Quistorff et al., 2008; van Hall, 2010; Schurr, 2014).

There is, therefore, a great deal of interest in the metabolic fate of peripherally derived lactate within the human brain as evidence emerges as to its role as a putative neuronal energy source (Pellerin and Magistretti, 1994; Bouzier-Sore et al., 2003; van Hall et al., 2009) and as a signaling molecule in neuronal plasticity (Yang et al., 2014). Whilst persistently elevated brain lactate may indicate pathology, transient increases are normal consequences of the energetic processes involved in vigorous exercise and are now also believed to be complimentary to healthy brain processes (Schurr, 2008; Dienel, 2012) and brain recovery (Bouzat et al., 2014; Brooks and Martin, 2015; Glenn et al., 2015).

It is now widely accepted that on-going cerebral activity results in the generation of lactate in the brain, with lactate produced within the astrocytes fuelling neuronal activities (Fox et al., 1988; Schurr et al., 1988; Pellerin and Magistretti, 1994) probably via the astrocyte-neuron lactate shuttle (ANLS) (Magistretti and Pellerin, 1999; Pellerin and Magistretti, 2012). Here, however, we are primarily interested in the fate of peripherally derived lactate generated during exercise. Lactate is both taken up and produced in the brain by reversible reactions (Hertz et al., 2014). In one direction, pyruvate is reduced to lactate while NADH is oxidized to NAD+. In the other direction, lactate is oxidized to pyruvate, and NAD+ is reduced to NADH. In this direction, pyruvate is hypothesized to be either fully oxidized, producing $6CO_2$ and $6H_2O$, or partially oxidized, to allow for carbon atoms to participate in exchange reactions (Cerdán et al., 2006; Massucci et al., 2013) resulting in *de novo* synthesis of amino acid neurotransmitters, particularly glutamate (Hertz and Dienel, 2004). It is therefore possible for the pyruvate derived from lactate to be both oxidized to fuel neuronal activity and act as a metabolic intermediate in exchange reactions, such as those involved in glutamate recycling.

Glutamate is a non-essential amino acid and is the main excitatory neurotransmitter of the cerebral cortex. It does not cross the blood-brain barrier and is therefore synthesized within the brain from glucose and a variety of other precursors such as lactate (Hertz and Fillenz, 1999). *In vivo* studies have established that the glutamate-glutamine cycle between glutamatergic neurons and glia is a major metabolic flux, reflecting synaptic glutamate release (Shen and Rothman, 2002). The glutamate-glutamine cycling flux is directly coupled to neuroenergetics (Sibson et al., 1998) and thus they are both important cerebral metabolites. The ability to measure glutamate and glutamine therefore will greatly increase our understanding of brain metabolic processes and aid in our understanding of brain lactate metabolism pathways.

Although there have been a number of studies measuring brain lactate changes following exercise (Ide et al., 2000; Dalsgaard et al., 2004; van Hall et al., 2009; Volianitis et al., 2011) these often involve invasive measures of venous blood from the dominant jugular vein and technology restricted to examining metabolites only present in blood leaving the brain. Proton Magnetic Resonance Spectroscopy (H^1 MRS) offers an attractive alternative to directly measuring cerebral blood measures as it is able to characterize brain tissues in terms of the relative concentration of many brain metabolites, including lactate, glutamate, and glutamine. 7 T ^{1}H MRS is non-invasive, non-ionizing, and has been widely used for human studies. Alternative methods exist which are capable of measuring changes in brain metabolites, but they have significant limitations. Positron Emission Tomography (PET) is able to quantify neurochemicals and their binding, but relies on ionizing radiation. ^{13}C MRS offers an alternative approach, where signal from ^{13}C can be recorded, either via an infusion of ^{13}C MRS or using hyperpolarization. However, although these techniques are perhaps the gold standard for this approach they involve both lengthy and expensive infusions or are still largely in development, neither of which would be appropriate to investigate the question here.

To date, only two studies have used ^{1}H MRS to investigate changes in brain metabolites with exercise (Dalsgaard et al., 2004; Maddock et al., 2011). Whilst Dalsgaard and colleagues (Dalsgaard et al., 2004) were unable to resolve to lactate peak, using similar methods Maddock et al. (2011) used MRS at 1.5 T to examine the change in lactate and a combined measure of the glutamate and glutamine (Glx) concentration following vigorous exercise. The authors reported a sustained increase in brain lactate following exercise together with a transient increase in brain Glx, suggesting that at least some of the lactate is only partially oxidized. Although these results provide important direct evidence for brain metabolite changes post-exercise in humans, there are some limitations to the study. For example, at lower field strengths, detection of the lactate signal is difficult (Dalsgaard et al., 2004), and it is not possible to distinguish between glutamate and glutamine, making it impossible to know which is driving any observed changes in the composite measure Glx.

The aim of this study was two-fold: to replicate the experiment conducted by Maddock et al. (2011) in a study of exercise-induced brain lactate uptake and to further examine the change in brain glutamate in the presence of increased lactate as a proof of principle for *in vivo* post exercise multi-metabolite measurements. Here we used MRS at 7T to measure the relative levels of lactate, glutamate, and glutamine before and after exercise in 11 volunteers. We hypothesized that exercise would lead to global cerebral lactate uptake which would be fully metabolized during recovery. We expected to be able to resolve the signal from glutamine and glutamate but did not expect any significant changes in other measureable metabolites.

MATERIALS AND METHODS

Participants

Eleven healthy, untrained, adult volunteers [mean age 30.0 years (range 22–41), 4 male] participated. The study was conducted in accordance with the Declaration of Helsinki and was approved by the Central Office for Research Ethics Committee [Oxford REC B (10/H0605/48)]. All participants gave their written informed consent prior to participation.

Experimental Design

Each subject underwent two experimental sessions: an exercise session and a control session. The order of the sessions was counterbalanced across the group. Sessions were conducted at the same time of day within subject. The experimental protocol for each session consisted of 20 min of baseline (*pre*) MRS measurements, after which subjects were removed from the scanner for the 15-min exercise or control intervention. They then returned to the scanner for 40 min of post-intervention (*post*) MRS measurement (**Figure 1**). During scanning, participants were instructed to lie awake but were not engaged in any task. Participants were asked to refrain from eating, drinking, or consuming caffeine in the 2 h prior to each session and to refrain from performing exhaustive exercise in the preceding 24 h.

In the exercise condition, subjects were required to perform a discontinuous, graded exercise paradigm to 85% of their predicted maximum heart rate (HR; HR_{max}) ($208-0.7 \times$ age, $\pm3\%$) on a cycle ergometer (Monarch, UK). This protocol was selected to be comparable with the previous MRS/exercise study in the literature (Maddock et al., 2011), to allow for blood lactate to be rapidly produced endogenously without inducing severe fatigue that would make it difficult for participants to lie still in the MRI scanner, and without resulting in dehydration that might affect brain MRS measurements. Exercise began at 60 W for females and 90 W for males, and increased by 30 W every 3 min until 85% HR_{max} was reached. HR was measured using a Polar heart rate monitor (Polar Electro 20, Finland) and was recorded in the last 30 s of every 3 min stage. The mean length of this intervention was 14 ± 3 min. In the control condition, participants sat in a quiet seating area where they were provided with some light reading material for 15 min.

A proxy measure of aerobic fitness, the Physical Work Capacity (PWC), was established *post-hoc* for each individual in line with the PWC at 150 beats per minute test (PWC150; Campbell et al., 2001). Work rate achieved in the final step of the exercise protocol was normalized by body weight to give an estimate of PWC, measured in W kg^{-1} at 85% maximal heart rate.

In both sessions, blood lactate was measured from a capillary sample from the big toe before the *pre* scans, at the end of the intervention session, and every 10 min *post* intervention. Blood lactate was measured using the Lactate-Pro electrochemical test strip (Lactate Pro, Arkray Japan). The toe was used as a measurement site as access to participants' fingers was impossible

when the participant was inside the 7T Magnetom scanner bore. Toe measurements were selected during exercise in order to match measurement site with those acquired in between MRS acquisitions. Measurements from the toe have been reported in the literature (Forsyth and Farrally, 2000; Garland and Atkinson, 2008) as a practical alternative site during exercise testing.

On reaching the end of the exercise test, participants were not afforded any time for active recovery. Continuing exercise at a lower intensity (active recovery) increases muscular blood flow (Bangsbo et al., 1994) facilitating the elimination of lactate. Instead, to maximize circulating lactate, subjects were returned to the scanner as soon as possible where they lay still for the duration of the post-exercise scans.

Magnetic Resonance Data Acquisition

Magnetic resonance (MR) data were acquired at the University of Oxford using a 7 T MRI scanner (Siemens Magnetom 7 T, Erlangen, Germany) with a 32-channel head coil (Nova Medical, MA, USA). Prior to MRS acquisition a high resolution T1-weighted sagittal structural scan [magnetization prepared rapid gradient echo (MPRAGE); Repetition time (TR) = 2200 ms; Echo time (TE) = 2.96 ms; Inversion time (TI) = 1050 ms; flip angle = $7°$; voxel size = 0.7 mm isotropic; 256 sagittal slices; Field of View (FoV) = 224 mm] was acquired for anatomical overlay of MRS voxel location.

MRS data were acquired using an ultra-short TE spin echo acquisition, the spin-echo full-intensity acquired localized (SPECIAL) sequence (60 averages; TR = 4500 ms; TE = 8.50 ms) (Mekle et al., 2009; Xin et al., 2013). VAPOR (variable power RF pulses with optimized relaxation delays) water suppression was used (Tkác et al., 1999), and outer volume suppression was used to eliminate signal contamination from outside the MRS voxel. Shimming was performed using the Siemens product manual shim and the mean linewidth for the acquired data were 0.03 (*SD* = 0.006). An 8 cm³ ($2 \times 2 \times 2$ cm) voxel of interest was positioned in the occipital cortex (identified using anatomical landmarks). This voxel position was selected as it has been demonstrated to provide good quality MRS spectra and as any metabolite changes resulting from exercise would be expected to be global (Mekle et al., 2009). The voxel was centered on the mid-sagittal plane with its posterior boundary positioned 6 mm anterior to the skull

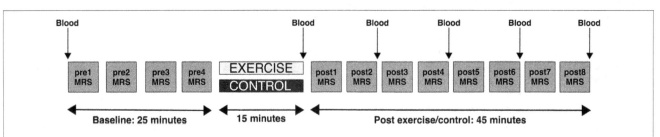

FIGURE 1 | Schematic depicting the study protocol. Participants underwent two 90-min scanning sessions on two different days. On one of the days they received an exercise intervention. On the other day, they received the control intervention (quiet reading). The order of the days were randomly assigned and counterbalanced. In both sessions participants first underwent a series of baseline (*pre*) scans involving four repeated MRS measurements (depicted by gray squares), came out of the scanner for the intervention, and then returned to the scanner for a series of post-intervention scans (*post*) involving eight repeated MRS measures. Blood lactate measurements (denoted as "Blood") were taken from the big toe before the pre-scan, at the end of the intervention period, and after post-MRS measurements 2, 4, 6, and 8.

at its point of closest proximity (**Figure 2**). Voxel placement was performed immediately after shimming on a rapidly acquired localiser scan prior to MRS measurement. Spectra were collected in blocks consisting of 60 acquired volumes, corresponding to a scan time of 4.5 min per block. Each scan session consisted of four *pre* time points and eight *post* time points. After the last MRS acquisition, a second T1-weighted structural scan was collected to allow registration of the *post* MRS voxels to those acquired at baseline.

MR Data Processing

MRS data pre-processing was conducted in Matlab and included removal of motion corrupted averages (typically only one or two were removed), and retrospective frequency and phase drift correction by spectral registration (Near et al., 2014). Spectra were quantified using LCModel (Provencher, 2001). The basis set used was generated in-house using the FID-A Simulation Toolbox (http://github.com/CIC-methods/FID-A). Simulations consisted of an ideal spin echo sequence at 7 T with an echo time equal to that of our MRS acquisition (8.5 ms). Only metabolites that could be quantified with Cramér-Rao lower bounds <25% were included in the analysis. The concentrations of all the metabolites were expressed relative to total creatine (tCr; creatine + phosphocreatine) as absolute quantification of metabolites has significant uncertainties, and we did not acquire simultaneous non-suppressed water spectra, so this approach may be misleading. However, in order to eliminate the chances of changes in metabolites being driven by change in creatine, statistics for absolute values are also reported.

To determine overlap between the *pre* and *post* voxels the two structural T1 scans were linearly registered using FLIRT (FMRIB's Linear Image Registration Tool; (Jenkinson and Smith, 2001) from the FMRIB software library (FSL; Smith et al., 2004). The *post* voxel masks were

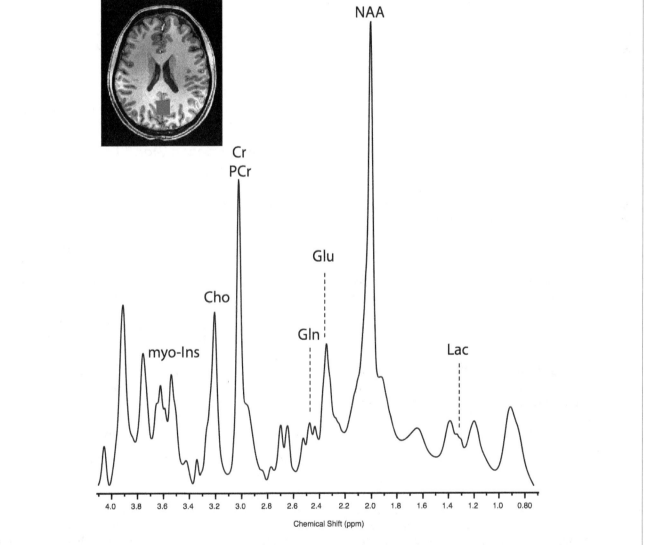

FIGURE 2 | Example of raw SPECIAL spectra acquired from one post-exercise block in a single subject. The lactate peak can be seen centered at 1.33 ppm, and glutamate (Glu) and glutamine (Gln) can be clearly separated.

transformed into the space of the *pre* scan and overlap was determined using the fslmaths tool from FSL 5.1 (www.fmrib.ox.ac.uk/fsl).

Statistical Analysis

Statistical analysis was conducted on all *pre* and *post* measures of blood and of brain lactate, glutamate, and glutamine. To compare the effects of exercise vs. control, a longitudinal Linear Mixed Effects (LME) modeling approach was used, implemented in the *nlme* package of the R statistical programming language (Singer and Willett, 2003; Pinheiro et al., 2013). LME is similar to hierarchical linear regression in that explanatory variables are sequentially added and tested to determine if they explain a statistically significant amount of the variance to warrant inclusion in the final model, but has the advantage of separately modeling variance due to within and between subject factors (Singer and Willett, 2003). LME models have become a popular tool for analysing longitudinal neuroimaging data because of their flexibility to account for correlation within subjects (Bernal-Rusiel et al., 2013; Guillaume et al., 2014). Due to potential time-varying confounds, such as scanner drift, our null model was a linear change with time regardless of intervention.

All blood lactate values were log-transformed as blood lactate has a highly skewed distribution (Foster et al., 1978). To compare baseline levels of blood lactate between sessions, paired *t*-tests were performed. To explore the relationship between metabolite concentration and PWC, correlation analysis with a standard Fisher transformation was used.

RESULTS

Subjects' mean ($\pm SD$) weight was 68.0 kg (±13.7) and height was 1.72 m (±0.10). In the exercise condition, subjects exercised to an average of 87% (±3.6) of their age-predicted maximal heart rate. Average maximum exercise intensity was 185 W (±35). Average time post-intervention to the beginning of the first MRS acquisition was 32 min (±10).

Good registration of *pre* and *post* voxels was achieved for all subjects. The *pre* and *post* voxels within individual subjects overlapped in volume by 67.1% (± 4.7). Consistent with previous reports, LCModel resolved the spectra of 20 different metabolites reliably (Mekle et al., 2009).

Exercise and Brain Creatine Concentration

Although not initially a metabolite of interest in the study, the metabolic nature of the paradigm deemed it necessary to examine the effect of exercise on creatine as this was the metabolite by which all others are expressed in relation to. Total creatine was successfully resolved at 3.03 ppm, with successful measurement for all time-points. Using the LME approach; the model including the post-exercise variable (0 or 1) explained significantly more of the variance than the null model (likelihood ratio = 15.90, $P = 0.0001$) demonstrating that brain creatine was significantly decreased from baseline after exercise but not after the control intervention (**Supplementary Figure 1**). Based on this finding, all subsequent statistical analysis were conducted on both the metabolite/Cr ratio and on the absolute concentrations in order

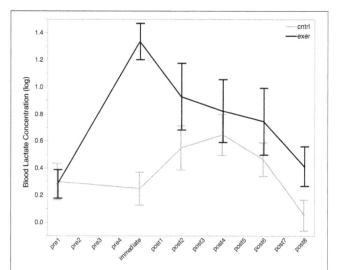

FIGURE 3 | Log blood lactate (log mmol/L) levels before (*pre*), immediately after, and *post* exercise (black line) and control (gray line) interventions. Blood lactate measurements were not taken at each MRS measurement (see **Figure 2**). All MRS time points are shown on the x-axis for ease of comparison with MRS data. All data are plotted as mean ± standard error. There was no significant difference in blood lactate levels between the baseline conditions, but a significant effect of exercise was seen after the intervention (likelihood ratio = 30.176, $P < 0.0001$).

to rule out the effect of decreasing creatine on the observed patterns in lactate, glutamate, and glutamine.

Exercise Increases Blood Lactate Concentration

Blood lactate was acquired in 91% of cases. Mean blood lactate concentration was 1.4 ± 0.6 mmol/L at baseline. Paired *t*-test revealed no significant difference between baseline blood lactate levels in the two sessions [$t_{(10)} = 0.12$, $P = 0.908$]. Following the exercise session, blood lactate levels were increased from baseline to 4.2 ± 2.1 mmol/L (**Figure 3**). To test this change statistically, we used a LME approach. We constructed a model to explain changes in blood lactate across all subjects, sessions, and time points using three explanatory variables: subject ID, session, time, and a variable indicating whether the data point was collected after the exercise session (0 or 1). This model provided a significantly better fit for the variance in blood lactate than the null model which included only subject ID, session, and time (likelihood ratio = 30.176, $P < 0.0001$) demonstrating that exercise significantly increased blood lactate level. Importantly, this increase in blood lactate was maintained for at least the first two blocks of the *post* MRS measurements.

Exercise Increases Brain Lactate Concentration

As has been demonstrated previously (Mekle et al., 2009; Schaller et al., 2013) brain lactate could be accurately quantified at 1.33 ppm within the SPECIAL spectra (see **Figure 2** for representative spectrum). Measurement of brain lactate was successful for 78% of MRS acquisitions. Using the same LME approach described above, we found that the model including the post-exercise variable (0 or 1) explained significantly more of the variance than the null model (ratio to Cr: likelihood ratio = 8.066, P = 0.005; absolute: likelihood ratio = 7.69, P = 0.006) demonstrating that brain lactate was significantly increased from baseline after exercise but not after the control intervention (**Figure 4A**). In a further analysis designed to assess the correlation between brain lactate and blood lactate, log blood lactate measures were added as a covariate into the LME model. Whilst this analysis did reduce the number of data points in the model (from 286 to 121) as blood lactate was measured after every other MRS acquisition after the intervention, this model provided a significantly better fit than the same model without log blood lactate included (ratio to Cr: Log likelihood = 3.839, P = 0.05; absolute: Log likelihood = 6.737, P = 0.0094). This indicates a correlation exists between blood and brain lactate measures.

Glutamate and Glutamine

Glutamate and glutamine were reliably resolved, with successful measurements at 99% of time points for glutamate and at 94% of time points for glutamine. There was no significant change in glutamate (**Figure 4B**) or glutamine (**Figure 4C**) in either session when normalized by creatine. The model including the exercise intervention was not a significantly better fit than the null model for glutamate (likelihood ratio = 1.158, P = 0.281) or glutamine (likelihood ratio = 1.759, P = 0.185), suggesting that exercise did not result in a significant change in either metabolite. However, when not normalizing by creatine, the models for both glutamate (likelihood ratio = 7.34, P = 0.007) and glutamine (likelihood ratio = 4.03, P = 0.045) showed a significantly better fit to the data when including the exercise variable.

Effect of Aerobic Fitness

It has previously been suggested that aerobic fitness modulates glutamatergic processing (Guezennec et al., 1998). In order to investigate this we first explored whether the mean baseline (*pre*) glutamate levels were related to the PWC150, a proxy measure of fitness. We demonstrated a significant negative correlation between baseline glutamate levels and fitness, such that fitter people had lower resting glutamate levels than less fit people (r = −0.627, P = 0.039, **Figure 5A**). We then went on to see whether this relationship could also be demonstrated immediately after exercise, i.e., whether any of the inter-subject variability in glutamate after the exercise condition could be explained by subject fitness. A correlational analysis revealed that brain glutamate immediately post-exercise and PWC were significantly negatively correlated (r = −0.726, P = 0.012; **Figure 5B**), such that fitter people had lower glutamate levels immediately post-exercise than less fit people. This relationship was not significantly different from that seen at baseline (Fisher's R-to-Z, Z = 0.12, P = 0.9).

DISCUSSION

This study investigated the effects of exercise-induced blood lactate increases on the levels of the brain metabolites lactate, glutamate, and glutamine in healthy adults. As in one previous study (Maddock et al., 2011), we have demonstrated

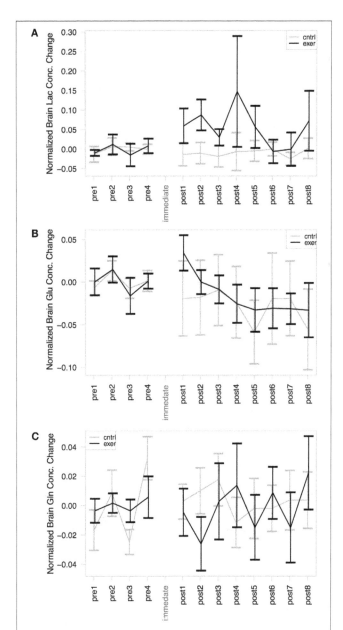

FIGURE 4 | MRS assessment of (A) Brain lactate/Cr; (B) Brain glutamate/Cr; and (C) Brain glutamine/Cr change from baseline within our voxel of interest. In each case the exercise session is shown in black and the control in gray. The mean baseline concentration for each session is subtracted from the values to illustrate change. A significant effect of exercise was demonstrated in the post-exercise lactate levels, compared with those from the control session (likelihood ratio = 8.066, P = 0.005). No significant changes were observed in glutamate or glutamine concentration with either the exercise or the control condition.

a transient increase in brain lactate after vigorous exercise as measured through ultra-high field strength MRS. In the brain at rest, metabolite concentrations are likely to be homeostatically controlled (Balaban et al., 1986; Hochachka, 2003). Whilst significant increases in brain-derived lactate have been reported in healthy subjects during prolonged visual and motor stimulations (Prichard et al., 1991; Sappey-Marinier et al.,

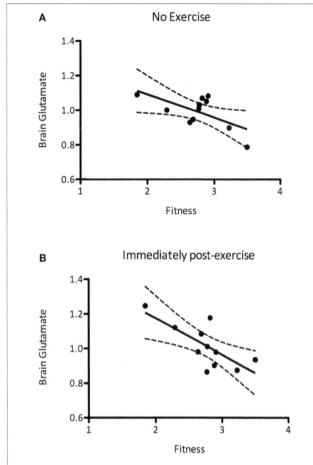

FIGURE 5 | (A) A significant negative correlation between brain glutamate levels at rest and fitness (*r* = −0.627, *P* = 0.039), such that fitter people had lower resting glutamate levels. **(B)** This correlation is also present immediately after exercise (*r* = −0.726, *P* = 0.012). The relationship between brain glutamate levels and fitness are not significantly altered after exercise (Fisher's R-to-Z, *Z* = 0.12, *P* = 0.9).

1992; Mangia et al., 2007; Schaller et al., 2014), such increases are transient and return to baseline within minutes. Therefore, there is no reason to expect an increase in brain tissue lactate between the *pre* and *post* scan in the current study, when neither acquisition required any task performance during data collection. We therefore believe our results support the hypothesis that lactate is taken up by the brain when available in high abundance in the plasma. However, unlike the previous study, we were able to resolve MRS peaks for both glutamine and glutamate. We did not observe any significant change in either amino acid following exercise, although we did observe a significant negative correlation between a proxy measure of aerobic fitness and glutamate.

The uptake and oxidization of lactate by the brain, heart, and muscle when available in the blood stream is not a newly discovered phenomenon, with a vast literature supporting its occurrence (Brooks, 1985, 2009; Schurr et al., 1997; Ide et al., 2000; van Hall et al., 2009; Bouzat et al., 2014). Here, for the first time, we present data from an ultra-high field

MR study of brain metabolite concentration changes following exercise. This is an important advance, since MRS at 7 T allows for the accurate, non-invasive quantification of a wide range of metabolites, most pertinently here including lactate, glutamate, and glutamine. Although proton MRS cannot provide information on cerebral flux of metabolites between cells, or on cerebral compartmentalization, it can provide valuable *in vivo* information about brain metabolism.

Interestingly, we also observed a significant decrease in brain creatine following exercise. This is an important finding given the prevalence in the literature to ratio metabolites to the usually stable metabolite creatine. Further studies interested in the fate of brain metabolites following exercise should consider reporting absolute concentrations based on normalization to unsuppressed water spectrum.

The Metabolic Fate of Peripherally-derived Brain Lactate in the Brain

A potential limitation with this type of experiment is that it is difficult to determine whether a change in lactate is due to increased brain uptake of plasma lactate or increases in locally produced lactate as a result of increased cerebral metabolism. However, results from our statistical analysis comparing brain lactate change were strengthened when blood lactate was added to the model, indicating a correlation exists between the brain and blood measures. This result, coupled with the absence of a change in glutamate and the temporal delay in acquiring our post-exercise measures, would be supportive of the increased uptake of plasma lactate. Thus, we believe our results support previous findings that lactate is taken up into the brain when it is in high supply in the bloodstream (Quistorff et al., 2008; van Hall et al., 2009). It has previously been shown that in the absence of exercise, all lactate taken up by the brain is oxidized, accounting for approximately 10% of cerebral energy requirements (Boumezbeur et al., 2010). During exercise, lactate accounts for 33% cerebral energy requirements (Overgaard et al., 2012), and may provide up to 66% of energy requirements when found in high concentration in the blood (Boumezbeur et al., 2010). Studies have suggested that the majority of plasma lactate is metabolized by the neurons (Boumezbeur et al., 2010). Whilst an interesting finding, and potentially in line with the hypothesis supporting a preferential use of lactate as a fuel source in exercising human subjects (Quistorff et al., 2008; van Hall, 2010), the MRS measurement is a total concentration and cannot dissociate between lactate within astrocytes and neurons; thus, we cannot conclude whether it is preferred to glucose following exercise. In addition, direct quantification of cerebral glucose levels was not possible with the MRS method used here and, therefore, we cannot comment on any changes in global brain glucose uptake.

In line with our hypothesis, but in contrast to a previous study in humans (Maddock et al., 2011), we did not observe any significant change in glutamate or glutamine following vigorous exercise, when the metabolites were normalized to creatine. When "absolute" quantification was performed, a significant decrease in both glutamate and glutamine after exercise was observed. As discussed earlier, presenting metabolites as a ratio to creatine is common practice as it is taken to provide a stable, simultaneously acquired reference metabolite, but here we see a significant decrease in creatine following exercise. In light of this, we also explored the changes in the absolute quantification of glutamate and glutamine, although we acknowledge there are uncertainties with this approach. With this analysis, a significant *decrease* in glutamate and glutamine was observed, in contrast to the increase observed by Maddock et al. (2011). It is not possible, therefore, given the discrepancy between these methods, to be confident as to whether there is a true decrease in glutamate and glutamine after exercise, but certainly our data do not support an *increase* in these metabolites, as previously observed.

Conceptually, glutamate concentration might be expected to increase in proportion to overall neuronal activity. During exercise, large global increases in cerebral metabolism are seen (van Praag, 2009). Evidence from the literature would suggest that non-oxidized carbohydrates, such as lactate, are only metabolized into glutamate when there is an increase in "brain work" demanding more glutamatergic neural activation, and an adequate source of ammonia (Hertz and Dienel, 2004). Therefore, measurements of glutamate, and lactate, taken *during* exercise may be expected to be elevated as a result of local production. However, our MRS measures were acquired some time after the cessation of exercise, and it is therefore unlikely that we would observe a heightened state of brain activity, and hence an increase in glutamate (MacIntosh et al., 2014).

Nevertheless, glutamate and glutamine changes may be observed in the presence of high brain lactate in some animal models (Waagepetersen et al., 1998; Hertz and Fillenz, 1999). For example, lactate may be partially oxidized in the TCA cycle allowing for glutamate to be oxidized to alpha-ketoglutarate, or for increased glutamate-glutamine cycling in the astrocytes in response to neural activity. However, these mechanisms largely depend on an increase in *brain-derived* lactate generated by the astrocytes in response to neural activation, and are not involved in response to an increase in plasma lactate. Studies of *peripherally derived* lactate uptake into the brain following either infusion of lactate or following exercise have reported virtually all (~87%) lactate taken up is recovered as CO_2 (Volianitis et al., 2008; van Hall et al., 2009), suggesting that there is little carbon being exchanged from lactate to other metabolites (van Hall et al., 2009).

Relationship Between Glutamate and Fitness

Whilst previous studies have reported differences in the NAA/Cr ratio in frontal gray matter and Cho/Cr ratios in occipitoparietal gray matter between aerobically trained and sedentary adults (Gonzales et al., 2013) and a correlation between aerobic fitness and the frontal NAA/Cr ratio (Erickson et al., 2012), currently no studies have reported differences in Glu/Cr ratios between trained and sedentary individuals (Gonzales et al., 2013), potentially due to the methodological difficulties in separating glutamate from glutamine.

The negative relationship we observed between fitness and glutamate may provide some support to the beneficial effects of regular exercise participation on brain health. For example, in rat models, exercise training results in decreased glutamatergic activity in response to oxygen and glucose deprivation in hippocampal slices (Mourão et al., 2014), and lowers the glutamatergic input to the rostro ventrolateral medulla (Zha et al., 2013), a phenomenon associated with lowering blood pressure. Therefore, our finding of lower glutamate levels in fitter subjects could be related to the neuro-protective benefits of regular physical exercise. It should be noted however, that the exercise paradigm was not designed as an exercise test and thus a subsequent proxy measure of fitness (PWC) was inferred from the available data. In light of the interesting relationship between PWC and glutamate, an established test of aerobic fitness or lactate threshold may provide a more comprehensive metric for examining the relationship between fitness and brain activity. It should also be noted that, whilst an interesting trend, further study of a population with a range of aerobic fitness levels would be necessary in order to elaborate on any proposed relation between fitness and resting brain glutamate levels.

Limitations

There are some limitations of the methods used in this study. The MRS technique allows for non-invasive measurement of neurochemicals *in vivo*, making it ideal for longitudinal studies in human populations. However, it has inherently lower signal-to-noise than more direct measures. MRS allows for measurement from a single ROI. The voxel in the visual cortex was selected based on the assumption that changes in brain lactate as taken up from the blood would be global and not regionally specific, and lactate peaks have previously been successfully resolved at 7 T in the visual cortex (Mangia et al., 2007; Mekle et al., 2009). However, this method required the voxel to be manually selected. Whilst every care was taken to ensure consistency, variations may have influenced the relative change in metabolites, though the reproducibility across the baseline and post-intervention time points suggests this is unlikely.

We only acquired an unsuppressed water spectrum at the beginning of the baseline scan and the post-intervention scan. We do not feel that this is an appropriate reference for the later post-exercise scans as hydration, as well as other physiological variables, might change. Secondly, there are significant uncertainties in calculating the "absolute" concentrations (highlighted in chapter 10 of the LCModel manual). Thirdly, we wished to extend the findings of Maddock et al. (2011), and so wished our results to be as comparable to that study, which used a creatine reference, as possible. However, given the discrepancy between our two quantification methods, future studies should include the appropriate scans to allow accurate absolute quantification to be performed.

It should also be acknowledged that the ROI approach gives us access to data from a specific region of the brain, which includes a number of constituents including brain tissue, CSF, and blood, and that in this voxel, with its proximity to the draining veins, the venous component might potentially be significant. However, we would argue strongly that the MRS measures we acquired here are not sensitive to signal from the blood within the voxel for a number of reasons. Whilst the initial excitation pulse will excite all the components of the ROI, the TE means that the vast majority of the blood that was in the voxel when the RF was applied will no longer be present, and therefore will not contribute to the signal acquired. This will be true of any arterial, arteriolar, and capillary supply within the voxel, where flow will be fast enough to remove a significant portion of the blood. Potentially, however, venous drainage in the sagittal sinus might be more sluggish than this. We were therefore careful to place the voxel sufficiently anterior of the sinuses to avoid this confound.

Whilst MRS offers an *in vivo* and non-invasive method for measuring brain metabolites, this "snapshot" measurement approach means only total, static measures are possible and measurement of flux is not. For information on metabolic flux, measures such as ^{13}C MRS would need to be employed.

Lastly, the time-interval between the ending of the exercise session and the start of the first post-exercise scan was variable. It should be noted however that blood lactate levels were still elevated from baseline during first post-exercise MRS acquisition maintaining the integrity of the protocol to examine peripherally derived lactate. Further study of the changes in brain lactate and glutamate immediately after exercise may shed further light on brain metabolism and activity changes in the immediate recovery period.

CONCLUSIONS

We observed a transient increase in brain lactate following vigorous exercise when blood lactate was elevated. We were also able to successfully measure brain glutamate and glutamine, and in line with our hypothesis, though contrary to previous findings (Maddock et al., 2011), we did not observe any change in either as a result of exercise. We did observe a negative correlation between brain glutamate and fitness, both after exercise and at

rest. These results provide support for the use of high-field MRS for measuring post-exercise brain metabolites.

FUNDING

The work was supported by the National Institute for Health Research (NIHR) Oxford Biomedical Research Center based at Oxford University Hospitals Trust, Oxford University. The views expressed are those of the author(s) and not necessarily those of the NHS, the NIHR, or the Department of Health. AT is supported by the NIMH Intramural Research Program based in Bethesda, MD. HJ is a Wellcome Trust Senior Research Fellow. CS holds a Sir Henry Dale Fellowship jointly funded by the Wellcome Trust and the Royal Society (Grant Number 102584/Z/13/Z).

ACKNOWLEDGMENTS

The authors are grateful to Anderson Winkler for statistical support, Isidro Hidalgo Arellano for assistance with R visualization, and to Martyn Morris for expert assistance.

REFERENCES

Balaban, R. S., Kantor, H. L., Katz, L. A., and Briggs, R. W. (1986). Relation between work and phosphate metabolite in the *in vivo* paced mammalian heart. *Science* 232, 1121–1123. doi: 10.1126/science.3704638

Bangsbo, J., Graham, T., Johansen, L., and Saltin, B. (1994). Muscle lactate metabolism in recovery from intense exhaustive exercise: impact of light exercise. *J. Appl. Physiol.* 77, 1890–1895.

Bernal-Rusiel, J. L., Greve, D. N., Reuter, M., Fischl, B., and Sabuncu, M. R. (2013). Statistical analysis of longitudinal neuroimage data with linear mixed effects models. *Neuroimage* 66, 249–260. doi: 10.1016/j.neuroimage.2012.10.065

Boumezbeur, F., Petersen, K. F., Cline, G. W., Mason, G. F., Behar, K. L., Shulman, G. I., et al. (2010). The contribution of blood lactate to brain energy metabolism in humans measured by dynamic 13C nuclear magnetic resonance spectroscopy. *J. Neurosci.* 30, 13983–13991. doi: 10.1523/JNEUROSCI.2040-10.2010

Bouzat, P., Sala, N., Suys, T., Zerlauth, J.B., Marques-Vidal, P., Feihl, F., et al. (2014). Cerebral metabolic effects of exogenous lactate supplementation on the injured human brain. *Intensive Care Med.* 40, 412–421. doi: 10.1007/s00134-013-3203-6

Bouzier-Sore, A.K., Voisin, P., Canioni, P., Magistretti, P. J., and Pellerin, L. (2003). Lactate is a preferential oxidative energy substrate over glucose for neurons in culture. *J. Cereb. Blood Flow Metab.* 23, 1298–1306. doi: 10.1097/01.WCB.0000091761.61714.25

Brooks, G. A. (2009). Cell-cell and intracellular lactate shuttles. *J. Physiol.* 587, 5591–5600. doi: 10.1113/jphysiol.2009.178350

Brooks, G. A. (1985). The lactate shuttle during exercise and recovery. *Med. Sci. Sport Exerc.* 18, 360–368. doi: 10.1249/00005768-198606000-00019

Brooks, G. A., and Martin, N. A. (2015). Cerebral metabolism following traumatic brain injury: new discoveries with implications for treatment. *Front. Neurosci.* 8:408. doi: 10.3389/fnins.2014.00408

Campbell, P. T., Katzmarzyk, P. T., Malina, R. M., Rao, D. C., Pérusse, L., and Bouchard, C. (2001). Prediction of physical activity and physical work capacity (PWC150) in young adulthood from childhood and adolescence with consideration of parental measures. *Am. J. Hum. Biol.* 13, 190–196. doi: 10.1002/1520-6300(200102/03)13:2<190::AID-AJHB1028>3.0.CO;2-N

Cerdán, S., Rodrigues, T. B., Sierra, A., Benito, M., Fonseca, L. L., Fonseca, C. P., et al. (2006). The redox switch/redox coupling hypothesis. *Neurochem. Int.* 48, 523–530. doi: 10.1016/j.neuint.2005.12.036

Chowdhury, G. M., Jiang, L., Rothman, D. L., and Behar, K. L. (2014). The contribution of ketone bodies to basal and activity-dependent neuronal oxidation *in vivo*. *J. Cereb. Blood Flow Metab.* 34, 1233–1242. doi: 10.1038/jcbfm.2014.77

Cruz, F., Villalba, M., García-Espinosa, M. A., Ballesteros, P., Bogónez, E., Satrústegui, J., et al. (2001). Intracellular compartmentation of pyruvate in primary cultures of cortical neurons as detected by (13)C NMR spectroscopy with multiple (13)C labels. *J. Neurosci. Res.* 66, 771–781. doi: 10.1002/jnr.10048

Dalsgaard, M. K., Ide, K., Cai, Y., Quistorff, B., and Secher, N. H. (2002). The intent to exercise influences the cerebral O2/carbohydrate uptake ratio in humans. *J. Physiol.* 540, 681–689. doi: 10.1113/jphysiol.2001.013062

Dalsgaard, M. K., Quistorff, B., Danielsen, E. R., Selmer, C., Vogelsang, T., and Secher, N. H. (2004). A reduced cerebral metabolic ratio in exercise reflects metabolism and not accumulation of lactate within the human brain. *J. Physiol.* 554, 571–578. doi: 10.1113/jphysiol.2003.055053

Dienel, G. A. (2012). Brain lactate metabolism: the discoveries and the controversies. *J. Cereb. Blood Flow Metab.* 32, 1107–1138. doi: 10.1038/jcbfm.2011.175

Erickson, K. I., Weinstein, A. M., Sutton, B. P., Prakash, R. S., Voss, M. W., Chaddock, L., et al. (2012). Beyond vascularization: aerobic fitness is associated with N-acetylaspartate and working memory. *Brain Behav.* 2, 32–41. doi: 10.1002/brb3.30

Forsyth, J. J., and Farrally, M. R. (2000). A comparison of lactate concentration in plasma collected from the toe, ear, and fingertip after a simulated rowing exercise. *Br. J. Sport Med.* 34, 35–38. doi: 10.1136/bjsm.34.1.35

Foster, K. J., Alberti, K. G., Hinks, L., Lloyd, B., Postle, A., Smythe, P., et al. (1978). Blood intermediary metabolite and insulin concentrations after an overnight fast: reference ranges for adults, and interrelations. *Clin. Chem.* 24, 1568–1572.

Fox, P. T., Raichle, M. E., Mintun, M. A., and Dence, C. (1988). Nonoxidative glucose consumption during focal physiologic neural activity. *Science* 241, 462–464. doi: 10.1126/science.3260686

Garland, S. W., and Atkinson, G. (2008). Effect of blood lactate sample site and test protocol on training zone prescription in rowing. *Int. J. Sport Physiol. Perform.* 3, 347–358.

Glenn, T. C., Martin, N. A., Horning, M. A., McArthur, D. L., Hovda, D. A., Vespa, P., et al. (2015). Lactate: brain fuel in human traumatic brain injury. A comparison to normal healthy control subjects. *J. Neurotrauma* 32, 820–832. doi: 10.1089/neu.2014.3483

Gonzales, M. M., Tarumi, T., Kaur, S., Nualnim, N., Fallow, B. A., Pyron, M., et al. (2013). Aerobic fitness and the brain: increased N-acetyl-aspartate and choline concentrations in endurance-trained middle-aged adults. *Brain Topogr.* 26, 126–134. doi: 10.1007/s10548-012-0248-8

Guezennec, C. Y., Abdelmalki, A., Merino, D., Bigard, X., Berthelot, M., Pierard, C., et al. (1998). Effects of prolonged exercise on brain ammonia and amino acids. *Physiol. Biochem.* 19, 323–327. doi: 10.1055/s-2007-971925

Guillaume, B., Hua, X., Thompson, P. M., Waldorp, L., and Nichols, T. E. (2014). Fast and accurate modelling of longitudinal and repeated measures neuroimaging data. *Neuroimage* 94, 287–302. doi: 10.1016/j.neuroimage.2014.03.029

Hertz, L., and Dienel, G. A. (2004). Lactate transport and transporters: general principles and functional roles in brain cells. *J. Neurosci. Res.* 79, 11–18. doi: 10.1002/jnr.20294

Hertz, L., and Fillenz, M. (1999). Does the "mystery of the extra glucose" during CNS activation reflect glutamate synthesis? *Neurochem. Int.* 34, 71–75. doi: 10.1016/S0197-0186(98)00071-0

Hertz, L., Gibbs, M. E., and Dienel, G. A., (2014). Fluxes of lactate into, from, and among gap junction-coupled astrocytes and their interaction with noradrenaline. *Front. Neurosci.* 8:261. doi: 10.3389/fnins.2014.00261

Hochachka, P. W. (2003). Intracellular convection, homeostasis and metabolic regulation. *J. Exp. Biol.* 206, 2001–2009. doi: 10.1242/jeb.00402

Ide, K., Schmalbruch, I. K., Quistorff, B., Horn, A., and Secher, N. H. (2000). Lactate, glucose and O2 uptake in human brain during recovery from maximal exercise. *J. Physiol.* 522(Pt 1), 159–164. doi: 10.1111/j.1469-7793.2000.t01-2-00159.xm

Jenkinson, M., and Smith, S. (2001). A global optimisation method for robust affine registration of brain images. *Med. Image Anal.* 5, 143–156. doi: 10.1016/S1361-8415(01)00036-6

MacIntosh, B. J., Crane, D. E., Sage, M. D., Rajab, A. S., Donahue, M. J., McIlroy, W. E., et al. (2014). Impact of a single bout of aerobic exercise on regional brain perfusion and activation responses in healthy young adults. *PLoS ONE* 9:e85163. doi: 10.1371/journal.pone.0085163

Maddock, R. J., Casazza, G. A., Buonocore, M. H., and Tanase, C. (2011). Vigorous exercise increases brain lactate and Glx (glutamate+glutamine): a dynamic 1H-MRS study. *Neuroimage* 57, 1324–1330. doi: 10.1016/j.neuroimage.2011.05.048

Magistretti, P. J., and Pellerin, L. (1999). Astrocytes couple synaptic activity to glucose utilization in the brain. *News Physiol. Sci.* 14, 177–182.

Mangia, S., Tkác, I., Gruetter, R., Van de Moortele, P.F., Maraviglia, B., and Uğurbil, K. (2007). Sustained neuronal activation raises oxidative metabolism to a new steady-state level: evidence from 1H NMR spectroscopy in the human visual cortex. *J. Cereb. Blood Flow Metab.* 27, 1055–1063. doi: 10.1038/sj.jcbfm.9600401

Massucci, F. A., DiNuzzo, M., Giove, F., Maraviglia, B., Castillo, I. P., Marinari, E., et al. (2013). Energy metabolism and glutamate-glutamine cycle in the brain: a stoichiometric modeling perspective. *BMC Syst. Biol.* 7:103. doi: 10.1186/1752-0509-7-103

Mekle, R., Mlynárik, V., Gambarota, G., Hergt, M., Krueger, G., and Gruetter, R. (2009). MR spectroscopy of the human brain with enhanced signal intensity at ultrashort echo times on a clinical platform at 3T and 7T. *Magn. Reson. Med.* 61, 1279–1285. doi: 10.1002/mrm.21961

Mourão, F. A., Leite, H. R., de Carvalho, L. E., Ferreira E Vieira, T. H., Pinto, M. C., de Castro Medeiros, D., et al. (2014). Neuroprotective effect of exercise in rat hippocampal slices submitted to in vitro ischemia is promoted by decrease of glutamate release and pro-apoptotic markers. *J. Neurochem.* 131, 65–73. doi: 10.1111/jnc.12786

Near, J., Edden, R., Evans, C. J., Paquin, R., Harris, A., and Jezzard, P. (2014). Frequency and phase drift correction of magnetic resonance spectroscopy data by spectral registration in the time domain. *Magn. Reson. Med.* 50, 44–50. doi: 10.1002/mrm.25094

Nybo, L., Møller, K., Pedersen, B. K., Nielsen, B., and Secher, N. H. (2003). Association between fatigue and failure to preserve cerebral energy turnover during prolonged exercise. *Acta Physiol. Scand.* 179, 67–74. doi: 10.1046/j.1365-201X.2003.01175.x

Overgaard, M., Rasmussen, P., Bohm, A. M., Seifert, T., Brassard, P., Zaar, M., et al. (2012). Hypoxia and exercise provoke both lactate release and lactate oxidation by the human brain. *FASEB J.* 26, 3012–3020. doi: 10.1096/fj.11-191999

Pellerin, L., and Magistretti, P. J. (1994). Glutamate uptake into astrocytes stimulates aerobic glycolysis: a mechanism coupling neuronal activity to glucose utilization. *Proc. Natl. Acad. Sci. U.S.A.* 91, 10625–10629. doi: 10.1073/pnas.91.22.10625

Pellerin, L., and Magistretti, P. J. (2012). Sweet sixteen for ANLS. *J. Cereb. Blood Flow Metab.* 32, 1152–1166. doi: 10.1038/jcbfm.2011.149

Pinheiro, J., Bates, D., DebRoy, S., Sarkar, D., and Team, R. C. (2013). *nlme: Linear and Nonlinear Mixed Effects Models.* Available online at: http://cran.r-project.org/package=nlme

Prichard, J., Rothmans, D., Novotny, E., Petroff, O., Kuwabara, T., Avisonf, M., et al. (1991). Lactate rise detected by 1H NMR in human visual cortex during physiologic stimulation. *Proc. Natl. Acad. Sci. U.S.A.* 88, 5829–5831.

Provencher, S. W. (2001). Automatic quantitation of localized *in vivo* 1H spectra with LCModel. *NMR Biomed.* 14, 260–264. doi: 10.1002/nbm.698

Quistorff, B., Secher, N. H., and Van Lieshout, J. J. (2008). Lactate fuels the human brain during exercise. *FASEB J.* 22, 3443–3449. doi: 10.1096/fj.08-106104

Sappey-Marinier, D., Calabrese, G., Fein, G., Hugg, J. W., Biggins, C., and Weiner, M. W. (1992). Effect of photic stimulation on human visual cortex lactate and phosphates using 1H and 31P magnetic resonance spectroscopy. *J. Cereb. Blood Flow Metab.* 12, 584–592. doi: 10.1038/jcbfm.1992.82

Schaller, B., Mekle, R., Xin, L., Kunz, N., and Gruetter, R. (2013). Net increase of lactate and glutamate concentration in activated human visual cortex detected with magnetic resonance spectroscopy at 7 tesla. *J. Neurosci. Res.* 91, 1076–1083. doi: 10.1002/jnr.23194

Schaller, B., Xin, L., O'Brien, K., Magill, A. W., and Gruetter, R. (2014). Are glutamate and lactate increases ubiquitous to physiological activation? A (1)H functional MR spectroscopy study during motor activation in human brain at 7Tesla. *Neuroimage* 93(Pt 1), 138–145. doi: 10.1016/j.neuroimage.2014.02.016

Schurr, A. (2008). Lactate: a major and crucial player in normal function of both muscle and brain. *J. Physiol.* 586, 2665–2666. doi: 10.1113/jphysiol.2008.155416

Schurr, A. (2014). Cerebral glycolysis: a century of persistent misunderstanding and misconception. *Front. Neurosci.* 8:360. doi: 10.3389/fnins.2014.00360

Schurr, A., Payne, R. S., Miller, J. J., and Rigor, B. M. (1997). Brain lactate is an obligatory aerobic energy substrate for functional recovery after hypoxia: further *in vitro* validation. *J. Neurochem.* 69, 423–426.

Schurr, A., West, C. A., and Rigor, B. M. (1988). Lactate-supported synaptic function in the rat hippocampal slice preparation. *Science* 240, 1326–1328.

Sharma, P., Karian, J., Sharma, S., Liu, S., and Mongan, P. D. (2003). Pyruvate ameliorates post ischemic injury of rat astrocytes and protects them against PARP mediated cell death. *Brain Res.* 992, 104–113. doi: 10.1016/j.brainres.2003.08.043

Shen, J., and Rothman, D. L. (2002). Magnetic resonance spectroscopic approaches to studying neuronal: glial interactions. *Biol Psychiatry* 52, 694–700. doi: 10.1016/S0006-3223(02)01502-0

Sibson, N. R., Dhankhar, A., Mason, G. F., Rothman, D. L., Behar, K. L., and Shulman, R. G. (1998). Stoichiometric coupling of brain glucose metabolism and glutamatergic neuronal activity. *Proc. Natl. Acad. Sci. U.S.A.* 95, 316–321.

Singer, J. D., and Willett, J. B. (2003). *Applied Longitudinal Data Analysis: Modeling Change and Event Occurrence.* New York, NY: Oxford University Press. doi: 10.1093/acprof:oso/9780195152968.001.0001

Smith, S. M., Jenkinson, M., Woolrich, M. W., Beckmann, C. F., Behrens, T. E., Johansen-Berg, H., et al. (2004). Advances in functional and structural MR image analysis and implementation as FSL. *Neuroimage* 23(Suppl. 1), S208–S219. doi: 10.1016/j.neuroimage.2004.07.051

Tkác, I., Starcuk, Z., Choi, I. Y., and Gruetter, R. (1999). In vivo 1H NMR spectroscopy of rat brain at 1 ms echo time. *Magn. Reson. Med.* 41, 649–656.

van Hall, G. (2010). Lactate kinetics in human tissues at rest and during exercise. *Acta Physiol. (Oxf).* 199, 499–508. doi: 10.1111/j.1748-1716.2010.02122.x

van Hall, G., Strømstad, M., Rasmussen, P., Jans, O., Zaar, M., Gam, C., et al. (2009). Blood lactate is an important energy source for the human brain. *J. Cereb. Blood Flow Metab.* 29, 1121–1129. doi: 10.1038/jcbfm.2009.35

van Praag, H. (2009). Exercise and the brain: something to chew on. *Trends Neurosci.* 32, 283–290. doi: 10.1016/j.tins.2008.12.007

Volianitis, S., Rasmussen, P., Seifert, T., Nielsen, H. B., and Secher, N. H. (2011). Plasma pH does not influence the cerebral metabolic ratio during maximal whole body exercise. *J. Physiol.* 589, 423–429. doi: 10.1113/jphysiol.2010.195636

Volianitis, S., Fabricius-Bjerre, A., Overgaard, A., Strømstad, M., Bjarrum, M., Carlson, C., et al. (2008). The cerebral metabolic ratio is not affected by oxygen availability during maximal exercise in humans. *J. Physiol.* 586, 107–112. doi: 10.1113/jphysiol.2007.142273

Waagepetersen, H. S., Bakken, I. J., Larsson, O. M., Sonnewald, U., and Schousboe, A. (1998). Comparison of lactate and glucose metabolism in cultured neocortical neurons and astrocytes using 13C-NMR spectroscopy. *Dev. Neurosci.* 20, 310–320.

Xin, L., Schaller, B., Mlynarik, V., Lu, H., and Gruetter, R. (2013). Proton T1 relaxation times of metabolites in human occipital white and gray matter at 7 T. *Magn. Reson. Med.* 69, 931–936. doi: 10.1002/mrm.24352

Yang, J., Ruchti, E., Petit, J. M., Jourdain, P., Grenningloh, G., Allaman, I., et al. (2014). Lactate promotes plasticity gene expression by potentiating NMDA signaling in neurons. *Proc. Natl. Acad. Sci. U.S.A.* 111, 12228–12233. doi: 10.1073/pnas.1322912111

Zha, Y. P., Wang, Y. K., Deng, Y., Zhang, R. W., Tan, X., Yuan, W. J., et al. (2013). Exercise training lowers the enhanced tonically active glutamatergic input to the rostral ventrolateral medulla in hypertensive rats. *CNS Neurosci. Ther.* 19, 244–251. doi: 10.1111/cns.12065

Conflict of Interest Statement: The authors declare that the research was conducted in the absence of any commercial or financial relationships that could be construed as a potential conflict of interest.

9

Dual-Energy X-Ray Absorptiometry, Skinfold Thickness, and Waist Circumference for Assessing Body Composition in Ambulant and Non-Ambulant Wheelchair Games Players

Annika Willems[1], Thomas A. W. Paulson[1], Mhairi Keil[2], Katherine Brooke-Wavell[3] and Victoria L. Goosey-Tolfrey[1]*

[1] The Peter Harrison Centre for Disability Sport, School of Sport, Exercise and Health Sciences, Loughborough University, Loughborough, UK, [2] Lilleshall National Sport Centre, English Institute of Sport, Sheffield, UK, [3] School of Sport, Exercise and Health Sciences, Loughborough University, Loughborough, UK

Edited by:
Vincent Pialoux,
University Lyon 1, France

Reviewed by:
Can Ozan Tan,
Harvard Medical School, USA
Jean Slawinski,
Université Paris Ouest Nanterre La
Défense, France

*Correspondence:
Victoria L. Goosey-Tolfrey
v.l.tolfrey@lboro.ac.uk

Field-based assessments provide a cost–effective and accessible alternative to dual-energy X-ray absorptiometry (DXA) for practitioners determining body composition in athletic populations. It remains unclear how the range of physical impairments classifiable in wheelchair sports may affect the utility of field-based body composition techniques. The present study assessed body composition using DXA in 14 wheelchair games players who were either wheelchair dependent (non-walkers; $n = 7$) or relied on a wheelchair for sports participation only (walkers; $n = 7$). Anthropometric measurements were used to predict body fat percentage with existing regression equations established for able-bodied persons by Sloan and Weir, Durnin and Womersley, Lean et al, Gallagher et al, and Pongchaiyakul et al. In addition, linear regression analysis was performed to calculate the association between body fat percentage and BMI, waist circumference, sum of 6 skinfold thickness and sum of 8 skinfold thickness. Results showed that non-walkers had significantly lower total lean tissue mass (46.2 ± 6.6 kg vs. 59.4 ± 8.2 kg, $P = 0.006$) and total body mass (65.8 ± 4.2 kg vs. 79.4 ± 14.9 kg; $P = 0.05$) than walkers. Body fat percentage calculated from most existing regression equations was significantly lower than that from DXA, by 2 to 9% in walkers and 8 to 14% in non-walkers. Of the anthropometric measurements, the sum of 8 skinfold thickness had the lowest standard error of estimation in predicting body fat content. In conclusion, existing anthropometric equations developed in able-bodied populations substantially underestimated body fat content in wheelchair athletes, particularly non-walkers. Impairment specific equations may be needed in wheelchair athletes.

Keywords: spinal cord injury, paralympic, total body mass, basketball, rugby

INTRODUCTION

Body composition measurement is vital in high performance sport because of the association of body fat and lean tissue mass with performance as well as health outcomes. Dual energy x-ray absorptiometry (DXA) is considered a relatively valid and reliable method to determine body composition in both able-bodied (Stewart and Sutton, 2012) and spinal cord injured (SCI) (Jones et al., 1998; Keil et al., 2014) individuals. However, the financial and logistical restrictions of DXA can limit accessibility for many practitioners and field-based body composition assessments are frequently employed as an alternative (e.g., waist circumference, skinfold thickness). Studies have shown body mass index (BMI), waist circumference and skinfold thickness to correlate well with total body fat and trunk fat and prediction equations have been developed to estimate body composition from these measurements (Eston et al., 2005; Weerarathna et al., 2008; Camhi et al., 2011). However, these relationships are population specific, differing according to gender and ethnicity due largely to different tissue distributions between these groups (Schreiner et al., 1996; Hill et al., 1999; Rahman et al., 2009; Camhi et al., 2011). Wheelchair game players present a range of lower and upper limb impairments that may also affect the relationships upon which such prediction equations are based. The accuracy of field-based methods for assessment of body composition in wheelchair game players is not known.

Lower limb paralysis and subsequent atrophy of lean mass following a SCI predisposes individuals to a decreased fat free mass (Maggioni et al., 2003; Stewart and Sutton, 2012), an increased fat mass (Spungen et al., 2003; Emmons et al., 2011) and a reduced resting metabolic rate (Buchholz and Pencharz, 2004). Previously, Spungen et al. (2003) observed comparable total lean and mass between individuals with thoracic and cervical level SCI. In contrast, some wheelchair games players with lower degrees of physical impairment remain ambulant in activities of daily life, only requiring a wheelchair for sports performance. The divergent fat distribution and lean mass profiles of individuals with varying degrees of physical impairments, and therefore modalities of daily ambulation, presents a challenge for cross-sectional and longitudinal body composition assessment. In addition, the standardized position to measure waist circumference and skinfolds in able-bodied persons is with the participant positioned in a standing anatomical reference position (Lohman et al., 1988). However, as this is not possible for most SCI-persons, waist circumference and skinfold thickness must be measured in supine or seated positions. These procedural differences might also affect the relationship between waist circumference, skinfold thickness and body fat and so affect the assessment of body composition by anthropometric techniques.

Two previous studies (Miyahara et al., 2008; Sutton et al., 2008) compared the body composition and fat distribution of male wheelchair athletes with able-bodied athletes and found a significantly lower lean body mass (Miyahara et al., 2008), higher body fat percentage (Miyahara et al., 2008; Sutton et al., 2008) and greater trunk fat mass (Sutton et al., 2008) in wheelchair athletes. In contrast, Sutton et al. (2009) did not find differences between the lean tissue mass and fat mass of the trunk when female SCI athletes and able-bodied non-athletic groups were compared. In addition, several studies (Bulbulian et al., 1987; Maggioni et al., 2003; Sutton et al., 2009) have investigated the applicability of using BMI, waist circumference, and skinfold thickness to estimate body fat percentage in wheelchair athletes using conventional regression-based body composition equations developed for able-bodied populations. These studies found that most regression equations (Sloan and Weir, 1970; Durnin and Womersley, 1974; Lean et al., 1996) underestimated body fat percentage for elite female wheelchair athletes (Sutton et al., 2009) and male paraplegic athletes (Bulbulian et al., 1987; Maggioni et al., 2003), with inaccuracy increasing with higher body fat percentages (Sutton et al., 2009). Interestingly, Sutton et al. (2009) suggested that regression equations that included the waist circumference appear to predict body fat percentage more accurately.

No distinction has yet been made between the body composition of athletes who are wheelchair dependent for daily activities and those that were ambulant yet eligible to compete in wheelchair sports using a sports wheelchair (Goosey-Tolfrey, 2010). The physical and disability characteristics are likely to influence the degree of relationship between field-based body composition assessment and DXA, as well as the accuracy of fat percentage prediction equations. The present study aimed to establish the accuracy of fat percentage prediction equations within wheelchair game players who were ambulant for daily living (walkers) and those who relied on wheelchair propulsion for daily ambulation (non-walkers). A secondary objective was to investigate the association between commonly employed field-based and DXA derived methods of determining body fat percentage in these two groups.

MATERIALS AND METHODS

Participants

Fourteen elite male wheelchair game players were recruited from national wheelchair basketball and national wheelchair rugby squads. All participants visited the laboratory once within the same competitive phase of their training schedule. The participants were divided into two groups; participants who were wheelchair independent during non-sporting activities (7 walkers) and daily wheelchair users (7 non-walkers). The participants' characteristics are shown in **Table 1**. The walkers comprised of five persons with single lower-limb amputations and two with lower limb deficiencies whilst the non-walkers comprised of all SCI-persons (motor complete SCI; C5–C7). All participants provided written informed consent prior to data collection and the study was approved by Loughborough University's Ethics Committee and the National Research Ethics Service.

Anthropometry

The anthropometric measurements performed were: height, body mass, waist circumference, and skinfold thickness. Height was measured in a standing position (walkers) or a supine

TABLE 1 | Participant characteristics, DXA-derived body composition, BMI, waist circumference, and sums of 6 and 8 skinfold thickness.

	Walkers (n = 7)	Non–Walkers (n = 7)	P-value (ES)
Age (years)	26 ± 8	32 ± 7	0.15 (0.8)
Time since injury (years)	19 ± 10	12 ± 7	0.16 (0.8)
Sport	WCB	WCR	n/a
Physical impairment	Amputee (n =5); Lower limb deficiency (n =2)	SCI (n =7)	n/a
Body mass (kg)	79.4 ± 14.9	65.8 ± 4.2	0.05* (1.1)
Fat mass (kg)	16.9 ± 7.6	16.3 ± 5.3	0.88 (0.8)
Fat percentage (%)	21.4 ± 5.9	26.2 ± 8.9	0.25 (0.6)
Lean tissue mass (kg)	59.4 ± 8.2	46.2 ± 6.6	0.01* (1.3)
Lean tissue percentage (%)	75.6 ± 5.5	70.2 ± 9.0	0.21 (0.7)
BMI	23 ± 4	21 ± 2	0.10 (0.9)
Waist circumference (cm)	85.5 ± 8.6	77.9 ± 7.8	0.11 (0.9)
Sum of 6 skinfold thicknesses (mm)	77.2 ± 18.6	85.0 ± 39.9	0.65 (0.3)
Sum of 8 skinfold thicknesses (mm)	102.2 ± 26.6	114.0 ± 47.0	0.57 (0.3)

*All date are mean ± standard deviation. ES, Effect size; WCB, Wheelchair Basketball; WCR, Wheelchair Rugby; SCI, Spinal Cord Injury; BMI, Body Mass Index; Significant differences are indicated with * at a significant level of P < 0.05.*

position (non-walkers), using a Luftkin measuring tape. Body mass was measured using a wheelchair accessible scale (Detecto 6550KGEU Portable, Detecto Scale Company, Webb City, Mo, USA). Participants who were not able to stand on the scale were weighed in their wheelchair, afterwards the wheelchair was weighed and its weight was subtracted from the total weight. Height (m) and body mass (kg) were used to calculate the BMI by the following formula:

$$BMI = bodymass/height^2$$

Waist circumference was measured directly to the skin using an inelastic tape at the narrowest part of the torso after normal expiration (Lohman et al., 1988; Buchholz and Bugaresti, 2005). For walkers, waist circumference was measured in a neutral standing position; for non-walkers, waist circumference was measured in a supine position with their arms at their sides. Waist circumference was measured three times and the average of these three measurements was taken for further analysis.

Skinfold thickness were measured at eight sites and were performed according to the guidelines from the ISAK (Lohman et al., 1988), having the same investigator measuring all skinfolds by using a set of Harpenden Skinfold Calipers (Baty International, West Sussex, UK). Skinfold sites included: biceps, triceps, subscapular, iliac crest, supraspinale, abdominal, anterior thigh, and medial calf. For the non-walkers, skinfolds were measured in a seated position, while the walkers were measured in a standing position. Each skinfold measurement was made in triplicate; true skinfold thickness was taken as the average of those three measures. However, in case of any outliers, the average

of two measurements was taken. Afterwards, skinfold thickness were used to calculate the sum of 6 skinfold thicknesses (biceps, triceps, subscapular, iliac crest, supraspinale, and abdominal) and the sum of 8 skinfold thicknesses (biceps, triceps, subscapular, iliac crest, supraspinale, abdominal, thigh, and calf).

Dual Energy X-ray Absorptiometry

Body composition was measured using DXA Lunar Prodigy Advance (GE Medical Systems, Madison, WI, USA) with Encore software version 13.2. The participants were instructed to wear loose fitting clothes without any metal and to remove all metal fixtures such as jewelry. Afterwards, the participants were positioned on the DXA-bed in a supine position as close as possible to standard positioning protocol, with Velcro straps used to help keep the legs still during measurement. Although some participants had muscular spasms during positioning, they were able to remain still once positioned. Scanning time varied between 6 and 10 min depending on the mass and height of the participants. The analyses of all scans were performed by the same operator to avoid any inter-observer variability. The total body scan was used to gain the outcome measures which were: total body fat mass, total body fat percentage, total lean tissue mass (with segmental data of the trunk, arms, and legs), lean tissue percentage and segmental fat mass of the trunk, arms, and legs.

Fat Percentage Predicting Regression Equations

To investigate whether traditional fat percentage predicting regression equations were applicable to elite male wheelchair game players the data acquired from the anthropometry measurements were used to predict body fat. The predicted body fat was than compared to the data resulting from the DXA scan. The regression equations to which the data were applied are from Sloan and Weir (1970), Durnin and Womersley (1974), Lean et al. (1996), Gallagher et al. (2000), and Pongchaiyakul et al. (2005).

Statistical Analyses

All statistical tests were performed using IBM SPSS Statics 22.0 and statistical significance was set a priori at $p < 0.05$. Firstly, the assumption of normal distribution was checked for all data by visual inspection of the box plot and q-q plot and also the Shapiro-Wilk test within the groups. Equality of variance was checked using the Levene's test. As all data were normally distributed, independent t-tests were used to compare body mass, DXA derived fat mass, body fat percentage, lean tissue mass, lean tissue percentage, and waist circumference, BMI and sum of 6 skinfold thickness and sum of 8 skinfold thickness between the walking and non-walking group. Further, segmental lean and fat mass for the trunk, arms, and legs were compared between groups. For all variables the 95% CI for the mean difference was determined and effect sizes were calculated for all variables using the method of Cohen (1992), where an effect size of 0.2 represents a small effect, 0.5 a moderate effect, and 0.8 a large effect. To test the agreement between the results of the fat percentage predicting regression equations and DXA outcomes, the statistical method of Bland and Altman (2012) was used.

Paired *t*-tests were performed for all five equations between the results of the DXA and equations to check for significant systematic errors. Also, Pearson's correlations were performed to check for proportional biases and heteroscedasticity. For the walkers and non-walkers, the association between body fat percentage and BMI, waist circumference, sum of 6 skinfold thicknesses and sum of 8 skinfold thicknesses was calculated by performing linear regression analysis and interpretation of slope and intercept.

RESULTS

Body Composition

There were no significant differences for age and time since injury between the two groups (**Table 1**). **Table 1** shows the physical characteristics of the two groups, where non-walkers were lighter than walkers ($P = 0.05$) with significantly lower lean tissue mass than the walking group ($P < 0.01$). Lean tissue mass was significantly lower ($P < 0.04$; effect size > 1.0) across the trunk, arms, and legs for non-walkers (**Figure 1**). For the other variables (fat mass, fat percentage, lean tissue percentage, segmental fat mass, BMI, waist circumference, sum of 6 skinfold thicknesses, and sum of 8 skinfold thicknesses) no significant differences between the two groups were found. However, the effect sizes of BMI and waist circumference were 0.9, indicating substantially, but not significantly, lower BMI and waist circumference in the non-walkers.

Fat Percentage Prediction Equations

The results of body fat percentage derived by DXA scan and the fat percentages calculated by the anthropometric prediction equations for walkers and non-walkers can be found in **Figure 2**. The agreement between the percent fat estimated from DXA and anthropometric predictions equations, displayed as mean percentage systematic error and 95% limits of agreement, are shown in **Table 2**. Pearson's correlations revealed that there were no proportional biases or heteroscedasticity within the walking group ($P \geq 0.93$) and non-walking group ($P \geq 0.142$). In the walking group, the equation of Lean et al. (1996) did not show a significant difference between the predicted body fat percentage and percent body fat measured by DXA. Also, this equation showed the lowest systematic error which was an underestimation of 2.1% of body fat percentage. The limits of agreements showed that the equation of Lean et al. (1996) will, 95% of the time, produce body fat percentage estimates between 9.7% less and 5.5% more than the DXA value. All other formulae showed significant differences between the equation outcomes and DXA measured body fat percentage ($P \leq 0.04$). For the non-walking group (see **Table 2**), all formulae showed significant differences between the equation outcomes and DXA measured body fat percentage, with underestimated body fat percentage and a large systematic errors (ranging from 8.3 to 13.7%).

Regression Analysis

Waist circumference was associated with percentage fat in walkers only (**Table 3**). However, the relationship appeared

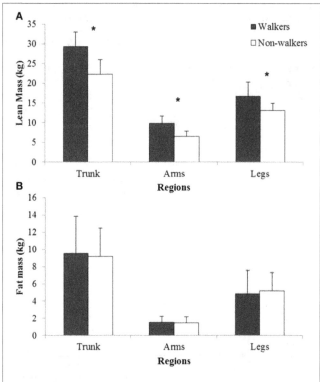

FIGURE 1 | Comparison of (A) segmental (trunks, arms, legs) lean tissue mass and (B) fat mass for walkers and non-walkers. * Significant difference between groups ($P < 0.04$).

different between the groups, particularly for waist circumference (**Table 3**). This is highlighted by the lower percentage fat, but higher waist circumference, in walkers than non-walkers (**Table 1**). BMI was not significantly associated with percentage fat in either group (**Table 3**) and the standard error of estimate of percentage fat from BMI was large, particularly in the non-walkers. The sums of 6 or 8 skinfold thickness were significantly associated with % fat in both groups, with standard errors of estimate within 5% in both groups. Also, the relationship between the sum of skinfold thicknesses and % fat did not seem to differ so substantially between groups (**Table 3**).

DISCUSSION

The estimation of body fat percentage in wheelchair game players is a difficult task due to the variety of disabilities and the consequent differences in distribution of body tissues from able-bodied persons. This may explain the paucity of studies that have evaluated the use of predictive equation techniques from anthropometric measurements in this population. The primary finding of our study is that fat percentage predicting regression equations, based on skinfold thickness, waist circumference, age, and sex, used in the able-bodied populations are not applicable to ambulant and non-ambulant wheelchair sportspersons. Due the strong correlations and positive association found for sum of 6 skinfold thicknesses and sum of 8 skinfold thicknesses in non-walkers and walkers with body fat percentage, respectively, these

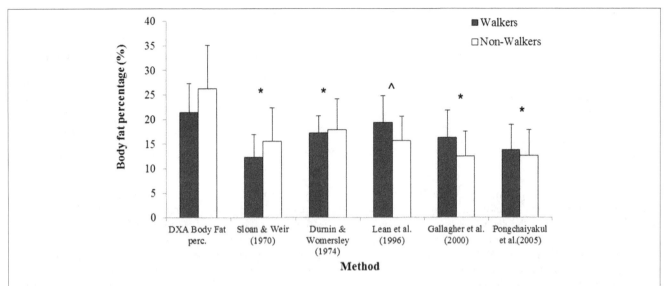

FIGURE 2 | Body fat percentage derived by DXA scan and the fat percentages calculated by the anthropometric prediction equations for walkers and non-walkers. * Both groups significantly lower than DXA ($P < 0.05$), ^ Non-walkers significantly lower than DXA ($P < 0.05$).

TABLE 2 | Agreement between DXA-determined percent body fat and values given by anthropometric equations for walkers ($n = 7$) and non-walkers ($n = 7$).

		Mean bias in % fat (anthropometry- DXA; mean ± SD)	p-value for bias	95% limits of agreement (Bland and Altman)		
				Lower	Upper	Range
Walkers	Sloan and Weir, 1970	−9.0 ± 2.6%	<0.01*	−14.0	−4.0	10.0
	Durnin and Womersley, 1974	−4.2 ± 3.8%	0.03*	−11.6	+3.3	14.9
	Lean et al., 1996	−2.1 ± 3.9%	0.21	−9.7	+5.5	15.3
	Gallagher et al., 2000	−5.1 ± 5.3%	0.04*	−15.5	+5.3	20.8
	Pongchaiyakul et al., 2005	−7.7 ± 5.0%	<0.01*	−17.5	+2.1	19.6
Non-walkers	Sloan and Weir, 1970	−10.6 ± 4.5%	<0.01*	−19.4	−1.78	17.6
	Durnin and Womersley, 1974	−8.3 ± 4.8%	<0.01*	−17.7	+1.1	18.8
	Lean et al., 1996	−10.6 ± 7.4%	<0.01*	−25.1	+3.9	29.0
	Gallagher et al., 2000	−13.7 ± 7.5%	<0.01*	−28.4	+1.0	29.4
	Pongchaiyakul et al., 2005	−13.6 ± 6.5%	<0.01*	−26.3	−0.9	25.5

*Eq., Equations; SD, Standard Deviation. Significant differences are indicated with * at a significant level of P < 0.05.*

variables could be useful to establish regression equations in the future for non-walking and walking wheelchair game players.

The results showed a difference in body mass between the groups, caused by a significantly lower lean tissue mass in the non-walkers as the fat mass was not significantly different between the groups. Segmental data for the trunk, arms, and legs showed lower lean tissue across all regions, representing the muscular atrophy associated with paralysis and impaired muscle innervation. These findings are in is line with findings of other studies who found significantly lower lean tissue mass in SCI-individuals (Maggioni et al., 2003; Miyahara et al., 2008; Stewart and Sutton, 2012). Previous studies showed a significantly higher body fat percentage for wheelchair athletes compared to able-bodied controls (Miyahara et al., 2008; Sutton et al., 2008). It could have been expected that this increased fat percentage in

wheelchair athletes is caused by the increased fat mass of the SCI-athletes, as people with SCI are previously reported to have a higher fat mass (Spungen et al., 2003; Emmons et al., 2011). However, our results showed that DXA derived body fat mass in the walkers is not significantly different form the non-walkers. The main difference in body composition between non-walkers and walkers is thus lean tissue mass and not a difference in fat mass. BMI and waist circumference showed no significant differences between the groups but the effect sizes were very high.

The equations that were applied in this study were all established for the able-bodied population. The results showed that they are not transferrable to the non-walking or the walking athletic wheelchair population. For the walkers, the equation of Lean et al. (1996) predicted a fat percentage that was not significantly different from DXA-measured fat percentage.

TABLE 3 | Linear regression analysis of anthropometric measures and DXA-derived percentage body fat.

	Correlation co-efficient (r)		SEE		Intercept		Slope (95% CI)	
	Walkers	Non-Walkers	Walkers	Non-Walkers	Walkers	Non-Walkers	Walkers	Non-Walkers
WC	0.79*	0.62	4.00	7.61	−24.7	−29.37	0.54 (0.05 to 1.21)	0.71 (−0.32 to 1.74)
BMI	0.49	0.59	5.65	7.83	2.5	−21.35	0.81 (−0.84 to 2.46)	2.32 (−1.2 to 5.93)
Sum of 6	0.84*	0.87*	3.54	4.78	0.81	9.75	0.27 (0.07 to 0.47)	0.19 (0.07 to 0.32)
Sum of 8	0.98*	0.88*	1.16	4.65	−0.95	7.32	0.22 (0.17 to 0.26)	0.17 (0.06 to 0.27)

WC, waist circumference; BMI, body mass index; SEE, standard error of the estimate. Significant correlations are indicated with * at a significant level of P < 0.05.

However, the limits of agreement were wide, making the prediction very inaccurate. Therefore, it is not advisable to use the equation for ambulant disabled wheelchair game players. All other equation based predictions for the non-walkers and walkers were significantly different from DXA-measured fat percentage, and are thus not usable to estimate body fat percentage in these populations. Our results are in agreement with the findings from Sutton et al. (2009), Maggioni et al. (2003), and Mojtahedi et al. (2009) who also concluded that the equations underestimate body fat percentage and are not accurate enough to use in daily practice.

No significant correlations between BMI and body fat percentage were found for either the walkers or non-walkers, in contrast to the results of Sutton et al. (2009) who found a strong correlation in female wheelchair athletes. The large standard error of estimation of percentage fat from BMI demonstrates that BMI is a particularly poor indicator of obesity in wheelchair athletes. Waist circumference correlated with body fat percentage in the walkers which is in agreement with the work of Sutton et al. (2009), however, no significant correlation was not found for the non-walkers. Despite the more centrally located fat mass in SCI (Spungen et al., 2003), non-walkers tended to have lower waist circumference at any given fat percentage than walkers, although the sample size was not sufficient to detect a significantly different relationship between the two groups. In contrast to Sutton et al. (2009) suggestion, the high SEE of fat percentage estimated from waist circumference suggests that waist circumference does not provide a better indicator of body fat content than skinfolds in this population.

The sums of 6 and 8 skinfold thickness showed the highest correlation with body fat content in this sample. A closer look at those correlations shows that for non-walkers, the correlation of sum of 6 skinfold thickness and sum of 8 skinfold thickness are similar, although the lower standard error of estimate with 8 skinfold thickness suggests this measure may provide most accuracy. Although existing skinfold thickness equations developed in able-bodied populations substantially underestimated body fat content, in this sample, the relatively low SEE for the regression of fat percentage and skinfold thickness suggests that it may be possible to derive population specific equations for wheelchair athletes based on skinfold thickness. Theoretically, it may be desirable to also include a variable that may reflect the atrophy of lean tissue, e.g., thigh circumference. Furthermore, given that height may be substantially affected in double amputees and also some SCI, an alternative index of

body size such as arm-span may be more appropriate in this population. However, one difficulty in developing such equations is the limited sample of wheelchair athletes, and a further difficulty is the heterogeneity of the population. Pending any future developments in body composition assessment in these groups, we suggest that body composition be assessed by DXA, and any estimates from anthropometric equations be adjusted accordingly.

In the present study DXA was used to assess body composition and not a four component model, which is standard better criterion measure for assessing body composition. Although some studies found very high precision of DXA in able-bodied persons (Stewart and Sutton, 2012) and in SCI individuals (Jones et al., 1998), the accuracy of DXA for assessing body composition is still debated (Van Loan and Mayclin, 1992; Glickman et al., 2004). Therefore, inaccuracies in body composition measurements might have occurred in this study. However, considering the reported accuracy of DXA (Jones et al., 1998; Stewart and Sutton, 2012), possible inaccuracies in assessing body composition should be relatively small. Another limitation of this study might be the small sample size. As the study deals with a highly specific population (Paralympic wheelchair athletes) it is hard to increase the sample size number. Despite the low participant number we were still able to uncover interesting results about the body composition of athletes classified as non-walkers and walkers. This study is the first study trying to assess body composition in wheelchair athletes with anthropometric measurements, differentiating between non-walkers and walkers. Given the interesting results of this study, further research into body composition assessment of non-walking and walking athletes should be able to establishing separate field-methods for body composition assessment within these populations.

CONCLUSION

In conclusion, there were notable differences for the total lean tissue mass between the non-walkers and walkers. Non-walkers displayed significantly lower segmental lean mass of the trunk, arms, and legs, resulting in significant differences in total body mass between groups. The regression equations developed from able-bodied populations using BMI, waist circumference, age, and skinfold thickness measurements substantially underestimated body fat content, particularly in non-walkers. All formulae, apart from that of Lean et al.'s (1996) in the walkers, showed significant differences between the equation outcomes and DXA-derived body fat percentage, with an underestimation in body fat percentage and large systematic errors across present in all equations (ranging from 8 to 14%). Due the strong correlation between sum of 8 skinfold thickness and body fat percentage, and the low SEE for walkers and non-walkers, this variable could be suitable to establish future impairment specific regression equations for wheelchair game players.

REFERENCES

Bland, J. M., and Altman, D. G. (2012). Agreed statistics: measurement method comparison. *Anesthesiology* 116, 182–185. doi: 10.1097/ALN.0b013e31823d7784

Buchholz, A. C., and Bugaresti, J. M. (2005). A review of body mass index and waist circumference as markers of obesity and coronary heart disease risk in persons with chronic spinal cord injury. *Spinal Cord* 43, 513–518. doi: 10.1038/sj.sc.3101744

Buchholz, A. C., and Pencharz, P. B. (2004). Energy expenditure in chronic spinal cord injury. *Curr. Opin. Clin. Nutr. Metab. Care* 7, 635–639. doi: 10.1097/00075197-200411000-00008

Bulbulian, R., Johnson, R. E., Gruber, J. J., and Darabos, B. (1987). Body composition in paraplegic male athletes. *Med. Sci. Sports Exerc.* 19, 195–201. doi: 10.1249/00005768-198706000-00002

Camhi, S. M., Bray, G. A., Bouchard, C., Greenway, F. L., Johnson, W. D., Newton, R. L., et al. (2011). The relationship of waist circumference and BMI to visceral, subcutaneous, and total body fat: sex and race differences. *Obesity* 19, 402–408. doi: 10.1038/oby.2010.248

Cohen, J. (1992). A power primer. *Psychol. Bull.* 112, 155–159. doi: 10.1037/0033-2909.112.1.155

Durnin, J., and Womersley, J. (1974). Body fat assessed from total body density and its estimation from skinfold thickness: measurements on 481 men and women aged from 16 to 72 years. *Br. J. Nutr.* 32, 77–97. doi: 10.1079/BJN19740060

Emmons, R. R., Garber, C. E., Cirnigliaro, C. M., Kirshblum, S. C., Spungen, A. M., and Bauman, W. A. (2011). Assessment of measures for abdominal adiposity in persons with spinal cord injury. *Ultrasound Med. Biol.* 37, 734–741. doi: 10.1016/j.ultrasmedbio.2011.02.002

Eston, R., Rowlands, A., Charlesworth, S., Davies, A., and Hoppitt, T. (2005). Prediction of DXA-determined whole body fat from skinfolds: importance of including skinfolds from the thigh and calf in young, healthy men and women. *Eur. J. Clin. Nutr.* 59, 695–702. doi: 10.1038/sj.ejcn.1602131

Gallagher, D., Heymsfield, S. B., Heo, M., Jebb, S. A., Murgatroyd, P. R., and Sakamoto, Y. (2000). Healthy percentage body fat ranges: an approach for developing guidelines based on body mass index. *Am. J. Clin. Nutr.* 72, 694–701.

Glickman, S. G., Marn, C. S., Supiano, M. A., and Dengel, D. R. (2004). Validity and reliability of dual-energy X-ray absorptiometry for the assessment of abdominal adiposity. *J. Appl. Physiol. (1985)* 97, 509–514. doi: 10.1152/japplphysiol.01234.2003

Goosey-Tolfrey, V. (2010). *Wheelchair Sport: A Complete Guide for Athletes, Coaches, and Teachers.* Champaign, IL: Human Kinetics.

Hill, J. O., Sidney, S., Lewis, C. E., Tolan, K., Scherzinger, A. L., and Stamm, E. R. (1999). Racial differences in amounts of visceral adipose tissue in young adults: the CARDIA (Coronary Artery Risk Development in Young Adults) study. *Am. J. Clin. Nutr.* 69, 381–387.

Jones, L., Goulding, A., and Gerrard, D. (1998). DEXA: a practical and accurate tool to demonstrate total and regional bone loss, lean tissue loss and fat mass gain in paraplegia. *Spinal Cord* 36, 637–640. doi: 10.1038/sj.sc.3100664

Keil, M., Totosy de Zepetnek, J. O., Brooke-Wavell, K., and Goosey-Tolfrey, V. L. (2014). Measurement precision of body composition variables in elite wheelchair athletes, using dual-energy X-ray absorptiometry. *Eur. J. Sport Sci.* doi: 10.1080/17461391.2014.966763. [Epub ahead of print].

Lean, M., Han, T. S., and Deurenberg, P. (1996). Predicting body composition by densitometry from simple anthropometric measurements. *Am. J. Clin. Nutr.* 63, 4–14.

Lohman, T. G., Roche, A. F., and Martorell, R. (1988). *Anthropometric Standardization Reference Manual.* Champaign, IL: Human Kinetics Books.

ACKNOWLEDGMENTS

The research was conducted in the absence of any commercial or financial relationships that could be construed as a potential conflict of interest. With thanks to the participants of the GB wheelchair basketball and rugby squads and Diane Harper for assisting with the DXA-scans and Dr. John Lenton with the skinfold measurements.

Maggioni, M., Bertoli, S., Margonato, V., Merati, G., Veicsteinas, A., and Testolin, G. (2003). Body composition assessment in spinal cord injury subjects. *Acta Diabetol.* 40, s183–s186. doi: 10.1007/s00592-003-0061-7

Miyahara, K., Wang, D.-H., Mori, K., Takahashi, K., Miyatake, N., Wang, B.-L., et al. (2008). Effect of sports activity on bone mineral density in wheelchair athletes. *J. Bone Miner. Metab.* 26, 101–106. doi: 10.1007/s00774-007-0789-1

Mojtahedi, M. C., Valentine, R. J., and Evans, E. M. (2009). Body composition assessment in athletes with spinal cord injury: comparison of field methods with dual-energy X-ray absorptiometry. *Spinal Cord* 47, 698–704. doi: 10.1038/sc.2009.20

Pongchaiyakul, C., Kosulwat, V., Rojroongwasinkul, N., Charoenkiatkul, S., Thepsuthammarat, K., Laopaiboon, M., et al. (2005). Prediction of percentage body fat in rural thai population using simple anthropometric measurements. *Obes. Res.* 13, 729–738. doi: 10.1038/oby.2005.82

Rahman, M., Temple, J. R., Breitkopf, C. R., and Berenson, A. B. (2009). Racial differences in body fat distribution among reproductive-aged women. *Metab. Clin. Exp.* 58, 1329–1337. doi: 10.1016/j.metabol.2009.04.017

Schreiner, P. J., Terry, J. G., Evans, G. W., Hinson, W. H., Crouse, J. R., and Heiss, G. (1996). Sex-specific associations of magnetic resonance imaging-derived intra-abdominal and subcutaneous fat areas with conventional anthropometric indices the atherosclerosis risk in communities study. *Am. J. Epidemiol.* 144, 335–345. doi: 10.1093/oxfordjournals.aje.a008934

Sloan, A., and Weir, J. B. (1970). Nomograms for prediction of body density and total body fat from skinfold measurements. *J. Appl. Physiol.* 28, 221–222.

Spungen, A. M., Adkins, R. H., Stewart, C. A., Wang, J., Pierson, R. N., Waters, R. L., et al. (2003). Factors influencing body composition in persons with spinal cord injury: a cross-sectional study. *J. Appl. Physiol.* 95, 2398–2407. doi: 10.1152/japplphysiol.00729.2002

Stewart, A. D., and Sutton, L. (2012). *Body Composition in Sport, Exercise and Health.* London: Routledge.

Sutton, L., Scott, M., Goosey-Tolfrey, V., Wallace, J., and Reilly, T. (2008). "Body composition of highly-trained wheelchair athletes measured by dual-energy X-ray absorptiometry," in *Kinanthropometry XI*, eds P. Hume and A. Stewart (Published electronically on behalf of the International Society for the Advancement of Kinanthropometry).

Sutton, L., Wallace, J., Goosey-Tolfrey, V., Scott, M., and Reilly, T. (2009). Body composition of female wheelchair athletes. *Int. J. Sports Med.* 30, 259–265. doi: 10.1055/s-0028-1105941

Van Loan, M. D., and Mayclin, P. L. (1992). Body composition assessment: dual-energy X-ray absorptiometry (DEXA) compared to reference methods. *Eur. J. Clin. Nutr.* 46, 125–130.

Weerarathna, T., Lekamwasam, S., and Rodrigo, M. (2008). Prediction of total and visceral fat contents using anthropometric measures of adiposity in women. *Ceylon Med. J.* 53, 128–132. doi: 10.4038/cmj.v53i4.281

Conflict of Interest Statement: The authors declare that the research was conducted in the absence of any commercial or financial relationships that could be construed as a potential conflict of interest.

10

Acute responses of circulating microRNAs to low-volume sprint interval cycling

Shu Fang Cui[1,2], Wei Li[3], Jie Niu[3], Chen Yu Zhang[1,2]*, Xi Chen[1,2]* and Ji Zheng Ma[1,2,3]*

[1] *State Key Laboratory of Pharmaceutical Biotechnology, NJU Advanced Institute for Life Sciences (NAILS), School of Life Sciences, Nanjing University, Nanjing, China,* [2] *Jiangsu Engineering Research Center for MicroRNA Biology and Biotechnology, Nanjing University, Nanjing, China,* [3] *The Lab of Military Conditioning and Motor Function Assessment, The PLA University of Science and Technology, Nanjing, China*

Edited by:
*Sergej Ostojic,
University of Novi Sad, Serbia*

Reviewed by:
*Henning Bay Nielsen,
Rigshospitalet, Denmark
Bryan Saunders,
University of São Paulo, Brazil*

*Correspondence:
*Chen Yu Zhang
cyzhang@nju.edu.cn;
Xi Chen
xichen@nju.edu.cn;
Ji Zheng Ma
mjz_mjj@163.com*

Low-volume high-intensity interval training is an efficient and practical method of inducing physiological responses in various tissues to develop physical fitness and may also change the expression of circulating microRNAs (miRNAs). The purpose of the present study was to examine whether miRNAs for muscle, heart, somatic tissue and metabolism were affected by 30-s intervals of intensive sprint cycling. We also examined the relationship of these miRNAs to conventional biochemical and performance indices. Eighteen healthy young males performed sprint interval cycling. Circulating miRNAs in plasma were detected using TaqMan-based quantitative PCR and normalized to Let-7d/g/i. In addition, we determined the levels of insulin-like growth factor-I, testosterone and cortisol, and anaerobic capacity. Compared to plasma levels before exercise muscle-specific miR-1 (0.12 ± 0.02 vs. 0.09 ± 0.02), miR-133a (0.46 ± 0.10 vs. 0.31 ± 0.06), and miR-133b (0.19 ± 0.02 vs. 0.10 ± 0.01) decreased (all $P < 0.05$), while miR-206 and miR-499 remained unchanged. The levels of metabolism related miR-122 (0.62 ± 0.07 vs. 0.34 ± 0.03) and somatic tissues related miR-16 (1.74 ± 0.27 vs. 0.94 ± 0.12) also decreased (both $P < 0.05$). The post-exercise IGF-1 and cortisol concentrations were significantly increased, while testosterone concentrations did not. Plasma levels of miR-133b correlated to peak power ($r = 0.712$, $P = 0.001$) and miR-122 correlated to peak power ratio ($r = 0.665$, $P = 0.003$). In conclusion sprint exercise provokes genetic changes for RNA related to specific muscle or metabolism related miRNAs suggesting that miR-133b and miR-122 may be potential useful biomarkers for actual physiological strain or anaerobic capacity. Together, our findings on the circulating miRNAs may provide new insight into the physiological responses that are being performed during exercise and delineate mechanisms by which exercise confers distinct phenotypes and improves performance.

Keywords: plasma microRNAs, biomarkers, blood lactate, blood hormones, anaerobic capacity

INTRODUCTION

Sprint interval training, interspersed with sufficient recovery periods (2–4 min), can produce the best possible average sprint performance over a series of sprints (<45 s; Weston et al., 2014). Therefore, sprint interval training is a commonly used intervention to maintain skeletal muscle health and to improve exercise performance, especially in individuals who require a high contribution of glycolytic energy (e.g., track-and-field sprint athletes and some team sport athletes; Buchheit and Laursen, 2013). Similarly, sprint interval cycling (SIC), which is modeled on the Wingate Anaerobic test, is extremely demanding and involves all-out 30-s sprints interspersed with 4 min active recovery periods with no resistance (Burgomaster et al., 2005). The high-intensity nature of SIC is thought to recruit all types of muscle fibers (Weston et al., 2014). However, repeated all-out 30-s bouts of exercise separated by 4 min of rest increasingly depend on aerobic metabolism (Burgomaster et al., 2005). Exercise intensity places mechanical and/or metabolic stress on contracting muscles (Laursen, 2010). The anabolic (e.g., growth hormone, testosterone, and insulin-like growth factor-1) and catabolic (e.g., cortisol) processes of tissue remodeling following exercise loading are typically reflected by acute changes in hormonal concentrations (Schoenfeld, 2012).

The microRNAs (miRNAs) are typically small, ~19–22 nucleotides long, non-coding RNA molecules that post-transcriptionally regulate gene expression by base-pairing with the 3′ untranslated region of complementary messenger RNA targets (Bartel, 2004). Recently, some miRNA species (particularly muscle-specific miRNAs and inflammatory-related miRNAs) have been found to change in human serum/plasma after acute prolonged endurance training, eccentric exercise, and strength exercise (Baggish et al., 2011, 2014; Aoi et al., 2013; Banzet et al., 2013; Gomes et al., 2014; Mooren et al., 2014; Uhlemann et al., 2014). Studies have suggested that they can be used as potential biomarkers for aerobic capacity and as markers or mediators of physiological adaptations (Baggish et al., 2011, 2014; Aoi et al., 2013; Banzet et al., 2013; Mooren et al., 2014; de Gonzalo-Calvo et al., 2015).

Exhaustive exercise has a deep effect on cellular, humoral, and metabolic processes of the body (Spencer et al., 2005; Meckel et al., 2011; Gibala et al., 2012). We hypothesized that a single session of low-volume sprint interval cycling can change the circulating miRNAs (c-miRNAs) profile. Accordingly, the levels of the myomiR family (miR-1, miR-133a, miR-133b, and miR-206) and other muscle-specific miRNA (miR-499), metabolism-related miRNA (miR-122), and somatic tissues-related miRNA (miR-16) were evaluated in response to extreme SIC. In addition, to provide insight into the potential roles of these c-miRNAs, we also determined whether alterations in the levels of these miRNAs in response to extreme SIC are correlated with changes in conventional anabolic-catabolic hormonal biomarkers or anaerobic capacity.

MATERIALS AND METHODS

Ethical Approval and Participants

Eighteen healthy young male participants (age, 20.23 ± 0.97 years; height, 1.75 ± 0.06 m; body mass, 68.90 ± 8.83 kg; and BMI, 22.39 ± 2.06 kg·m^{-2}) who were habituated to a regular exercise regimen were recruited to participate in this study. University cadets were contacted to volunteer for this study who led similar lives and who had the same dietary habits for 2 years prior to the study. None of the subjects had any current or prior chronic disease, a history of smoking or current use of any medications. Written informed consent was obtained from all of the participants. Ethical approval for this study conformed to the standards of the Declaration of Helsinki, and the protocol was approved by the Institutional Review Board of Nanjing University.

Study Design

Before the SIC session, the participants refrained from exercise for at least 72 h. Sprint interval cycling was performed on a mechanically braked stationary cycle ergometer (Monark Ergomedic 839E, Monark, Sweden) against a pre-determined force load of approximately 7.5% of the subject's body weight in kilograms. Sprint interval cycling involved two 30-s all-out sprints (Sprint 1 and Sprint 2) with 4 min of active recovery between them (Burgomaster et al., 2005). The tests were conducted between 10:00 am and 11:30 am.

Anaerobic Capacity

The first 30 s of Wingate data for each participant were used to assess anaerobic power. Fatigue index was calculated as ([Peak Power − Minimum Power]/Peak Power) × 100%. The change in Wingate data for Sprint 1 and Sprint 2 were used to assess the ability to maintain anaerobic power.

Plasma Sampling

Venous blood was collected at two different time points during the acute exercise test. Five milliliters of blood was collected in standard anticoagulant (EDTA)-treated Vacutainer tubes prior to acute exercise testing (Pre) and within 1 min of exercise testing completion (Post). All of the blood samples were centrifuged at 1500 × g for 10 min to pellet cellular elements immediately after each blood draw and were then centrifuged at 10,000 × g for 5 min at 4°C to completely remove cell debris. To minimize freeze–thaw degradation, the supernatant plasma was then aliquoted and immediately frozen at −80°C.

Blood Lactate and Hormones

The blood lactate (LA) concentration was measured with an automatic lactate analyzer (EKF Diagnostic, Germany). Blood samples were analyzed for conventional physiological markers, including lactate, insulin-like growth factor-1 (IGF-1), testosterone, and cortisol. The IGF-1 level was measured with an IMMULITE 2000 Analyzer (EuroDPC Med Limited, Llanberis, UK). The assays were conducted using the solid-phase, enzyme-labeled, chemiluminescent immunometric method in accordance with the manufacturer's instructions. The testosterone and cortisol levels in the plasma were determined by a chemiluminescence immunoassay (UniCel DxI 800, Access Immunoassay System, Beckmann Coulter GmbH, Krefeld, Germany). The IGF-1, testosterone and cortisol levels were considered normal according to the reference ranges for ages provided by the kit manufacturer.

miRNA Isolation and RT-qPCR

Total RNA, including miRNAs, was isolated from the plasma samples using a 1-step phenol/chloroform purification protocol as previously described (Liu et al., 2011). A panel of miRNAs was investigated that are related to either skeletal/heart muscle (miR-1, miR-133a, miR-133b, miR-206, and miR-499) or to metabolism and somatic tissue (miR-122 and miR-16; Aoi et al., 2013; Boettger et al., 2014; Bandiera et al., 2015). To quantify the abundance of mature miRNAs, real time quantitative polymerase chain reaction (RT-qPCR) was performed. RT-qPCR was performed using a TaqMan PCR Kit and an Applied Biosystems 7300 Sequence Detection System as previously described (Wu et al., 2014). The cycle threshold (Ct) data were determined using default threshold settings, and the mean Ct was determined from triplicate PCRs. In addition, we calculated the Ct values of Let-7d, Let-7g, and Let-7i because the use of this combination of reference genes (Chen et al., 2013) in human serum for normalization has been demonstrated to be superior to that of the other commonly used single reference genes. The relative levels of miRNAs were normalized to a Let-7d/g/i trio and were calculated using the $2^{-\Delta\Delta Ct}$ method. ΔCt was calculated by subtracting the Ct values of Let-7d/g/i from the average Ct values of the target miRNAs. ΔCt values were then compared ($\Delta\Delta Ct$) with each participant's own resting baseline at the Pre time point (normalized to fold change of 1).

Statistical Analyses

GraphPad Prism 5 and SigmaPlot 10.0 packages were used. Subject characteristics, exercise testing data and blood parameters were reported as the mean ± standard deviation, and c-miRNA data were presented as the mean ± standard error of the mean (SEM). Paired variables were compared in Student's t-test or a Wilcoxon's matched pairs test as appropriate for the data distribution. Correlation analyses were performed using the Spearman or Pearson's method as appropriate for the data distribution. Values of $P < 0.05$ were considered significant.

RESULTS

Wingate Performance

After the SIC, Wingate peak power was significantly decreased by 11% following two 30-s periods of all-out SIC (659.48 ± 217.64 W vs. 562.78 ± 146.38 W, $P = 0.006$). The average power was also significantly decreased by 16%. The average power of Sprint 1 was 6.69 ± 0.78 W·kg^{-1} and that of Sprint 2 was 5.58 ± 0.80 W·kg^{-1} ($P < 0.001$). There was no significant difference in the fatigue index between the first and second 30-s sprint (62.87 ± 11.22% vs.

60.26 ± 12.44%, $P = 0.820$). In addition, there was no significant difference in maximum speed between the first and second sprint (151.96 ± 16.83 rpm vs. 150.57 ± 20.04 rpm, $P = 0.740$).

Blood Lactate

After exercise, the LA concentration significantly increased (1.56 ± 1.90 mmol·L^{-1} vs. 11.27 ± 1.90 mmol·L^{-1}, $P < 0.001$).

Plasma Hormones

Compared to plasma levels before exercise, the post-exercise IGF-1 concentration was significantly increased by 13% following two 30-s periods of all-out SIC (298.94 ± 50.13 ng·mL^{-1} vs. 332.72 ± 57.76 ng·mL^{-1}, $P < 0.001$). Testosterone concentrations were similar between pre- and post-exercise (40.59 ± 8.45 nmol·L^{-1} vs. 41.74 ± 11.57 nmol·L^{-1}, $P = 0.608$). The cortisol concentration increased by 45% (216 ± 87 nmol·L^{-1} vs. 278 ± 91 nmol·L^{-1}, $P = 0.028$) and a decrease in testosterone/cortisol ratio tended to be statistical significant.

The Plasma miRNA Levels in Response to an Acute Bout of Sprint Interval Cycling

The Ct values of Let-7d/g/i at pre- and post-SIC show low variability (**Figure 1**; $P = 0.280$). Acute sprint interval cycling significantly decreased the levels of miR-1, miR-133a, miR-133b, miR-122, and miR-16 (**Figure 2**). Levels of miR-206 and miR-499 were not significantly changed by acute sprint interval cycling (**Figure 3**).

Correlations between Blood, Anaerobic Parameters and c-miRNA Levels

To explore the feasibility of using c-miRNAs as biomarkers of an acute exercise response, the association of specific changes

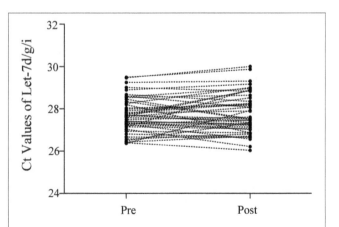

FIGURE 1 | The Ct values of Let-7d/g/i in plasma samples before and after the sprint interval cycling. The total amount of Lot 7d/g/i trio was simultaneously measured in a same RT-qPCR reaction. Let-7d, Let-7g, and Let-7i were reverse-transcribed in a single reaction using a mixture of stem-loop primers of Let-7d, Let-7g, and Let-7i (in the ratio of 1:1:1). Accordingly, real-time PCR was performed using a TaqMan miRNA probe pool of Let-7d, Let-7g and Let-7i (in the ratio of 1:1:1). Ct values of every individual's Let-7d/g/i before (Pre) and after (Post) the exercise almost remained unchanged.

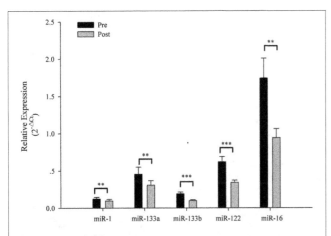

FIGURE 2 | The plasma miRNA levels in response to sprint interval cycling. Plasma levels of miR-1, miR-133a, miR-133b, miR-122, and miR-16 decreased significantly after an acute bout of sprint interval cycling. Values represent the mean ± SEM obtained from 18 subjects. **$P < 0.01$, ***$P < 0.001$.

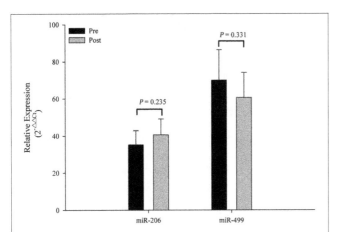

FIGURE 3 | Changes in circulating miR-206 and miR-499 in response to acute exercise. Plasma levels of miR-206 and miR-499 showed no significant difference after an acute bout of sprint interval cycling. Values represent the mean ± SEM obtained from 18 subjects.

in c-miRNA was examined in relation to the changes in blood hormonal and anaerobic parameters. No correlations were found between the changes in the plasma IGF-1, testosterone, and cortisol levels, or the testosterone/cortisol ratio and the changes in the miR-1, miR-133a, miR-133b, miR-122, and miR-16 levels (**Table 1**).

There were not correlations among the levels of peak power, average power and fatigue index and levels of plasma miR-133a, miR-1, and miR-16 levels (**Table 1**). However, there was a significant correlation between the levels of peak power of Sprint 1 and levels of plasma miR-133b (**Figure 4A**). These results suggest a potential role for plasma miR-133b as a marker of anaerobic capacity. Furthermore, there was a significant correlation between the levels of the peak power ratio of Sprint 1/Sprint 2 and plasma miR-122 level (**Figure 4B**), suggesting a potential

role of plasma miR-122 as a restriction marker of anaerobic capacity.

DISCUSSION

Sprint interval cycling is one of the most frequently used training methods in anaerobic sports. Our data indicated that several miRNA species in plasma responded to sprint interval cycling. These acute responses may be more critical to tissue growth and remodeling than chronic changes in resting concentrations (Kraemer and Ratamess, 2005). Exercise rapidly and transiently regulates several miRNA species in circulation, suggesting that they could be used to precisely monitor physiological acute responses to exercise.

Sprint interval exercise involves very high intensity, and the myosin heavy chain (MHC) IIa and IIx fibers are highly responsive to intense exercise at the transcriptional level for genes involved with muscle growth and remodeling (Trappe et al., 2015). miR-1 and miR-133a are expressed in both skeletal and cardiac muscles (Boettger et al., 2014). miR-133b and miR-206 are specific to skeletal muscle and preferentially detected in slow myofibers (Boettger et al., 2014). Pervious study has shown that circulating plasma miR-1 levels were significantly decreased in patients with supraventricular tachycardia, while miR-133 significantly increased in patients with ventricular tachycardia (Sun et al., 2015). The interactions of miRNAs (such as miR-1 and miR-133) with ion channel-encoding genes and calmodulin regulate cardiac contractility, rhythm and excitement (Terentyev et al., 2009). However, cardiac contraction during exercise is the physiological process most sensitive to calmodulin integrity, which can be affected by acute exercise (Sondergaard et al., 2015). Moreover, extracellular miRNAs are dynamic indices of pathophysiological processes in skeletal muscle (Roberts et al., 2013). Endurance also increased the miR-1 and miR-133a levels both in plasma and skeletal muscle (Nielsen et al., 2010; Baggish et al., 2014; Gomes et al., 2014; Mooren et al., 2014). During high intensity exercise the heart rate can greatly increase. In the present study, miR-1 and miR-133a levels in plasma decreased, and miR-1 and miR-133a expression in adult mice decreased during skeletal muscle hypertrophy (Mccarthy and Esser, 2007). These results indicate that these miRNAs may partly reflect the cardiac or skeletal muscle responses induced by exercise or a temporal regulation controlled by miRNAs during exercise.

Furthermore, miR-133b, miR-206, and miR-499 levels in plasma decreased or remained unchanged in the current study but significantly increased after acute endurance exercise in a previous study (Mooren et al., 2014). Training with high intensity exercise induces expression of fast-twitch fibers. Therefore, no change of circulating miR-206 and miR-499 observed in the present work, associated with slow myofibers or oxidative red fibers (Gan et al., 2013; Boettger et al., 2014), might reflect a non-predominance of slow-twitch fibers in SIC. However, at present, specific miRNAs related to fast-twitch fibers in human, such as MHC IIa and MHC IIx muscle fibers, have not been found.

Two miRNAs not restricted to muscle in origin (miR-122 and miR-16) also deceased in plasma following acute high intensity exercise. A previous study has shown that miR-122 is a key factor

TABLE 1 | Correlations between changes in exercise-related blood parameters and anaerobic parameters and changes in plasma levels of miRNAs (*n* = 18).

	IGF-1		Testosterone		Cortisol		Testosterone/ Cortisol		Peak Power of Sprint 1		Average Power of Sprint 1		Peak Power Ratio of Sprint1/Sprint2		Fatigue Index	
	r	*P*	*r*	*P*	*r*	*P*	*r*	*P*	*r*	*P*	*r*	*P*	*r*	*P*	*r*	*P*
miR-1	−0.101	ns	−0.060	ns	−0.111	ns	0.165	ns	0.410	ns	−0.018	ns	−0.057	ns	0.201	ns
miR-133a	−0.379	ns	0.078	ns	−0.155	ns	0.060	ns	0.441	ns	−0.145	ns	−0.078	ns	−0.087	ns
miR-133b	−0.179	ns	0.086	ns	0.284	ns	−0.118	ns	0.712	0.001	0.076	ns	−0.053	ns	−0.059	ns
miR-122	−0.045	ns	0.023	ns	0.037	ns	0.009	ns	0.257	ns	−0.132	ns	0.655	0.003	0.012	ns
miR-16	0.066	ns	−0.137	ns	−0.143	ns	0.102	ns	0.189	ns	0.050	ns	−0.104	ns	0.096	ns

ns, not significant.

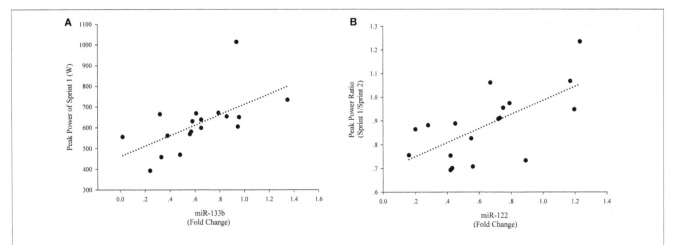

FIGURE 4 | Correlations of plasma miRNAs and exercise-related anaerobic parameters. For each participant, baseline c-miRNAs levels before the exercise were assigned a fold change of 1, to which measurements obtained after the exercise were compared. A direct correlation was observed between levels of peak power of Sprint 1 and levels of plasma miR-133b (Post exercise) **(A)** A direct correlation was also observed between the peak power ratio of Sprint 1/Sprint 2 and levels of miR-122 (Post exercise) **(B)**.

in liver development, differentiation, homeostasis, and metabolic function (Bandiera et al., 2015). The peroxisome proliferator-activated receptor (PPAR) γ coactivator 1-α (PGC-1α) plays a pivotal role in the regulation of the expression of mitochondrial proteins cytochrome c and cytochrome oxidase subunit I in the liver in response to a single exercise bout (Haase et al., 2011). Exercise induced beneficial alterations in the liver mitochondrial morphology and increased mitochondrial biogenesis (PGC-1α and mitochondrial transcription factor A) (Santos-Alves et al., 2015), and liver AMP-activated protein kinase (AMPK) activity increased during heavy exercise (Carlson and Winder, 1999). The putative effectors of miR-122-mediated metabolic control in the liver may be involved in both circadian metabolic regulators of the PPAR family and AMPK (Bandiera et al., 2015). Thus, the currently observed decrease of circulating miR-122 might reflect a liver cellular temporal regulation controlled by miRNAs during exercise. In addition, circulating miR-16 level also decreased, suggesting that non-muscle tissue is also needed to cope with this stress.

Exercise is a potent stimulus for the release of many hormones in response to the specific demands of the particular exercise type (Stokes et al., 2013). Changes in the anabolic-catabolic hormonal balance were found following brief sprint interval exercise training, may be used to gauge training adaptation to different anaerobic exercises (Kraemer and Ratamess, 2005; Meckel et al., 2011). But in the present study, there was no significant correlation between the change in these plasma hormone levels and the change in the c-miRNAs levels. Given their different physiological roles, it is likely that the c-miRNAs would show different expression patterns induced by SIC. However, in our study a negative correlation was observed between the reduced magnitudes in miR-133b and peak power and between the reduced magnitudes in miR-122 and the ability to maintain anaerobic power. In this case, the reduction in miR-133b and miR-122 in circulation may be considered a biomarker that reflects internal physiological stress caused by SIC.

At present, the mechanism(s) and clinical significance of an exercise-induced decrease in specific c-miRNAs remains poorly understood. An exercise-induced miRNA uptake by certain recipient cells has been postulated (Aoi et al., 2013; Aoi and Sakuma, 2014). Given the transportability of vesicles, the role of miRNAs in exosomes is gaining increasing attention. In the present study, high-intensity exercise may destroy exosomes, leading to degradation of miRNAs by RNases. However, the miR-206 and miR-499 in circulation remained unchanged, suggesting that significant degradation of exosomes did not occur as a result of SIC (Aoi et al., 2013; Aoi and Sakuma, 2014). The miRNAs in the exosomes are selectively packaged rather than included indiscriminately (Etheridge et al., 2013; Zhang et al., 2015). Moreover, the exosomal miRNA expression levels are altered under different physiological conditions (Etheridge et al., 2013; Zhang et al., 2015). It is reasonable to consider that acute high-intensity exercise may promote the uptake of some c-miRNAs into certain recipient cells (Aoi et al., 2013; Aoi and Sakuma, 2014). Further investigation is required to validate this hypothesis.

In conclusion, our data demonstrate that extreme sprint interval cycling affects the expression patterns of plasma miRNAs. Selective c-miRNAs, such as miR-133b and miR-122, may be potentially suitable for use as novel biomarkers to monitor training-induced acute changes within diverse tissues in response to low-volume sprint interval cycling.

AUTHOR CONTRIBUTIONS

SC designed the study, performed the experiments, collected and analyzed the data, and revised the final version of the manuscript. WL and JN recruited participants, collected samples and performed the experiments. CZ and XC designed the study and critically revised the final version of the manuscript. JM designed the study, recruited participants, analyzed the data and wrote the final version of the manuscript. All authors read and approved the final version of the manuscript.

FUNDING

The authors acknowledge that this work was supported by the National Basic Research Program of China (2014CB542300), the National Natural Science Foundation of China (81101330, 31271378, 81250044), the Natural Science Foundation of Jiangsu Province (BK2012014) and the Research Special Fund for Public Welfare Industry of Health (201302018). This work was also supported by the Program for New Century Excellent Talents in University from Ministry of Education of China (NCET-12-0261).

REFERENCES

Aoi, W., Ichikawa, H., Mune, K., Tanimura, Y., Mizushima, K., Naito, Y., et al. (2013). Muscle-enriched microRNA miR-486 decreases in circulation in response to exercise in young men. Front. Physiol. 4:80. doi: 10.3389/fphys.2013.00080

Aoi, W., and Sakuma, K. (2014). Does regulation of skeletal muscle function involve circulating microRNAs? Front. Physiol. 5:39. doi: 10.3389/fphys.2014.00039

Baggish, A. L., Hale, A., Weiner, R. B., Lewis, G. D., Systrom, D., Wang, F., et al. (2011). Dynamic regulation of circulating microRNA during acute exhaustive exercise and sustained aerobic exercise training. J. Physiol. 589, 3983–3994. doi: 10.1113/jphysiol.2011.213363

Baggish, A. L., Park, J., Min, P. K., Isaacs, S., Parker, B. A., Thompson, P. D., et al. (2014). Rapid upregulation and clearance of distinct circulating microRNAs after prolonged aerobic exercise. J. Appl. Physiol. (1985) 116, 522–531. doi: 10.1152/japplphysiol.01141.2013

Bandiera, S., Pfeffer, S., Baumert, T. F., and Zeisel, M. B. (2015). miR-122–a key factor and therapeutic target in liver disease. J. Hepatol. 62, 448–457. doi: 10.1016/j.jhep.2014.10.004

Banzet, S., Chennaoui, M., Girard, O., Racinais, S., Drogou, C., Chalabi, H., et al. (2013). Changes in circulating microRNAs levels with exercise modality. J. Appl. Physiol. (1985) 115, 1237–1244. doi: 10.1152/japplphysiol.00075.2013

Bartel, D. P. (2004). MicroRNAs: genomics, biogenesis, mechanism, and function. Cell 116, 281–297. doi: 10.1016/S0092-8674(04)00045-5

Boettger, T., Wüst, S., Nolte, H., and Braun, T. (2014). The miR-206/133b cluster is dispensable for development, survival and regeneration of skeletal muscle. Skelet. Muscle 4, 23. doi: 10.1186/s13395-014-0023-5

Buchheit, M., and Laursen, P. B. (2013). High-intensity interval training, solutions to the programming puzzle. Part II: anaerobic energy, neuromuscular load and practical applications. Sports Med. 43, 927–954. doi: 10.1007/s40279-013-0066-5

Burgomaster, K. A., Hughes, S. C., Heigenhauser, G. J., Bradwell, S. N., and Gibala, M. J. (2005). Six sessions of sprint interval training increases muscle oxidative potential and cycle endurance capacity in humans. J. Appl. Physiol. (1985) 98, 1985–1990. doi: 10.1152/japplphysiol.01095.2004

Carlson, C. L., and Winder, W. W. (1999). Liver AMP-activated protein kinase and acetyl-CoA carboxylase during and after exercise. J. Appl. Physiol. (1985) 86, 669–674.

Chen, X., Liang, H., Guan, D., Wang, C., Hu, X., Cui, L., et al. (2013). A combination of Let-7d, Let-7g and Let-7i serves as a stable reference for normalization of serum microRNAs. PLoS ONE 8:e79652. doi: 10.1371/journal.pone.0079652

de Gonzalo-Calvo, D., Dávalos, A., Montero, A., García-González, Á., Tyshkovska, I., Gonzalez-Medina, A., et al. (2015). Circulating inflammatory miRNA signature in response to different doses of aerobic exercise. J. Appl. Physiol. (1985) 119, 124–134. doi: 10.1152/japplphysiol.00077.2015

Etheridge, A., Gomes, C. P., Pereira, R. W., Galas, D., and Wang, K. (2013). The complexity, function and applications of RNA in circulation. Front. Genet. 4:115. doi: 10.3389/fgene.2013.00115

Gan, Z., Rumsey, J., Hazen, B. C., Lai, L., Leone, T. C., Vega, R. B., et al. (2013). Nuclear receptor/microRNA circuitry links muscle fiber type to energy metabolism. J. Clin. Invest. 123, 2564–2575. doi: 10.1172/JCI67652

Gibala, M. J., Little, J. P., Macdonald, M. J., and Hawley, J. A. (2012). Physiological adaptations to low-volume, high-intensity interval training in health and disease. J. Physiol. 590, 1077–1084. doi: 10.1113/jphysiol.2011.224725

Gomes, C. P., Oliveira-Jr, G. P., Madrid, B., Almeida, J. A., Franco, O. L., and Pereira, R. W. (2014). Circulating miR-1, miR-133a, and miR-206 levels are increased after a half-marathon run. Biomarkers 19, 585–589. doi: 10.3109/1354750X.2014.952663

Haase, T. N., Ringholm, S., Leick, L., Biensø, R. S., Kiilerich, K., Johansen, S., et al. (2011). Role of PGC-1alpha in exercise and fasting-induced adaptations in mouse liver. Am. J. Physiol. Regul. Integr. Comp. Physiol. 301, R1501–R1509. doi: 10.1152/ajpregu.00775.2010

Kraemer, W. J., and Ratamess, N. A. (2005). Hormonal responses and adaptations to resistance exercise and training. Sports Med. 35, 339–361. doi: 10.2165/00007256-200535040-00004

Laursen, P. B. (2010). Training for intense exercise performance: high-intensity or high-volume training? Scand. J. Med. Sci. Sports 20(Suppl. 2), 1–10. doi: 10.1111/j.1600-0838.2010.01184.x

Liu, R., Zhang, C., Hu, Z., Li, G., Wang, C., Yang, C., et al. (2011). A five-microRNA signature identified from genome-wide serum microRNA expression profiling serves as a fingerprint for gastric cancer diagnosis. *Eur. J. Cancer* 47, 784–791. doi: 10.1016/j.ejca.2010.10.025

McCarthy, J. J., and Esser, K. A. (2007). MicroRNA-1 and microRNA-133a expression are decreased during skeletal muscle hypertrophy. *J. Appl. Physiol.* *(1985)* 102, 306–313. doi: 10.1152/japplphysiol.00932.2006

Meckel, Y., Nemet, D., Bar-Sela, S., Radom-Aizik, S., Cooper, D. M., Sagiv, M., et al. (2011). Hormonal and inflammatory responses to different types of sprint interval training. *J. Strength Cond. Res.* 25, 2161–2169. doi: 10.1519/JSC.0b013e3181dc4571

Mooren, F. C., Viereck, J., Krüger, K., and Thum, T. (2014). Circulating microRNAs as potential biomarkers of aerobic exercise capacity. *Am. J. Physiol. Heart Circ. Physiol.* 306, H557–H563. doi: 10.1152/ajpheart.00711.2013

Nielsen, S., Scheele, C., Yfanti, C., Akerström, T., Nielsen, A. R., Pedersen, B. K., et al. (2010). Muscle specific microRNAs are regulated by endurance exercise in human skeletal muscle. *J. Physiol.* 588, 4029–4037. doi: 10.1113/jphysiol.2010.189860

Roberts, T. C., Godfrey, C., McClorey, G., Vader, P., Briggs, D., Gardiner, C., et al. (2013). Extracellular microRNAs are dynamic non-vesicular biomarkers of muscle turnover. *Nucleic Acids Res.* 41, 9500–9513. doi: 10.1093/nar/gkt724

Santos-Alves, E., Marques-Aleixo, I., Rizo-Roca, D., Torrella, J. R., Oliveira, P. J., Magalhães, J., et al. (2015). Exercise modulates liver cellular and mitochondrial proteins related to quality control signaling. *Life Sci.* 135, 124–130. doi: 10.1016/j.lfs.2015.06.007

Schoenfeld, B. J. (2012). Does exercise-induced muscle damage play a role in skeletal muscle hypertrophy? *J. Strength Cond. Res.* 26, 1441–1453. doi: 10.1519/JSC.0b013e31824f207e

Søndergaard, M. T., Sorensen, A. B., Skov, L. L., Kjaer-Sorensen, K., Bauer, M. C., Nyegaard, M., et al. (2015). Calmodulin mutations causing catecholaminergic polymorphic ventricular tachycardia confer opposing functional and biophysical molecular changes. *FEBS J.* 282, 803–816. doi: 10.1111/febs.13184

Spencer, M., Bishop, D., Dawson, B., and Goodman, C. (2005). Physiological and metabolic responses of repeated-sprint activities:specific to field-based team sports. *Sports Med.* 35, 1025–1044. doi: 10.2165/00007256-200535120-00003

Stokes, K. A., Gilbert, K. L., Hall, G. M., Andrews, R. C., and Thompson, D. (2013). Different responses of selected hormones to three types of exercise in young men. *Eur. J. Appl. Physiol.* 113, 775–783. doi: 10.1007/s00421-012-2487-5

Sun, L., Sun, S., Zeng, S., Li, Y., Pan, W., and Zhang, Z. (2015). Expression of circulating microRNA-1 and microRNA-133 in pediatric patients with tachycardia. *Mol. Med. Rep.* 11, 4039–4046. doi: 10.3892/mmr.2015.3246

Terentyev, D., Belevych, A. E., Terentyeva, R., Martin, M. M., Malana, G. E., Kuhn, D. E., et al. (2009). miR-1 overexpression enhances Ca(2+) release and promotes cardiac arrhythmogenesis by targeting PP2A regulatory subunit B56alpha and causing CaMKII-dependent hyperphosphorylation of RyR2. *Circ. Res.* 104, 514–521. doi: 10.1161/CIRCRESAHA.108.181651

Trappe, S., Luden, N., Minchev, K., Raue, U., Jemiolo, B., and Trappe, T. A. (2015). Skeletal muscle signature of a champion sprint runner. *J. Appl. Physiol. (1985)* 118, 1460–1466. doi: 10.1152/japplphysiol.00037.2015

Uhlemann, M., Möbius-Winkler, S., Fikenzer, S., Adam, J., Redlich, M., Möhlenkamp, S., et al. (2014). Circulating microRNA-126 increases after different forms of endurance exercise in healthy adults. *Eur. J. Prev. Cardiol.* 21, 484–491. doi: 10.1177/2047487312467902

Weston, K. S., Wisløff, U., and Coombes, J. S. (2014). High-intensity interval training in patients with lifestyle-induced cardiometabolic disease: a systematic review and meta-analysis. *Br. J. Sports Med.* 48, 1227–1234. doi: 10.1136/bjsports-2013-092576

Wu, C., Wang, C., Guan, X., Liu, Y., Li, D., Zhou, X., et al. (2014). Diagnostic and prognostic implications of a serum miRNA panel in oesophageal squamous cell carcinoma. *PLoS ONE* 9:e92292. doi: 10.1371/journal.pone.0092292

Zhang, J., Li, S., Li, L., Li, M., Guo, C., Yao, J., et al. (2015). Exosome and exosomal microRNA: trafficking, sorting, and function. *Genomics Proteomics Bioinformatics* 13, 17–24. doi: 10.1016/j.gpb.2015.02.001

Conflict of Interest Statement: The authors declare that the research was conducted in the absence of any commercial or financial relationships that could be construed as a potential conflict of interest.

11

Individualized Internal and External Training Load Relationships in Elite Wheelchair Rugby Players

Thomas A. W. Paulson*, Barry Mason, James Rhodes and Victoria L. Goosey-Tolfrey

The Peter Harrison Centre for Disability Sport, School of Sport, Exercise and Health Sciences, Loughborough University, Loughborough, UK

Aim: The quantification and longitudinal monitoring of athlete training load (TL) provides a scientific explanation for changes in performance and helps manage injury/illness risk. Therefore, accurate and reliable monitoring tools are essential for the optimization of athletic performance. The aim of the present study was to establish the relationship between measures of internal [heart rate (HR) and session RPE (sRPE)] and external TL specific to wheelchair rugby (WR).

Methods: Fourteen international WR athletes (age $= 29 \pm 7$ years; body mass $= 58.9 \pm 10.9$ kg) were monitored during 18 training sessions over a 3 month period during the competitive phase of the season. Activity profiles were collected during each training session using a radio-frequency based indoor tracking system (ITS). External TL was quantified by total distance (m) covered as well as time spent and distance covered in a range of classification-specific arbitrary speed zones. Banister's TRIMP, Edwards's summated HR zone (SHRZ), and Lucia's TRIMP methods were used to quantify physiological internal TL. sRPE was calculated as the product of session duration multiplied by perceived exertion using the Borg CR10 scale. Relationships between external and internal TL were examined using correlation coefficients and the 90% confidence intervals (90% CI).

Results: sRPE ($r = 0.59$) and all HR-based ($r > 0.80$) methods showed large and very large relationships with the total distance covered during training sessions, respectively. Large and very large correlations ($r = 0.56 - 0.82$) were also observed between all measures of internal TL and times spent and distances covered in low and moderate intensity speed zones. HR-based methods showed very large relationships with time ($r = 0.71 - 0.75$) and distance ($r = 0.70 - 0.73$) in the very high speed zone and a large relationship with the number of high intensity activities (HIA) performed ($r = 0.56 - 0.62$). Weaker relationships ($r = 0.32 - 0.35$) were observed between sRPE and all measures of high intensity activity. A large variation of individual correlation co-efficient was observed between sRPE and all external TL measures.

Conclusion: The current findings suggest that sRPE and HR-based internal TL measures provide a valid tool for quantifying volume of external TL during WR training but may underestimate HIA. It is recommended that both internal and external TL measures are employed for the monitoring of overall TL during court-based training in elite WR athletes.

Keywords: paralympic, performance, perceived exertion, exercise prescription, heart rate, speed zones

Edited by:
Davide Malatesta,
Université de Lausanne, Switzerland

Reviewed by:
Melissa L. Bates,
University of Wisconsin–Madison, USA
Gianluca Vernillo,
University of Milan, Italy
Matthew Weston,
Teesside University, UK

*Correspondence:
Thomas A. W. Paulson
t.paulson@lboro.ac.uk

INTRODUCTION

Coaches and sports science practitioners continue to take an increasingly scientific approach to the prescription and monitoring of athlete training (Malone et al., 2015; McLaren et al., 2015). The longitudinal monitoring of individual training load (TL) provides a quantifiable explanation for changes in performance, ensures target doses are achieved, and helps manage illness/injury risk. External TL describes the work completed by the athlete in terms of distance, speed or power using micro-technologies including time-motion analysis, accelerometers or power-meters, respectively (Lambert and Borresen, 2010; Halson, 2014; McLaren et al., 2015). The resultant physiological or psychological stress imposed, described as internal TL, drives adaptation in the relevant metabolic, cardiovascular and neurological systems (Halson, 2014). The outcome of any training intervention is therefore the consequence of both external and internal stimuli and reliable monitoring tools are vital for the optimization of athletic performance.

Like basketball and its wheelchair-based equivalent, wheelchair rugby (WR) is a court-based, intermittent sport characterized by frequent high intensity accelerations and decelerations (Barfield et al., 2010; Rhodes et al., 2015a). Eligibility for WR classification requires a functional impairment in all four limbs and encompasses a range of physical impairments including cervical level spinal cord injury (SCI), amputees, and cerebral palsy. Recently a novel radio-frequency based indoor tracking system (ITS) has been employed to quantify the external demands of competition (Rhodes et al., 2015a) and key determinants of successful performance during WR match-play (Rhodes et al., 2015b). Athletes typically cover distances ranging between 3500–4600 m during matches (Sarro et al., 2010; Rhodes et al., 2015a) with the majority of time spent (~75%) performing low intensity activities interspersed with short, frequent bouts of high intensity activity (Rhodes et al., 2015a). The ability to reach high peak speeds and perform a greater number of high intensity activities (HIA) are key indicators of mobility associated with successful performance, as determined by team rank (Rhodes et al., 2015b).

WR squads are characterized by a large heterogeneity in athlete impairment which may result in a range of internal TL responses to the same dose of external load. Yet, training within a team sport environment is frequently prescribed on a squad-basis to develop sport-specific, technical, and tactical competences, thereby increasing the risk of non-functional over-reaching or under-training. Currently no research has investigated the use of internal TL measures during WR training in relation to commonly used measures of external TL. Barfield et al. (2010) attempted to quantify the exercise intensity of WR training sessions for a group of athletes with a cervical SCI using heart rate (HR) as a measure of internal load. However, HR is considered an ineffective tool for monitoring TL in some athletes with a cervical level SCI due the reduction in maximal HR responses (120–150 bpm^{-1}) associated with impaired autonomic function (Valent et al., 2007; Paulson et al., 2013). An increasing number of non-SCI athletes now compete in WR, therefore, HR-based methods

maybe suitable for these individuals. Banister's TRIMP, Edwards' summated HR zone (SHRZ), and Lucia's TRIMP are HR-based methods that have been utilized to quantify physiological load in able-bodied sports (Banister, 1991; Edwards, 1993; Lucia et al., 2003; Waldron et al., 2011; Scanlan et al., 2014). However, the use of these HR-based methods in intermittent sports may underestimate near maximal short high and very high intensity efforts due to the heavy reliance on anaerobic metabolism (Alexiou and Coutts, 2008; Akubat and Abt, 2011).

The session rating of perceived exertion (sRPE) provides an alternative method of quantifying internal TL, which describes a subjective, global rating of intensity and is the product of training duration, and perceived exertion using Borgs CR10 scale (Borg, 1998; Foster et al., 2001). Very large linear relationships are observed between HR and RPE-based methods in field and indoor intermittent sports supporting sRPE as a valid alternative for the quantification of internal TL (Impellizzeri et al., 2004; Manzi et al., 2010; Waldron et al., 2011; Scott et al., 2013; Lupo et al., 2014; Scanlan et al., 2014). Lovell et al. (2013) and Scott et al. (2013) have also observed large relationships between sRPE and external TL indices, including total distance covered, during elite Rugby League and Football training, respectively. In contrast, Weston et al. (2015) report only small relationships between overall match RPE and GPS-derived measures of external load in Australian League Football. Currently no "gold standard" method currently exists for the quantification of internal TL during high intensity/intermittent activities representative of WR. The aim of this study was to establish the relationship between traditional measures of internal TL (HR and sRPE) and external TL measures specific to WR.

METHODS

Participants

Fourteen international WR players (age = 29 ± 7 years; body mass = 58.9 ± 10.9 kg; time in sport = 9 ± 2 years; training hours = 9 ± 2 h.wk^{-1}; n = 1 female) with a cervical SCI (n = 9) and non-SCI (n = 5) volunteered to participate in the current study. Ethical approval for the study was obtained through Loughborough University's ethics committee. Prior to participation, all players provided their written, informed consent.

Design

The study employed a single cohort observation with data collected during a total of 18 WR training sessions performed over a 3 month period during the competitive phase of the season. Prior to the training phase all participants performed an initial laboratory exercise test for the determination of resting (HR$_{rest}$) and peak (HR$_{peak}$) HR and peak oxygen uptake ($\dot{V}O_{2peak}$). During training sessions external and internal TL data were collected for all athletes using the ITS and sRPE, respectively. HR was only collected during training from the non-SCI players. All training sessions were performed at the same indoor venue on wooden sprung flooring. Data were only analyzed for individuals completing whole training sessions.

Submaximal Test and Graded-Exercise Test to Exhaustion (GXT)

HR_{rest} was determined following a 10-min rest in a semi-supine position using radio telemetry (Polar PE 4000, Kempele, Finland). All participants' performed the tests in their competition sports wheelchair on a motorized treadmill (HP Cosmos, Traunstein, Germany). The submaximal test and GXT were performed according to the protocols described by Leicht et al. (2012). Briefly, participants performed six to eight submaximal constant-load 4-min exercise blocks at ascending speeds at a fixed gradient of 1.0%, in order to elicit physiological responses covering a range from 40 to 80% $\dot{V}O_{2peak}$ (Leicht et al., 2012). This was followed by a 15-min passive recovery. The gradient at the start of the GXT was 1.0% with subsequent increases of 0.1% every 40 s to ensure a minimum GXT duration of $\sim$8 min. After the GXT, participants recovered actively at a low intensity (1.2 ms^{-1}) at a 1.0% gradient for 5 min. Participants then performed a verification test, designed as a test to exhaustion at the same constant speed but 0.1% higher than the maximal gradient achieved during the GXT. The GXT and the verification test were terminated when participants were unable to maintain the speed of the treadmill. HR was measured throughout the test with the highest 5 s rolling average used to establish HR_{peak}. On-line respiratory gas analysis was carried out throughout the GXT and verification stage via a breath-by-breath system (Cortex metalyser 3B, Cortex, Leipzig, Germany). Before the test, gases were calibrated according to the manufacturer's recommendations using a 2-point calibration ($O_2 = 17.0\%$, $CO_2 = 5.0\%$ against room air) and volumes with a 3-L syringe at flow rates of 0.5–3.0 L·s^{-1}. Breath-by-breath data allowed the highest 30 s rolling average $\dot{V}O_2$ value recorded and was taken as the $\dot{V}O_{2peak}$.

External TL

Activity profiles were quantified during each training session using a radio-frequency based ITS (Ubisense, Cambridge, UK) described previously (Rhodes et al., 2014; Perrat et al., 2015). Each participant was equipped with a small lightweight tag (25 g), which was attached on or near the foot-strap of athletes own rugby wheelchairs. Tags communicate wirelessly at a frequency of 8 Hz via ultra wideband radio signals with six sensors elevated around the perimeter of the court (28 $\times$ 15 m) to provide time and location data in three dimensions. The reliability of tags operating at this sampling frequency range between a coefficient of variation of 0.5% for distance covered and mean speed reached and never exceeded 2.0% for peak speed detection (Rhodes et al., 2014).

External TL was quantified by the total distance (m) covered during each training session. The time spent and distance covered in a range of classification-specific arbitrary speed zones, determined by the mean, peak speed (V_{max}) of each class, as previously defined by Rhodes et al. (2015a) were also reported. These speed zones were based on a percentage of the peak speed (%V_{max}) for each classification group and were categorized as the following intensities: zone 1 = very low speed ($\leq$20%V_{max}), zone 2 = low speed (21–50%V_{max}), zone 3 = moderate speed (51–80%V_{max}), zone 4 = high speed (81–95%V_{max}), and zone 5 = very high speed ($>$95%V_{max}). The number of HIA, as defined by the frequency of bouts performed in both high and very high speed zones, were also recorded.

Internal TL
HR-Based Methods

During training HR was collected via a Polar team system (Polar Team^2, Kempele, Finland) sampling at 5 s intervals. This HR data were incorporated into the Banister's TRIMP (Banister, 1991), Edwards SHRZ (Edwards, 1993) and Lucia's TRIMP to provide physiological measures of internal TL and are quantified in arbitrary units (AU). Banisters' TRIMP combines predetermined, individualized HR_{peak} and HR_{rest} measures, as well as the average HR during training (HR_{ex}). The activity intensity is weighted using a fixed exponential relationship between changes in HR and blood lactate concentration during incremental exercise (Banister, 1991). The formula to determine TL in males using the TRIMP model proposed by Banister is as follows:

$$TRIMP\ training\ load\ (AU) = [duration\ (min)](HR_{ex} - HR_{rest})/$$
$$(HR_{peak} - HR_{rest}) \times 0.64e^{1.92x}$$
$$where \quad e = 2.712, and\ x = (HR_{ex} - HR_{rest})/$$
$$(HR_{peak} - HR_{rest}).$$

The SHRZ model proposed by Edwards determines internal TL by multiplying the accumulated training duration in five discrete HR zones relative to HR_{peak} by a coefficient relative to each zone and summating the results. The formula to determine TL using the SHRZ model is represented as:

$$SHRZ\ training\ load\ (AU) = (duration\ in\ zone\ 1 \times 1)$$
$$+(duration\ in\ zone\ 2 \times 2)$$
$$+(duration\ in\ zone\ 3 \times 3)$$
$$+(duration\ in\ zone\ 4 \times 4)$$
$$+(duration\ in\ zone\ 5 \times 5)$$
$$where \quad zone\ 1 - 50 - 60\% HR_{peak};$$
$$zone\ 2 = 60 - 70\% HR_{peak};$$
$$zone\ 3 = 70 - 80\% HR_{peak};$$
$$zone\ 4 = 80 - 90\% HR_{peak};$$
$$and \quad zone\ 5 = 90 - 100\% HR_{peak}.$$

Lucia's TRIMP method was calculated by multiplying the time spent in three different HR zones (zone 1 = below the ventilatory threshold, zone 2 = between the ventilatory threshold and the compensation point, zone 3 = above the respiratory compensation point) by a co-efficient for each zone (zone 1 = 1, zone 2 = 2, zone 3 = 3) and summating the results. HR zones are therefore defined on individual parameters obtained in the laboratory (Lucia et al., 2003). Lactate thresholds were employed as previously indicated (Impellizzeri et al., 2004) due to the more frequent threshold determination using BLa over ventilatory data in wheelchair athletes reported by Leicht et al. (2014).

Session RPE

The session RPE represents a single global rating of the intensity of a training session as described previously by Foster et al. (2001). Prior to the study all training participants were familiarized with the Borg CR10 scales and the associated verbal anchors (Borg, 1998). Within 30 min of a training session being completed participants were shown the scale and asked to provide a rating of the overall perceived intensity of the session. The sRPE was then calculated by multiplying the duration of the session in minutes by the individual RPE for that training session and was again presented as AU.

Statistical Analyses

Participants completing <5 training sessions were excluded from the statistical analysis leaving a total number of 78 observations from nine participants ($n = 6$ cervical SCI). All data were analyzed using the Statistical package for the Social Sciences (SPSS version 21.0, Chicago, Illinois, USA). The mean ± SD were calculated for each measure of external and internal TL. A within-measures design was used to determine if high internal load measures (Banister's, Edwards, Lucia's, sRPE) were associated with higher ITS-derived TL measures for the whole group as described previously (Bland and Altman, 1995). Confidence intervals (90% CI) for the within-player correlations were calculated. Individual relationships between external and internal TL measures were examined using Pearson correlation coefficients and the 90% CI. The magnitude of all correlations were categorized as trivial ($r < 0.1$), small ($r = 0.1$–0.3), moderate ($r = 0.3$–0.5), large (0.5–0.7), very large ($r = 0.7$–0.9), nearly perfect ($r > 0.9$), and perfect ($r = 1$; Hopkins et al., 2009). Statistical significance was set at $P < 0.05$.

RESULTS

The mean duration of all training sessions was 143 ± 40 min and ranged from 84 to 230 min. The mean external load measures of all training sessions are presented in **Table 1**. Mean internal TL was 97 ± 38 AU (Banisters), 310 ± 119 AU (Edwards), 247 ± 74 (Lucia's), and 934 ± 359 AU (sRPE). A large correlation was found between sRPE and both Banisters TRIMP ($r = 0.62$), Edwards SHRZ ($r = 0.64$). In addition, a very large correlation was found between sRPE and Lucia's TRIMP ($r = 0.81$).

HR and sRPE-based methods of internal TL showed a very large and large correlation with the total distance covered during training sessions, respectively. **Table 2** demonstrates the relationship between measures of external TL associated with exercise intensity and internal TL. Very large correlations were observed between Banisters TRIMP, Edwards SHRZ and Lucia's TRIMP and the times spent and distances covered in speed zones 2, 3, and 5. Large, significant correlations were observed between sRPE and the time spent and distance covered in zones 2 and 3. All HR-based methods demonstrated a large relationship (0.56–0.62) with the number of HIA performed. No significant correlation was identified between the number of HIA performed and sRPE.

Individual correlation coefficients between sRPE and measures of external TL are presented in Table 3. The only measures of external TL that demonstrated a positive correlation with sRPE for all individuals were the times spent in speed zone 2 and the distances covered in speed zones 1 and 2.

DISCUSSION

The individualization of athlete training is vital to optimize physical preparation within a team environment. Reliable and valid tools are required to accurately quantify intermittent, court-based TL involving athletes with the range of physical impairments displayed in WR. An interesting finding of the current study was the large relationships between all internal TL measures and total distance covered during training as previously observed in the able-bodied sports of elite football (Casamichana et al., 2013; Scott et al., 2013) and rugby league (Lovell et al., 2013). All internal TL measures demonstrated large or very large correlations with time spent and distance covered in speed zones 2 (low) and 3 (moderate). Also in accordance with previous findings (Casamichana et al., 2013; Scott et al., 2013), weaker relationships were observed between internal TL and external TL measures of high intensity training, including the number of HIA performed. The current observations suggest sRPE and HR-based measures of internal TL provide a valid tool for quantifying volume measures of external TL during WR training but sRPE may underestimate high intensity training doses. Large ranges in within-individual sRPE-external TL relationships suggest a variety of perceptual cues are responsible for determining sRPE during WR training. It is recommended that both internal and external TL measures are employed for the monitoring of overall TL during court-based training in elite WR athletes.

Coaches and Sport Science practitioners prescribe external TLs to replicate or exceed competition intensities and induce physiological and/or psychological stress (i.e. internal TL) that drives subsequent training adaptation. The use of HR in intermittent sports is less straightforward than for endurance/aerobic-based sports, due to the heavy reliance on

TABLE 1 | Descriptive statistics of external load measures during wheelchair rugby training sessions measured by the ITS ($n = 9$).

	Mean (SD)	Range	% of training session
Total distance (m)	4511 (1666)	1678–8694	–
Time in Zone 1	24:23 (12:13)	05:27–52:51	38.4
Time in Zone 2	24:05 (11:01)	07:41–54:21	38.0
Time in Zone 3	11:49 (04:08)	04:02–25:12	18.6
Time in Zone 4	02:23 (01:22)	00:34–06:00	3.8
Time in Zone 5	00:38 (00:33)	00:00–02:46	1.0
Distance in Zone 1	458 (193)	113–962	10.2
Distance in Zone 2	1781 (851)	589–4113	39.5
Distance in Zone 3	1655 (597)	569–3463	36.7
Distance in Zone 4	462 (269)	107–1164	10.2
Distance in Zone 5	147 (134)	0–674	3.3
HIA (n)	53 (29)	14–127	–

All distances (m) and times (mm:ss).

TABLE 2 | Within-individual correlation coefficients (90% confidence interval) for relationship between intensity measures of external load and internal training load.

External load	Internal load			
	Banisters TRIMP ($n = 31$)	Edwards SHRZ ($n = 31$)	Lucias TRIMP ($n = 31$)	sRPE ($n = 78$)
Total Distance	0.81** (0.67–0.89)	0.84** (0.72–0.91)	0.82** (0.69–0.90)	0.59* (0.47–0.70)
Time in Zone 1	0.37 (0.08–0.60)	0.40 (0.22–0.63)	0.39 (0.10–0.62)	0.37 (0.20–0.53)
Time in Zone 2	0.85* (0.74–0.92)	0.87** (0.77–0.93)	0.83** (0.69–0.90)	0.56* (0.42–0.68)
Time in Zone 3	0.66* (0.46–0.81)	0.72** (0.53–0.84)	0.75** (0.59–0.86)	0.59* (0.45–0.70)
Time in Zone 4	0.41 (0.12–0.63)	0.41 (0.13–0.63)	0.37 (0.08–0.60)	0.22 (0.03–0.39)
Time in Zone 5	0.75** (0.58–0.86)	0.75** (0.57–0.85)	0.71** (0.52–0.83)	0.33 (0.15–0.49)
Distance in Zone 1	0.52* (0.26–0.71)	0.52* (0.26–0.71)	0.51* (0.25–0.71)	0.45 (0.28–0.59)
Distance in Zone 2	0.82** (0.69–0.90)	0.84** (0.72–0.91)	0.81** (0.67–0.89)	0.56* (0.42–0.68)
Distance in Zone 3	0.67* (0.46–0.81)	0.72** (0.53–0.84)	0.74** (0.56–0.85)	0.58* (0.55–0.69)
Distance in Zone 4	0.43 (0.15–0.65)	0.43 (0.15–0.65)	0.39 (0.10–0.62)	0.22 (0.03–0.39)
Distance in Zone 5	0.72** (0.53–0.84)	0.73** (0.54–0.84)	0.70* (0.10–0.62)	0.35 (0.18–0.51)
No. of HIA	0.62* (0.39–0.78)	0.61* (0.38–0.77)	0.56* (0.50–0.83)	0.32 (0.14–0.48)

*Large within-individual correlation ($r = 0.5–0.7$).
**Very large within-individual correlation ($r = 0.7–0.9$).

TABLE 3 | Individual correlation coefficients between sRPE and measures of external training load.

Participant			Time in speed zones					Distance in speed zones					
	n	TD	1	2	3	4	5	1	2	3	4	5	HIA
1	8	0.44	0.81	0.65	−0.22	−0.43	0.32	0.80	0.63	−0.25	−0.42	0.29	−0.54
2	11	0.52	0.50	0.46	0.54	0.04	0.44	0.59	0.41	0.55	0.04	0.53	0.07
3	7	−0.03	0.62	0.43	−0.03	−0.69	0.12	0.42	0.41	−0.28	−0.69	0.02	−0.70
4	8	0.82	0.26	0.79	0.77	0.76	0.82	0.27	0.79	0.79	0.77	0.78	0.72
5	7	0.39	0.49	0.62	0.46	−0.58	−0.13	0.56	0.58	0.40	−0.58	0.06	−0.55
6	7	0.61	0.83	0.71	0.47	−0.39	0.60	0.81	0.72	0.43	−0.40	0.62	−0.09
7	16	0.38	0.23	0.24	0.56	0.04	−0.08	0.19	0.25	0.57	0.04	−0.05	0.17
8	9	0.70	0.71	0.74	0.55	0.28	0.33	0.72	0.73	0.43	0.25	0.33	0.16
9	5	0.82	0.97	0.67	0.68	0.85	0.67	0.96	0.67	0.69	0.83	0.67	0.68
Min	5	−0.03	0.23	0.24	−0.22	−0.69	−0.13	0.19	0.25	−0.28	−0.69	−0.05	−0.70
Max	16	0.82	0.97	0.79	0.77	0.85	0.82	0.96	0.79	0.79	0.83	0.78	0.72
Range	11	0.85	0.74	0.55	0.99	1.54	0.95	0.77	0.54	1.07	1.52	0.83	1.42

anaerobic metabolism and the associated delay in HR response with short duration, high intensity efforts (Alexiou and Coutts, 2008; Akubat and Abt, 2011). sRPE has been proposed as a cost-effective alternative to HR-based methods as a global measure of training intensity that may more accurately quantify internal TL in intermittent sports. In accordance with previous findings in football (Impellizzeri et al., 2004; Alexiou and Coutts, 2008), rugby union (Waldron et al., 2011), and basketball (Manzi et al., 2010), **Table 2** displays large and very large relationships between sRPE and Banisters TRIMP, Edward's SHRZ, and Lucia's TRIMP.

An interesting finding of the present study was the large relationships between all internal TL measures and total distance covered during intermittent, court-based WR training. Scott et al. (2013) previously observed very large ($r = 0.71–0.84$) correlations between internal TL measures (sRPE, Bansiters

TRIMP, Edwards SHRZ) and total distance covered and volume of low speed activity during in-season training of 15 professional football players. Similarly, Casamichana et al. (2013) found large to very large associations between total distance and both sRPE and Edwards SHRZ in 28 semi-professional football players over 44 training sessions. Lovell et al. (2013) investigated the validity of sRPE for quantifying overall TL in 32 professional rugby league players. A very large correlation was observed between sRPE and total distance ($r = 0.69–0.80$) in conditioning, skills-conditioning, and speed-based training (Lovell et al., 2013). A large significant correlation was also observed in the present study between the time spent and distance covered in low and moderate speed zones, with stronger relationships between HR-based methods ($r = 0.63–0.84$) than sRPE ($r = 0.54–0.59$). The present findings support both internal TL variants as a marker of volume (total distance covered) and low/moderate intensity activity. This is significant as WR match-play and training are frequently characterized by large volumes of low intensity movements (~75%) interspersed with short, frequent bouts of high intensity activity (Sarro et al., 2010; Rhodes et al., 2015a).

Weaker relationships were observed between sRPE (~0.30) distance covered and time spent in high (zone 4) and very high (zone 5) speed zones vs. all HR-based methods. Previously, sRPE has been found to display weaker relationships to high/very high speed running activity ($r = 0.40$–0.67) in professional football (Scott et al., 2013) and high intensity-based measures of rugby league TL (Lovell et al., 2013). As the criterion speed of external TL increases, the strength of relationship to sRPE becomes weaker (Scott et al., 2013). This may represent the small window in which RPE can change (1–10) and the lack of sensitivity to small manipulations in training intensity. Also high speed activities interspersed with long periods of rest may reduce RPE despite high activity levels. Typically less than 5% of time during WR match-play is spent at speeds above 80% Vmax (Rhodes et al., 2015a,b). However, the sRPE-based relationships described above may under-estimate large volumes of time spent/distance covered in high or very high speed zones that accumulate during intensive training periods.

A novel finding of the present work was the large variation observed in individual relationships between sRPE and all external TL measures times spent in low intensity speed zones (zone 2) and the distances covered in very low (zone 1) and low intensity speed zones (zone 2). Perceived exertion is a subjective global rating of intensity governed by a multitude of physiological, psychological, and environmental perceptual cues (Hampson et al., 2001). While the subjective range of intensity (from min to max effort) is known to be equal between individuals, the dominant cues determining perceptions of effort may differ greatly (Lambert and Borresen, 2010). Interestingly, Weston et al. (2015) observed only small to moderate relationships between differentiated and overall sRPE and match-play movement demands in Australian League Football. By analysing the intra-individual correlation co-efficient it is clear a wide range of relationships are present between sRPE and external load measures (i.e. total distance $r = -0.03$–0.82). All participants were familiarized in using the scale prior to the study using standardized instructions (Borg, 1998). However, factors including technical role on court,

accumulated fatigue, or psychological stress could all influence an individual athlete's perception of effort during a training session. As previously described, players performing very defensive roles on court may spend a large portion of training performing low-volume activity, including blocking maneuvers, with a high physiological cost. Therefore, baselines of RPE for distinct training intensities should be established by practitioners prior to any longitudinal monitoring in order to gain an insight into intra-individual variations in RPE.

A limitation of the current methodology was that no distinction was made between on-court training modes during the correlation analysis. Weaving et al. (2014) recently employed principle component analysis to explore the influence of training modality on relationships between TL measures during sport-specific training modes 32 rugby league players. For skills training, external measures of body load and total impacts explained the greatest proportion of variance in TL (Weaving et al., 2014). Internal measures of sRPE and Banisters TRIMP explained the greatest variance in speed-based training (Weaving et al., 2014). HIA including jumping, turning, physical contact, or resistance training may be recorded as low speed activity but demand a high physiological load (Scott et al., 2013; Weaving et al., 2014). The metabolic cost of sport-specific skills, including dribbling and kicking in football and tackling in rugby, is also greater than running alone at the same speed (Scott et al., 2013). It is therefore recommended that external TL data are considered within the context of the training environment and a combination of internal and external load measures employed to accurately quantify across training modes (Weaving et al., 2014). Future research should explore the individual internal TL responses to external TL doses experienced during individual WR-specific training drills with a larger cohort of participants.

In conclusion, methods for quantifying external TL, particularly the no. of HIA performed, should always be employed for monitoring overall TL in elite WR athletes. sRPE provides a valid alternative to HR-based methods for assessing distance covered and low to moderate intensity activity in individuals with an impaired HR response. However, sRPE-based measures may underestimate the dose of external TL performed at high or very high intensities. The intra-individual relationships between external TL measures and sRPE should be assessed for each athlete prior to performing any systematic longitudinal monitoring.

REFERENCES

Akubat, I., and Abt, G. (2011). Intermittent exercise alters the heart rate–blood lactate relationship used for calculating the training impulse (TRIMP) in team sport players. *J. Sci. Med. Sport* 14, 249–253. doi: 10.1016/j.jsams.2010.12.003

Alexiou, H., and Coutts, A. J. (2008). A comparison of methods used for quantifying internal training load in women soccer players. *Int. J. Sports Physiol. Perform.* 3, 320–330.

Banister, E. W. (1991). "Modelling elite athletic performance," in *Physiological Testing of Elite Athletes*, eds H. Green, J. McDougal, and H. Wenger (Champaign, IL: Human Kinetics), 403–424.

Barfield, J. P., Malone, L. A., Arbo, C., and Jung, A. P. (2010). Exercise intensity during wheelchair rugby training. *J. Sport Sci.* 28, 389–398. doi: 10.1000/026104110903500039

Bland, J. M., and Altman, D. G. (1995). Calculating correlation coefficients with repeated observations: part 2—correlation between subjects. *BMJ* 310:633. doi: 10.1136/bmj.310.6980.633

Borg, G. (1998). *Borg's Perceived Exertion and Pain Scales*. Champaign, IL: Human Kinetics Publishers.

Casamichana, D., Castellano, J., Calleja-Gonzalez, J., San Román, J., and Castagna, C. (2013). Relationship between indicators of training load in soccer players. *J. Strength Cond. Res.* 27, 369–374. doi: 10.1519/JSC.0b013e318 2548af1

Edwards, S. (1993). "High performance training and racing," in *The Heart Rate Monitor Book*, ed S. Edwards (Sacramento, CA: Feet Fleet Press), 113–123.

Foster, C., Florhaug, J. A., Franklin, J., Gottschall, L., Hrovatin, L. A., and Parker, S. (2001). A new approach to monitoring exercise training. *J. Strength Cond. Res.* 15, 109–115. doi: 10.1519/00124278-200102000-00019

Halson, S. (2014). Monitoring training load to understand fatigue in athletes. *Sports Med.* 44, S139–S147. doi: 10.1007/s40279-014-0253-z

Hampson, D. B., Gibson, A. S. C., Lambert, M. I., and Noakes, T. D. (2001). The influence of sensory cues on the perception of exertion during exercise and central regulation of exercise performance. *Sports Med.* 31, 935–952. doi: 10.2165/00007256-200131130-00004

Hopkins, W. G., Marshall, S. W., Batterham, A. M., and Hanin, J. (2009). Progressive statistics for studies in sports medicine and exercise science. *Med. Sci. Sports Exerc.* 41, 3–13. doi: 10.1249/MSS.0b013e31818cb278

Impellizzeri, F. M., Rampinini, E., Coutts, A. J., Sassi, A., and Marcora, S. M. (2004). Use of RPE-based training load in soccer. *Med. Sci. Sports Exerc.* 36, 1042–1047. doi: 10.1249/01.MSS.0000128199.23901.2F

Lambert, M. I., and Borresen, J. (2010). Measuring training load in sports. *Int. J. Sports Physiol. Perform.* 5, 406–411.

Leicht, C. A., Bishop, N. C., and Goosey-Tolfrey, V. L. (2012). Submaximal exercise responses in tetraplegic, paraplegic and non spinal cord injured elite wheelchair athletes. *Scand. J. Med. Sci. Sports* 22, 729–736. doi: 10.1111/j.1600-0838.2011.01328.x

Leicht, C. A., Griggs, K. E., Lavin, J., Tolfrey, K., and Goosey-Tolfrey, V. L. (2014). Blood lactate and ventilatory thresholds in wheelchair athletes with tetraplegia and paraplegia. *Eur. J. Appl. Physiol.* 114, 1635–1643. doi: 10.1007/s00421-014-2886-x

Lovell, T. W. J., Sirotic, A. C., Impellizzeri, F. M., and Coutts, A. J. (2013). Factors affecting perception of effort (session rating of perceived exertion) during rugby league training. *Int. J. Sports Physiol. Perform.* 8, 62–69.

Lucia, A. J., Hoyos, A., Santalla, C., Earnest, C., and Chicharro, J. L. (2003). Tour de France versus Vuelta a Espana: which is harder? *Med. Sci. Sports Exerc.* 35, 872–878. doi: 10.1249/01.MSS.0000064999.82036.B4

Lupo, C., Capranica, L., and Tessitore, A. (2014). The validity of the session-RPE method for quantifying training load in water polo. *Int. J. Sports Physiol. Perform.* 9, 656–660. doi: 10.1123/IJSPP.2013-0297

Malone, J. J., Di Michele, R., Morgans, R., Burgess, D., Morton, J. P., and Drust, B. (2015). Seasonal training-load quantification in elite English premier league soccer players. *Int. J. Sports Physiol. Perform.* 10, 489–497. doi: 10.1123/ijspp.2014-0352

Manzi, V., D'Ottavio, S., Impellizzeri, F. M., Chaouachi, A., Chamari, K., and Castagna, C. (2010). Profile of weekly training load in elite male professional basketball players. *J. Strength Cond. Res.* 24, 1399–1406. doi: 10.1519/JSC.0b013e3181d7552a

McLaren, S. J., Weston, M., Smith, A., Cramb, R., and Portas, M. D. (2015). Variability of physical performance and player match loads in professional rugby union. *J. Sci. Med. Sport.* doi: 10.1016/j.jsams.2015.05.010. [Epub ahead of print].

Paulson, T. A. W., Bishop, N. C., Leicht, C. A., and Goosey-Tolfrey, V. L. (2013). Perceived exertion as a tool to self-regulate exercise in individuals with tetraplegia. *Eur. J. Appl. Physiol.* 113, 201–209. doi: 10.1007/s00421-012-2426-5

Perrat, B., Smith, M., Rhodes, J., Mason, B., and Goosey-Tolfrey, V. L. (2015). Quality assessment of an UWB positioning system for indoor wheelchair court sports. *J. Sports Eng. Technol.* 229, 81–91. doi: 10.1177/1754337115581111

Rhodes, J., Mason, B., Perrat, B., Smith, M., and Goosey-Tolfrey, V. (2014). The validity and reliability of a novel indoor tracking system for use within wheelchair court sports. *J. Sports Sci.* 32, 1639–1647. doi: 10.1080/02640414.2014.910608

Rhodes, J. M., Mason, B. S., Malone, L. A., and Goosey-Tolfrey, V. L. (2015b). Effect of team rank and player classification on activity profiles of elite wheelchair rugby players. *J. Sports Sci.* 33, 2070–2078. doi: 10.1080/02640414.2015.1028087

Rhodes, J. M., Mason, B. S., Perrat, B., Smith, M. J., Malone, L. A., and Goosey-Tolfrey, V. L. (2015a). Activity profiles of elite wheelchair rugby players during competition. *Int. J. Sports Physiol. Perform.* 10, 318–324. doi: 10.1123/ijspp.2014-0203

Sarro, K. J., Misuta, M. S., Burkett, B., Malone, L. A., and Barros, M. L. (2010). Tracking of wheelchair rugby players in the 2008 Demolition Derby final. *J. Sport Sci.* 28, 192–200. doi: 10.1080/02640410903428541

Scanlan, A. T., Wen, N., Tucker, P. S., Borges, N. R., and Dalbo, V. J. (2014). Training mode's influence on the relationships between training-load models during basketball conditioning. *Int. J. Sports Physiol. Perform.* 9, 851–856. doi: 10.1123/ijspp.2013-0410

Scott, B. R., Lockie, R. G., Knight, T. J., Clark, A. C., and Janse de Jonge, X. A. K. (2013). A comparison of methods to quantify the in-season training load of professional soccer players. *Int. J. Sports Physiol. Perform.* 8, 195–202.

Valent, L. J. M., Dallmeijer, A. J., Houdijk, H., Slootman, J., Janssen, T. W. J., Hollander, A. P., et al. (2007). The individual relationship between heart rate and oxygen uptake in people with tetraplegia during exercise. *Spinal Cord* 45, 104–111. doi: 10.1038/sj.sc.3101946

Waldron, M., Twist, C., Highton, J., Worsfold, P., and Daniels, M. (2011). Movement and physiological match demands of elite rugby league using portable global positioning systems. *J. Sport Sci.* 29, 1223–1230. doi: 10.1080/02640414.2011.587445

Weaving, D., Marshall, P., Earle, K., Nevill, A., and Abt, G. (2014). Combining internal and external training-load measures in professional rugby league. *Int. J. Sports Physiol. Perform.* 9, 905–912. doi: 10.1123/ijspp.2013-0444

Weston, M., Siegler, J., Bahnert, A., McBrien, J., and Lovell, R. (2015). The application of differential ratings of perceived exertion to Australian Football League matches. *J. Sci. Med. Sport* 18, 704–705. doi: 10.1016/j.jsams.2014.09.001

Conflict of Interest Statement: The authors declare that the research was conducted in the absence of any commercial or financial relationships that could be construed as a potential conflict of interest.

12

Simulated Firefighting Task Performance and Physiology Under Very Hot Conditions

Brianna Larsen[1]*, Rod Snow[1,2], Michael Williams-Bell[3] and Brad Aisbett[1,2]

[1] School of Exercise and Nutrition Sciences, Faculty of Health, Deakin University, Melbourne, VIC, Australia, [2] Centre for Physical Activity and Nutrition Research, Faculty of Health, Deakin University, Melbourne, VIC, Australia, [3] Faculty of Health Sciences, University of Ontario Institute of Technology, Oshawa, ON, Canada

Purpose: To assess the impact of very hot (45°C) conditions on the performance of, and physiological responses to, a simulated firefighting manual-handling task compared to the same work in a temperate environment (18°C).

Methods: Ten male volunteer firefighters performed a 3-h protocol in both 18°C (CON) and 45°C (VH). Participants intermittently performed 12 × 1-min bouts of raking, 6 × 8-min bouts of low-intensity stepping, and 6 × 20-min rest periods. The area cleared during the raking task determined work performance. Core temperature, skin temperature, and heart rate were measured continuously. Participants also periodically rated their perceived exertion (RPE) and thermal sensation. Firefighters consumed water *ad libitum*. Urine specific gravity (USG) and changes in body mass determined hydration status.

Results: Firefighters raked 19% less debris during the VH condition. Core and skin temperature were 0.99 ± 0.20 and 5.45 ± 0.53°C higher, respectively, during the VH trial, and heart rate was 14–36 beats.min^{-1} higher in the VH trial. Firefighters consumed 2950 ± 1034 mL of water in the VH condition, compared to 1290 ± 525 in the CON trial. Sweat losses were higher in the VH (1886 ± 474 mL) compared to the CON trial (462 ± 392 mL), though both groups were hydrated upon protocol completion (USG < 1.020). Participants' average RPE was higher in the VH (15.6 ± 0.9) compared to the CON trial (12.6 ± 0.9). Similarly, the firefighters' thermal sensation scores were significantly higher in the VH (6.4 ± 0.5) compared to the CON trial (4.4 ± 0.4).

Conclusions: Despite the decreased work output and aggressive fluid replacement observed in the VH trial, firefighters' experienced increases in thermal stress, and exertion. Fire agencies should prioritize the health and safety of fire personnel in very hot temperatures, and consider the impact of reduced productivity on fire suppression efforts.

Keywords: work output, heat, hydration, thermal stress, exertion

Edited by:
Gregoire P. Millet,
University of Lausanne, Switzerland

Reviewed by:
Naoto Fujii,
University of Ottawa, Canada
Henning Bay Nielsen,
Rigshospitalet, Denmark

*Correspondence:
Brianna Larsen
b.larsen@deakin.edu.au

INTRODUCTION

Performing physical work under very hot ambient conditions has been documented as dangerous, potentially even fatal, for wildland fire personnel (Cuddy and Ruby, 2011; Baldwin and Hales, 2012). Given future climate predictions, it is likely that firefighters will be exposed to such hazardous conditions on a more regular basis (Liu et al., 2010; Hanna et al., 2011; Coumou and Rahmstorf, 2012). For instance, the 2009 Black Saturday bushfires (in Victoria, Australia) were accompanied by temperatures of 46.4°C and extremely low humidity levels, and were preceded by a record-breaking heat wave of 3 days above 43°C (Teague et al., 2010). Even so, little policy exists in the fire industry around extreme heat and wildland firefighting practice in Australia. An operations bulletin was released by the Victorian Country Fire Authority (CFA) in 2012, which provides generalized guidelines around the management of heat stress in "extreme" weather conditions (e.g., rotate crews where possible, drink fluids at regular intervals; Country Fire Authority, 2012). However, the document reflects "common-sense" recommendations, rather than policy derived from a scientific evidence-base. Thus, rigorous research into the effects of high ambient heat on firefighters' and their work performance is warranted, as such research could underpin future heat policies for fire agencies.

There is a breadth of knowledge surrounding heat and exercise physiology (Cheuvront et al., 2010; Nybo et al., 2014). However, most research has focused on temperatures ranging from 30 to 40°C; fewer have explored the more "extreme" ambient conditions (e.g., 45°C) firefighters may be exposed to on the fireground. Select groups who have researched extremely hot ambient temperatures (e.g., 41.8–125°C) have done so over very short durations (≤15 min) (Duncan et al., 1979), have used modes of exercise far removed from firefighting work (e.g., cycling; Caldwell et al., 2012), or have not compared their findings to a more temperate control condition (Bennett et al., 1993; Walker et al., 2014). The small body of relevant research suggests that heart rate (Rowell et al., 1966; Wilson et al., 1975; Sköldström, 1987), perceived exertion (Sköldström, 1987), core temperature (Rowell et al., 1966; Wilson et al., 1975; Sköldström, 1987), skin temperature (Sköldström, 1987), sweat rate (Wilson et al., 1975), and fluid intake (Wilson et al., 1975) are all elevated when treadmill walking in extremely hot ambient conditions (40–50°C) when compared to temperate ambient environments (15–25.6°C). However, wildland firefighting work is also characterized by manual handling actions such as dig, rake, and drag (Phillips et al., 2012), and thus, treadmill walking may not serve as the best proxy when quantifying the effect of high heat on the performance and physiological responses during fire suppression work. In an urban structure firefighting protocol, ambient temperatures of up to 89°C significantly increased heart rate, tympanic temperature, and perceived exertion compared with performing the same fire drills under cool conditions (13°C) (Smith et al., 1997). Conversely, construction workers in the United Arab Emirates have been observed to maintain steady heart rate, tympanic temperature, fluid intake, and urine specific gravity (USG) values when working in temperatures ranging from 32.5 to 49°C (Bates and Schneider, 2008). However, work productivity was not monitored during these studies (Smith et al., 1997; Bates and Schneider, 2008), which prohibits understanding of the potential trade-off between physiological homeostasis and the maintenance of work performance in very hot ambient conditions.

The aim of the present study was to assess the impact of very hot (45°C) and dry conditions on the performance of, and physiological and subjective responses to, a wildland firefighting manual-handling task when compared to the same work in a temperate environment (18°C). It is extremely likely that, in concert with past research, significant increases in thermal stress (e.g., core and skin temperature) and exertion (e.g., heart rate) will be observed in the heat. However, quantifying the magnitude of these changes when performing intermittent, firefighting-specific work tasks is paramount when developing evidence-based health and safety policy. Further, no research to date has utilized a moderate duration, intermittent manual-handling protocol to investigate the performance changes that may occur during very hot conditions. Therefore, the true novelty of the study lies in understanding the impact of very hot ambient environments on simulated wildland firefighting work performance. Though research investigating manual-handling work performance in very hot temperatures is not yet available to support a firm hypothesis, the current authors predict that firefighters work performance will be reduced in the "very hot" condition. Acquiring information on the productivity of personnel in various ambient conditions may be vital for fire agencies in managing their human resources, and ensuring wildfires are controlled as efficiently and safely as possible.

MATERIALS AND METHODS

Participants

Ten healthy male volunteer wildland firefighters participated in the study. Participants provided written informed consent, and filled out a medical questionnaire to ensure they were physically able to perform the work protocol. Ethical approval was obtained from the Deakin University Human Ethics Committee. Participant's height was measured and recorded without shoes using a stadiometer (Fitness Assist, England). Semi-nude body mass (i.e., in underwear only) was measured using an electronic scale (Tanita, USA) pre- and post-exercise. In all trials, participants wore their own firefighting protective clothing, including a two-piece jacket and trouser set made from Proban® cotton fabric (Protex®, Australia), suspenders, boots, gloves, and helmet (amounting to ~5 kg). All testing took place during the winter months to limit heat acclimatization, which could have potentially confounded results.

Experimental Protocol

Participants were familiarized with the physical tasks, as well as the rating of perceived exertion (RPE) and thermal sensation scales, in a separate session within a week of testing (in 18°C) in order to minimize the chance of a learning effect (Hopkins et al., 2001). During the familiarization session, participants performed two sets of the 60-s rake bout (and thereafter provided practice RPE and thermal sensation ratings), and one 8-min step test (see *Raking task* and *Step test*). In the 24 h prior to testing, participants documented their activities (e.g., diet, sleep, and exercise behaviors), and were asked to replicate the same behaviors as closely as possible prior to both trials. Participants were instructed to abstain from alcohol and hard exercise, and to ensure they received adequate fluid intake and sleep, in order to minimize the risk of heat illness (Armstrong et al., 2007).

Participants ingested a core temperature capsule (Jonah, Minimitter, Oregon), a method of core temperature measurement that has been validated against both rectal and esophageal temperature (O'Brien et al., 1998), 6–8 h prior to testing. This allowed adequate time for the pill to pass through the stomach into the intestines to minimize inaccurate readings occurring as a result of ingested food or liquid (Lee et al., 2000). Core temperature results recorded on a data logger (worn in firefighters' jacket pocket) at 1-min epochs throughout the testing period (VitalSense, Minimitter, Oregon). Firefighters were also instructed to slowly consume water ($\sim$5–7 mL.kg^{-1}) in the 4 h prior to testing, to promote adequate hydration (Sawka et al., 2007). Upon arrival to the testing facility, participants had heart rate monitors (Polar, Finland), and skin temperature patches (VitalSense/Jonah, Minimitter, Oregon) affixed. Skin temperature was recorded at four sites on the left side of the body; the chest, thigh, upper arm, and calf (Payne et al., 1994).

Participants performed the protocol on two separate occasions, separated by at least 1 week to allow full recovery between trials. One session was conducted in a temperate environment (CON), and the other under very hot and dry conditions (VH). Trial order was counterbalanced. All testing was conducted in a climate chamber (Vötsch, Germany) which displayed ambient temperature and humidity readings (recorded at 10-min intervals). The climate chamber temperature was $18.0 \pm 0.0°C$ in the CON trial and $45.0 \pm 0.3°C$ in the VH trial ($P < 0.001$). Ambient humidity was $55.7 \pm 1.2\%$ in the CON trial, compared to $26.9 \pm 2.0\%$ in the VH condition ($P < 0.001$). A fan was used to provide a light breeze, to more realistically simulate an outdoor environment. Wind speed (measured at four sites in the chamber, and averaged) was maintained at <1 m.s^{-1} across both trials. Participants performed 3 h of intermittent, simulated rakehoe work (see *Raking task*) interspersed with a low-intensity stepping test (Siconolfi et al., 1985). A 3-h protocol was used as a compromise between simulating long-duration wildland firefighting work, and ensuring participants safety when performing physical work in very hot temperatures. Participants consumed water *ad libitum* throughout testing. Drinking water was maintained at 14.7 ± 0.6 and $15.2 \pm 0.5°C$ in the CON and VH conditions, respectively ($P = 0.074$).

Raking Task

The raking task simulated building a firebreak using a rakehoe. Rakehoe work was chosen due to its prevalence in different types of wildland firefighting (Phillips et al., 2011). Job task analysis research describes this task as short but intense, typically lasting 38–461 s on average (Budd et al., 1997; Phillips et al., 2011). The task simulation involved raking 29 kg of rubber tire crumb from one end of a rectangular (2 × 0.9 m) wooden box to the other repetitively, using a rakehoe. One "repetition" comprised participants raking the vast majority of the tire crumb from one half of the box (over a dividing line in the middle) into the other half. Participants had to wait until the researcher was satisfied that they had cleared enough material before progressing to the next end. The same researcher counted the repetitions

for each participant, to ensure a consistent standard was being met. Rakehoe work performance was evaluated and compared between the CON and VH trials based on the number of repetitions participants were able to complete within the work periods (to the nearest quarter). Repetitions were converted to area (m^2) for analysis.

Step Test

The present research utilized a modified version of a sub-maximal step test (Siconolfi et al., 1985), to simulate the lighter intensity activity (e.g., periodic walking/hiking) performed on the fireground (Aisbett and Nichols, 2007; Raines et al., 2013). Only the lowest intensity phase of the test was utilized, as the energy expenditure of walking "with purpose" has been estimated at 4 METs (Powers and Howley, 2008). The test comprised repeatedly stepping up and down a 25-cm platform at a rate of 17 steps.min^{-1} (Siconolfi et al., 1985), as timed by a metronome. Participants who completed both trials were able to perform all of the prescribed stepping bouts in full. Thus, stepping performance was not included in the analysis.

Work to Rest Ratios

Over the course of a work shift, wildfire fighters have been observed to have periods of predominantly sedentary activity interspersed with brief spurts of moderate/vigorous activity (Cuddy et al., 2007; Raines et al., 2013). For example, mean time spent in the sedentary range for any given 2-h block of a 12-h workday has been observed to be 60.9–79.5 min.2 h^{-1} (Cuddy et al., 2007; Raines et al., 2013), which equates to spending 51–66% in the sedentary range. Further, 43.2 ± 24.2 min of any 2-h period is spent performing light intensity activity (Raines et al., 2013), with only 3.9–8.3 min.2 h^{-1} spent in the moderate/vigorous intensity range (Cuddy et al., 2007; Raines et al., 2013).

In order to simulate the varied-intensity, intermittent nature of wildland firefighting work (Aisbett and Nichols, 2007; Cuddy et al., 2007), the current protocol was broken up into three 1-h bouts (T1, T2, and T3). During each hour, participants spent 4 min intermittently performing the rakehoe task (4 × 1-min bouts), 16 min intermittently performing the stepping task (2 × 8-min bouts), and 40 min resting in the testing environment (2 × 20 min). These rest breaks equate to spending 67% in the sedentary range, which is close to the upper limit observed during fire suppression work (Cuddy et al., 2007; Raines et al., 2013). However, previous research investigating work intensity on the fireground was conducted in more mild ambient conditions (e.g., peak temperatures ranging from 18.6 to 33.9°C; Raines et al., 2013). It is reasonable to assume that rest periods could increase in hotter ambient temperatures. Similarly, the present study employed only 1-min raking bouts, as it is likely that rest breaks could be taken more frequently when performing this task under very hot environmental conditions.

Participants were allowed to remove their helmet and jacket during the 20-min rest periods, as is common during rest breaks on the fireground (Raines et al., 2012). Participants left the climate chamber only to go to the toilet, or if heat illness symptoms presented. Any time spent outside of the environmental condition was recorded.

Physiological and Subjective Measurements

Core temperature, skin temperature, and heart rate were recorded continuously throughout testing. Mean skin temperature was calculated using the formula $0.3(t_{chest} + t_{arm}) + 0.2(t_{thigh} + t_{leg})$ (Ramanathan, 1964). Fluid intake was recorded across the testing period. Urine was sampled pre-, during-, and post-exercise, and USG analyzed (using a portable refractometer; Atago, Japan), to approximate changes in hydration status. Pre- and post-body weight was recorded (and adjusted for ingested and expelled liquids) to determine changes in body mass (%) and to estimate sweat loss. Participants were also asked to provide RPE (on a 6–20 point scale; Borg, 1998) and thermal sensation (on a 0–8 point scale; Young et al., 1987) ratings after each rake bout.

Statistical Analysis

All statistical tests were carried out using the IBM Statistical Package for the Social Sciences (SPSS V.22.0.0, Champaign, Illinois). The distribution of the data was evaluated using Shapiro–Wilk tests. All data (with the exception of "time spent outside" the climate chamber and the total number of rake bouts completed) were normally distributed. The difference between conditions in total area raked, ambient temperature and humidity, and drinking water temperature was analyzed using t-tests. Repeated measures analysis of variance (ANOVA) were performed for all other normally distributed variables, with condition (CON or VH) and time as the two within-participant factors. Where the ANOVA revealed a significant interaction, simple effects analyses were used to detect at which point the significant difference occurred. The "time spent outside" and "bouts completed" data was not normally distributed, and this could not be corrected via transformation of the data. Thus, Wilcoxin-Signed Rank tests were used to assess the difference in these variables between conditions. These data are presented as median (inter-quartile range), whereas all other data are presented as mean ± SD. Significance was set at $p < 0.05$. For the data analyzed using t-tests, t-values were converted into effect sizes (r) using the method described by Field (2013). For the non-parametric data analyzed using Wilcoxin-Signed Rank test, effect sizes (r) were calculated by converting the z-score into an effect size estimate (Field, 2013). For both of these types of data, 0.1, 0.3, and 0.5 are considered small, medium, and large effect sizes (Field, 2013). For all normally distributed variables analyzed using ANOVA, partial eta-squared (η_p^2) effect sizes are presented (Lakens, 2013). When interpreting partial eta-squared results, 0.01, 0.06, and 0.14 are considered small, medium, and large effect sizes, respectively (Richardson, 2011).

RESULTS

Participant details are reported in **Table 1**. There was no difference between conditions ($P = 0.357$; $r = 0.21$) in the "time

spent outside" data, with firefighters spending a median of 0 (2) and 2 (2) min outside the climate chamber (for toilet breaks) in the CON and VH trials, respectively.

Work Performance

All participants were able to complete the 3-h protocol in the CON trial, whereas two participants withdrew from the study due to heat illness symptoms in the VH condition after performing 9 and 10 (out of a possible 12) rake bouts, respectively. The difference in the number of bouts completed between conditions did not reach statistical significance ($P = 0.180$; $r = 0.30$). However, participants were able to clear 19% more total debris during the rakehoe task in the CON (23.45 ± 3.59 m^2) compared to the VH trial (19.08 ± 4.24 m^2; $P < 0.001$; $r = 0.88$). An interaction was also observed when the 12×60-s rake bouts were analyzed individually ($P = 0.014$; $\eta_p^2 = 0.11$), with firefighters raking significantly more in the CON compared to the VH condition during bout 4, and during all bouts from 6 onwards ($P < 0.014$; **Figure 1**).

Core and Skin Temperature

Firefighters' baseline core and mean skin temperatures were not different between the CON (37.45 ± 0.31 and $31.09 \pm 0.90°C$) and VH (37.37 ± 0.18 and $31.59 \pm 1.34°C$) trials ($P \geq 0.240$). There was, however, a significant interaction for hourly core temperature between conditions ($P < 0.001$; $\eta_p^2 = 0.62$). While there was no difference at T1 ($P = 0.721$), T2 and T3 reached $0.53 \pm 0.18°C$ and $0.95 \pm 0.17°C$ higher in the VH trial, respectively ($P < 0.001$; **Figure 3A**). Similarly, a significant interaction was observed for the peak core temperature reached

TABLE 1 | Participant details.

N	10
Age (years)	41 ± 17
Height (cm)	180.4 ± 9.0
Weight (kg)	89.4 ± 8.8
BMI	27.6 ± 3.1
Firefighting experience (years)	12 ± 12

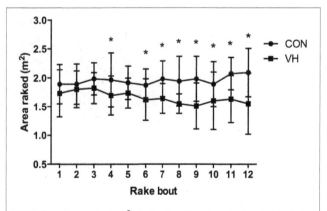

FIGURE 1 | Rake output (m^2) during the 12 × 60-s rake bouts. * Indicates that VH significantly lower ($P < 0.05$) than CON at individual time points.

each hour ($P < 0.001$; $\eta_p^2 = 0.50$). Again, the increase observed in the VH condition fell short of reaching significance during T1 ($0.16 \pm 0.21°C$; $P = 0.109$), but was on average 0.63 ± 0.21 and $0.99 \pm 0.20°C$ higher during T2 and T3 ($P < 0.001$; **Table 2**) when compared to the CON trial. There was no interaction between conditions for hourly mean skin temperature ($P = 0.072$; $\eta_p^2 = 0.11$), however there was a main effect observed for condition, such that firefighters mean skin temperature was on average $5.14 \pm 0.48°C$ hotter across the VH compared to the CON trial ($P < 0.001$; $\eta_p^2 = 0.98$; **Figure 3B**). Conversely, a significant interaction was observed for the peak mean skin temperature reached each hour ($P = 0.044$; $\eta_p^2 = 0.13$). In this instance, the increase observed in the VH condition was significant at all time-points ($P < 0.001$), with participants reaching 4.57 ± 0.53, 5.07 ± 0.53, and 5.45 ± 0.53 higher during T1, T2, and T3 in the VH when compared to the CON trial (**Table 2**). Individual core temperature data was also plotted in **Figure 2**.

Heart Rate

There was a significant interaction observed for mean hourly heart rate ($P < 0.001$; $\eta_p^2 = 0.41$), such that participants' heart rate was 100 ± 16, 98 ± 16, and 97 ± 15 beats.min^{-1} over T1, T2, and T3 during the CON trial, compared to 114 ± 16, 126 ± 18, and 133 ± 14 beats.min^{-1} in the VH condition ($P < 0.001$),

respectively. Conversely, no interaction ($P = 0.118$; $\eta_p^2 = 0.09$) and no main effect for time ($P = 0.271$; $\eta_p^2 = 0.06$) were observed for firefighters' peak hourly heart rate. However, a main effect for condition highlighted that participants' peak heart rate was on average 19 ± 8 beats.min^{-1} higher across the VH compared to the CON trial ($P < 0.001$; $\eta_p^2 = 0.68$; **Table 2**). Heart rate data was also analyzed according to the periods of "work" (including both the rakehoe and stepping tasks) and rest. Time × condition interactions were observed for firefighters' heart rate during both the work and rest phases of the protocol ($P < 0.001$; $\eta_p^2 = 0.46$ and 0.33, respectively). Firefighters' heart rate was, on average, 22 ± 6 beats.min^{-1} and 27 ± 7 beats.min^{-1} higher in the VH compared to the CON trial for the periods of work (**Figure 3C**) and rest (**Figure 3D**), respectively.

Perceptual Responses

An interaction was observed for participants' RPE ratings ($P < 0.001$; $\eta_p^2 = 0.27$), such that participants' RPE was significantly higher during the VH compared to the CON trial after each of the 12 rake bouts ($P < 0.001$; **Figure 3E**). The average RPE for the rake task in the VH condition was 15.6 ± 0.9 and categorized as "hard/heavy," compared to 12.6 ± 0.9 ("somewhat hard") in the CON trial. Similarly, an interaction was observed for participants' thermal sensation ratings ($P < 0.001$; $\eta_p^2 = 0.16$). Again, this difference was statistically significant at each of the 12 time points

TABLE 2 | Peak core temperature, skin temperature, and heart rate over the 3-h work period.

Variable	T1		T2		T3	
	CON	VH	CON	VH	CON	VH
Peak core temperature (°C)	37.71 ± 0.26	37.89 ± 0.21	37.73 ± 0.25	$38.35 \pm 0.21^*$	37.67 ± 0.21	$38.65 \pm 0.24^*$
Peak mean skin temperature (°C)	33.20 ± 1.05	$37.77 \pm 0.31^*$	32.98 ± 0.84	$38.04 \pm 0.43^*$	32.55 ± 0.80	$38.12 \pm 0.55^*$
Peak heart rate (beats.min^{-1})	148 ± 22	$162 \pm 21^{\#}$	148 ± 21	$168 \pm 18^{\#}$	147 ± 21	$167 \pm 18^{\#}$

*Indicates that VH significantly higher (P < 0.05) than CON at individual time points.
#Indicates VH higher than CON (main effect; P < 0.001).

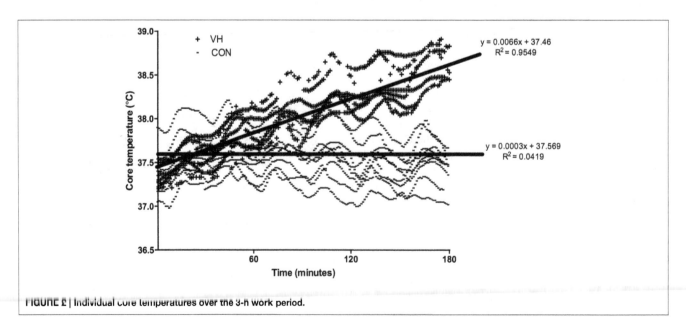

FIGURE 2 | Individual core temperatures over the 3-h work period.

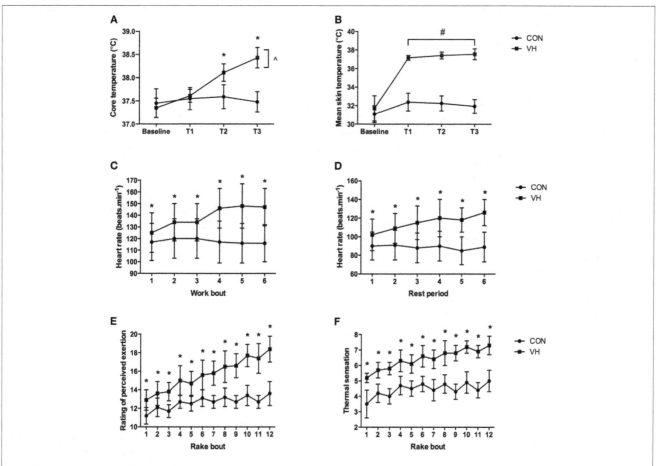

FIGURE 3 | Differences between the CON and VH conditions in: (A) hourly core temperature, (B) hourly mean skin temperature, (C) heart rate during the 10-min work bouts, (D) heart rate during the 20-min rest periods, (E) RPE after the 60-s rake bouts, and (F) thermal sensation after the 60-s rake bouts. *Indicates that VH significantly higher (*P* < 0.05) than CON at individual time points. ^Indicates significant increase from T1 to T2, and T2 to T3 (*P* ≤ 0.004) in the VH. #Indicates VH higher than CON (main effect; *P* < 0.001).

(*P* < 0.001; **Figure 3F**). Firefighters felt hotter during the VH condition, rating their thermal sensation on average as 6.4 ± 0.5, compared to 4.4 ± 0.4 during the CON trial. The average thermal sensation in the VH trial signified "hot-very hot," whereas average thermal sensation in the CON trial was "comfortable-warm."

Hydration
Firefighters consumed 2950 ± 1034 mL of water in the VH condition, compared to only 1290 ± 525 in the CON trial (*P* = 0.001). Conversely, there was no difference in urine output between conditions (*P* = 0.126), with firefighters producing 930 ± 783 and 634 ± 414 mL of urine in the CON and VH conditions, respectively. Firefighters in the VH condition did, however, have higher (*P* < 0.001) estimated sweat losses, reaching 1886 ± 474 mL compared to only 462 ± 392 mL when in the CON environment. There was no interaction (*P* = 0.506; η_p^2 = 0.04), and no main effects for condition (*P* = 0.170; η_p^2 = 0.06) or time (*P* = 0.269; η_p^2 = 0.02), observed for participants' USG scores pre-, during-, and post-work. Firefighters elicited pre-work USG scores of 1.014 ± 0.008 in both trials. During- and post-work USG scores reached 1.011 ± 0.005 and 1.016 ± 0.006 in the CON trial, compared to 1.017 ± 0.008 and 1.018 ± 1.007 in the

VH condition. Thus, firefighters in both conditions were in the "hydrated" range (<1.020) at all time-points measured (Sawka et al., 2007). Further, there was no difference in the percentage body mass change between trials (*P* = 0.265). Participants in the CON trial lost 0.1 ± 0.9% of their body mass across the course of the protocol, whereas participants in the VH condition gained 0.5 ± 1.0%.

DISCUSSION

As predicted, firefighters' self-selected work output was reduced in the VH compared to the CON trial, which was reflected during both the individual rake bouts and the total amount of debris raked across the course of the protocol. Further, all measures of thermal stress (including core temperature, skin temperature, and thermal sensation) were elevated in the VH compared to the CON trial. Participants' heart rate and RPE were also significantly higher in the VH condition. However, firefighters' hydration status in the VH trial was not significantly different (in terms of their percentage body mass change and USG scores) than the CON trial, despite having higher sweat losses. This difference was offset by increased fluid intake in the VH environment.

To the current authors' knowledge, no previous research has evaluated the effects of very hot ambient temperatures (45°C) on self-paced, manual handling work performance (such as firefighting). Previous heat research investigating self-paced work (albeit usually employing different modes of exercise to firefighting) has typically observed one of two phenomena; either work output remains the same and physiological measures are elevated, or work output is decreased in an attempt to maintain thermal homeostasis (Cheung and Sleivert, 2004; Nybo et al., 2014). However, though participants in the current study performed 19% less work on the rakehoe task in the VH trial, significant increases across all measures of thermal strain (core temperature, skin temperature, thermal sensation) and exertion (heart rate, RPE) were recorded. It is possible, then, that the limits of self-pacing for modulating physiology were reached in the current protocol. Skin temperature, heart rate, RPE, and thermal sensation were significantly higher at all points during the VH trial, though participants remained hydrated throughout. Core temperature, on the other hand, was not significantly higher in the VH trial until T2 and T3. Given that the lower rake output was observed only in bout 4 and from bout 6 onwards, it is not unreasonable to assume that the increase in core temperature (in concert with the cardiovascular adjustments accompanying high skin temperatures) was the "trigger" behind firefighters self-selecting a lower work output relative to the CON trial. The interplay between increasing skin temperature, core temperature, and cardiovascular variables has been previously described as the primary explanation for impaired exercise performance in the heat (Cheuvront et al., 2010).

It must also be noted that, although not significant between conditions, two (of 10) participants in the VH trial withdrew before the end of the protocol due to experiencing heat illness symptoms (headaches and nausea). If, hypothetically, 20% of firefighters in the field were unable to complete their allocated shift length due to illness, this would have significant adverse follow-on consequences for the fire-suppression effort, as well as straining health support resources. This issue may be of particular concern for older firefighters, as they have been shown to have a reduced heat loss capacity relative to their younger counterparts (Kenny et al., 2015). However, unlike the current study, firefighters in the field would often be able to modify the length of their work bouts as well as their work intensity, which could further assist their ability to stave off heat illness symptoms. Nevertheless, the fire industry must consider the possibility of firefighter illness and "dropout" when operating under very hot fire weather conditions.

In addition to understanding the effect of very hot conditions on work performance, it is vital that the concurrent physiological changes are also quantified in order to develop policy that promotes and preserves the health and safety of personnel. Participants' core temperature was significantly increased in the VH compared to the CON trial, but perhaps not to the level that was expected based on the previous (albeit extremely limited) research in very hot temperatures (Rowell et al., 1966; Sköldström, 1987). Firefighters in the current protocol reached a peak core temperature of 38.63 ± 0.24°C in the third

hour of testing. Conversely, Rowell et al. (1966) observed core temperatures of 39.4°C after 2 h of intermittent treadmill walking in 43.3°C, and Sköldström (1987) reported core temperatures of 38.7°C after just 1-h of low-intensity (3.5 km.h^{-1}) treadmill walking in 45°C, while wearing PPC and breathing apparatus (BA). It is likely that the 1:2 work to rest ratio employed in the current protocol somewhat blunted the rise in core temperature, which may partially explain the differences when compared to the 1:1 and continuous work protocols utilized by Rowell et al. (1966) and Sköldström (1987), respectively. Firefighters also removed their helmet and opened their jacket during each of the 20-min rest periods, which would have helped reduce the thermal burden when compared to the fully-encapsulating PPC and BA utilized in the Sköldström (1987) study. Further, wind speed in these two studies was described as either "minimal" or <0.2 m.s^{-1}; thus it is possible that the breeze provided by the fan in the present research (<1 m.s^{-1}), in concert with participants' removal of helmets and opening of jackets, would have aided convective heat losses (Nybo et al., 2014).

The increased fluid intake observed in the VH trial also allowed for significantly higher estimated sweat losses, which in turn would have assisted in modulating core body temperature (Cheuvront et al., 2010). Indeed, firefighters managed to more than double their fluid intake in the VH condition, which also allowed them to maintain their body mass across the course of the trial. The USG findings also show that firefighters in both ambient conditions were classified as hydrated (<1.020) before, during, and after the work protocol. Firefighters in the field have also been observed to self-regulate fluid intake in order to complete their shift in a euhydrated state (Raines et al., 2012).

Despite the somewhat encouraging core temperature and hydration findings, participants' heart rate values were as much as 36 beats.min^{-1} higher in the VH when compared to the CON trial, despite performing significantly less work in the heat. Heart rate peaked at 168 ± 18 beats.min^{-1} in T2, which equated to 94 ± 12% of participants age predicted maximum heart rate (using the formula 207−0.7 × age) (Gellish et al., 2007). This is high given that the most intense task was performed in only 1-min bouts, and totaled only 4-min each hour. Recent research has shown that 37% of male volunteer firefighters in Victoria, Australia are considered at "high risk" of developing coronary heart disease in the next 10 years (Wolkow et al., 2013). Cardiovascular disease related fatalities are the leading cause of on-duty deaths in US firefighters, the majority of which occur in individuals with pre-existing risk factors (Wolkow et al., 2012). While regular physical activity may reduce the risk of mortality arising from cardiovascular events, vigorous exercise inducing high heart rates has been shown to increase the risk of acute cardiovascular events in untrained or at-risk populations (Dyer et al., 1980; Siscovick et al., 1984; Cobb and Weaver, 1986; Thompson et al., 2007). Thus, the high levels of physiological exertion experienced in the present study clearly illustrates that close monitoring of firefighter health is necessary and warranted during very hot wildfire conditions.

It is important to note that the current study may have some limitations that prevent direct extrapolation to the fireground.

Firstly, the focus of this research was on ambient heat, whereas firefighters in the field would also be exposed to radiant heat from the sun, and in some cases, the fire. If anything, this means that the present findings may underestimate the thermal stress placed on personnel when on duty. Secondly, the wind speed utilized in the current protocol may not reflect the variations in wind speed/direction that would be experienced in an outdoor environment. Finally, though long in duration relative to past research in very hot temperatures, the 3-h protocol used may not serve as the perfect proxy for a firefighting shift. Although firefighters may not be exposed to ambient temperatures as high as 45°C for longer than a few hours, it is likely that they would perform physical work in hot conditions throughout the course of the day, and would begin their work in the "extreme" conditions (typically in the afternoon) with a higher starting core temperature and some level of physical or mental fatigue. While participants' core temperature in the VH condition perhaps rose more gradually than expected, it did not plateau; core temperature each hour was significantly hotter than the previous hour (**Figure 3A**). Thus, it is not unreasonable to assume that firefighters' performing a similar workload over a longer period would reach core temperatures likely to lead to heat exhaustion. For instance, if the trend line equation from **Figure 2** was used to extrapolate the data, it is predicted that core temperatures could reach 39.84°C in the VH condition after 6 h of work. The wildland firefighting industry must continue to consider and evaluate strategies (e.g., shorter shift lengths, progressively longer rest periods between work bouts) in order to maximize the effectiveness of wildfire suppression efforts in very hot temperatures, while also preserving the health and safety of fire personnel.

CONCLUSIONS

Firefighters in the present study recorded significantly lower performance values, and higher levels of thermal stress and exertion, in the 45°C condition. However, firefighters were able to self-regulate their water intake to prevent changes in body mass and USG (which serve as a proxy for hydration status). Further, the observed elevations in core temperature were relatively moderate when compared to previous research in similar ambient environments. It is likely that the frequent rest breaks employed in the current protocol aided in blunting the rise in core temperature, along with providing the firefighters with ample fluid replacement opportunities. However, given that core temperatures did not plateau over the course of the protocol, it is unlikely that the firefighters would have been able to continue at that rate of work over more extended periods. Fire agencies need to consider how they are going to manage the observed decline in work output in very hot conditions, in order to maximize the effectiveness of fire suppression operations and manage individual health and safety.

ACKNOWLEDGMENTS

Deakin University funded this research. The authors would also like to thank the Bushfire CRC for their support of this research.

REFERENCES

Aisbett, B., and Nichols, D. (2007). Fighting fatigue whilst fighting bushfire: an overview of factors contributing to firefighter fatigue during bushfire suppression. *Aust. J. Emerg. Manage.* 22, 31–39.

Armstrong, L. E., Casa, D. J., Millard-Stafford, M., Moran, D. S., Pyne, S. W, and Roberts, W. O. (2007). American College of Sports Medicine position stand: exertional heat illness during training and competition. *Med. Sci. Sports Exerc.* 39, 556–572. doi: 10.1249/MSS.0b013e3 1802fa199

Baldwin, T., and Hales, T. (2012). *Wildland Fire Fighter Dies from Hyperthermia and Exertional Heatstroke While Conducting Mop-up Operations - Texas.* Cincinnati, OH: NIOSH Fire Fighter Fatality Investigation Team.

Bates, G. P., and Schneider, J. (2008). Hydration status and physiological workload of UAE construction workers: a prospective longitudinal observational study. *J. Occup. Med. Toxicol.* 3, 1–10. doi: 10.1186/1745-6673-3-21

Bennett, B. L., Hagan, R. D., Banta, G., and Williams, F. (1993). Physiological responses during shipboard firefighting. *Aviat. Space Environ. Med.* 66, 225–231.

Borg, G. (1998). *Borg's Perceived Exertion and Pain Scales.* Champaign, IL: Human Kinetics.

Budd, G., Brotherhood, J., Hendrie, A., Jeffery, S., Beasley, F., Costin, B., et al. (1997). Project Aquarius 5. Activity distribution, energy expenditure, and productivity of men suppressing free-running wildland fires with hand tools. *Int. J. Wildland Fire* 7, 105–118. doi: 10.1071/WF9970105

Caldwell, J., Patterson, M., and Taylor, N. (2012). Exertional thermal strain, protective clothing and auxiliary cooling in dry heat: evidence for physiological but not cognitive impairment. *Eur. J. Appl. Physiol.* 112, 3597–3606. doi: 10.1007/s00421-012-2340-x

Cheung, S. S., and Sleivert, G. G. (2004). Multiple triggers for hyperthermic fatigue and exhaustion. *Exerc. Sport Sci. Rev.* 32, 100–106. doi: 10.1097/00003677-200407000-00005

Cheuvront, S. N., Kenefick, R. W., Montain, S. J., and Sawka, M. N. (2010). Mechanisms of aerobic performance impairment with heat stress and dehydration. *J. Appl. Physiol.* 109, 1989–1995. doi: 10.1152/japplphysiol.00367.2010

Cobb, L. A., and Weaver, W. D. (1986). Exercise: a risk for sudden death in patients with coronary heart disease. *J. Am. Coll. Cardiol.* 7, 215–219. doi: 10.1016/S0735-1097(86)80284-4

Coumou, D., and Rahmstorf, S. (2012). A decade of weather extremes. *Nature* 2, 491–496. doi: 10.1038/nclimate1452

Country Fire Authority (2012). "Management of heat stress," in *Operations Bulletin*, ed CFA Fire and Emergency Management (Melbourne, VIC: Fire and Emergency Management), 1–5.

Cuddy, J. S., Gaskill, S. E., Sharkey, B. J., Harger, S. G, and Ruby, B. C. (2007). Supplemental feedings increase self-selected work output during wildfire suppression. *Med. Sci. Sports Exerc.* 39, 1004–1012. doi: 10.1249/mss.0b013e318040b2fb

Cuddy, J. S., and Ruby, B. C. (2011). High work output combined with high ambient temperatures caused heat exhaustion in a wildland firefighter despite high fluid intake. *Wilderness Environ. Med.* 22, 122–125. doi: 10.1016/j.wem.2011.01.008

Duncan, H. W., Gardner, G. W., and Barnard, R. J. (1979). Physiological responses of men working in fire fighting equipment in the heat. *Ergonomics* 22, 521–527. doi: 10.1080/00140137908924636

Dyer, A. R., Persky, V., Stamler, J., Paul, O., Shekelle, R. B., Berkson, D. M., et al. (1980). Heart rate as a prognostic factor for coronary heart disease and mortality: findings in three Chicago epidemiologic studies. *Am. J. Epidemiol.* 112, 736–749.

Field, A. (2013). *Discovering Statistics Using IBM SPSS Statistics.* London, UK: Sage Publications Ltd.

Gellish, R. L., Goslin, B. R., Olson, R. E., McDonald, A., Russi, G. D., and Moudgil, V. (2007). Longitudinal modeling of the relationship between age and maximal heart rate. *Med. Sci. Sports Exerc.* 39, 822–829. doi: 10.1097/mss.0b013e31803349c6

Hanna, E. G., Kjellstrom, T., Bennett, C., and Dear, K. (2011). Climate change and rising heat: population health implications for working people in Australia. *Asia Pac. J. Public Health* 23, 14–26. doi: 10.1177/10105395103 91457

Hopkins, W. G., Schabort, E. J., and Hawley, J. A. (2001). Reliability of power in physical performance tests. *Sports Med.* 31, 211–234. doi: 10.2165/00007256-200131030-00005

Kenny, G. P., Larose, J., Wright-Beatty, H. E., Boulay, P., Sigal, R. J., and Flouris, A. D. (2015). Older firefighters are susceptible to age-related impairments in heat dissipation. *Med. Sci. Sports Exerc.* 47, 1281–1290. doi: 10.1249/MSS.0000000000000537

Lakens, D. (2013). Calculating and reporting effect sizes to facilitate cumulative science: a practical primer for t-tests and ANOVAs. *Front. Psychol.* 4:863. doi: 10.3389/fpsyg.2013.00863

Lee, S., Williams, W., and Schneider, S. (2000). *Core Temperature Measurement during Submaximal Exercise: Esophageal, Rectal, and Intestinal Temperatures.* Houston, TX: National Aeronautics and Space Administration.

Liu, Y., Stanturf, J., and Goodrick, S. (2010). Trends in global wildfire potential in a changing climate. *For. Ecol. Manage.* 259, 685–697. doi: 10.1016/j.foreco.2009.09.002

Nybo, L., Rasmussen, P., and Sawka, M. (2014). Performance in the heat—physiological factors of importance for hyperthermia-induced fatigue. *Compr. Physiol.* 4, 657–689. doi: 10.1002/cphy.c130012

O'Brien, C., Hoyt, R. W., Buller, M. J., Castellani, J. W., and Young, A. J. (1998). Telemetry pill measurement of core temperature in humans during active heating and cooling. *Med. Sci. Sports Exerc.* 30, 468–472. doi: 10.1097/00005768-199803000-00020

Payne, W. R., Portier, B., Fairweather, I., Zhou, S., and Snow, R. (1994). Thermoregulatory response to wearing encapsulated protective clothing during simulated work in various thermal environments. *Am. Ind. Hyg. Assoc. J.* 55, 529–536. doi: 10.1080/15428119491018808

Phillips, M., Netto, K., Payne, W., Nichols, D., Lord, C., Brooksbank, N., et al. (2011). "Frequency, intensity and duration of physical tasks performed by Australian rural firefighters during bushfire suppression," *Bushfire CRC and AFAC Conference,* ed R. P. Thornton (Sydney, NSW).

Phillips, M., Payne, W., Lord, C., Netto, K., Nichols, D., and Aisbett, B. (2012). Identification of physically demanding tasks performed during bushfire suppression by Australian rural firefighters. *Appl. Ergon.* 43, 435–441. doi: 10.1016/j.apergo.2011.06.018

Powers, S., and Howley, E. (2008). *Exercise Physiology: Theory and Application to Fitness and Performance.* Baltimore, MD: McGraw-Hill.

Raines, J., Snow, R., Petersen, A., Harvey, J., Nichols, D., and Aisbett, B. (2012). Pre-shift fluid intake: effect on physiology, work and drinking during emergency wildfire fighting. *Appl. Ergon.* 43, 532–540. doi: 10.1016/j.apergo.2011.08.007

Raines, J., Snow, R., Petersen, A., Harvey, J., Nichols, D., and Aisbett, B. (2013). The effect of prescribed fluid consumption on physiology and work behavior of wildfire fighters. *Appl. Ergon.* 44, 404–413. doi: 10.1016/j.apergo.2012.10.002

Ramanathan, N. L. (1964). A new weighting system for mean surface temperature of the human body. *J. Appl. Physiol.* 19, 531–533.

Richardson, J. (2011). Eta squared and partial eta squared as measures of effect size in educational research. *Educ. Res. Rev.* 6, 135–147. doi: 10.1016/j.edurev.2010.12.001

Rowell, L. B., Marx, H. J., Bruce, R. A., Conn, R. D., and Kusumi, F. (1966). Reductions in cardiac output, central blood volume, and stroke volume with thermal stress in normal men during exercise. *J. Clin. Invest.* 45, 1801–1816. doi: 10.1172/JCI105484

Sawka, M. N., Burke, L. M., Eichner, E. R., Maughan, R. J., Montain, S. J., and Stachenfeld, N. S. (2007). American College of Sports Medicine position stand: exercise and fluid replacement. *Med. Sci. Sports Exerc.* 39, 377–390. doi: 10.1249/mss.0b013e31802ca597

Siconolfi, S. F., Garber, C. E., Lasater, T. M., and Carleton, R. A. (1985). A simple, valid step test for estimating maximal oxygen uptake in epidemiologic studies. *Am. J. Epidemiol.* 121, 382–390.

Siscovick, D. S., Weiss, N. S., Fletcher, R. H., and Lasky, T. (1984). The incidence of primary cardiac arrest during vigorous exercise. *New Engl. J. Med.* 311, 874–877. doi: 10.1056/NEJM198410043111402

Sköldström, B. (1987). Physiological responses of fire fighters to workload and thermal stress. *Ergonomics* 30, 1589–1597. doi: 10.1080/001401387089 66049

Smith, D. L., Petruzzello, S. J., Kramer, J. M., and Misner, J. E. (1997). The effects of different thermal environments on the physiological and psychological responses of firefighters to a training drill. *Ergonomics* 40, 500–510. doi: 10.1080/001401397188125

Teague, B., McLeoud, R., and Pascoe, S. (2010). *2009 Victorian Bushfires Royal Commission.* Melbourne, VIC: Parliament of Victoria.

Thompson, P. D., Franklin, B. A., Balady, G. J., Blair, S. N., Corrado, D., Estes, N. A. M., et al. (2007). Exercise and acute cardiovascular events placing the risks into perspective: a scientific statement from the American Heart Association Council on Nutrition, Physical Activity, and Metabolism and the Council on Clinical Cardiology. *Circulation* 115, 2358–2368. doi: 10.1161/CIRCULATIONAHA.107.181485

Walker, A., Driller, M., Brearley, M., Argus, C., and Rattray, B. (2014). Cold-water immersion and iced-slush ingestion are effective at cooling firefighters following a simulated search and rescue task in a hot environment. *Appl. Physiol. Nutr. Metab.* 39, 1159–1166. doi: 10.1139/apnm-2014-0038

Wilson, B. D., Gisolfi, C. V., and Smith, T. F. (1975). Thermal responses to intermittent work in selected environments. *Am. Ind. Hyg. Assoc. J.* 36, 648–652. doi: 10.1080/0002889758507310

Wolkow, A., Netto, K., Langridge, P., Green, J., Nichols, D., Sergeant, M., et al. (2012). "Cardiovascular risk screening of volunteer firefighters," in *Proceedings of Bushfire CRC and AFAC 2012 Conference Research Forum* (Melbourne, VIC), 170–184.

Wolkow, A., Netto, K., Langridge, P., Green, J., Nichols, D., Sergeant, M., et al. (2013). Coronary heart disease risk in volunteer firefighters in Victoria, Australia. *Arch. Environ. Occup. Health* 69, 112–120. doi: 10.1080/19338244.2012.750588

Young, A. J., Sawka, M. N., Epstein, Y., Decristofano, B., and Pandolf, K. B. (1987). Cooling different body surfaces during upper and lower body exercise. *J. Appl. Physiol.* 63, 1218–1223.

Conflict of Interest Statement: The authors declare that the research was conducted in the absence of any commercial or financial relationships that could be construed as a potential conflict of interest.

13

Comparison Between 30-15 Intermittent Fitness Test and Multistage Field Test on Physiological Responses in Wheelchair Basketball Players

Thierry Weissland[1,2]*, Arnaud Faupin[3,4], Benoit Borel[5] and Pierre-Marie Leprêtre[1]

[1] *Laboratoire de Recherche Adaptations Physiologiques à L'exercice et Réadaptation à L'effort, EA-3300, UFR-STAPS, Université de Picardie Jules Verne, Amiens, France,* [2] *Institut d'Ingénierie de la Santé, UFR de Médecine, Université de Picardie Jules Verne, Amiens, France,* [3] *Laboratoire Motricité Humaine Education Sport Santé, EA-6312, UFR-STAPS, Université de Toulon, La Garde, France,* [4] *Laboratoire Motricité Humaine Education Sport Santé, EA-6312, Université Nice Sophia Antipolis, Nice, France,* [5] *Laboratoire Handicap, Activité, Vieillissement, Autonomie, Environnement, EA-6310, Département STAPS, Université de Limoges, Limoges, France*

Edited by:
Olivier Girard,
University of Lausanne, Switzerland

Reviewed by:
Peter Hofmann,
University of Graz, Austria
Javier Yanci,
University of the Basque Country,
Spain

*Correspondence:
Thierry Weissland
thierry.weissland@u-picardie.fr

The intermittent nature of wheelchair court sports suggests using a similar protocol to assess repeated shuttles and recovery abilities. This study aimed to compare performances, physiological responses and perceived rating exertion obtained from the continuous multistage field test (MFT) and the 30-15 intermittent field test ($30\text{-}15_{IFT}$). Eighteen trained wheelchair basketball players (WBP) (WBP: 32.0 ± 5.7 y, IWBF classification: 2.9 ± 1.1 points) performed both incremental field tests in randomized order. Time to exhaustion, maximal rolling velocity (MRV), VO_{2peak} and the peak values of minute ventilation (V_{Epeak}), respiratory frequency (RF) and heart rate (HR_{peak}) were measured throughout both tests; peak and net blood lactate ($\Delta[\text{Lact}^-] = \text{peak–rest}$ values) and perceived rating exertion (RPE) values at the end of each exercise. No significant difference in VO_{2peak}, VE_{peak}, and RF was found between both tests. $30\text{-}15_{IFT}$ was shorter (12.4 ± 2.4 vs. 14.9 ± 5.1 min, $P < 0.05$) but induced higher values of MRV and $\Delta[\text{Lact}^-]$ compared to MFT (14.2 ± 1.8 vs. 11.1 ± 1.9 km·h^{-1} and 8.3 ± 4.2 vs. 6.9 ± 3.3 mmol·L^{-1}, $P < 0.05$). However, HR_{peak} and RPE values were higher during MFT than $30\text{-}15_{IFT}$ (172.8 ± 14.0 vs. 166.8 ± 13.8 bpm and 15.3 ± 3.8 vs. 13.8 ± 3.5, respectively, $P < 0.05$). The intermittent shuttles intercepted with rest period occurred during the $30\text{-}15_{IFT}$ could explain a greater anaerobic solicitation. The higher HR and overall RPE values measured at the end of MFT could be explained by its longer duration and a continuous load stress compared to $30\text{-}15_{IFT}$. In conclusion, $30\text{-}15_{IFT}$ has some advantages over MFT for assess in addition physical fitness and technical performance in WBP.

Keywords: wheelchair, basketball, field test, aerobic fitness, evaluation

INTRODUCTION

Wheelchair basketball (WB) attracts many persons with different physical impairment and has great success at the Paralympic Games since 1960. WB has been described as intermittent aerobic-based sport scattered with short anaerobic bouts (Coutts, 1992; Bloxham et al., 2001). In their game analysis, Sporner et al. (2009) reported that the wheelchair basketball players (WBP) on average traveled 2679 ± 1103 m cut off by 239.8 ± 60.6 stops and starts during a match. Wheeling tasks including sprint, endurance, and slalom were strongly correlated with aerobic fitness in WBP (Hutzler, 1993; Vanlandewijck et al., 1999). WBP presented larger cardiac dimensions, greater power output and peak oxygen uptake (VO_{2peak}) values compared to untrained counterparts (Huonker et al., 1998; Schmid et al., 1998). Thus, maximal oxygen uptake was correlated to functional capacity and competition level in WBP (Schmid et al., 1998; De Lira et al., 2010).

Cardiorespiratory adaptation to exercise provided valuable information on training status. VO_{2peak} is generally assessed in laboratory condition during graded exercise performed on a wheelchair rolling on a motor driven treadmill and on an arm cycle ergometer. However, low correlations are obtained between peak cardiorespiratory values measured while pushing on the wheelchair and those measured with arm cranking on ergometer or in selected wheeling task (Hutzler, 1993; Rotstein et al., 1994). Standardized laboratory protocol tests can also provide higher VO_{2peak} reached at the end of test compared to field tests (Cunningham et al., 2000; Goosey-Tolfrey and Tolfrey, 2008). However, laboratory conditions did not take into account the natural environment (floor surface, specific wheelchair equipment) and not relate specific skills at the environment and ability to maneuver the wheelchair (Bernardi et al., 2010; Molik et al., 2010; De Groot et al., 2012; Goosey-Tolfrey and Leicht, 2013). Several authors adapted continuous (Vinet et al., 1996; Vanderthommen et al., 2002; Bernardi et al., 2010) and shuttle (Vanlandewijck et al., 1999; Cunningham et al., 2000; Goosey-Tolfrey and Tolfrey, 2008) tests for able-bodied players to assess aerobic fitness and predict the VO_{2peak} of disabled players. To assess agility, sprint recovery and endurance characteristics of WBP, Yanci et al. (2015) and Gil et al. (2015) also proposed a modified Yo-Yo intermittent recovery test (10-m instead of 20-m shuttle run). Yanci et al. (2015) showed a good test—retest reliability (ICC = 0.74–0.94; CV: ranged from 2.6 to 7.2%).

Buchheit (2008) developed for able-bodied athletes the 30-15 Intermittent Field Test (30-15$_{IFT}$), which aims to evaluate the maximal aerobic velocity in court sport players and acute responses to high-intensity intermittent shuttle-runs. The main interests of this test is the final speed reached at the end of the test which is well suited for training prescription and the rest time is longer than the Yo-Yo intermittent recovery test and more representative of defensive phase of WP (Buchheit and Rabbani, 2014). Nevertheless, wheelchair sports are distinct from those able-bodied due to functional impairment of the disabled and the displacement imposed by wheelchair (Goosey-Tolfrey and Leicht, 2013).

Previously, an incremental multistage field test (MFT) specific for disabled body wheelchair subjects was validated

(Vanderthommen et al., 2002). It was observed that a slightly MFT adaptation—as alternating right and left turns vs. single direction—increase VO_{2peak} and peak minute ventilation (V_{Epeak}) responses without any significant differences in perceived exertion and maximal rolling velocity (MRV) reached at the end of the test (Weissland et al., 2015). These adjustments have no correspondence with the intermittent nature and the metabolic and cardio-respiratory responses induced by pivots, sprints and dribbles requested in WBP. Moreover, it has been observed, in able-bodied team sport players, that higher peak velocity were reached with a shorter time to exhaustion in intermittent shuttle vs. continuous running tests, with no significant difference in peak values of heart rate (HR$_{peak}$) and blood lactate (Carminatti et al., 2013).

Hence, the aim of the study was (i) to assess the aerobic fitness derived from an able-bodied intermittent field test in WBP (Buchheit, 2008) and (ii) to compare with a continuous and validated wheelchair field test. This study aimed to examine the end-test rolling velocity, the physiological responses and perceived exertion obtained from the continuous MFT and with the 30-15 intermittent field test (30-15$_{IFT}$).

METHODS

Subjects

Eighteen national WBP were recruited and all were engaged in national WB competitions every week, with several training sessions per week. Skinfolds thickness at four sites (triceps, subscapular, suprailiac, and abdominal) was measured using a Harpenden caliper. A summary of their characteristics, pathology and international classification (International Wheelchair Basketball Federation Web site, 2009) is presented in **Table 1**. For both tests, all players always used their own wheelchair. Before each test, the tire pressure was checked (Sawatzky et al., 2005). All procedures were conducted in accordance with approval of the "Fédération Française Handisport" medical committee, and in accordance with the Helsinki Declaration. All participants are fully informed of any risk giving and provided written informed consent.

Experimental Design

Testing for this study was conducted during the competitive period, in the middle of the season. Both tests replaced technical and physical training sessions during a week between competitive matches. Training load was reduced on the day preceding each test, which was performed between 9:00 a.m. and 4:00 p.m. Each WBP performed both tests within 48 h in a randomized order, in the same indoor hall: (i) the MFT which is an incremental continuous test (Vanderthommen et al., 2002) and (ii) the 30-15 intermittent fitness test (30-15$_{IFT}$) (Buchheit, 2008). Briefly, the MFT included wheeling around an octagon (15×15 m) at an initial speed of 6 km·h^{-1} during 1 min. Then, the speed increased by 0.37 km·h^{-1} every minute until exhaustion (Vanderthommen et al., 2002). The 30-15$_{IFT}$ consisted of 40-m shuttle runs during 30-s with 15-s of passive recovery. The initial velocity was set at 8 km·h^{-1} (instead of 8 km·h^{-1} in the original protocol) for the first 30-s trial and was increased by 0.5 km·h^{-1} every 45-s

TABLE 1 | Individual Wheelchair basketball players' characteristics (gender, age, disability, sum of four skinfolds) according to International Wheelchair Basketball Federation classification (IWBF).

Player	Sex	Age (years)	Disability	IWBF classification	ΣSK (mm)
P1	M	29	Poliomyelitis	1.0	45.1
P2	F	28	Lower limb agenesis	1.0	76.2
P3	M	27	Spinal cord injury	1.5	52.2
P4	M	30	Spinal cord injury	2.0	42.9
P5	M	41	Spinal cord injury	2.0	27.2
P6	M	39	Spina bifida	2.5	33.7
P7	M	35	Hemiplegia	2.5	45.0
P8	M	36	Agenesis	3.0	44.9
P9	M	22	Larsen syndrome	3.0	30.8
P10	M	39	Spinal cord injury	3.0	39.1
P11	M	23	Spinal cord injury	3.0	37.9
P12	M	29	Cerebral palsy	3.0	44.1
P13	M	36	Spinal cord injury	4.0	48.3
P14	M	36	Spina bifida	4.0	54.5
P15	M	27	Cerebral palsy	4.0	23.1
P16	M	30	Above knee amputation	4.0	56.9
P17	F	38	Above knee amputation	4.5	34.1
P18	M	31	Orthopedic impairments	4.5	44.6
mean ± SD		32.0 ± 5.7		2.9 ± 1.1	43.5 ± 12.3

ΣSK represents the sum of four skinfolds (biceps, triceps, subscapular, supra-iliac).

(Buchheit, 2008). During the 15-s recovery period, the subjects rolled in the forward direction to join the closest line (at the middle or at one end of the area, depending on where they stopped) from where they started the next stage. No indication for the propulsion strategy was given for the two tests and WBP freely used their push rate and modality (synchronous and/or asynchronous).

All participants were instructed to complete as many stages as possible. The test ended when the participant could no longer be located within the turning zone (MFT) or consecutively to reach a 2-m zone around each line (30-15$_{\text{IFT}}$) at beep signal despite verbal encouragement. The time to exhaustion (TTE) was the longer time maintaining to the speed imposed on the last stage during each respective test. MRV was the velocity at the end of test reached at the TTE.

All subjects were advised to keep the same meals between both tests and to refrain from smoking and caffeinated drinks during the 2 h prior to testing.

Physiological and Perceived Responses Measurements

The resting oxygen uptake (VO_2), carbon dioxide production (VCO_2), respiratory frequency (RF), and minute ventilation (V_E) were measured breath-by-breath at rest and throughout both tests using Cosmed K4b^2 or Metamax 3B portable spirometric systems. To reduce the duration of the test time and the turnover subjects, two portable measurement systems were used. A previous study showed a satisfactory comparison between the two measuring devices with able-bodied cyclists (Leprêtre et al.,

2012). Participants always used the same analyzer for both tests to repeat the mistake device. The turbines flow meters (with a 3-L syringe) and analysers were calibrated before each test, according to the constructor instruction manuals using a two-point calibration (calibration gas O_2 = 16% and CO_2 = 5% against room air). Then we used the software of each device to automatically eliminate ectopic values and average the data every 5 s. Heart rate (HR) was continuously recorded beat-to-beat (Polar RS800, Polar Electro, Kempele, Finland) and averaged every 5 s.

Small capillary blood samples (0.5 μL) were collected from finger to assess basal lactate concentration. A sample of lactate at rest was taken upon arrival of the player and before warm-up, immediately after the test and 3 min after during the passive recovery period. Net blood lactate values (Δ[Lact$^-$]) were calculated by the difference between the peak [Lact$^-$] values and rest values. All blood samples were analyzed using a portable lactate analyzer (Lactate Pro, Arkray, Japan) calibrated before each test using a standard strip of provided by the manufacturer (Pyne et al., 2000).

Immediately after the end of both tests, participants individually rated their overall perceived exertion (RPE) using the Borg's 6–20 scale (Borg, 1990).

Statistical Analysis

Descriptive data are presented as mean and standard deviation (mean ± SD). Normality and homogeneity of the distribution were verified via Shapiro Wilks and Levene tests, respectively. Student's t-test was used to compare the resting and peak values measured during MFT and 30-15$_{IFT}$. The determination of the Pearson correlation coefficients (R) were used to examine the relationship between TTE, MRV, $VO2peak$, and condition test. Absolute effect size (ES) and 95% confidence intervals of the differences (95% CI) were computed. An ES of 0.2 refers to a small effect, 0.5 a moderate effect, and 0.8 a large effect according to Cohen (Cohen, 1992). Agreements were sought by the Bland and Altman' method (Bland and Altman, 1986) between the peak values of VO_2 and V_E between the both tests. In all statistical analyses, the (alpha) level of significance was set at $P < 0.05$.

RESULTS

Peak values of cardiorespiratory responses and performance measured during MFT and 30-15$_{IFT}$ are shown in **Table 2**. Higher MRV values (14.2 ± 1.8 vs. 11.1 ± 1.9 km·h^{-1}, $P < 0.05$, $ES = 0.6$) and shorter TTE (12.4 ± 2.4 vs. 14.9 ± 5.1 min, $P < 0.05$, $ES = 0.3$) were observed during 30-15$_{IFT}$ compared to MFT. HR$_{peak}$ and RPE values were significantly lower during 30-15$_{IFT}$ compared to MFT (166.8 ± 13.8 vs. 172.8 ± 14.0 bpm, $ES = 0.4$, and 13.8 ± 3.5 vs. 15.3 ± 3.8, $ES = 0.5$, $P < 0.05$, respectively). 30-15$_{IFT}$ induced a higher Δ[Lact$^-$] values compared to MFT (8.3 ± 4.2 vs. 6.9 ± 3.3 mmol·L^{-1}, $P < 0.05$, $ES = 0.4$) without any significant difference between rest ($P = 0.88$) and peak [Lact$^-$] values (9.8 ± 4.4 mmol·L^{-1} vs. 8.5 ± 3.1, $P = 0.2$, $ES = 0.3$). No significant difference was found for VO_{2peak}, V_{Epeak}, and RF peak values between both tests.

A significant relationship for MRV ($r = 0.57$, $P < 0.05$) TTE ($r = 0.64$, $P < 0.05$), and $VO2peak$ ($r = 0.84$, $P < 0.01$) was found between MFT and 30-15$_{IFT}$ (**Figure 1**). The Bland–Altman plots showed that, for VO_{2peak} and V_{Epeak} measurements, the bias ± random error was acceptable with an acceptable agreement between both tests ($-0.27 ± 6.81$ ml.min.kg^{-1}; **Figure 2A** and 2.6 ± 34.8 L.min^{-1}; **Figure 2B**, respectively). Differences between MFT and 30-15$_{IFT}$ HR$_{peak}$ and Δ[Lact$^-$] per WBP were reported in **Figure 3**. Individual responses have reflected significant changes measured in HR (**Figure 4**) and Δ[Lact$^-$] for 30-15$_{IFT}$.

DISCUSSION

The aim of this study was to compare a modified able-bodied field intermittent test with a validated standardized wheelchair-users field test. The observed performances at 30-15$_{IFT}$ were better with higher MRV associated with a shorter time to exhaustion ($P < 0.05$). However, no significant difference for peak oxygen uptake and ventilation values was noted between both tests (**Table 2**).

MFT is a validated field test to estimate VO_{2peak} for disabled body wheelchair subjects in indoor conditions (Vanderthommen et al., 2002). No significant difference was found for VO_{2peak} between MFT and 30-15$_{IFT}$ and a significant relationship for VO_{2peak} were found between the both tests ($r = 0.84$, $P < 0.01$) (**Figure 1**). We used Bland-Altman plots to graphically display the variability of VO_{2peak} and V_{Epeak} variables (**Figure 2**). In each case, the systematic bias is close to zero and the 95% limits of agreements are acceptable.

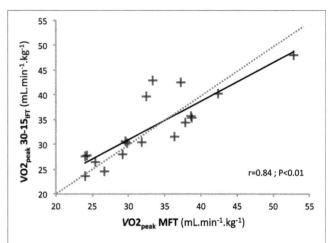

FIGURE 1 | Correlation between VO_{2peak} reached during MFT and 30-15$_{IFT}$ tests ($r = 0.54$, $r^2 = 0.71$, $P < 0.01$).

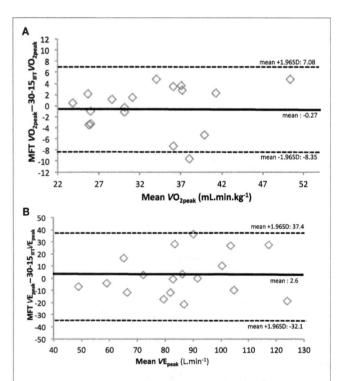

FIGURE 2 | Analysis of the individual difference by Bland-Altman method between MFT and 30-15$_{IFT}$ test and (A) peak oxygen consumption (VO_{2peak}) and (B) peak ventilation (V_{Epeak}).

Thus, we can conclude that the 30-15$_{IFT}$ is comparable to VO_{2peak} and V_{Epeak} encountered during the end of the test. Nevertheless, it would be necessary in the future to investigate the reliability and validity of the 30-15$_{IFT}$ with a standardized test on a wheelchair ergometer in the laboratory. However, the only valid option to confirm whether a "true" VO_{2max} has been reached during both tests is currently in a verification phase (VER) (Leicht et al., 2013), absent in our protocol.

TABLE 2 | Peak values and 95% confidence interval (CI) measured during the MFT and the 30-15$_{IFT}$, Mean ± SD.

	TTE min:s	MRV km.h^{-1}	RF b·min^{-1}	V_{Epeak} L·min^{-1}	VO_{2peak} mL·min^{-1}·kg^{-1}	HR$_{peak}$ bpm	peak [Lact$^-$] mmol·L^{-1}	Δ[Lact$^-$] mmol·L^{-1}	RPE
MFT	14:53 ± 5:04	11.1 ± 1.9	49.9 ± 11.4	87.0 ± 22.8	33.0 ± 7.5	172.8 ± 14.0	8.5 ± 3.1	6.9 ± 3.3	15.3 ± 3.8
CI	12:32–17:13	10.3–12.0	44.7–55.2	76.5–97.6	29.5–36.5	166.3–179.2	7.1–9.9	5.4–8.4	13.5–17
30-15$_{IFT}$	12:25 ± 2:21*^{γ}	14.2 ± 1.8*^{θ}	48.4 ± 12.8^θ	84.4 ± 20.1	33.3 ± 7	166.8 ± 13.8*^{θ}	9.8 ± 4.4^2	8.3 ± 4.2*^{θ}	13.5 ± 3.5*^{θ}
CI	11:19–13:31	13.4–15.1	42.5–54.3	75.1–93.7	30.1–36.5	160.5–173.2	7.7–11.8	6.3–10.2	11.9–15.1

TTE, indicates Time To Exhaustion; MRV, Maximal Rolling Velocity; RF, peak respiratory frequency; V_{Epeak}, peak values of ventilation; VO_{2peak}, peak oxygen uptake; HR$_{peak}$, peak heart rate; peak [La$^-$], peak blood lactate value; Δ[La$^-$], the difference between rest and maximal blood lactate values; RPE, the rating of perceived exertion.
*Significantly different from MFT (P < 0.05); ^{θ}moderate effect size; ^{γ}small effect size (Cohen, 1992).

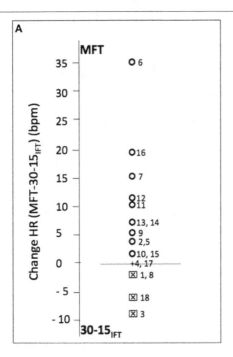
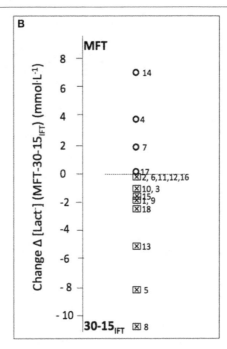

FIGURE 3 | Individual wheelchair basketball players difference in peak heart rate and blood lactate values between continuous multistage field test (MFT) and 30-15 intermittent field test (30-15$_{IFT}$) (n = 18). (A) Difference HR (bpm) and **(B)** Difference Δ[Lact$^-$], respectively represented the difference in peak values of heart rate (bpm) and Δ blood lactate (peak-rest values [La$^-$] mmol·L^{-1}). A circle plots indicated a difference between MFT and 30-15$_{IFT}$ values in favor of MFT; a square worth the 30-15$_{IFT}$.

TTE to reach VO_{2peak} is shorter during 30-15$_{IFT}$ than MFT (12.4 ± 2.4 vs. 14.9 ± 5.1 min, P < 0.05, ES = 0.3) and a significant correlation between both TTE tests was found (r = 0.64, P < 0.05). To reach VO_{2max}, Buchfuhrer et al. (1983) recommended a time span of 10 ± 2 min for an incremental ramp protocol. This widely cited recommendation is applied for incremental protocols with able-bodied participants but also for upper body exercises and disabled subjects. With 16 untrained able-bodied men, Smith et al. (2006) observed, during an incremental arm crank ergometry, the effects of two ramp rates (12W·min^{-1} vs. 6W·min^{-1}) on the attainment of peak physiological responses and power output (Smith et al., 2006). In this study, TTE was shorter for the 12W·min^{-1} protocol (within the range of 8–12 min) whereas, for the 6W·min^{-1} protocol, TTE extends to 15 ± 4 min. However, no significant difference was found for VO_2, V_E, and HR$_{peak}$ between both protocols. In wheelchair athletes, Vinet et al. (1997) adjusted the velocity increment from a progressive treadmill test to be within the limits defined by Buchfuhrer et al. (8:50 ± 1:24 min). The Modified Yo-Yo intermittent recovery test (10 m shuttle run) provides higher TTE (16.96 ± 1.14 min), as reported by Yanci et al. (2015) in WBP. Considering the recommendations of time span (between 8 and 12 min) and given the absence of differences in the peak physiological responses, IFT$_{30-15}$ would be more appropriate than MFT for the trained participants, due to the shorter TTE required for reaching VO_{2peak}.

The difference in HR$_{peak}$ measured at the end during both tests (166.8 ± 13.8 vs. 172.8 ± 14.0 bpm for 30-15$_{IFT}$ and MFT, respectively, ES = 0.4, P < 0.05) can be explained by the intermittent nature of the 30-15$_{IFT}$, which is based on

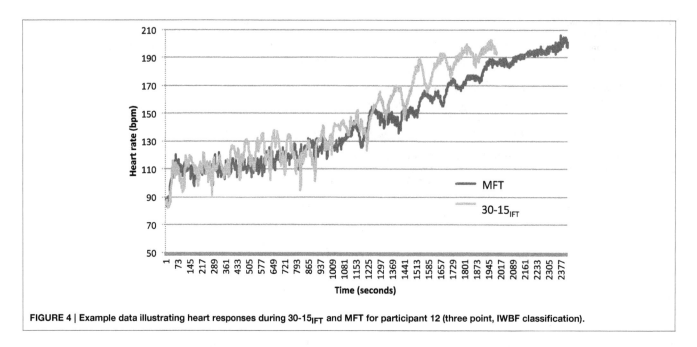

FIGURE 4 | Example data illustrating heart responses during 30-15$_{IFT}$ and MFT for participant 12 (three point, IWBF classification).

the use of 15-s passive rest periods between each stage. HR responses represented as an example in **Figure 4** for the 12 WBP clearly show the difference in HR evolution between the two tests. 30-15$_{IFT}$ therefore allows a discontinuous load stress for WBP. 30-15$_{IFT}$ does not elicit maximal HR and the maximal capabilities of the cardiovascular system while some other criteria for the attainment of a maximal exercise (like VO_2 plateau, RER > 1.1, lactate concentration accumulates > 8 mmol.L^{-1}) were achieved. A peripheral limitation may explain the submaximal values for HR$_{peak}$. Vanlandewijck et al. (1999) has supported that shuttle test is not a direct measure of aerobic capacity but rather reflects ability and specific skills using the wheelchair. Indeed, Goosey-Tolfrey and Tolfrey (2008) showed that cardiorespiratory responses during a continuous shuttle multi-stage fitness test did not fully reflect those obtained during an exercise on arm crank ergometer. With WBP population, Yanci et al. (2015) reported greater HR$_{peak}$ values (+4.7%) with a longest time (+36%) with Yo-Yo intermittent recovery test than the 30-15$_{IFT}$. One other explanation can be the disruption of the autonomic control of the HR in three subjects with high spinal cord lesion, which would control the cardiovascular function during exercise and rest (West et al., 2014).

Peak RPE measured during MFT are consistent with the level of cardio-respiratory solicitations but RPE should be used cautiously for spinal cord injury athletes and differentiated for high and low lesion (Goosey-Tolfrey et al., 2010). Test duration and monotony of continuous displacement in MFT could increase the overall rate of perceived exertion during MFT in comparison with 30-15$_{IFT}$ (15.3 ± 3.8 vs. 13.8 ± 3.5 ES = 0.5, P < 0.05). Turning in the same direction during MFT could induce premature tiredness and muscle fatigue in the upper limb of the external curve. This could be in relation to the great push power output and high arm frequency and the centrifugal force exerted on the wheelchair in the curve. With novice wheelchair users, Paulson et al. (2013) showed self-regulation

of intermittent exercises based on the overall or peripheral perceptions. Dissociating muscular and respiratory RPE in order to analyze match load is a feasible method of quantification in monitoring the training of WBP (Iturricastillo et al., 2015). In our study, overall RPE did not provide information of the muscular load perceived by the succession of starts and changes of direction in the 30-15$_{IFT}$'s protocol. An evaluation of peripheral RPE would certainly have given additional information between the two tests.

Higher MRV values were reached in a shorter time during 30-15$_{IFT}$ compared to MFT (14.2 ± 1.8 vs. 11.1 ± 1.9 km·h^{-1}, P < 0.05, ES = 0.6). 30-15$_{IFT}$ adaptation by initially starting at 6 km·h^{-1} allowed to extend the standard protocol of 3-min, in order to have the same initial velocity between MFT and 30-15$_{IFT}$. Despite this modification, 30-15$_{IFT}$ induces shorter TTE. It is explained by the difference in less than 15-s and in addition to 0.13 km·h^{-1} per stage in detriment to MFT between the both tests. Also for these reasons, MRV attained higher values at 30-15$_{IFT}$that MFT for similar VO_{2peak}.

Higher 30-15$_{IFT}$'s MRV could explain the higher peak blood lactate values. Smith et al. (2006) measured higher peak [Lact$^-$] for 12 W·min^{-1} ramp protocol and had argued that the higher workload increment than 6 W·min^{-1} was linked with higher lactactes concentration. In this study, the workload during the graded exercise has an impact on the muscular component. Thus, compared with continuous octagonal line rolling in MFT, 30-15$_{IFT}$ with direction changes and multiple acceleration phases could present a greater physiological load, as supported by relative blood lactate concentration and the extra energy expended. Δ[Lact$^-$] 30-15$_{IFT}$ values compared to MFT were higher (8.3 ± 4.2 vs. 6.9 ± 3.3 mmol·L^{-1}, P < 0.05, ES = 0.4). The significant increase of velocity per 0.5 km·h^{-1} at IFT after rest period, added to direction changes, deceleration and acceleration phase generate significant muscular efforts and greater anaerobic solicitation. However, Yanci et al.

(2015) reported, for the modified Yo-Yo protocol, lower peak [Lact$^-$] values than our data (7.21 ± 2.4 mmol·L^{-1} vs. 9.8 ± 4.4 mmol·L^{-1}). Intermittent field tests correspond to the nature of the court sport in WB. Comparing Yo-Yo and 30-15$_{IFT}$ with young soccer players, Buchheit and Rabbani (2014) have noted a large correlation ($r = 0.75$) between both tests, with 30-15$_{IFT}$ being more related to maximal sprinting speed and Yo-Yo being more associated with aerobic endurance. Bloxham et al. (2001) showed with the Canadian team that 28% of the WB playtime was spent at high anaerobic intensities and estimated 20% above the ventilatory threshold. But, 48.3% of playtime concerns recovery and low-speed replacement periods. Considering these aspects, 30-15$_{IFT}$ could be closer to the WB conditions than the Yo-Yo intermittent test. Intermittent field testing would also have the advantage in determining the BLa threshold rather than ventilatory data collection (Leicht et al., 2014) with the sample blood lactate at each level.

Using able-bodied field tests to assess the physical condition of athletes with disabilities remains difficult and even imperfect (Goosey-Tolfrey and Leicht, 2013). First, pushing for inducing wheelchair rolling is not comparable to running. The amount of energy required for the inertia of the wheelchair are different, especially to start, to turn or to glide at half turn. Secondly, the initial rolling velocity is often inappropriate and the increment may be too important. In these conditions, shuttle protocols need a great technique or ability to maneuver the wheelchair and could limit the wheelchair novices and players with a low classification point (IWBF) that have more significant disabilities than the others. Shuttle tests could be more disadvantageous for athletes with greater disabilities than MFT in which the participants determine their preferred direction of rotation (Vanlandewijck et al., 1999). Functional asymmetry with a dominant side and contralateral side deficit in strength, imbalance had low impact for the physiological responses and MRV that are related between both tests ($r = 0.57$, $P < 0.05$). Heterogeneity of pathologies and residual functional capabilities represented in our study provide individual responses as shown in **Figure 3**.

Maneuvering a wheelchair during acceleration-deceleration phases, slide and half turns requires specific skills, considering individual muscular impairments and trunk imbalance. A moderate to high level of expertise of these techniques is essential for not stopping prematurely in 30-15$_{IFT}$. It would be useful to compare our results during 30-15$_{IFT}$ with other untrained or novice wheelchair users in order to determine if 30-15$_{IFT}$ is also adaptable to various populations like MFT. Sprinting ability and

wheelchair maneuverability are probably important predictors of performance in WBP (Vanlandewijck et al., 1999; Granados et al., 2015; Yanci et al., 2015). Thus, the 30-15$_{IFT}$ has the advantage to assess, in addition to physical fitness, the technical performance to maintain wheeling velocity with succession of alternating turns. MFT was originally developed to assess aerobic fitness of the wheelchair users without a GTX laboratory protocol. MFT is validated and the VO_{2peak} extrapolation equation from MFT-score is reliable, repeatable and similar to VO_{2peak} measured (Vanderthommen et al., 2002; Weissland et al., 2015). However, MFT protocol is not representative of the WB nature while intermittent field tests are more similar but would need assessment to determine their level of reliability, validity and sensitivity.

As a take home message, the MFT test is more appropriate for the determination of maximal physiological capacities of WBP and the associated MRV can be used for the individualization of pre-season training programs. However, with a shorter time to exhaustion, 30-15$_{IFT}$ is also really interesting and relevant for the evaluation of the WBP. This intermittent field test allows reaching VO_{2peak} with a higher contribution of the anaerobic metabolism, while also assessing and taking into account the specific technical characteristics of WB. The important differences for peak HR, [Lact$^-$] and MRV values between both tests emphasize the importance of an adequate and relevant test selection, according to the parameter of interest.

CONCLUSION

The 30-15 Intermittent Fitness Test induced a higher MRV with a greater blood lactate value but lower heart rate and perceived exertion compared to the original continuous MFT. Moreover, time of exhaustion is shorter for 30-15$_{IFT}$ with similar peak oxygen uptake reached at the end of both test. Intermittent field test has some advantages over MFT for jointly assessing physical fitness and technical ability of WBP. It would be necessary in the future to investigate the reliability and validity from a standardized test on wheelchair ergometer in the laboratory.

ACKNOWLEDGMENTS

The authors also thank the athletes and their coaches for their participation to this study. We warmly thank ≪ Fédération Française Handisport ≫ collaborating for this study. The authors wish to thank Clare Doyle for his participation.

REFERENCES

Bernardi, M., Guerra, E., Di Giacinto, B., Di Cesare, A., Castellano, V., and Bhambhani, Y. (2010). Field evaluation of paralympic athletes in selected sports: implications for training. *Med. Sci. Sports Exerc.* 42, 1200–1208. doi: 10.1249/MSS.0b013e3181c67d82

Bland, J. M., and Altman, D. G. (1986). Statistical methods for assessing agreement between two methods of clinical measurement. *Lancet* 1, 307–310.

Bloxham, L. A., Bell, G. J., Bhambhani, Y., and Steadward, R. D. (2001). Time motion analysis and physiological profile of canadian world cup

wheelchair basketball players. *Sports Med. Train. Rehabil.* 10, 183–198. doi: 10.1080/1057831021039

Borg, G. (1990). Psychophysical scaling with applications in physical work and the perception of exertion. *Scand. J. Work Environ. Health* 16, 55–58.

Buchfuhrer, M. J., Hansen, J. E., Robinson, T. E., Sue, D. Y., Wasserman, K., and Whipp, B. J. (1983). Optimizing the exercise protocol for cardiopulmonary assessment. *J. Appl. Physiol. Respir. Environ. Exerc. Physiol.* 55, 1558–1564.

Buchheit, M. (2008). The 30-15 intermittent fitness test: accuracy for individualizing interval training of young intermittent sport players. *J. Strength Cond. Res.* 22, 365–374. doi: 10.1519/JSC.0b013e3181635b2e

Buchheit, M., and Rabbani, A. (2014). The 30-15 Intermittent Fitness Test versus the Yo-Yo Intermittent Recovery Test Level 1: relationship and sensitivity to training. *Int. J. Sports Physiol. Perform.* 9, 522–524. doi: 10.1123/ijspp.2012-0335

Carminatti, L. J., Possamai, C. A. P., de Moraes, M., da Silva, J. F., de Luacs, R. D., Dittrich, N., et al. (2013). Intermittent versus continuous incremental field tests: Are maximal variables interchangeable. *J. Sports Sci. Med.* 12, 165–170.

Cohen, J. (1992). A power primer. *Psychol. Bull.* 112, 155–159.

Coutts, K. D. (1992). Dynamics of wheelchair basketball. *Med. Sci. Sports Exerc.* 24, 231–234.

Cunningham, T. K., McCann, G. P., Nimmo, M. A., and Hillis, W. S. (2000). A comparison of the multistage fitness test with ergometer derived peak VO2 in paraplegic athletes. *Br. J. Sports Med.* 34, 148–152.

De Groot, S., Balvers, I., Kouwenhoven, S., and Janssen, T. (2012). Validity and reliability of tests determining performance-related components of wheelchair basketball. *J. Sports Sci.* 30, 879–887. doi: 10.1080/02640414.2012.675082

De Lira, C. A., Vancini, R. L., Minozzo, F. C., Sousa, B. S., Dubas, J. P., Andrade, M. S., et al. (2010). Relationship between aerobic and anaerobic parameters and functional classification in wheelchair basketball players. *Scand. J. Med. Sci. Sport* 20, 638–643. doi: 10.1111/j.1600-0838.2009.00934.x

Gil, S. M., Yanci, J., Otero, M., Olasagasti, J., Badiola, A., Bidaurrazaga-Letona, I., et al. (2015). The functional classification and field test performance in wheelchair basketball players. *J. Hum. Kinet.* 46, 219–230. doi: 10.1515/hukin-2015-0050

Goosey-Tolfrey, V., Lenton, J., Goddard, V., Oldfield, V., Tolfrey. K., and Eston, R. (2010). Regulating intensity using perceived exertion in spinal cord–injured participants. *Med. Sci. Sports Exerc.* 42, 608–613. doi: 10.1249/MSS.0b013e3181b72cbc

Goosey-Tolfrey, V. L., and Leicht, C. A. (2013). Field-based physiological testing of wheelchair athletes. *Sports Med.* 43, 77–91. doi: 10.1007/s40279-012-0009-6

Goosey-Tolfrey, V. L., and Tolfrey, K. (2008). The multi-stage fitness test as a predictor of endurance fitness in wheelchair athletes. *J. Sports Sci.* 26, 511–517. doi: 10.1080/02640410701624531

Granados, C., Yanci, J., Badiola, A., Iturricastillo, A., Otero, M., Olasagasti, J., et al. (2015). Anthropometry and performance in wheelchair basketball. *J. Strength Cond. Res.* 29, 1812–1820. doi: 10.1519/JSC.0000000000000817

Huonker, M., Schmid, A., Sorichter, S., Schmidt-Trucksäb, A., Mrosek, P., and Keul, J. (1998). Cardiovascular differences between sedentary and wheelchair-trained subjects with paraplegia. *Med. Sci. Sports Exerc.* 30, 609–613.

Hutzler, Y. (1993). Physical performance of elite wheelchair basketball players in armcranking ergometry and in selected wheeling tasks. *Paraplegia* 31, 255–261.

International Wheelchair Basketball Federation Web site (2009). *International Wheelchair Basketball Federation Web site [Internet] IWBF Player Classification for Wheelchair Basketball.* Available online at: http://www.iwbf.org (Accessed Dec 28, 2014).

Iturricastillo, A., Yanci, J., Granados, C., and Goosey-Tolfrey, V. (2015). Quantifying wheelchair basketball match load:a comparison of heart rate and perceived exertion methods. *Int. J. Sports Physiol. Perform.* doi: 10.1123/ijspp.2015-0257. [Epub ahead of print].

Leicht, C. A., Griggs, K. E., Lavin, J., Tolfrey, K., and Goosey-Tolfrey, V. L. (2014). Blood lactate and ventilatory thresholds in wheelchair athletes with tetraplegia and paraplegia. *Eur. J. Appl. Physiol.* 114, 1635–1643. doi: 10.1007/s00421-014-2886-x

Leicht, C. A., Tolfrey, K., Lenton, J. P., Bishop, N. C., and Goosey-Tolfrey, V. L. (2013). The verification phase and reliability of physiological parameters in peak testing of elite wheelchair athletes. *Eur. J. Appl. Physiol.* 113, 337–345. doi: 10.1007/s00421-012-2441-6

Leprêtre, P. M., Weissland, T., Paton, C., Jeanne, M., Delanaud, S., and Ahmaidi, S. (2012). Comparison of 2 portable respiratory gas analysers. *Int. J. Sports Med.* 33, 728–733. doi: 10.1055/s-0031-1301316

Molik, B., Kosmol, A., Laskin, J.-J., Morgulec-Adamowicz, N., Skucas, K., Dabrowska, A., et al. (2010). Wheelchair basketball skill tests: differences

between athletes functional classification level and disability type. *Fizyo. Rehabil.* 21, 11–19.

Paulson, T. A., Bishop, N. C., Eston, R. G., and Goosey-Tolfrey, V. L. (2013). Differentiated perceived exertion and self-regulated wheelchair exercise. *Arch. Phys. Med. Rehabil.* 94, 2269–2276. doi: 10.1016/j.apmr.2013.03.018

Pyne, D. B., Boston, T., Martin, D. T., and Logan, A. (2000). Evaluation of the lactate pro blood lactate analyser. *Eur. J. Appl. Physiol.* 82, 112–116. doi: 10.1007/s004210050659

Rotstein, A., Sagiv, M., Ben-Sira, D., Werber, G., Hutzler, J., and Annenburg, H. (1994). Aerobic capacity and anaerobic threshold of wheelchair basketball players. *Paraplegia* 32, 196–201.

Sawatzky, B. J., Miller, W. C., and Denison, I. (2005). Measuring energy expenditure using heart rate to assess the effects of wheelchair tyre pressure. *Clin. Rehabil.* 19, 182–187. doi: 10.1191/0269215505 cr823oa

Schmid, A., Huonker, M., Stober, P., Barturen, J.-M., Schmidt-Trucksäss, A., Dürr, H., et al. (1998). Physical performance and cardiovascular and metabolic adaptation of elite female wheelchair basketball players in wheelchair ergometry and in competition. *Am. J. Phys. Med. Rehabil.* 77, 527–533.

Smith, P. M., Amaral, I., Doherty, M., Price, M. J., and Jones, A. (2006). The influence of ramp rate on VO$_{2peak}$ and "excess" VO$_2$ during arm crank ergometry. *Int. J. Sports. Med.* 27, 610–616. doi: 10.1055/s-2005-865857

Sporner, M. L., Grindle, G. G., Kelleher, A., Teodorski, E. E., Cooper, R. and Cooper, R. A. (2009). Quantification of activity during wheelchair basketball and rugby at the national veterans wheelchair games: a pilot study. *Prosthet. Orthot. Int.* 33, 210–217. doi: 10.1080/03093640903051816

Vanderthommen, M., Francaux, M., Colinet, C., Lehance, C., Lhermerout, C., Crielaard, J. M., et al. (2002). A multistage field test of wheelchair users for evaluation of fitness and prediction of peak oxygen consumption. *J. Rehabil. Res. Dev.* 39, 685–692.

Vanlandewijck, Y. C., Daly, D. J., and Theisen, D. M. (1999). Field test evaluation of aerobic, anaerobic, and wheelchair basketball skill performances. *Int. J. Sports Med.* 20, 548–554. doi: 10.1055/s-1999-9465

Vinet, A., Bernard, P.-L., Poulain, M., Varray, A., Le Gallais, D., and Micallef, J. P. (1996). Validation of an incremental field test for the direct assessment of peak oxygen uptake in wheelchair-dependent athletes. *Spinal Cord* 34, 228–293.

Vinet, A., Le Gallais, D., Bernard, P. L., Poulain, M., Varray, A., Mercier, J., et al. (1997). Aerobic metabolism and cardioventilatory responses in paraplegic athletes during an incremental wheelchair exercise. *Eur. J. Appl. Physiol.* 76, 455–461.

Weissland, T., Faupin, A., Borel, B., Berthoin, S., and Leprêtre, P. M. (2015). Effects of modified multistage field test on performance and physiological responses in wheelchair basketball players. *BioMed. Res. Int.* 2015:245378. doi: 10.1155/2015/245378

West, C. R., Wong, S. C., and Krassioukov, A. V. (2014). Autonomic cardiovascular control in paralympic athletes with spinal cord injury. *Med. Sci. Sports Exerc.* 46, 60–68. doi: 10.1249/MSS.0b013e31829e46f3

Yanci, J., Granados, C., Otero, M., Badiola, A., Olasagasti, J., Bidaurrazaga-Letona, I., et al. (2015). Sprint, agility, strength and endurance capacity in wheelchair basketball players. *Biol. Sport* 32, 71–78. doi: 10.5604/20831862.1127285

Conflict of Interest Statement: The authors declare that the research was conducted in the absence of any commercial or financial relationships that could be construed as a potential conflict of interest.

14

Performance changes and relationship between vertical jump measures and actual sprint performance in elite sprinters with visual impairment throughout a Parapan American games training season

Irineu Loturco[1]*, Ciro Winckler[2], Ronaldo Kobal[1], Cesar C. Cal Abad[1], Katia Kitamura[1], Amaury W. Veríssimo[2], Lucas A. Pereira[1] and Fábio Y. Nakamura[1,3]

[1] Nucleus of High Performance in Sport, São Paulo, Brazil, [2] Brazilian Paralympic Committee, Brasilia, Brazil, [3] Department of Physical Education, State University of Londrina, Londrina, Brazil

Edited by:
Thomas Janssen,
VU University Amsterdam,
Netherlands

Reviewed by:
Naoto Fujii,
University of Ottawa, Canada
Alvaro N. Gurovich,
Indiana State University, USA

*Correspondence:
Irineu Loturco
irineu.loturco@terra.com.br

The aims of this study were to estimate the magnitude of variability and progression in actual competitive and field vertical jump test performances in elite Paralympic sprinters with visual impairment in the year leading up to the 2015 Parapan American Games, and to investigate the relationships between loaded and unloaded vertical jumping test results and actual competitive sprinting performance. Fifteen Brazilian Paralympic sprinters with visual impairment attended seven official competitions (four national, two international and the Parapan American Games 2015) between April 2014 and August 2015, in the 100- and 200-m dash. In addition, they were tested in five different periods using loaded (mean propulsive power [MPP] in jump squat [JS] exercise) and unloaded (squat jump [SJ] height) vertical jumps within the 3 weeks immediately prior to the main competitions. The smallest important effect on performances was calculated as half of the within-athlete race-to-race (or test-to-test) variability and a multiple regression analysis was performed to predict the 100- and 200-m dash performances using the vertical jump test results. Competitive performance was enhanced during the Parapan American Games in comparison to the previous competition averages, overcoming the smallest worthwhile enhancement in both the 100- (0.9%) and 200-m dash (1.43%). In addition, The SJ and JS explained 66% of the performance variance in the competitive results. This study showed that vertical jump tests, in loaded and unloaded conditions, could be good predictors of the athletes' sprinting performance, and that during the Parapan American Games the Brazilian team reached its peak competitive performance.

Keywords: Paralympics, track and field, muscle power, physical disability, blind athletes

INTRODUCTION

In general, the public is astonished by the performance of Paralympic athletes, given their extreme physical and technical capacities in spite of the presence of mild to severe physical disabilities. Although it is known that sprinting performance in Paralympic Track and Field has improved at a higher rate than the Olympic results (Grobler et al., 2015), there has been no systematic analysis of the variability and progression in competitive performance of successful teams in the months of preparation leading up to a main competition (e.g., Parapan American Games).

It has been suggested that the smallest important effect in performance at a target international event is one-half of the typical within-athlete random variability between events (Hopkins et al., 1999). An important performance progression to enhance the chances of a medal for Olympic and Paralympic swimmers in the year leading up to the main competition has been estimated to be ≈1–2% (Pyne et al., 2004; Fulton et al., 2009). In addition, in elite Olympic track athletes (including sprinters), an improvement of as little as 0.3–0.5% is considered meaningful (Hopkins, 2005). Calculating the smallest important change in Paralympic sprinters may help coaches to define targets for performance improvements in the year of preparation for the upcoming Paralympic Games.

Importantly, although the actual performance is considered the "gold standard" to assess elite athletes, simple and field based tests assessing key components of competitive outcomes can be considered as important evaluation and monitoring tools. For instance, it has been shown that loaded and unloaded vertical jumping performances are largely correlated with sprinting speed in elite sprinters (Loturco et al., 2015a,b). Confirmation of these associations between loaded/unloaded jumps (or even in combination) and sprinting performance in Paralympic athletes may help coaches to choose appropriate tests in order to evaluate and monitor Paralympic sprinters. This is particularly relevant to athletes with visual impairments as vertical jumping tests may be executed without the need for much assistance, enabling easy implementation in the training routines.

In this regard, it is important to know the within-athlete variability and progression in vertical jumping performance, to allow coaches to effectively decide whether a given change in testing performance might be considered meaningful or within the trivial variation caused by biological and/or technical factors. Based on this information, coaches can better select training strategies to optimize athletes' sports form, without necessarily assessing the actual competitive performance. Furthermore, simple tests can be used on a daily basis, thus providing fine feedback for training adjustments.

Therefore, the aim of this study was to estimate the magnitude of variability and progression in actual competitive and field vertical jump test performances in elite Paralympic sprinters with visual impairment in the year leading up to the 2015 Parapan American Games. Furthermore, we aimed to investigate the relationships between loaded and unloaded vertical jumping test results and the actual competitive sprinting performance, through the use of simple and multiple linear regression analyses.

MATERIALS AND METHODS

Seven official competitions were analyzed (four national, two international and the Parapan American Games 2015) between April 2014 and August 2015. The competitions were sanctioned by the Brazilian Paralympic Committee (CPB), International Paralympic Committee (IPC), and Americas Paralympic Committee (APC), respectively. The physical assessments were performed close to the competitions (up to 3 weeks prior to the main competitions) in five different periods (between April 2014 and July 2015) scheduled by the High Performance Programs of CPB, as part of the athletes' monitoring during the competitive season. Fifteen Brazilian Paralympic sprinters with visual impairment, from 18 to 36 years old, took part of the study (seven men and eight women, classes: T11 [$n = 9$]; T12 [$n = 3$]; and T13 [$n = 3$]). All athletes were part of the permanent Brazilian team, frequently involved in national and international competitions. This elite sample comprised four world champions, two Paralympic champions, four world record holders, two Paralympic record holders, eight world medalists, 11 Paralympic medalists, 12 top-five athletes and two top-ten athletes in the 2015 world ranking, thus attesting their high level of competitiveness.

For analysis purposes, only the times attained in the finals were retained. Across the seven competitions, a total of 120 official times (68 from the 100-m and 52 from the 200-m dash) were included in the analyses. Additionally, 192 test results in the five different periods using loaded (mean propulsive power [MPP] in jump squat [JS] exercise) and unloaded (squat jump [SJ] height) vertical jumps were analyzed. All the athletes had been previously familiarized with the testing procedures. This study was approved by the Ethics Committee of the Bandeirantes Anhanguera University. Prior to study participation, all the athletes signed an informed consent form.

Vertical Jumping Ability

Vertical jumping ability was assessed using SJ. To perform the SJ, a static position with a 90° knee flexion angle was maintained for 2-s before every jump attempt. No preparatory movement was allowed and an experienced researcher visually inspected for proper technique. Five attempts were performed interspersed by 15-s intervals. All attempts were executed with the hands on the hips. The jumps were performed on a contact platform (Smart Jump; Fusion Sport, Coopers Plains, Australia) with the obtained flight time (t) being used to estimate the height of the rise of the body's center of gravity (h) during the vertical jump (i.e., h = $gt^2/8$, where $g = 9.81$ m·s^{-2}. The best attempt was used for data analysis purposes. The athletes executed the attempts without assistance.

Bar Mean Propulsive Power in Jump Squat

Bar MPP in the JS exercise was assessed on a customized Smith machine (adapted by Hammer Strength, Rosemont, IL, USA). The athletes were instructed to execute three repetitions at maximal velocity for each load, starting at 40% of their body mass (BM). The athletes with visual impairment executed a knee flexion until the thigh was parallel to the ground (≈100°

knee angle for 2-s) and, after a command, jumped as fast as possible without losing contact between their shoulder and the bar. A load of 10% BM was gradually added in each set until a decrease in MPP was observed. A 5-min interval was provided between sets. All athletes attained their maximum values of MPP during the execution of the tests, within 4–5 attempts. Of note, the athletes achieved their highest MPP outputs at a load corresponding to ≈100% BM. To determine MPP, a linear transducer (T-Force, Dynamic Measurement System; Ergotech Consulting S.L., Murcia, Spain) was attached to the Smith machine bar. The finite differentiation technique was used to calculate bar velocity (Sanchez-Medina et al., 2010). As Sanchez-Medina et al. (2010) demonstrated that mean mechanical values during the propulsive phase better reflect the differences in the neuromuscular potential between two given individuals, MPP rather than peak power was used in the JS. The bar maximum MPP value obtained was considered for data analysis purposes. In order to consider the differences in BM between the athletes and avoid misinterpretation of the power outputs, these values were normalized by dividing the absolute power value by the BM (i.e., relative power = W.kg^{-1}) (MPP REL). All the tests were performed by the athletes with no assistance.

Statistical Analysis

The normality of data was confirmed using the Shapiro-Wilk test. Data are presented as means ± standard deviations (SD). The smallest important effect on performances was calculated as half of the within-athlete race-to-race (or test-to-test) variability (Hopkins et al., 1999). Additionally, the within-subject coefficient of variation (CV), with 90% confidence intervals (CI), was calculated as a measure of competitive and testing performance variability. A Pearson product-moment coefficient of correlation was used to analyze the relationships between SJ and MPP REL in the JS and sprinting time in the 100- and 200-m. The vertical jumping tests took place in close proximity to five of the seven competitions. A multiple regression analysis was performed using the vertical jump test results as predictors of 100- and 200-m dash performances. The possibility of collinearity between the predictive variables in multiple regression models was examined using variance inflation factor (VIF) and tolerance (i.e., VIF < 10 and tolerance > 0.2; Kennedy, 1992; Hair et al., 1995; Tabachnick and Fidell, 2001). Intraclass correlation coefficients (ICCs) were used to indicate the relationship within SJ and JS for, respectively, jumping height and MPP. The significance level was set as $P < 0.05$.

RESULTS

All data presented herein showed normal distribution. The VIF and tolerance values were 2.43 and 0.42, respectively, attesting that the independent variables (i.e., SJ and JS) were not collinear. The characteristics of the subjects are presented in the **Table 1**. The BM of the athletes did not vary substantially across the five evaluation moments (varying from 61.41 ± 9.76 to 63.84 ± 10.66). **Figure 1A** displays the means of the 100-m dash performances in the seven competitions. The mean CV (90% CI) over the competitions was 1.79% (1.47; 2.24). Meanwhile, **Figure 1B** depicts the mean performance in the 200-m events. The mean CV (90% CI) across the seven competitions was 1.35% (0.83; 1.88). The performance variation in the SJ and JS over the five moments is displayed in **Figures 2A,B**, respectively. Importantly, the ICC was 0.94 for the SJ and 0.92 for the loaded JS. The mean CVs (90% CI) for SJ and JS were 5.58% (4.18; 6.99) and 7.97% (5.91; 10.02), respectively.

The correlations (90% CI) between SJ and JS test results and 100- and 200-m dash performances were −0.80 (−0.71; −0.88) and −0.71 (−0.61; −0.81) for SJ and JS with 100-m, respectively, and; −0.81 (−0.72; −0.89) and −0.65 (−0.48; −0.79) for SJ and JS with 200-m, respectively ($P < 0.01$ for all correlations; **Figure 3**). The multiple regression analysis using SJ and JS test results as predictors of 100- and 200-m dash performances is presented in **Table 2**. The SJ and JS explained 66% of the performance variance in both 100- and 200-m dash performances.

DISCUSSION

This is the first study to investigate the relationships between loaded/unloaded vertical jump tests and the actual performance obtained by top-level Paralympic sprinters in 100 and 200 m dash events. The main finding reported herein is that, providing they are executed only a few weeks before the official tournaments (i.e., from 1 to 3 weeks), SJs and loaded JSs—when combined in a multiple linear regression model—can be good predictors of the actual competitive performance of top-level athletes with visual impairment. In addition, during a given training period, the dynamics of the performance in these specific jump tests seem to be analogous to the dynamics of the actual results obtained in 100 and 200 m dash events.

Another study has already reported strong correlations between sprinting performance (i.e., measured in time) and SJ height ($r = -0.82$) in elite sprinters who compete in 100 m dash events (Loturco et al., 2015b). This "close relationship" can be explained when analyzing the mechanical aspects of unloaded SJs. In order to jump higher, an athlete has to apply a substantial amount of force against the ground—and against his/her own BM (Loturco et al., 2015a,b). Thus, this measurement is already normalized by the subject's weight, being able to express his/her relative neuromuscular potential (i.e., relative values of muscle force and muscle power; Bosco et al., 1983; Copi et al., 2014). Furthermore, from a mechanical perspective, athletes with better performances in vertical jumps are possibly more efficient at overcoming the inertia and accelerating their bodies vertically (Bunton et al., 1993; Loturco et al., 2015b). Importantly, as the ground reaction forces increase, the vertical jump height increases (Loturco et al., 2015b). The same occurs in sprinting, during the transition from lower to higher velocities

TABLE 1 | Characteristics of the subjects (mean ± SD).

Age (years)	Weight (kg)	Height (cm)
26.5 ± 6.2	63.3 ± 10.6	169 ± 0.9

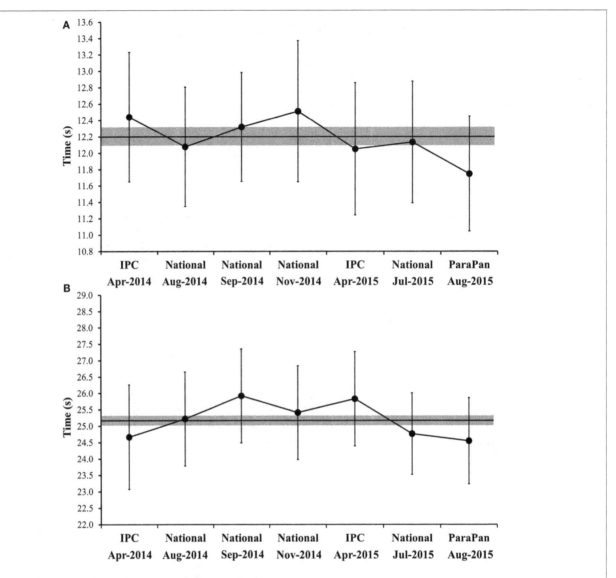

FIGURE 1 | Variation in 100- (A) and 200-m (B) dash performances across seven official competitions. The black line represent the mean individual performances, and the gray area represent the smallest important effect on performances (i.e., calculated as half of the within-athlete race-to-race variability). *National* corresponds to competitions organized by the local Paralympic Committee; *IPC* corresponds to international competitions organized by the International Paralympic Committee; *ParaPan* corresponds to the ParaPan American Games.

(i.e., top-speed sprinting), which results in shorter support phases with simultaneous increases in vertical peak force (Nilsson and Thorstensson, 1989). Curiously, even in sprinters with visual impairment, this mechanical similarity seems to be capable of influencing the specific performance in 100 and 200 m dash events. Certainly, the user-friendly characteristic and practicality of SJ facilitates its execution by athletes with visual impairment, thus reinforcing its use as a tool to control/monitor the variation in sprinting performance presented by this specific group of Paralympics.

Loaded JSs are usually performed with moderate training loads, moved as rapidly as possible (Cormie et al., 2011; Loturco et al., 2015d). In this study, the athletes executed an *optimal loading test* in order to determine their individual *optimal power loads* (i.e., loads capable of generating higher values of muscle power). The maximal JS power has been extensively related to a variety of specific sports measures, including speed and acceleration abilities (Sleivert and Taingahue, 2004; Cronin and Hansen, 2005; Loturco et al., 2015a,b,d). Interestingly, the athletes also presented significant correlations between MPP and actual sprinting time, both in 100 and 200 m dash events ($r = -0.71$ and -0.65, for 100- and 200-m). Of note, the athletes reached their highest MPP at $\approx 100\%$ of their BM, which represents a substantial amount of external overloading. At this loading condition, movement performance is possibly associated with maximum dynamic strength (i.e., ability to apply high force at low velocity; Baker and Nance, 1999; Young et al., 2001; Stone et al., 2003). Similarly, to start from

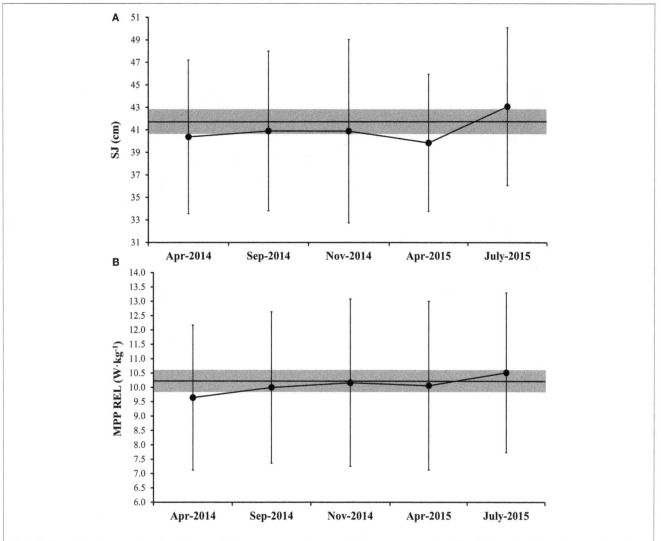

FIGURE 2 | Variation in squat jump (SJ) (A) and relative mean propulsive power in jump squat exercise (MPP REL JS) (B) test results across the five periods. The black line represents the mean individual performances, and the gray area represents the smallest important effect on performances (i.e., calculated as half of the within-athlete test-to-test variability).

zero-velocity and achieve higher accelerations in very-short periods, the athletes have to apply greater amounts of force (at lower velocities) against the ground (Wisløff et al., 2004; Loturco et al., 2014). More importantly, based on the parametric relationship between force and velocity (Cronin et al., 2002; Loturco et al., 2015c), these higher rates of acceleration can only be attained if the accelerated mass (i.e., athlete's BM) represents a relatively low resistance for the athlete involved (when compared to his/her maximum dynamic strength; Moss et al., 1997; Cormie et al., 2007; Loturco et al., 2014). Therefore, although we did not have the "partial times" of the actual competitions to perform additional correlational analysis in this study, it is highly conceivable that the more powerful athletes presented superior performance in the acceleration phases of sprinting, in both the 100 and 200 m dash. Undoubtedly, this issue should receive priority in future investigations, in spite of the difficulty in obtaining partial times in official competitions.

In this study, the possibility of combining two independent variables (i.e., SJ and JS) in a multiple linear regression model to more accurately predict the athletes' actual performance was considered due to the distinct importance of each one of these measures in sprinting mechanics and due to the high levels of competitiveness found in Paralympic track and field competitions. As aforementioned, whereas JS is probably more related to the accelerating phases of sprinting (Wisløff et al., 2004; Loturco et al., 2014), SJ may be more associated with the "top-speed" phases of both the 100- and 200-m dash (Loturco et al., 2015b). Therefore, since individual performance in top-level sports depends on very fine adjustments, it is worth considering novel and better models/strategies to predict results and enhance performance. Still, although the use of multiple

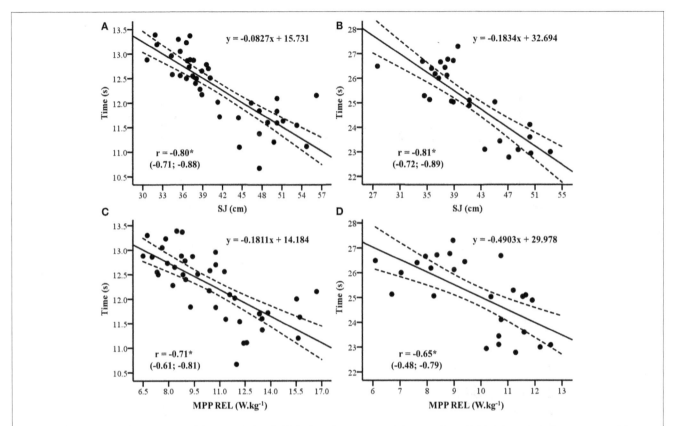

FIGURE 3 | Linear regression between 100 (A,C) and 200-m (B,D) dash performances and the squat jump (SJ) height and relative mean propulsive power (MPP REL) in the jump squat (JS) exercise; *$P < 0.01$.

regression models have increased only (on average) ∼1.2% of the explained variance between dependent (actual sprint times) and independent variables (SJ and JS), we considered relevant to carry out this calculation, since slight differences between individuals in 100- and 200-m dash events might significantly affect their competitive results. Observing the data reported here, from this point on, Paralympic coaches can better estimate the actual performance of their top-level athletes in official sprint competitions. Furthermore, by understanding the importance of this specific "mechanical combination" (i.e., SJ and JS) in sprinting performance, they will be able to develop more effective and specific training programs.

Concerning the within-subject variability, the smallest worthwhile enhancements in the 100- (0.9%) and 200-m dash (1.43%) were comparable to those reported in Olympic and Paralympic swimmers (Pyne et al., 2004). However, these values were higher than the estimates provided by elite track athletes without disabilities (Hopkins, 2005). The greater variability in athletes with visual impairment's performances may be associated with their disabilities (Fulton et al., 2009) and the possible influence of their respective guides on the individuals' sprinting mechanics (unpublished data). Importantly, the smallest worthwhile enhancement provides the coach with an idea of the meaningfulness of a given change in an athlete's performance. In general, an enhancement needs to be higher than the smallest worthwhile enhancement to affect the results

TABLE 2 | Predictions of 100- and 200-m dash performances using multiple regression analysis.

	R^2	Equation
100-m	0.66*	$y = 15.558 - (0.063 \times SJ) - (0.061 \times JS)$
200-m	0.66*	$y = 32.918 - (0.167 \times SJ) - (0.098 \times JS)$

*SJ, squat jump; JS, jump squat; *$P < 0.01$.*

(i.e., medal prospects; Fulton et al., 2009). Curiously, in the 100-m dash, the athletes presented worse sprinting times than their mean times during the period of observation, but during the Parapan American Games they achieved their "performance peak." Although in the 200-m the times were close to the mean performance throughout the observation, during the Parapan American Games, they reached a meaningful performance change (in comparison to the previous analyzed competitions). To some extent, this explains the outstanding results obtained by the Brazilian team during the 2015 Pan American Games (three gold, six silver, and two bronze medals in the 100- and 200-m races).

The jumping test results were substantially more variable than the actual competitive performances in the 100- and 200-m dash (CV of SJ = 5.58% and JS = 7.97%), which implies the need for larger improvements in jumping tests, in order to consider these enhancements as meaningful. The general dynamics of the vertical jumping performance were similar to the sprinting performance; nevertheless, only SJ (change > 2.79%) attained a meaningful enhancement prior to the Parapan American Games. Accordingly, while monitoring SJ and JS in Paralympic athletes, coaches need to be aware that the meaningful performance changes should be greater than ≈2.79–3.98%; smaller changes can be considered within the range of the inherent measurement variability. The advantage of these practical and timesaving tests is that they can be easily implemented in the athletes' routines, for finely adjusting the training strategies and, therefore, improving sprinting performance (e.g., stretch-shortening cycle efficiency).

Future studies are necessary in order to determine other factors involved in the non-explained variance of sprinting ability in athletes with visual impairment (e.g., anthropometric characteristics of the subjects and coordination between the athletes with visual impairment and their respective guides, etc). Possibly, some factors related to jumping and running mechanics will reveal more movement similarities and additional associations between their respective kinetic and kinematic parameters.

CONCLUSION

Performance in Paralympic elite sprinting depends on a series of neuromuscular, physiological and technical factors. This study showed that vertical jump tests, in loaded and unloaded conditions, could be good predictors of athletes' sprinting performance, mainly when combined in a multiple linear regression equation. Furthermore, in this specific group of top-level Paralympic athletes, the dynamics of SJ and JS performances seem to follow the same variation as 100- and 200-m actual times. These findings may have important implications in athletes with visual impairment's training and testing methodology, since vertical jump tests can be easily performed by subjects with total or partial visual impairments. In addition, Paralympic track and field coaches can use these simple field assessments to specifically monitor their elite athletes close to official competitions, adjusting the training contents in order to optimize each athlete's performance peak. Finally, further studies should be conducted to investigate the chronic effects of training athletes with visual impairment using exclusively loaded and unloaded vertical jumps.

REFERENCES

Baker, D., and Nance, S. (1999). The relation between strength and power in professional rugby league players. *J. Strength Cond. Res.* 13, 224–229.

Bosco, C., Luhtanen, P., and Komi, P. V. (1983). A simple method for measurement of mechanical power in jumping. *Eur. J. Appl. Physiol. Occup. Physiol.* 50, 273–282. doi: 10.1007/BF00422166

Bunton, E. E., Pitney, W. A., Cappaert, T. A., and Kane, A. W. (1993). The role of limb torque, muscle action and proprioception during closed kinetic chain rehabilitation of the lower extremity. *J. Athl. Train.* 28, 10–20.

Ćopić, N., Dopsaj, M., Ivanović, J., Nešić, G., and Jarić, S. (2014). Body composition and muscle strength predictors of jumping performance: differences between elite female volleyball competitors and nontrained individuals. *J. Strength Cond. Res.* 28, 2709–2716. doi: 10.1519/JSC.0000000000000468

Cormie, P., McCaulley, G. O., and McBride, J. M. (2007). Power versus strength-power jump squat training: influence on the load-power relationship. *Med. Sci. Sports Exerc.* 39, 996–1003. doi: 10.1097/mss.0b013e3180408e0c

Cormie, P., McGuigan, M. R., and Newton, R. U. (2011). Developing maximal neuromuscular power: part 2 - training considerations for improving maximal power production. *Sports Med.* 41, 125–146. doi: 10.2165/11538500-000000000-00000

Cronin, J. B., and Hansen, K. T. (2005). Strength and power predictors of sports speed. *J. Strength Cond. Res.* 19, 349–357. doi: 10.1519/14323.1

Cronin, J. B., McNair, P. J., and Marshall, R. N. (2002). Is velocity-specific strength training important in improving functional performance? *J. Sports Med. Phys. Fitness.* 42, 267–273.

Fulton, S. K., Pyne, D., Hopkins, W., and Burkett, B. (2009). Variability and progression in competitive performance of Paralympic swimmers. *J. Sports Sci.* 27, 535–539. doi: 10.1080/02640410802641418

Grobler, L., Ferreira, S., and Terblanche, E. (2015). Paralympic Sprint Performance Between 1992 and 2012. *Int. J. Sports Physiol. Perform.* doi: 10.1123/ijspp.2014-0560. [Epub ahead of print].

Hair, J. F. Jr., Anderson, R. E., Tatham, R. L., and Black, W. C. (1995). *Multivariate Data Analysis.* New York, NY: Macmillan.

Hopkins, W. G. (2005). Competitive performance of elite track-and-field athletes: variability and smallest worthwhile enhancements. *Sportscience* 9, 17–20.

Hopkins, W. G., Hawley, J. A., and Burke, L. M. (1999). Design and analysis of research on sport performance enhancement. *Med. Sci. Sports Exerc.* 31, 472–485. doi: 10.1097/00005768-199903000-00018

Kennedy, P. (1992). *A Guide to Econometrics.* Oxford: Blackwell.

Loturco, I., D'Angelo, R. A., Fernandes, V., Gil, S., Kobal, R., Cal Abad C. C., et al. (2015a). Relationship between sprint ability and loaded/unloaded jump tests in elite sprinters. *J. Strength Cond. Res.* 29, 758–764. doi: 10.1519/JSC.0000000000000660

Loturco, I., Kobal, R., Gil, S., Pivetti, B., Kitamura, K., Pereira, L. A., et al. (2014). Differences in loaded and unloaded vertical jumping ability and sprinting performance between Brazilian elite under-20 and senior soccer players. *Am. J. Sports Sci.* 2, 8–13. doi: 10.11648/j.ajss.s.2014020601.12

Loturco, I., Nakamura, F. Y., Artioli, G. G., Kobal, R., Kitamura, K., Cal Abad, C. C., et al. (2015d). Strength and power qualities are highly associated with punching impact in elite amateur boxers. *J. Strength Cond. Res.* doi: 10.1519/JSC.0000000000001075. [Epub ahead of print].

Loturco, I., Nakamura, F. Y., Kobal, R., Gil, S., Cal Abad, C. C., Cuniyochi, R., et al. (2015c). Training for power and speed: effects of increasing or decreasing jump-squat velocity in elite young soccer players. *J. Strength Cond. Res.* 29, 2771–2779. doi: 10.1519/JSC.0000000000000951

Loturco, I., Pereira, L. A., Cal Abad, C. C., D'Angelo, R. A., Fernandes, V., Kitamura, K., et al. (2015b). Vertical and horizontal jump tests are strongly associated with competitive performance in 100-m dash events. *J. Strength Cond. Res.* 29, 1966–1971. doi: 10.1519/JSC.0000000000000849

Moss, B. M., Refsnes, P. E., Abildgaard, A., Nicolaysen, K., and Jensen, J. (1997). Effects of maximal effort strength training with different loads on dynamic strength, cross-sectional area, load-power and load-velocity relationships. *Eur. J. Appl. Physiol. Occup. Physiol.* 75, 193–199. doi: 10.1007/s004210050147

Nilsson, J., and Thorstensson, A. (1989). Ground reaction forces at different speeds of human walking and running. *Acta Physiol. Scand.* 136, 217–227. doi: 10.1111/j.1748-1716.1989.tb08655.x

Pyne, D., Trewin, C., and Hopkins, W. (2004). Progression and variability of competitive performance of olympic swimmers. *J. Sports Sci.* 22, 613–620. doi: 10.1080/02640410310001655822

Sanchez-Medina, L., Perez, C. E., and Gonzalez-Badillo, J. J. (2010). Importance of the propulsive phase in strength assessment. *Int. J. Sports Med.* 31, 123–129. doi: 10.1055/s-0029-1242815

Sleivert, G., and Taingahue, M. (2004). The relationship between maximal jump-squat power and sprint acceleration in athletes. *Eur. J. Appl. Physiol.* 91, 46–52. doi: 10.1007/s00421-003-0941-0

Stone, M. H., O'Bryant, H. S., McCoy, L., Coglianese, R., Lehmkuhl, M., and Schilling, B. (2003). Power and maximum strength relationships during performance of dynamic and static weighted jumps. *J. Strength Cond. Res.* 17, 140–147.

Tabachnick, B. G., and Fidell, L. S. (2001). *Using Multivariate Statistics.* Boston, MA: Allyn and Bacon.

Wisløff, U., Castagna, C., Helgerud, J., Jones, R., and Hoff, J. (2004). Strong correlation of maximal squat strength with sprint performance and vertical jump height in elite soccer players. *Br. J. Sports Med.* 38, 285–288. doi: 10.1136/bjsm.2002.002071

Young, W., Benton, D., and Pryor, J. M. (2001). Resistance training for short sprints and maximum-speed sprints. *Strength Cond. J.* 23, 7. doi: 10.1519/00126548-200104000-00001

Conflict of Interest Statement: The authors declare that the research was conducted in the absence of any commercial or financial relationships that could be construed as a potential conflict of interest.

15

Low Intensity Exercise Training Improves Skeletal Muscle Regeneration Potential

Tiziana Pietrangelo [1, 2, 3, 4], *Ester S. Di Filippo* [1, 3, 4], *Rosa Mancinelli* [1, 3, 4]*, *Christian Doria* [1, 2, 4], *Alessio Rotini* [1, 4], *Giorgio Fanò-Illic* [2, 3, 4] and *Stefania Fulle* [1, 2, 3, 4]

[1] Department of Neuroscience, Imaging and Clinical Sciences, University "G. d'Annunzio" Chieti-Pescara, Chieti, Italy, [2] Laboratory of Functional Evaluation, "G. d'Annunzio" University of Chieti-Pescara, Chieti, Italy, [3] Centre for Aging Sciences, d'Annunzio Foundation, Chieti, Italy, [4] Department of Neuroscience, Imaging and Clinical Sciences, Interuniversity Institute of Myology, Chieti, Italy

Purpose: The aim of this study was to determine whether 12 days of low-to-moderate exercise training at low altitude (598 m a.s.l.) improves skeletal muscle regeneration in sedentary adult women.

Methods: Satellite cells were obtained from the *vastus lateralis* skeletal muscle of seven women before and after this exercise training at low altitude. They were investigated for differentiation aspects, superoxide anion production, antioxidant enzymes, mitochondrial potential variation after a depolarizing insult, intracellular Ca^{2+} concentrations, and micro (mi)RNA expression (miR-1, miR-133, miR-206).

Results: In these myogenic populations of adult stem cells, those obtained after exercise training, showed increased Fusion Index and intracellular Ca^{2+} concentrations. This exercise training also generally reduced superoxide anion production in cells (by 12–67%), although not in two women, where there was an increase of ~15% along with a reduced superoxide dismutase activity. miRNA expression showed an exercise-induced epigenetic transcription profile that was specific according to the reduced or increased superoxide anion production of the cells.

Conclusions: The present study shows that low-to-moderate exercise training at low altitude improves the regenerative capacity of skeletal muscle in adult women. The differentiation of cells was favored by increased intracellular calcium concentration and increased the fusion index. This low-to-moderate training at low altitude also depicted the epigenetic signature of cells.

Keywords: low-to-moderate intensity exercise training, satellite cells, superoxide anion, oxidative status, miRNA, women

Edited by:
Barbara Morgan,
University of Wisconsin-Madison, USA

Reviewed by:
Naoto Fujii,
University of Ottawa, Canada
Shane A. Phillips,
University of Illinois at Chicago, USA

*Correspondence:
Rosa Mancinelli
r.mancinelli@unich.it

INTRODUCTION

Satellite cells are myogenic cells that are responsible for postnatal skeletal muscle growth. In normal adult muscle, satellite cells account for differently activated peripheral sub-sarcolemmal nuclei, which depend on the metabolic properties of the muscle fiber and the age of the person (Verdijk et al., 2014). In response to various stimuli, satellite cells can enter the mitotic cycle, proliferate, and fuse, thereby contributing to muscle regeneration for repair or hypertrophy of postnatal skeletal muscle (Lorenzon et al., 2004; Snijders et al., 2012; Ceafalan et al., 2014). Satellite cells are specifically involved in skeletal muscle adaptation to different types of exercise, such as with strength (Kvorning et al., 2014; Verdijk et al., 2014) and endurance (Kadi et al., 2004) training, whereby the intensity and duration of muscle stimulation is crucial for satellite cell activation. Indeed, although it has been demonstrated that satellite cells are not activated in response to a single bout of exercise (Kadi et al., 2004), they can modulate specific factor content after 9 h of combined resistance–endurance exercise (Verdijk, 2014). Furthermore, even if it is currently accepted that exercise has positive effects on skeletal muscle regeneration, the fitness level of subjects and the type and intensity of exercise protocols have crucial roles in satellite cell activation. In fact, a number of study demonstrated that both resistance and endurance training increased satellite cells content (Kadi et al., 2005). At the ultrastructural level, it has been observed that the endurance-training programme induced the formation of new myotubes (Appell et al., 1988). However, there are many points to be addressed at molecular level. The $[Ca^{2+}]i$ increase is a prerequisite for fusion process due to specific signaling it activates (Millay et al., 2013; Hindi et al., 2013). In fact, many studies have shown that myoblast fusion is regulated by $[Ca^{2+}]i$ increase (Constantin et al., 1996) that may depend on cholinergic (Bernareggi et al., 2012), stretch-activated and KCa channels activation (Pietrangelo et al., 2006; Shin et al., 1996).

Another molecular messenger influenced by exercise is reactive oxygen species (ROS) production (Abruzzo et al., 2013). The ROS include: superoxide anions, hydroxyl radicals, oxide anions, hydrogen peroxide, nitric oxide, peroxynitrite, lipid peroxyls, and lipid alkoxyls. ROS production is related to with the term oxidative stress, which was originally defined as "a disturbance in the pro-oxidant/anti-oxidant balance in favor of the former" (Siens and Cadenas, 1985). However, due to the complexity of the cellular redox balance, this was refined to "an imbalance between oxidants and anti-oxidants in favor of the oxidants, leading to a disruption of redox signaling and control and/or molecular damage" (Siens and Jones, 2007; Powers et al., 2011).

The cellular antioxidant system consists on the activity of scavengers as vitamin C and E, for instance, and enzymes as glutathione peroxidase, superoxide dismutase (SOD), catalase (Cat). In particular, the SOD reduces the superoxide anion to hydrogen peroxide and in turn the Cat reduces this to water. There are several studies accounting for the involvement of antioxidant enzymes in exercise-induced muscle plasticity and also in vitamin supplementation (Cumming et al., 2014; Nikolaidis et al., 2015). However, it is not well understood the role of antioxidants in human myogenesis.

In mitochondria the cellular aerobic metabolism reduces around 1–2% of oxygen to superoxide anions, which represent the most abundant free radicals produced. The superoxide reactivity could last for days in absence of enzymatic removal and it can spread out into also outside the cell, and undergo reactions far from its site of production, thus provoking cellular and general oxidative stress. However, a gender distinguish has to be considered, as female subjects are more protected than men against oxidative stress thanks to their estrogen hormone. The estrogen level in young woman exerts an antioxidant effect, as demonstrated by four-fold less DNA and lipid oxidation in female with respect to male subjects (Mecocci et al., 1999; Green and Simpkins, 2000).

Skeletal muscle contraction during exercise produces variable amounts of ROS, which depend on exercise intensity and duration (Fisher-Wellman and Bloomer, 2009; Powers et al., 2011). ROS can activate specific signaling pathways at the plasma membrane and/or stimulate gene transcription (Gundersen, 2011; Baar, 2014). In particular, recent literature suggests that both exercise and ROS can activate muscle-specific microRNAs (myo-miRs; small post-transcriptional RNAs), and regulate the differentiation levels of satellite cells (Eisenberg et al., 2009; Crippa et al., 2012; Huang et al., 2012). Among the myo-miRs of value for satellite cells, there are miR-1, miR-133, and miR-206 (Kwon et al., 2005; McCarthy and Esser, 2007; La Rovere et al., 2014).

The aim of this study was to determine whether 12-day exercise training at low altitude (598 m a.s.l.) can improve skeletal muscle regeneration in adult women. In particular, we investigated whether this kind of exercise could affect some molecular actor of the differentiation process as the fusion index, the intracellular calcium level, the redox balance, the mitochondrial activation, and the miRNA expression.

METHODS

Subjects

Seven healthy women of childbearing age (mean age, 36.3 ± 7.1 years old) who were generally used to a sedentary life-style (at 110 m altitude sea level, a.s.l.) were enrolled to serve as subjects to the study known as GOKYO KHUMBU/AMA DABLAM TREK 2012. None of these women suffered from any metabolic or skeletal muscle diseases. The women were not engaged in any specific trekking or exercise training protocols within a few months of their enrolment, except two of them who occasionally went trekking. All of the subjects provided written, informed consent before participating in the study. The study was conducted according to the Helsinki Declaration, and it was approved by Ethic Committee of "G. d'Annunzio" University of Chieti-Pescara, Italy (protocol no. 773 COET).

Experimental Design and Training

Trekking consisted of a 12- day walking at low-altitude on mountain paths in central Italy (L'Aquila, Abruzzo, Italy). The average altitude was 598 m ± 561 and a range of difference in elevation between consecutive days was 250–1000 m. The total covered distance was 139000 m. The total ascent and descent

---

Abbreviations: a.s.l., altitude sea level; $[Ca^{2+}]i$, intracellular calcium concentration; Cat, catalase; DCF-DA, 2′,7′ Dichlorodihydrofluorescein diacetate; JC-1,5,5′,6,6′-Tetrachloro-1,1′,3,3′ tetraethylbenzimidazolylcarbocyanine; H_2O_2, hydrogen peroxide; iodide/chloride; MHC, Myosin Heavy Chain; miRNA, micro ribonucleic acid; $O_2^{\bullet-}$, superoxide anion; PBS, Dulbecco's phosphate-buffered saline; ROS, Reactive oxygen species; SOD, superoxide dismutase.

were 5500 m (458 m d^{-1}; range: 0–1000 m d^{-1}) and 5350 m (445 m d^{-1}; range: 0–1000 m d^{-1}), respectively. The total walking time was 149580 s $\pm$ 27.06, on average 3 h and 28 min per day, and the average speed was 0.93 m s^{-1}. The total number of steps was 182372 $\pm$ 77.43. The volunteers freely choose their intensity of exercise also considering the general recommendations to approach physical exercise with a load adapted to personal capacity (guidelines of American College Sport Medicine, Garber et al., 2011). The exercise intensity of the training was monitored with a heart rate monitor for each subject (POLAR®, Kempele, Finland). The average heart rate of the seven subjects in the 12 day of exercise training period was 111 $\pm$ 10 bpm, which was classified as light-to-moderate intensity (Tam et al., 2015). The subjects did not perform other exercise outside the trekking protocol.

Skeletal Muscle Needle Biopsy

Tiny percutaneous needle biopsies from the *vastus lateralis* muscle were performed at the Laboratory of Functional Evaluation, "G. d'Annunzio" University of Chieti-Pescara, as described by Pietrangelo et al. (2011), a week before initiating the exercise training (PRE-Ex), and 9 days after the specific planned light-to-moderate exercise training at low altitude (POST-Ex). Specifically, after the training period, the subjects stayed at rest for a couple of days, then they were engaged in functional evaluations described in (Tam et al., 2015), that lasted 5 days, and after a couple of days of recovering, they had the needle biopsies.

Satellite Cell Population and Myogenicity

The satellite cells were obtained, expanded as myoblasts in growth medium, and differentiated as previously described (Fulle et al., 2005; Mancinelli et al., 2011). Briefly, the percentages of myogenicity of the cell cultures were obtained using an immunocytochemistry assay, with the marker desmin (Kaufman and Foster, 1988; Behr et al., 1994), and with biotinylated streptavidin-AP kits (LSAB + System-AP Universal kits; Cat. No. K0678; DAKO, Dakocytomation, Glostrup, Denmark). Differentiation of the cell populations was determined by counting the numbers of nuclei in the myotubes after 7 days of differentiation, as percentages with respect to the total number of nuclei, with the ratio between these two values (nuclei in myotubes/total nuclei × 100%) giving the Fusion Index. We only considered myotubes that were positive to the primary antibody against myosin heavy chain (MHC), using the MF20 anti-MHC monoclonal antibody (diluted 1:50; Developmental Studies Hybridoma Bank, University of Iowa, Iowa City, IA, USA), and that contained three or more nuclei (Pietrangelo et al., 2009).

Intracellular Calcium Concentration Measurement

The cells were loaded with Fura2-AM at the final concentration of 5 μM for 30 min, which was then de-esterificated for 20 min at 37°C. The experiments were performed and images were acquired using the procedures and set-up described by Pietrangelo et al. (2002).

Reactive Oxygen Species

The general analysis of ROS, specifically the cellular peroxidation end products, was conducted using the dye 2,7-dichlorofluorescein diacetate (DCF; Cat.No. D6883; Sigma). The cells were plated and grown in 96-well microplates (1000 cells 0.32 cm^{-1}), and incubated with 10 μM DCF for 30 min at 37°C in sterile normal extracellular solution (140 mM NaCl, 2.8 mM KCl, 2 mM $CaCl_2$, 2 mM $MgCl_2$, 10 mM glucose, 10 mM Hepes, pH 7.3). The fluorescence of the dye accumulated in the cytoplasm (i.e., 2,7-dichlorofluorescein) was determined at 530 nm (excitation, 490 nm) using a fluorometer (SPECTRAmax Gemini XS; Molecular Devices Toronto, ON, Canada). The analysis was conducted using the SOFTmax Pro software. The cells were stimulated with 100 nM hydrogen peroxide (H_2O_2) to evaluate their response to an oxidant (Menghini et al., 2011).

To determine the superoxide anion ($O_2^{\bullet-}$), we used an assay based on the dye nitroblue tetrazolium chloride (NBT; Cat. No. N6639; Sigma-Aldrich) and its reduction into formazan $O_2^{\bullet-}$ (Sozio et al., 2013). The absorbance at 550 nm was determined using a spectrophotometer (SPECTRAmax 190 microplate 257; Molecular Devices, Sunnyvale, CA, USA), such that the greater the $O_2^{\bullet-}$ level, the greater the absorbance. The cells (1 × 10^6 cells) were detached, centrifuged at 170 × g for 5 min, resuspended in 1 ml NBT at 1 mg ml^{-1} in 0.9% aqueous NaCl, and incubated for 3 h at 37°C. Then, the cells were centrifuged at 100 × g for 10 min, resuspended in 1 ml DMSO, and left for 20 min at 37°C. Finally, the NBT absorbance was determined.

Transmembrane Mitochondrial Potential

The mitochondrial membrane potential was determined using the JC-1 dye (5,5′,6, 6′-tetracloro-1,1′,3,3′-tetraethylbenzimidazolylcarbocianine iodide/chloride; Molecular Probes). JC-1 is a cationic dye that accumulates in the mitochondria. When the mitochondrial potential is high, as in normal cells, JC-1 aggregates into dimers that emit red fluorescence (aggregated J: excitation/ emission, 560/595 nm). When the membrane potential is low, as in the presence of oxidative stress, JC-1 forms monomers that emit green fluorescence (excitation/emission, 488/522 nm), with concomitant decreased red fluorescence. The ratio of the red/green fluorescence depends exclusively on the mitochondrial potential, with no effects of other factors (such as mitochondrial dimension, volume, shape, or density). The cells were plated into 96-well plates, incubated with 10 μg ml^{-1} JC-1 for 15 min at 37°C, and assayed using a fluorometer (SPECTRAmax Gemini XS; Molecular Devices Toronto, ON, Canada) equipped with the SoftMax Pro software (Gemini XS, Molecular Devices Toronto, ON, Canada) (Nuydens et al., 1999). The fluorescence is reported as means $\pm$SEM of the red/green fluorescence ratios of samples with respect to control, as $f(r/g)/f(r/g)_c$ (Morabito et al., 2010), and is here given as $\Delta\Psi_{mit}$. The dye ratio for JC-1 between the inner and outer mitochondrial membrane potentials was related to the mitochondrial depolarization after an oxidant insult, such as with (H_2O_2).

Antioxidant Enzyme Activity

The antioxidant enzymes analyzed were superoxide dismutase and catalase, The assays were performed using the cells cytosolic fraction.

Superoxide Dismutase

The activity of superoxide dismutase (SOD) is direct against $O_2^{\bullet-}$. SOD catalyzes a disproportionation reaction where a first $O_2^{\bullet-}$ is oxidized and the second molecule is reduced, turning two molecules of superoxide into O_2 and H_2O_2. The enzymatic activity was determined according to Fulle et al. (2000) The final assay volume was 1 ml and contained 20 mM Na_2CO_3 buffer pH 10, 10 mM Cytochrome c, 1 mM Xanthine and Xanthine Oxidase. Xanthine-xanthine oxidase is the $O_2^{\bullet-}$ generation system. As the xanthine oxidase activity varies, the amount used for the assay was such that produced a rate of cytochrome c reduction, at 550 nm, of 0.025 per minute without SOD addiction. The assay was performed at 550 nm for 10 min. The SOD units were calculated considering that 1 SOD unit is defined as the quantity that inhibits the rate of cytochrome c reduction by 50%.

Catalase

The reaction for which catalase (Cat) is best known is the "catalatic" reaction, in which H_2O_2 oxidizes the heme iron of the resting enzyme to form an oxyferryl group with a π-cationic porphyrin radical (Kirkman and Gaetani, 2006). This step is followed by oxidation of a second molecule of H_2O_2. Catalase forms two molecules of H_2O and O_2, starting from two molecules of H_2O_2. Catalase activity was determined, according to Greenwald (1985), by the decrease in absorbance due to H_2O_2 consumption ($\varepsilon = -0.04\,mM^{-1}\,cm^{-1}$) measured at 240 nm. The final reaction volume was 1 ml and contained 100 mM Na-phosphate buffer pH 7.0, 12 μM H_2O_2 and 70 μg of sample proteins. The reaction was followed for 1 min and the Cat activity was expressed in μmol/minute/mg proteins.

miRNA Expression

PureLink miRNA Isolation kits were used for the miRNA extractions (Cat. No. K1570-01, Invitrogen, Life Technologies, Molecular Devices, Sunnyvale, USA). About 800,000 cells were resuspended in 300 μl binding buffer (from the PureLink miRNA kits), and 300 μl 70% alcohol was added to the lysate. This was forced into the spin cartridges of the PureLink miRNA Isolation kits, which were then centrifuged at 12000 × g for 1 min. After washing with 100% alcohol, these were centrifuged again, as before. Then 500 μl wash buffer was added to the spin cartridges, which were centrifuged again at 12000 × g for 1 min. This procedure was performed twice, and then the spin cartridges were centrifuged at 12000 × g for 3 min, to remove residual buffer. Finally, they were eluted with 50 μl RNase-free sterile water. The RNA concentrations were determined using a NanoDrop™ spectrophotometer.

Retro-transcription and real-time PCR were carried out according to the Applied Biosystems TaqMan miRNA assay kit protocols. Briefly, the retro-transcription involved 20 ng of a "small" RNA, as the "stem loop" primer that was specific for each miRNA, dNTPs, and inverse transcriptase RNAse inhibitors (according to the Applied Biosystems high capacity cDNA reverse transcription kit, part N° 4368814), using a thermocycler (30 min at 16°C, 30 min at 42°C, 5 min at 85°C, then at 4°C). Then, the real-time PCR for the miRNA expression levels was performed using TaqMan probes and specific TaqMan® Universal Master Mix II, without UNG, in 96-well plates (Part No.: 4440040, Applied Biosystems) with a sequence detection system (Applied Biosystems PRISM 7900 HT), in triplicate. MiR-16 was used as the endogenous control. The specific miRNA sequence probes used were (Applied Biosystems):

(i) has-miR-1 (UGGAAUGUAAAGAAGUAUGUAU; #002222);

(ii) has-miR-206 (UGGAAUGUAAGGAAGUGUGUGG; #000510);

(iii) has-miR-133b (UUUGGUCCCCUUCAACCAGCUA; #002247);

(iv) has-miR-16-5p (UAGCAGCACGUAAAUAUUGGCG; #000391).

The relative quantification of the miRNA targets was carried out using the ΔCt formula, according to the Ct method.

Statistical Analysis

The statistical analysis was carried out using GraphPad Prism Software, version 5 (GraphPad Software, La Jolla, CA, USA). The data are reported as means ± standard error (SE). Unpaired and paired t-tests (for different group of cells and for the same cells with specific treatment, respectively) were used to reveal the statistical differences.

RESULTS

Subjects

Seven healthy women of childbearing age who were generally used to a sedentary life-style were enrolled to study the skeletal muscle regeneration potential after low to moderate intensity training as trekking at low altitude. **Table 1** summarize their anthopometric and physiological features.

TABLE 1 | Anthropometric and physiological characteristics of the subjects before (PRE-Exercise) and after (POST-Exercise) 12-days training period.

	PRE-exercise	POST-exercise
BW (Kg)	65.7 ± 4.4	65.1 ± 4.0
BMI (Kg m^{-2})	24.3 ± 1.5	24.1 ± 1.4
BF (%)	27.2 ± 2.6	25.9 ± 2.7
VO$_{2max}$ (L min^{-1})	2.13 ± 0.13	2.16 ± 0.12

BW, body weight; BMI, body mass index; BF (%), body fat percentage; VO$_{2max}$, maximum oxygen consumption.

TABLE 2 | Characteristics of myogenicity and differentiation of the satellite cell populations isolated from the seven women after trekking in the Abruzzo hills (central Italy).

Subject code	PRE-exercise			POST-exercise		
	%Desmin$^+$	Fusion Index (%)	%Desmin$^+$ unfused	%Desmin$^+$	Fusion Index (%)	%Desmin$^+$ unfused
#1	68.5	38.0	75.0	70.5	33.3	75.8
#2	66.0	23.3	73.9	77.3	60.2	22.4
#3	76.2	28.2	91.3	87.0	30.0	87.0
#4	90.4	14.6	82.1	88.8	67.9	28.5
#5	70.0	19.8	71.8	46.7	44.5	37.2
#6	67.0	23.5	58.4	34.5	42.6	25.7
#7	48.1	18.0	49.2	–	–	–

POST-Exercise Fusion Index differs significantly from the PRE-Exercise Fusion Index (p < 0.05, one tailed); POST-Exercise %Desmin$^+$ unfused differs significantly from the PRE-Exercise %Desmin$^+$ unfused (p < 0.05, one tailed).

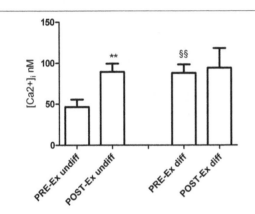

FIGURE 1 | Intracellular Ca^{2+} concentrations as basal levels for undifferentiated and differentiated (as indicated) cells obtained from skeletal muscle of female subjects for PRE-Ex and POST-Ex (as indicated). **$p < 0.01$ vs. undifferentiated PRE-Ex cells; §§$p < 0.01$ vs. undifferentiated PRE-Ex cells. The total analyzed cells were 90 myoblasts and 70 myotubes.

Myogenic Characteristics and Analysis of Cell Differentiation After Exercise Training

We obtained myogenic populations of adult stem cells, myoblasts, from percutaneous needle biopsies from the *vastus lateralis* muscle of female volunteers before (PRE-Ex) and after (POST-Ex) low altitude exercise training in the Abruzzo mountains. The characteristics of the cell differentiation are reported in **Table 2**.

The analysis of desmin-positive undifferentiated cells suggested that there were no significant difference in the myogenicity between the PRE-Ex and POST-Ex conditions. Of note, the Fusion Index, which represents the percentage of myoblasts that can fuse over 7 days of differentiation forming myotubes, was significantly increased at POST-Ex ($p < 0.05$). The percentage of desmin-positive cells in the differentiation media (after 7 days of differentiation) significantly decreased ($p < 0.05$).

Intracellular Ca^{2+} Concentrations of Cells

Figure 1 shows the basal levels of the intracellular Ca^{2+} concentrations ([Ca^{2+}]$_i$) of the undifferentiated and

differentiated cells. The undifferentiated POST-Ex myoblasts had [Ca^{2+}]$_i$ that were significantly higher than PRE-Ex myoblasts ($p \leq 0.01$). In the comparison of the differentiated PRE-Ex cells with respect to the undifferentiated PRE-Ex cells, these also showed an increase in [Ca^{2+}]$_i$ ($p \leq 0.01$). There were, however, no differences for the [Ca^{2+}]$_i$ between the differentiated and undifferentiated POST-Ex cells and among the differentiated ones.

Superoxide Production and General Oxidation State

The myoblasts showed different level of superoxide production (**Table 3**). While the myoblasts from subject #1 maintained the same O$_2^{\bullet-}$ levels, those from subjects #2, #3, and #4 showed significant decreases ($p \leq 0.0001$); conversely, those from subjects #5 and #6 showed significant increases in O$_2^{\bullet-}$ production ($p \leq 0.0001$) after the exercise training. The increases in O$_2^{\bullet-}$ production here were about 15% with respect to the control production, while the decreases ranged from 12 to 67% (**Table 3**).

The analysis of general oxidation state was conducted using DCF fluorescence. The addition of 100 nM H$_2$O$_2$ to the myoblasts loaded with DCF resulted in rapid increases in fluorescence that returned to basal level within 5 min, in the samples with both decreased and increased O$_2^{\bullet-}$ production (**Figure 2**). Of note, the POST-Ex cell populations showing reduced superoxide anion production showed also a less amount of ROS at basal level, as revealed by 10% less DCF fluorescence with respect to that measured at PRE-Ex, even if not significant. In fact, the DCF fluorescence of POST-Ex vs. PRE-Ex at 0 min was 5.4 ± 0.7 vs. 6.0 ± 0.9 (**Figure 2**, confront **Figure 2B** vs. **Figure 2A**). The POST-Ex myoblasts showing increased superoxide anion production showed similar amounts of DCF fluorescent dye with respect to the PRE-Ex (4.6 ± 0.6 vs. 4.3 ± 0.7, not significant, **Figures 2C,D**).

Antioxidant Enzyme Activity

The activity of antioxidant enzymes Superoxide dismutase and Catalase were determined on cytosolic fractions of PRE-Ex and POST-Ex undifferentiated cells both in population with reduced and increased superoxide anion production (**Figure 3**). The myoblasts with increased O$_2^{\bullet-}$ production (empty bars) showed no variation of both enzyme activity while those with decreased

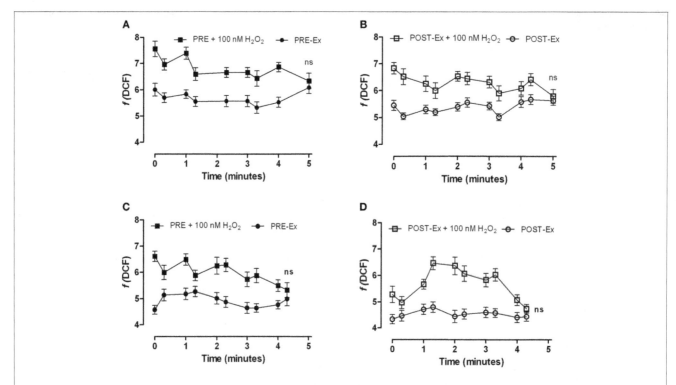

FIGURE 2 | Kinetics of DCF fluorescence in the control (PRE-Ex; A, C) and POST-Ex (B, D) myoblasts obtained from the skeletal muscle of the women that saw both decreased (A, B) and increased (C, D) $O_2^{\bullet-}$ production, without and with addition of 100 nM H_2O_2 (as indicated). The H_2O_2 was added at 0 min in dedicated samples (+100 nM H_2O_2). Data came from three independent experiments. All of the ±H_2O_2 data points were significantly different ($p \leq 0.0001$), except after 5 min ns, not significant.

TABLE 3 | Superoxide anion detection in the control (PRE-exercise) and after the low-moderate exercise conditioned (POST-exercise) satellite cells, as revealed by NBT dye fluorescence.

Subject	NBT dye fluorescence (mean ±SD)		Variation[a](%)
	PRE-exercise	**POST-exercise**	
#1	0.170 ± 0.030	0.180 ± 0.011	0
#2	0.132 ± 0.012	0.114 ± 0.006 §§	−14
#3	0.139 ± 0.004	0.045 ± 0.001 §§	−67
#4	0.080 ± 0.004	0.070 ± 0.002 §§	−12.5
#5	0.060 ± 0.002	0.070 ± 0.003 §§	+16
#6	0.106 ± 0.003	0.125 ± 0.004 §§	+18

[a]*percentage of variation with respect to PRE-Ex data (assumed as 100%), § significantly decreased or increased $O_2^{\bullet-}$ radical level for POST-Ex vs. PRE-Ex ($p < 0.001$).*

$O_2^{\bullet-}$ production (dotted bars) showed a significant reduction of Superoxide dismutase activity ($p \leq 0.05$) and no significant change of Catalase activity.

Transmembrane Mitochondrial Potential

The undifferentiated and differentiated PRE-Ex and POST-Ex cells showed stable transmembrane mitochondrial potentials (measured as the f[r/g]/f[r/g]$_c$ ratio for JC-1; $\Delta\Psi_{mit}$), which was reversibly depolarized (in a range of 10–20%) under the oxidative stimulus of 100 nM H_2O_2 (data not shown). Acute stimulation with the H_2O_2 induced less mitochondrial

depolarization of the POST-Ex myotubes than was seen PRE-Ex, even if the depolarization levels were not significantly different (data not shown). The transmembrane mitochondrial potential of the myoblasts producing more superoxide anion provided an exception here: the PRE-Ex $\Delta\Psi_{mit}$ showed H_2O_2-dependent depolarization, as previously described, while the POST-Ex $\Delta\Psi_{mit}$ was stable with this addition of H_2O_2 (**Figure 4**).

Epigenetic Profile Induced by Exercise Training

The analysis of the expression of miRNAs in the POST-Ex myoblasts showed an up-regulation of miR-1, miR133b, and miR206 respect to PRE-Ex in samples with decreased $O_2^{\bullet-}$ production conversely we found a down-regulation of all miRNAs tested in samples with increased $O_2^{\bullet-}$ production (**Figure 5**).

DISCUSSION

We have analyzed here skeletal muscle regeneration in adult women after low-to-moderate exercise training with specific attention paid to oxidative status. Recently, molecular studies in humans, highlighted that fusion of myogenic cells is triggered by endurance exercise-induced muscle plasticity (Frese et al., 2015)

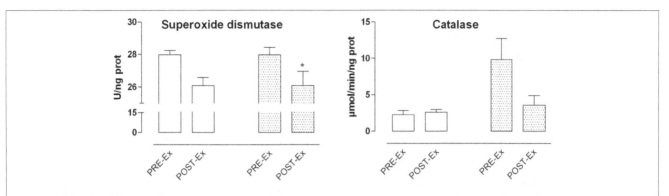

FIGURE 3 | Superoxide dismutase and Catalase activity. In the Figure is shown a representative example of enzyme activities. The activity of Superoxide dismutase showed similar level on myoblasts with decreased $O_2^{\bullet-}$ production (empty bars) while it was reduced in myoblasts showing increased $O_2^{\bullet-}$ production (dotted bars) with respect to PRE-Ex (*$p \leq 0.05$). The Catalase activity was similar among the PRE-Ex and POST-Ex cells, despite the $O_2^{\bullet-}$ production.

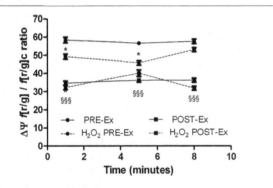

FIGURE 4 | Kinetics of the JC1 red/green fluorescence ratio variations as indirect measures of the transmembrane mitochondrial potential (ΔΨ) of myotubes obtained from skeletal muscle of female subjects for PRE-Ex and POST-Ex, without and with addition of 100 nM H_2O_2 (as indicated). Data came from three independent experiments. The treatment with H_2O_2 produced significant ΔΨ variation only in PRE-Ex cells (*$p \leq 0.05$). The condition PRE-Ex vs. POST-Ex resulted significant only in untreated cells (§§§, $p \leq 0.0001$).

At the cellular level, the fusion process is characterized by the alignment/fusion of myoblast membranes and cytoskeleton/cytoplasm rearrangements which results in the formation of nascent myotubes. Many studies of in vitro skeletal myogenesis have shown that myoblast fusion is regulated by calcium-increase in myoblasts before myotube formation (Constantin et al., 1996). We recorded an increased $[Ca^{2+}]_i$ in the POST-Ex myoblats that could be at the base of their increased ability to fuse to each other to form myotubes (Antigny et al., 2014). In fact, the fusion index significantly increased after the exercise training (POST-Ex) despite the $O_2^{\bullet-}$ production, along with a trend to a reduction in the levels of desmin-positive cells that did not fuse in the differentiation media.

The data from the literature are consistent with the observation that intracellular ROS generation by contracting skeletal muscle increases by two-four–fold during contraction (Jackson et al., 2007). These ROS are derived through different biochemical pathways, and in particular by mitochondrial activity.

In fact, during aerobic training, the enzymatic activity of this electron transfer shifts from complex IV to complex III (maximal ADP-stimulated respiration), which improves the efficiency of the mitochondria for the production of ATP and the reduction of $O_2^{\bullet-}$ (Di Meo and Venditti, 2001; Muller et al., 2004; Kozlov et al., 2005; Quinlan et al., 2013).

The results here for the satellite cell populations obtained after this low altitude exercise training suggested that the exercise linked to training provoked redox imbalance in some manner, mainly reducing $O_2^{\bullet-}$ production. These data thus showed that in the satellite cell populations of three of the six subjects there was significantly reduced $O_2^{\bullet-}$ production, for one of the six there was no change, and for two of the six there was about a 15% increase in the $O_2^{\bullet-}$ production, as a relatively small amount. Albeit the myoblasts from two subjects increased cellular $O_2^{\bullet-}$ production, this was linked to reduced superoxide dismutase activity. This reduction could be due to both the involvement of the enzyme in the oxidant reduction activity or in the partial inhibition of the dismutase enzyme.

The ROS species produced physiologically during exercise can stimulate important physiological mechanisms. For instance, there can be reversible oxidation of exposed protein thiols of the amino-acid cysteine in the ryanodine receptor, which governs correct excitation-contraction coupling (Fulle et al., 2007). Other examples include stimulation of mitochondrial biogenesis (Powers et al., 2011), up-regulation of antioxidant defenses (Gomez-Cabrera et al., 2008), expression of several genes for muscle hypertrophy (Powers et al., 2010), management of optimum muscle contractility (Reid et al., 1985), and muscle fatigue (Morillas-Ruiz et al., 2005).

Moreover, the data on general cellular peroxidation performed using DCF fluorescence, revealed that the presence of increased $O_2^{\bullet-}$ production did not match with an establishment of oxidative stress. In fact, the POST-Ex cell populations showing increased $O_2^{\bullet-}$ production, showed similar amount of DCF fluorescence with respect to PRE-Ex while those with reduced $O_2^{\bullet-}$ production showed about 10% less amounts of the fluorescent dye DCF with respect to the PRE-Ex, albeit

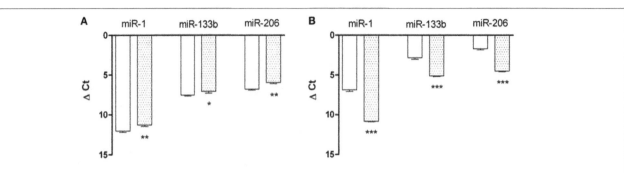

FIGURE 5 | Epigenetic signatures of miRNA expression. Relative expression of miR-1, miR-133b, and miR-206 (as indicated) in undifferentiated cells obtained from skeletal muscle of female subjects that saw both decreased **(A)** and increased **(B)** $O_2^{\bullet-}$ production before (empty bars) and after (dotted bars) exercise training. Data came from three independent experiments, each performed in triplicate. *, $p < 0.05$; **, $p < 0.01$; ***, $p < 0.0001$.

it not reached significant statistical differences. After the addition of H_2O_2 as external oxidant to mimic acute oxidative stress, all the cells completely reduced the ROS at the control levels in 5 min, as shown by the kinetics of DCF fluorescence.

The $O_2^{\bullet-}$ radical is rapidly converted into the cell by the superoxide dismutases, to the more stable H_2O_2 (Abele et al., 2002). This H_2O_2 then undergoes specific degradation by catalase (Sullivan-Gunn and Lewandowski, 2013). The measurement of Catalase activity showed no significant differences among cell populations despite the level of $O_2^{\bullet-}$ production, suggesting that probably the cells did not undergo the oxidative stress. The mitochondria are the main source of $O_2^{\bullet-}$ production; in addition there are other intracellular sources, such as the sarcoplasmic reticulum-associated and plasma-membrane-associated NAD(P)H oxidases, whereby the latter release $O_2^{\bullet-}$ mainly into the extracellular space, so they would be less important for intracellular $O_2^{\bullet-}$ production. Although we cannot exactly distinguish the sources of increased $O_2^{\bullet-}$ in our samples, we think that it could depend on the decreased superoxide dismutase activity and not on the impaired electron transfer shifts from mitochondrial complexes. In fact, the analysis of the mitochondrial transmembrane potential, $\Delta\Psi_{mit}$, suggested that the cell populations with decreased superoxide production after the exercise training showed the same levels of $\Delta\Psi_{mit}$ under the PRE-Ex and POST-Ex conditions. Acute stimulation with the H_2O_2 induced less mitochondrial depolarization of the POST-Ex myotubes than was seen PRE-Ex, which demonstrates potentially more efficient mitochondrial regulation. The investigation of $\Delta\Psi_{mit}$ in the cell populations with increased superoxide production showed that albeit some POST-Ex myotubes were more depolarized than their PRE-Ex controls, the depolarizing insult with H_2O_2 did not provoke further variations. It could be that these mitochondrial potential were fixed as in a protective asset (Starkov, 1997). This might be linked to the effectiveness of the exercise training, which would adapt the myotubes to counteract oxidation-dependent depolarization and thus avoid its eventual negative consequences. In this manner, the mitochondrial functionality and the ATP production would remain optimal.

The miRNA analysis of myoblasts revealed a particular signature of this low-to-moderate training at low altitude in relation to the oxidant production. In fact, the increased accumulation of $O_2^{\bullet-}$ in myoblasts occurred along with down-regulation of miR-1, miR-133b, and miR-206 expression while these miRNAs were up-regulated in samples with increased $O_2^{\bullet-}$ production. miR-1 pushes cells toward apoptosis by inhibiting the heat shock proteins 60 and 70 which inhibit the mitochondrial apoptosis pathway, miR-133 acts in an opposite way through the repression of caspase nine. Interestingly, the coherent up- or down-regulation of miR-1 and miR-133b, as found in all our samples despite the $O_2^{\bullet-}$ production, suggested that apoptosis was switched off (Xu et al., 2007). Moreover, we noted that when miRNA-1, miRNA-133b and miRNA-206 were up-regulated the cells showed decreased level of $O_2^{\bullet-}$ production, on the contrary when down-regulated, increased level of $O_2^{\bullet-}$ production. It could be possible that in female human myoblasts these miRNAs are specifically sensible to $O_2^{\bullet-}$ presence. Moreover, the down-regulation of miRNA-1, miRNA-133b, and miRNA-206 has been correlated with skeletal muscle inflammatory (Georgantas et al., 2014). We think that in this muscle condition among oxidant species it could be present increased $O_2^{\bullet-}$ production that could be responsible for these miRNA regulation and this scenario could be managed during female low training intensity session.

CONCLUSIONS

The low to moderate intensity training has been able to stimulate the regeneration of female skeletal muscle. It induced mainly a decrease of $O_2^{\bullet-}$ production, an increase of human myoblasts fusion index along with $[Ca^{2+}]_i$ increase. The $O_2^{\bullet-}$ production could regulate the miRNA-1, miRNA 133b, and miRNA-206 expression without affecting the myoblast differentiation.

AUTHOR CONTRIBUTIONS

TP designed the project, realised calcium imaging experiments, wrote the manuscript, analyzed and discussed the data.

ED performed experiments on oxidative status and miRNA regulation. RM managed cell cultures, performed experiments on oxidative status, analyzed and discussed the data. CD trained the volunteers and discussed the data. AR performed experiments on oxidative status. GF discussed the data. SF analyzed and discussed the data.

ACKNOWLEDGMENTS

The authors would like to thank all of the volunteers for their collaboration. This study was funded by a "G. d'Annunzio" University grant, the 2012N8YJC3_003 and the 2010R8JK2X_007 PRIN national grants to PT and SF, respectively; the RBFR12BUMH_005 FIRB national grant to MR.

REFERENCES

Abele, D., Heise, K., Pörtner, H. O., and Puntarulo, S. (2002). Temperature dependence of mitochondrial function and production of reactive oxygen species in the intertidal mud clam *Mya arenaria. J. Exp. Biol.* 205, 1831–1841.

Abruzzo, P. M., Esposito, F., Marchionni, C., di Tullio, S., Belia, S., Fulle, S., et al. (2013). Moderate exercise training induces ROS-related adaptations to skeletal muscles. *Int. J. Sports Med.* 34, 676–687. doi: 10.1055/s-0032-1323782

Antigny, F., Konig, S., Bernheim, L., and Frieden, M. (2014). Inositol 1,4,5 trisphosphate receptor 1 is a key player of human myoblast differentiation. *Cell Calcium* 56, 513–521. doi: 10.1016/j.ceca.2014.10.014

Appell, H. J., Forsberg, S., and Hollmann, W. (1988). Satellite cell activation in human skeletal muscle after training: evidence for muscle fiber neoformation. *Int. J. Sports Med.* 9, 297–299. doi: 10.1055/s-2007-1025026

Baar, K. (2014). Nutrition and the adaptation to endurance training. *Sports Med.* 44(Suppl. 1), S5–S12. doi: 10.1007/s40279-014-0146-1

Behr, T., Fischer, P., Müller-Felber, W., Schmidt-Achert, M., and Pongratz, D. (1994). Myofibrillogenesis in primary tissue cultures of adult human skeletal muscle: expression of desmin, titin, and nebulin. *Clin. Investig.* 72, 150–155. doi: 10.1007/BF00184594

Bernareggi, A., Luin, E., Formaggio, E., Fumagalli, G., and Lorenzon, P. (2012). Novel role for prepatterned nicotinic acetylcholine receptors during myogenesis. *Muscle Nerve* 46, 112–121. doi: 10.1002/mus.23284

Ceafalan, L. C., Popescu, B. O., and Hinescu, M. E. (2014). Cellular players in skeletal muscle regeneration. *BioMed Res. Int.* 2014:957014. doi: 10.1155/2014/957014

Constantin, B., Cognard, C., and Raymond, G. (1996). Myoblast fusion requires cytosolic calcium elevation but not activation of voltage-dependent calcium channels. *Cell Calcium* 19, 365–374. doi: 10.1016/S0143-4160(96)90109-8

Crippa, S., Cassano, M., and Sampaolesi, M. (2012). Role of miRNAs in muscle stem cell biology: proliferation differentiation and death. *Curr. Pharm. Des.* 18, 1718–1729. doi: 10.2174/138161212799859620

Cumming, K. T., Raastad, T., Holden, G., Bastani, N. E., Schneeberger, D., Paronetto, M. P., et al. (2014). Effects of vitamin C and E supplementation on endogenous antioxidant systems and heat shock proteins in response to endurance training. *Physiol. Rep.* 2:e12142 doi: 10.14814/phy2.12142

Di Meo, S., and Venditti, P. (2001). Mitochondria in exercise-induced oxidative stress. *Biol. Signals Recept.* 10, 125–140. doi: 10.1159/000046880

Eisenberg, I., Alexander, M. S., and Kunkel, L. M. (2009). miRNAS in normal and diseased skeletal muscle. *J. Cell. Mol. Med.* 13, 2–11. doi: 10.1111/j.1582-4934.2008.00524.x

Fisher-Wellman, K., and Bloomer, J. (2009). Acute exercise and oxidative stress: a 30 year history. *Dyn. Med.* 8:1. doi: 10.1186/1476-5918-8-1

Frese, S., Ruebner, M., Suhr, F., Konou, T. M., Tappe, K. A., Toigo, M., et al. (2015). Long-term endurance exercise in humans stimulates cell fusion of myoblasts along with fusogenic endogenous retroviral genes *in vivo*. *PLoS ONE* 10:e0132099. doi: 10.1371/journal.pone.0132099

Fulle, S., Di Donna, S., Puglielli, C., Pietrangelo, T., Beccafico, S., Bellomo, R., et al. (2005). Age-dependent imbalance of the antioxidative system in human satellite cells. *Exp. Gerontol.* 40, 189–197. doi: 10.1016/j.exger.2004.11.006

Fulle, S., Mecocci, P., Fanó, G., Vecchiet, I., Vecchini, A., Racciotti, D., et al. (2000). Specific oxidative alterations in vastus lateralis muscle of patients with the diagnosis of chronic fatigue syndrome. *Free Radic. Biol. Med.* 29, 1252–1259. doi: 10.1016/S0891-5849(00)00419-6

Fulle, S., Pietrangelo, T., Mancinelli, R., Saggini, R., and Fanò, G. (2007). Specific correlations between muscle oxidative stress and chronic fatigue syndrome: a working hypothesis. *J. Muscle Res. Cell Motil.* 28, 355–362. doi: 10.1007/s10974-008-9128-y

Garber, C. E., Blissmer, B., Deschenes, M. R., Franklin, B. A., Lamonte, M. J., Lee, I. M., et al. (2011). American college of sports medicine position stand. Quantity and quality of exercise for developing and maintaining cardiorespiratory, musculoskeletal, and neuromotor fitness in apparently healthy adults: guidance for prescribing exercise. *Med. Sci. Sports Exerc.* 43, 1334–1359. doi: 10.1249/MSS.0b013e318213fefb

Georgantas, R. W., Streicher, K., Greenberg, S. A., Greenlees, L. M., Zhu, W., Brohawn, P. Z., et al. (2014). Inhibition of myogenic microRNAs 1, 133, and 206 by inflammatory cytokines links inflammation and muscle degeneration in adult inflammatory myopathies. *Arthritis Rheumatol.* 66, 1022–1033. doi: 10.1002/art.38292

Gomez-Cabrera, M. C., Domenech, E., and Viña, J. (2008). Moderate exercise is an antioxidant: upregulation of antioxidant genes by training. *Free Radic. Biol. Med.* 44, 126–131. doi: 10.1016/j.freeradbiomed.2007.02.001

Green, P. S., and Simpkins, J. W. (2000). Neuroprotective effects of estrogens: potential mechanisms of action. *Int. J. Dev. Neurosci.* 18, 347–358. doi: 10.1016/S0736-5748(00)00017-4

Greenwald, R. A. (1985). Therapeutic benefits of oxygen radical scavenger treatments remain unproven. *J. Free Radic. Biol. Med.* 1, 173–177.

Gundersen, K. (2011). Excitation-transcription coupling in skeletal muscle: the molecular pathways of exercise. *Biol. Rev. Camb. Philos. Soc.* 86, 564–600. doi: 10.1111/j.1469-185X.2010.00161.x

Hindi, S. M., Tajrishi, M. M., and Kumar, A. (2013). Signaling mechanisms in mammalian myoblast fusion. *Sci. Signal.* 6:re2. doi: 10.1126/scisignal.2003832

Huang, Z.-P., Espinoza-Lewis, R., and Wang, D.-Z. (2012). Determination of miRNA targets in skeletal muscle cells. *Methods Mol. Biol. Clifton N.J.* 798, 475–490. doi: 10.1007/978-1-61779-343-1_28

Jackson, M. J., Pye, D., and Palomero, J. (2007). The production of reactive oxygen and nitrogen species by skeletal muscle. *J. Appl. Physiol.* 102, 1664–1670. doi: 10.1152/japplphysiol.01102.2006

Kadi, F., Charifi, N., Denis, C., Lexell, J., Andersen, J. L., Schjerling, P., et al. (2005). The behaviour of satellite cells in response to exercise: what have we learned from human studies? *Pflugers Arch Eur. J. Physiol.* 451, 319–327. doi: 10.1007/s00424-005-1406-6

Kadi, F., Johansson, F., Johansson, R., Sjöström, M., and Henriksson, J. (2004). Effects of one bout of endurance exercise on the expression of myogenin in human quadriceps muscle. *J. Histochem. Cell Biol.* 121, 329–334. doi: 10.1007/s00418-004-0630-z

Kaufman, S. J., and Foster, R. F. (1988). Replicating myoblasts express a muscle-specific phenotype. *Proc. Natl. Acad. Sci. U.S.A.* 85, 9606–9610.

Kirkman, H. N., and Gaetani, G. F. (2006). Mammalian catalase: a venerable enzyme with new mysteries. *Trends Biochem. Sci.* 32, 44–50. doi: 10.1016/j.tibs.2006.11.003

Kozlov, A. V., Szalay, L., Umar, F., Koprik, K., Staniek, K., Niedermuller, H., et al. (2005). Skeletal muscles, heart, and lung are the main sources of oxygen radicals in old rats. *Biochim. Biophys. Acta* 1740, 382–389. doi: 10.1016/j.bbadis.2004.11.004

Kvorning, T., Kadi, F., Schjerling, P., Andersen, M., Brixen, K., Suetta, C., et al. (2014). The activity of satellite cells and myonuclei following 8 weeks of strength training in young men with suppressed testosterone levels. *Acta Physiol. (Oxf.)* 213, 676–687. doi: 10.1111/apha.12404

Kwon, C., Han, Z., Olson, E. N., and Srivastava, D. (2005). MicroRNA1 influences cardiac differentiation in Drosophila and regulates Notch signaling. *Proc. Natl. Acad. Sci. U.S.A.* 102, 18986–18991. doi: 10.1073/pnas.0509535102

La Rovere, R. M., Quattrocelli, M., Pietrangelo, T., Di Filippo, E. S., Maccatrozzo, L., Cassano, M., et al. (2014). Myogenic potential of canine craniofacial satellite cells. *Front. Aging Neurosci.* 6:90. doi: 10.3389/fnagi.2014.00090

Lorenzon, P., Bandi, E., de Guarrini, F., Pietrangelo, T., Schäfer, R., Zweyer, M., et al. (2004). Ageing affects the differentiation potential of human myoblasts. *Exp. Gerontol.* 39, 1545–1554. doi: 10.1016/j.exger.2004.07.008

Mancinelli, R., Pietrangelo, T., La Rovere, R., Toniolo, L., Fanò, G., Reggiani, C., et al. (2011). Cellular and molecular responses of human skeletal muscle exposed to hypoxic environment. *J. Biol. Regul. Homeost. Agents* 25, 635–645.

McCarthy, J. J., and Esser, K. A. (2007). MicroRNA-1 and microRNA-133a expression are decreased during skeletal muscle hypertrophy. *J. Appl. Physiol.* 102, 306–313. doi: 10.1152/japplphysiol.00932.2006

Mecocci, P., Fanó, G., Fulle, S., MacGarvey, U., Shinobu, L., Polidori, M. C., et al. (1999). Age-dependent increases in oxidative damage to DNA, lipids and proteins in human skeletal muscle. *Free Radic. Biol. Med.* 26, 303–308. doi: 10.1016/s0891-5849(98)00208-1

Menghini, L., Leporini, L., Scanu, N., Pintore, G., La Rovere, R., Di Filippo, E. S., et al. (2011). Effect of phytochemical concentrations on biological activities of cranberry extracts. *J. Biol. Regul. Homeost. Agents* 25, 27–35.

Millay, D. P., O'Rourke, J. R., Sutherland, L. B., Bezprozvannaya, S., Shelton, J. M., Bassel-Duby, R., et al. (2013). Myomaker is a membrane activator of myoblast fusion and muscle formation. *Nature* 499, 301–305. doi: 10.1038/nature12343

Morabito, C., Rovetta, F., Bizzarri, M., Mazzoleni, G., Fanò, G., and Mariggiò, M. A. (2010). Modulation of redox status and calcium handling by extremely low frequency electromagnetic fields in C2C12 muscle cells: a real-time, single-cell approach. *Free Radic. Biol Med.* 48, 579–589. doi: 10.1016/j.freeradbiomed.2009.12.005

Morillas-Ruiz, J., Zafrilla, P., Almar, M., Cuevas, M. J., Lopez, F. J., bellan, P., et al. (2005). The effects of an anti-oxidant-supplemented beverage on exercise-induced oxidative stress: results from a placebo-controlled double-blind study in cyclists. *Eur. J. Appl. Physiol.* 95, 543–549. doi: 10.1007/s00421-005-0017-4

Muller, F. L., Liu, Y., and Van Remmen, H. (2004). Complex III releases superoxide to both sides of inner mitochondrial membrane. *J. Biol. Chem.* 279, 49064–49073. doi: 10.1074/jbc.M407715200

Nikolaidis, M. G., Margaritelis, N. V., Paschalis, V., Theodorou, A. A., Kyparos, A., and Vrabas, I. S. (2015). "Common questions and tentative answers on how to assess oxidative stress after antioxidant supplementation and exercise," in *Antioxidants in Sport Nutrition*, ed M. Lamprecht (Boca Raton, FL: CRC Press).

Nuydens, R., Novalbos, J., Dispersyn, G., Weber, C., Borgers, M., and Geerts, H. (1999). A rapid method for the evaluation of compounds with mitochondria-protective properties. *J. Neurosci. Methods* 92, 153–159. doi: 10.1016/S0165-0270(99)00107-7

Pietrangelo, T., D'Amelio, L., Doria, C., Mancinelli, R., Fulle, S., and Fanò, G. (2011). Tiny percutaneous needle biopsy: an efficient method for studying cellular and molecular aspects of skeletal muscle in humans. *Int. J. Mol. Med.* 27, 361–367. doi: 10.3892/ijmm.2010.582

Pietrangelo, T., Fioretti, B., Mancinelli, R., Catacuzzeno, L., Franciolini, F., Fanò, G., et al. (2006). Extracellular guanosine-5′-triphosphate modulates myogenesis via intermediate Ca(2+)-activated K+ currents in C2C12 mouse cells. *J. Physiol.* 572, 721–733. doi: 10.1113/jphysiol.2005.102194

Pietrangelo, T., Mariggiò, M. A., Lorenzon, P., Fulle, S., Protasi, F., Rathbone, M., et al. (2002). Characterization of specific GTP binding sites in C2C12 mouse skeletal muscle cells. *J. Muscle Res. Cell Motil.* 23, 107–118. doi: 10.1023/A:1020288117082

Pietrangelo, T., Puglielli, C., Mancinelli, R., Beccafico, S., Fanò, G., and Fulle, S. (2009). Molecular basis of the Myogenic profile of aged human skeletal muscle satellite cells during differentiation. *Exp. Geront.* 44, 523–531. doi: 10.1016/j.exger.2009.05.002

Powers, S. K., Duarte, J., Kavazis, A. N., and Talbert, E. E. (2010). Reactive oxygen species are signaling molecules for skeletal muscle adaptation. *Exp. Physiol.* 95, 1–9. doi: 10.1113/expphysiol.2009.050526

Powers, S. K., Nelson, W. B., and Hudson, M. B. (2011). Exercise-induced oxidative stress in humans: cause and consequences. *Free Radic. Biol. Med.* 51, 942–950. doi: 10.1016/j.freeradbiomed.2010.12.009

Quinlan, C. L., Perevoshchikova, I. V., Hey-Mogensen, M., Orr, A. L., and Brand, M. D. (2013). Sites of reactive oxygen species generation by mitochondria oxidizing different substrates. *Redox Biol.* 1, 304–312. doi: 10.1016/j.redox.2013.04.005

Reid, M. B., Khawli, F. A., and Moody, M. R. (1985). Reactive oxygen in skeletal muscle. III. Contractility of unfatigued muscle. *J. Appl. Physiol.* 75, 1081–1087.

Shin, K. S., Park, J. Y., Ha, D. B., Chung, C. H., and Kang, M.-S. (1996). Involvement of KCa channels and stretch-activated channels in calcium influx, triggering membrane fusion of chick embryonic myoblasts. *Dev. Biol.* 175, 14–23. doi: 10.1006/dbio.1996.0091

Siens, H., and Cadenas, E. (1985). Oxidative stress: damage to intact cells and organs. *Philos. Trans. R. Soc. Lond. Ser. B Biol. Sci.* 311, 617–631. doi: 10.1098/rstb.1985.0168

Siens, H., and Jones, D. P. (2007). "Oxidative stress," in *Encyclopedia of Stress*, ed G. Fink (Victoria: Elsevier); 45–48.

Snijders, T., Verdijk, L. B., Beelen, M., McKay, B. R., Parise, G., Kadi, F., et al. (2012). A single bout of exercise activates skeletal muscle satellite cells during subsequent overnight recovery. *Exp. Physiol.* 97, 762–773. doi: 10.1113/expphysiol.2011.063313

Sozio, P., Cerasa, L. S., Laserra, S., Cacciatore, I., Cornacchia, C., Di Filippo, E. S., et al. (2013). Memantine-sulfur containing antioxidant conjugates as potential prodrugs to improve the treatment of Alzheimer's disease. *Eur. J. Pharm. Sci.* 49, 187–198. doi: 10.1016/j.ejps.2013.02.013

Starkov, A. A. (1997). "Mild" uncoupling of mitochondria. *Biosci. Rep.* 17, 273–279. doi: 10.1023/A:1027380527769

Sullivan-Gunn, M. J., and Lewandowski, P. A. (2013). Elevated hydrogen peroxide and decreased catalase and glutathione peroxidase protection are associated with aging sarcopenia. *BMC Geriatr.* 13:104. doi: 10.1186/1471-2318-13-104

Tam, E., Bruseghini, P., Calabria, E., Sacco, L. D., Doria, C., Grassi, B., et al. (2015). Gokyo Khumbu/Ama Dablam Trek 2012: effects of physical training and high-altitude exposure on oxidative metabolism, muscle composition, and metabolic cost of walking in women. *Eur. J. Appl. Physiol.* doi: 10.1007/s00421-015-3256-z. [Epub ahead of print].

Verdijk, L. B. (2014). Satellite cells activation as a critical step in skeletal muscle plasticity. *Exp. Physiol.* 99, 1449–1450. doi: 10.1113/expphysiol.2014.081273

Verdijk, L. B., Snijders, T., Drost, M., Delhaas, T., Kadi, F., and van Loon, L. J. (2014). Satellite cells in human skeletal muscle; from birth to old age. *Age* 36, 545–547. doi: 10.1007/s11357-013-9583-2

Xu, C., Lu, Y., Pan, Z., Chu, W., Luo, X., Lin, H., et al. (2007). The muscle-specific microRNAs miR-1 and miR-133 produce opposing effects on apoptosis by targeting HSP60, HSP70 and caspase-9 in cardiomyocytes. *J. Cell Sci.* 120(Pt 17), 3045–3052. doi: 10.1242/jcs.010728

Conflict of Interest Statement: The authors declare that the research was conducted in the absence of any commercial or financial relationships that could be construed as a potential conflict of interest.

16

Cardiac autonomic responses after resistance exercise in treated hypertensive subjects

Gabriela A. Trevizani[1], Tiago Peçanha[2], Olivassé Nasario-Junior[1], Jeferson M. Vianna[3], Lilian P. Silva[4] and Jurandir Nadal[1*]

[1] Biomedical Engineering Program COPPE, Universidade Federal do Rio de Janeiro, Rio de Janeiro, Brazil, [2] Exercise Hemodynamic Laboratory, School of Physical Education and Sport, Universidade de São Paulo, São Paulo, Brazil, [3] Faculty of Physical Education and Sports, Universidade Federal de Juiz de Fora, Juiz de Fora, Brazil, [4] Faculty of Physiotheraphy, Universidade Federal de Juiz de Fora, Juiz de Fora, Brazil

Edited by:
Sergej Ostojic,
University of Novi Sad, Serbia

Reviewed by:
Yu-Chieh Tzeng,
University of Otago, Wellington,
New Zealand
Caroline Alice Rickards,
The University of North Texas Health
Science Center, USA
Naoto Fujii,
University of Ottawa, Canada

*Correspondence:
Jurandir Nadal,
Biomedical Engineering Program
COPPE, Universidade Federal do Rio
de Janeiro, 2030 Horácio Macedo
Ave., Block H, PO Box 68510, Rio de
Janeiro, 21941-972 RJ, Brazil
jn@peb.ufrj.br

The aim of this study was to assess and to compare heart rate variability (HRV) after resistance exercise (RE) in treated hypertensive and normotensive subjects. Nine hypertensive men [HT: 58.0 ± 7.7 years, systolic blood pressure (SBP) = 133.6 ± 6.5 mmHg, diastolic blood pressure (DBP) = 87.3 ± 8.1 mmHg; under antihypertensive treatment] and 11 normotensive men (NT: 57.1 ± 6.0 years, SBP = 127 ± 8.5 mmHg, DBP = 82.7 ± 5.5 mmHg) performed a single session of RE (2 sets of 15–20 repetitions, 50% of 1 RM, 120 s interval between sets/exercise) for the following exercises: leg extension, leg press, leg curl, bench press, seated row, triceps push-down, seated calf flexion, seated arm curl. HRV was assessed at resting and during 10 min of recovery period by calculating time (SDNN, RMSSD, pNN50) and frequency domain (LF, HF, LF/HF) indices. Mean values of HRV indices were reduced in the post-exercise period compared to the resting period (HT: lnHF: 4.7 ± 1.4 vs. 2.4 ± 1.2 ms^2; NT: lnHF: 4.8 ± 1.5 vs. 2.2 ± 1.1 ms^2, $p < 0.01$). However, there was no group vs. time interaction in this response ($p = 0.8$). The results indicate that HRV is equally suppressed after RE in normotensive and hypertensive individuals. These findings suggest that a single session of RE does not bring additional cardiac autonomic stress to treated hypertensive subjects.

Keywords: heart rate variability, autonomic nervous system, parasympathetic activity, sympathetic activity, resistance exercise

Introduction

Resistance exercise (RE) has been widely used as an adjunct to aerobic exercise in a comprehensive exercise training program oriented to health (Williams et al., 2007; Garber et al., 2011). Several studies have demonstrated the benefits of RE for increasing muscle mass, strength, balance, and quality of life in older adults or other frail populations (Cheema et al., 2014; Joshua et al., 2014; Silva-Batista et al., 2014; Vechin et al., 2015) and more recent evidence also indicate positive effects of RE in cardiovascular function and regulation (Queiroz et al., 2010; Grizzo Cucato et al., 2011).

Despite these recommendations, a single session of RE promotes a great cardiac autonomic stress, characterized by a reduction in cardiac vagal modulation and an increase in sympathetic activity that persist during the post-exercise period (Heffernan et al., 2006; Rezk et al., 2006; Kingsley and Figueroa, 2014). This autonomic stress promoted by RE has been claimed to be greater than that promoted by aerobic exercise (Heffernan et al., 2006), a fact that can acutely increase the risks of cardiovascular events after RE, particularly in subjects with cardiovascular diseases, such as hypertension (Thompson et al., 2007).

Hypertension (HTN) is a highly prevalent chronic disease (Mozaffarian et al., 2015), characterized by increased levels of blood pressure, end-organ damage, and increased cardiovascular risks (Chobanian et al., 2003). Autonomic dysfunction is one of the main pathophysiological mechanisms of HTN, since it is related both to the development and also the complications of this disease (Mancia and Grassi, 2014). The autonomic dysfunction of HTN has been mainly demonstrated in rest, either by increased levels of sympathetic nerve firing (Schlaich et al., 2004) or reduced heart rate variability (HRV; Singh et al., 1998), but also during physiological maneuvres, such as exercise (Rondon et al., 2006). Accordingly, some recent studies have demonstrated a slower autonomic recovery after aerobic exercise in hypertensives in comparison with normotensives (Erdogan et al., 2011; Aneni et al., 2014).

Given that a single session of RE promotes significant autonomic disturbances, and that autonomic recovery after aerobic exercise is suggested to be slower in hypertensives compared with normotensives, it seems reasonable to expect that autonomic recovery from RE will be further slowed in hypertensives in comparison with normotensives. Thus, the aim of this study was to assess and to compare the cardiac autonomic recovery, assessed by HRV, after RE in treated hypertensive and normotensive subjects.

Methods

Sample
Eleven normotensive (NT) and nine hypertensive men (HT) under regular antihypertensive treatment (period of treatment = 9.7 ± 4.9 years; **Table 1**) participated in this study. Inclusion criteria were: age greater than 50 years old, no smoking for at least 1 year, no practicing of regular physical exercise (frequency up to one session per week) for at least 1 year. None of the study subjects had a history of musculoskeletal injury or cardiovascular diseases that could affect results, no arrhythmias were detected in the resting electrocardiography and none were using beta blockers. All of the subjects provided written voluntary informed consent, which was approved by the University Human Ethics Review Board and followed the recommendations from the Declaration of Helsinki.

Preliminary Assessment
Preliminary evaluations were performed on non-consecutive days. On the first day, the volunteers performed a clinical evaluation, anamneses (personal data, lifestyle questionnaires, previous diseases history, and cardiovascular risk parameters) and physical measurements were taken, such as height and body mass for subsequent calculation of the body mass index (BMI = mass/height^2; kg/m^2), waist and hip circumferences

TABLE 1 | Antihypertensive medication.

Pharmacological class	Number of volunteers	Percentage (%)
1. Not on medication	1	11.1
2. Under medication use	8	88.9
2.1. Monotherapy	5	55.6
Diuretics	1	11.1
Calcium channel blockers	1	11.1
Angiotensin receptor antagonist	3	33.3
2.2. Combination of therapies	3	33.3
Angiotensin receptor antagonist and diuretics	1	11.1
Angiotensin receptor antagonist and calcium channel blockers	1	11.1
Angiotensin receptor antagonist, calcium channel blockers and diuretics	1	11.1

for the calculation of waist–hip ratio and percentage of body fat. Single measurements of systolic (SBP) and diastolic (DBP) blood pressures were taken by an experienced evaluator using a calibrated sphygmomanometer after 10 and 20 min of supine resting. The average of these two measurements was retained for analysis. Additionally, mean blood pressure (MBP) was calculated through the sum of the DBP and one-third of the pulse pressure. From the second to the fourth day, the subjects underwent three RE sessions to become familiar with the equipment and exercise techniques. On the fifth and sixth day, individuals performed the test and retest of one-repetition maximum (1 RM) to evaluate the maximum dynamic muscle strength. During the 1 RM assessment, participants were allowed to perform up to five attempts to reach the maximal load for each exercise (see experimental protocol), with rest intervals of 5 min between exercises. Differences lower than 5% between tests were accepted and the greatest 1 RM-value was considered for the prescription of exercise sessions.

Experimental Protocol
The experimental protocol consisted of three phases: rest, RE session, and recovery. All participants were advised not to ingest caffeinated or alcoholic drinks, and not to practice vigorous physical activity in the 24 h prior to the experiments. Initially, the volunteers remained seated for 10 min (rest stage). Then, they were submitted to a RE session in which they performed two sets of 20 repetitions at 50% of 1 RM on the following exercises: leg extension, leg press, leg curl, bench press, and seated row; and 15 repetitions at: triceps push-down, seated calf flexion, and seated arm curl. The rest interval between the sets and exercises was set to 2 min. Finally, individuals returned to the seated position, remaining in recovery for 10 min. At rest and during the recovery phases, heart rate (HR) was recorded beat-to-beat (RR-intervals) by an HR monitor (Polar® RS800CX, Kempele, Finland, sampling frequency = 1000 Hz; Nunan et al., 2009).

Procedures

Heart Rate Measures

The series of RR-intervals (RRi) recorded during rest and recovery were directed to a microcomputer, by infrared transmission to the Polar Precision Performance software (Polar Inc., Kempele, Finland). After a visual inspection, ectopic beats and artifacts were manually corrected by an expert (J.N.). Then, trend component removal of the time series was carried out according to the "*a priori*" smoothing method (Tarvainen et al., 2002), and interpolation using cubic splines at a frequency of 4 Hz was thus applied to extract equally spaced samples, thereby ensuring series of normal RR-intervals (NN). In sequence, the HR average value of the initial 5 min (rest) and HR-values in each 30-s window during the initial 5 min of recovery were calculated.

Heart Rate Variability Analysis: First 5 Min of Recovery

Since the behavior of the RRi signal in the first 5 min of recovery is non-linear (Goldberger et al., 2006), for the analysis of the HRV in such a period the time-varying vagal-related index RMSSD (square root of the mean of the sum of the squares of differences between adjacent normal R–R intervals) was calculated on subsequent 30 s non-overlapped segments (RMSSD30s), as proposed by Goldberger et al. (2006). To smooth out any transient outliers in the RMSSD30s plots, a median filter operation was applied, where each outlier value was replaced with the median of the value as well as the preceding and following values. The first and last values were not median filtered (Goldberger et al., 2006).

Heart Rate Variability Analysis: Resting and 5–10 Min of Recovery

The resting and late recovery period (5–10 min) HRV was analyzed according to the HRV Task Force (Task-Force, 1996) in the Kubios software (v 2.0, Biomedical Signal Analysis Group, Department of Applied Physics, University of Kuopio, Finland). The following time domain indices were calculated: the standard deviation of NN (SDNN), the square root of the mean square differences of successive NN (RMSSD) and the ratio between the number of times in which the difference between successive NN presented a duration higher than 50 ms in relation to the total number of NN (pNN50). The SDNN reflects the participation of all the rhythmic components responsible for variability, and is related to the joint action of both branches of the autonomous nervous system for the control of heart rate, whereas the RMSSD and pNN50 reflect the contributions of variations in high frequencies, which are related to the vagal action on the sinoatrial node (Task-Force, 1996). The frequency domain indices were calculated by the power spectral density function (PSD) using the Fast Fourier Transform (FFT; Malik and Camm, 1990; Task-Force, 1996). Prior to this transformation, the time series were detrended (smoothing priors) and resampled to 4 Hz sampling rate using cubic spline interpolation. For the spectral analysis, the following indices were calculated: the power of the spectral bands of low frequencies (LF; 0.04–0.15 Hz) in absolute units (ms^2), which represents the set of sympathetic and vagal influences on the sinoatrial node, and in normalized units (nu), which predominantly represents the cardiac sympathetic modulation (Task-Force, 1996); the power of the spectral bands of high frequencies (HF; 0.15–0.4 Hz) in absolute (ms^2) and normalized (nu) units, which represents the cardiac vagal modulation (Task-Force, 1996); and the LF/HF ratio, whose value is interpreted as a sympathetic-vagal balance indicator (Pagani et al., 1986; Task-Force, 1996).

Statistical Analysis

The results of this study are reported as mean ± standard deviation and the Alpha level was set at 5%. Following the use of the Shapiro–Wilk test, the hypothesis of normality was rejected for SDNN, RMSSD30s, RMSSD, HF, and LF indices, so variables were natural log-transformed (ln). The Student-t-test for independent samples and the Mann–Whitney tests were used to compare demographic, anthropometric and haemodynamic variables, and the measures of maximum dynamic muscle strength between the groups. A Two-Way ANOVA (group vs. time), followed by Tukey's *post hoc*-test, were employed to compare the HRV variables between the groups.

Results

Table 2 presents the demographic, anthropometric, and haemodynamic characteristics of the experimental groups. There were no differences between groups in any of these variables. There were also no differences in maximum dynamic muscle strength in each exercise between groups (**Table 3**).

The HR and RMSSD30s values in the post-exercise period were, respectively, increased and decreased in comparison to their resting values in both groups (time effect: $p < 0.01$ for all analyses), however, there were no differences in these responses between NT and HT (group vs. time interactions: $p = 0.10$ and 0.83, for HR and RMSSD30s, respectively; **Figure 1**).

The mean values of the HRV time-domain indices were reduced in the post-exercise period compared to the resting

---

TABLE 2 | Sample characterization: demographic, anthropometric, and haemodynamic variables.

	HT	NT	*p*-value
DEMOGRAPHIC VARIABLES			
Age (years)	58.0 ± 7.7	56.5 ± 6.3	0.65
	(50–65 years)	(50–74 years)	
ANTHROPOMETRIC VARIABLES			
BMI (kg/m^2)	29.0 ± 3.9	24.8 ± 3.5	0.06
Waist–hip ratio	0.93 ± 0.1	0.88 ± 0.1	0.08
% BF	26.8 ± 7.0	22.7 ± 6.0	0.27
HAEMODYNAMIC VARIABLES			
SBP (mmHg)	133.6 ± 6.5	127.0 ± 8.5	0.09
DBP (mmHg)	87.3 ± 8.1	82.7 ± 5.5	0.10
MBP (mmHg)	102.8 ± 6.9	96.2 ± 7.8	0.08

Values described as mean ± standard deviation.

HT, hypertensive group; NT, normotensive group; BMI, body mass index; % BF, percentage of body fat; SBP, systolic blood pressure; DBP, diastolic blood pressure; MBP, mean blood pressure.

period in both groups (time effect: $p < 0.01$ for all analyses), however there was no difference in this response between NT and HT (group vs. time interactions: $p = 0.2–0.4$ depending on the index analyzed; **Figure 2**). Regarding the frequency domain indices, we observed a significant reduction in the LF (ms^2) and HF (ms^2 and nu) and an increase in the LF (nu) and LF/HF in the post-exercise period in comparison to resting values (time effect: $p < 0.01$ for all analyses), with no differences between groups in these responses (group vs. time interactions: $p = 0.2–0.8$ depending on the index analyzed; **Figure 3**).

Discussion

The main findings of this study were the suppression of the HRV after RE and the lack of influence of hypertension in this response.

It has been demonstrated that an increase in sympathetic and decrease in parasympathetic activity in the post-exercise period underlies the increased risk of acute cardiovascular events in this period (Smith et al., 2005; Thompson et al., 2007). In this context, several studies have been conducted in order to understand which aspects of the exercise could influence the

autonomic responses after exercise. Accordingly, the type of exercise seems to play an important role on the post-exercise autonomic recovery. In this regard, Heffernan et al. (2006) compared the HRV after a session of resistance or aerobic exercise, demonstrating a greater reduction of HRV after the RE. Similar results were found by Niemelä et al. (2008), who observed a delayed autonomic recovery after heavy-resistance exercise in comparison with aerobic and light-resistance exercises. Despite the absence of comparisons between resistance and aerobic exercise, the present results are in line with the previous ones (Heffernan et al., 2006) since a significant reduction was observed in parasympathetic activity (reduction in RMSSD and HF) and an increase in sympathetic balance [increase of LF (nu) and LF/HF], leading to an increase in HR and a suppression of HRV during the entire recovery period after the RE session in both groups. These findings spark an alert for the potential risks that could be brought by the practice of RE in subjects more prone to developing cardiovascular abnormalities after exercise, such as individuals with HTN (Thompson et al., 2007).

Hypertension is a chronic highly prevalent disease that is characterized mainly by increased levels of blood pressure, leading to higher rates of cardiovascular morbidity and mortality (Chobanian et al., 2003). The degenerative process of this disease is mediated by some pathophysiological mechanisms and autonomic dysfunction has been advocated as being a crucial one (Mancia and Grassi, 2014). Indeed, studies have already identified an increased sympathetic drive to the kidneys and muscles (Schlaich et al., 2004), and a reduced HRV (Guzzetti et al., 1988; Pagani and Lucini, 2001; Mancia and Grassi, 2014) in hypertensive individuals and it seems that these responses are even worse in more complicated hypertensive states (Grassi et al., 1998a, 2004). Recently, some studies with aerobic exercise have also demonstrated that this autonomic dysfunction in hypertensive subjects is also present in the post-exercise period (Erdogan et al., 2011; Aneni et al., 2014; Best et al., 2014). Accordingly, Erdogan et al. (2011) have demonstrated a slower heart rate recovery after aerobic exercise in hypertensives in comparison to normotensives, and Aneni et al. (2014) observed that this reduction in heart rate recovery accompanies the progression of HTN.

TABLE 3 | Measures of maximum dynamic muscle strength for each exercise.

Exercises	Maximum dynamic muscle strength (kg)		
	HT	NT	p-value
Leg extension	127.7 ± 41.2	130.9 ± 33.8	0.72
Leg press	122.2 ± 37.0	148.4 ± 39.7	0.56
Leg curl	78.4 ± 29.2	92.2 ± 18.3	0.28
Bench press	52.4 ± 15.7	59.6 ± 12.8	0.16
Seated row	99.1 ± 18.4	102.1 ± 16.6	0.75
Triceps push-down	51.0 ± 14.0	54.6 ± 10.1	0.71
Seated calf flexion	34.7 ± 9.3	37.5 ± 5.8	0.43
Seated arm curl	50.0 ± 10.0	55.0 ± 7.8	0.30

Values described as mean ± standard deviation.
HT, Hypertensive group; NT, Normotensive group.

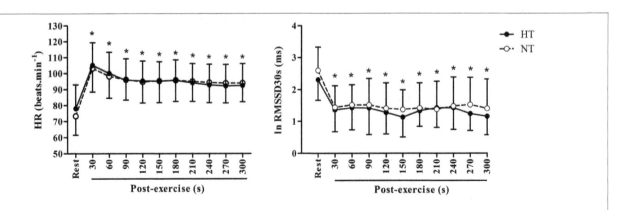

FIGURE 1 | Heart rate (HR) and heart rate variability (RMSSD30s index) at rest and during 5 min of recovery (post-exercise). HT, hypertensive group; NT, normotensive group; * significantly different from rest in both groups ($p < 0.05$).

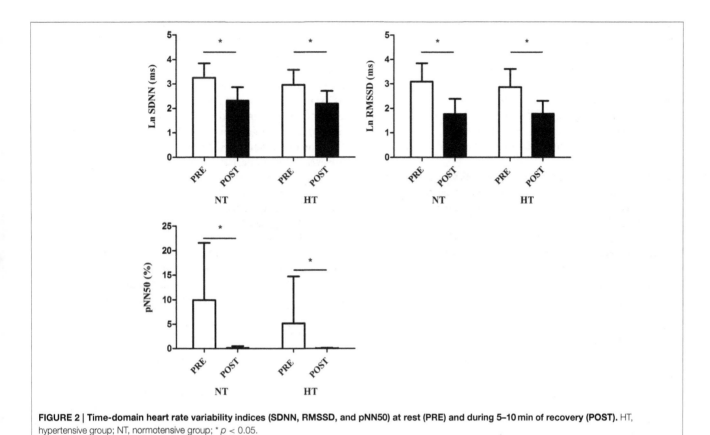

FIGURE 2 | Time-domain heart rate variability indices (SDNN, RMSSD, and pNN50) at rest (PRE) and during 5–10 min of recovery (POST). HT, hypertensive group; NT, normotensive group; * $p < 0.05$.

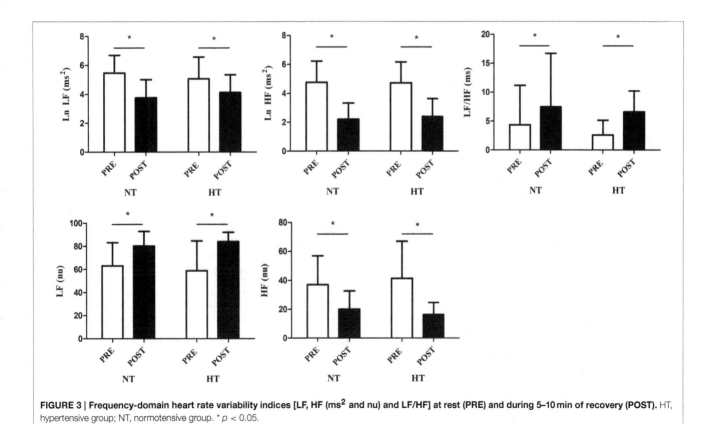

FIGURE 3 | Frequency-domain heart rate variability indices [LF, HF (ms^2 and nu) and LF/HF] at rest (PRE) and during 5–10 min of recovery (POST). HT, hypertensive group; NT, normotensive group. * $p < 0.05$.

Given that RE is known to produce high levels of autonomic stress, and that hypertensive subjects are supposed to present autonomic dysfunction in the post-exercise period, the hypothesis of this study was that treated hypertensives would present a reduced HRV in the post-exercise period in comparison with normotensives. Despite that, this study did not observe any influence of HTN status on post-exercise HR or HRV. This finding suggests that the autonomic stress imposed by the RE is not different between normotensive and treated hypertensive subjects.

It should be highlighted that the hypertensive subjects in this study were under medication treatment and well-controlled, a factor that is known to improve autonomic function (Kailasam et al., 1995; Ye et al., 2002). This could have prevented a greater post-exercise autonomic stress after RE in this group. Accordingly, most of studies that have shown the presence of autonomic dysfunction in hypertensives have used never-treated subjects (Rondon et al., 2006; Erdogan et al., 2011) or employed a wash-out period before the exercise intervention (Schlaich et al., 2004). Indeed, in the present study HRV-values showed no differences between treated hypertensives and normotensives even in the resting state (i.e., pre-exercise values), a fact that suggests that they did not present autonomic dysfunction in their baseline. The hypertensive subjects of the present study were also free of associated comorbidities and HTN-related complications, factors which are known to negatively influence autonomic function (Grassi et al., 1998b, 2004). Therefore, it seems likely that at least in well-controlled hypertensive subjects with no additional comorbidities and complications, the autonomic stress posed by RE is similar to that of normotensive ones.

The absence of standardization of the antihypertensive drugs among the hypertensive subjects could be viewed as a limitation of this study. However, the modification of the antihypertensive drugs, particularly in well-controlled hypertensives may be problematic, since it could worsen their blood pressure control, thus hampering the treatment. For this reason, the decision to maintain their original prescribed medication was taken in order to warrant the best treatment for each subject. It should also be emphasized that despite each individual using a specific antihypertensive drug (**Table 1**), no one was under the use of beta blockers, a class of drugs known to directly influence the autonomic nervous system (Frishman, 2003). Another potential limitation of this study could be the reduced number of subjects. However, a *post hoc* power analysis revealed a power >0.7 in most of the statistical comparisons, indicating that the sample size of the current study was adequate for the analysis performed. Finally, it should be emphasized that HRV provides information regarding the cardiac autonomic modulation rather than cardiac autonomic tone *per se*. This means that the tools of the present study did not allow an assessment of the degree of the sympathetic and parasympathetic drives to the heart, but rather its balanced responses to variations in respiration, blood pressure, and temperature, among other factors (Saul, 1990).

Conclusion

The results of the present study indicate that RE promotes a significant suppression of HRV after exercise, a fact that can potentially increase the cardiovascular risks of the practice of this exercise. However, this response was similar between normotensives and treated hypertensives, suggesting that a controlled hypertension does not bring additional cardiovascular risks to the practice of RE.

Acknowledgments

This study received financial support from FAPEMIG (APQ – 02800-11) and CNPq.

References

Aneni, E., Roberson, L. L., Shaharyar, S., Blaha, M. J., Agatston, A. A., Blumenthal, R. S., et al. (2014). Delayed heart rate recovery is strongly associated with early and late-stage prehypertension during exercise stress testing. *Am. J. Hypertens.* 27, 514–521. doi: 10.1093/ajh/hpt173

Best, S. A., Bivens, T. B., Dean Palmer, M., Boyd, K. N., Galbreath, M. M., Okada, Y., et al. (2014). Heart rate recovery after maximal exercise is blunted in hypertensive seniors. *J. Appl. Physiol.* 117, 1302–1307. doi: 10.1152/japplphysiol.00395.2014

Cheema, B. S., Chan, D., Fahey, P., and Atlantis, E. (2014). Effect of progressive resistance training on measures of skeletal muscle hypertrophy, muscular strength and health-related quality of life in patients with chronic kidney disease: a systematic review and meta-analysis. *Sports Med.* 44, 1125–1138. doi: 10.1007/s40279-014-0176-8

Chobanian, A. V., Bakris, G. L., Black, H. R., Cushman, W. C., Green, L. A., Izzo, J. L. Jr., et al. (2003). The seventh report of the joint national committee on prevention, detection, evaluation, and treatment of high blood pressure: the JNC 7 report. *JAMA* 289, 2560–2571. doi: 10.1001/jama.289.19.2560

Erdogan, D., Gonul, E., Icli, A., Yucel, H., Arslan, A., Akcay, S., et al. (2011). Effects of normal blood pressure, prehypertension, and hypertension on autonomic nervous system function. *Int. J. Cardiol.* 151, 50–53. doi: 10.1016/j.ijcard.2010.04.079

Frishman, W. H. (2003). Beta-adrenergic blockers. *Circulation* 107, e117–e119. doi: 10.1161/01.CIR.0000070983.15903.A2

Garber, C. E., Blissmer, B., Deschenes, M. R., Franklin, B. A., Lamonte, M. J., Lee, I. M., et al. (2011). American College of Sports Medicine position stand. Quantity and quality of exercise for developing and maintaining cardiorespiratory, musculoskeletal, and neuromotor fitness in apparently healthy adults: guidance for prescribing exercise. *Med. Sci. Sports Exerc.* 43, 1334–1359. doi: 10.1249/MSS.0b013e318213fefb

Goldberger, J. J., Le, F. K., Lahiri, M., Kannankeril, P. J., Ng, J., and Kadish, A. H. (2006). Assessment of parasympathetic reactivation after exercise. *Am. J. Physiol. Heart Circ. Physiol.* 290, H2446–H2452. doi: 10.1152/ajpheart.01118.2005

Grassi, G., Cattaneo, B. M., Seravalle, G., Lanfranchi, A., and Mancia, G. (1998a). Baroreflex control of sympathetic nerve activity in essential and secondary hypertension. *Hypertension* 31, 68–72. doi: 10.1161/01.HYP.31.1.68

Grassi, G., Colombo, M., Seravalle, G., Spaziani, D., and Mancia, G. (1998b). Dissociation between muscle and skin sympathetic nerve activity in essential hypertension, obesity, and congestive heart failure. *Hypertension* 31, 64–67. doi: 10.1161/01.HYP.31.1.64

Grassi, G., Seravalle, G., Dell'oro, R., Facchini, A., Ilardo, V., and Mancia, G. (2004). Sympathetic and baroreflex function in hypertensive or heart failure patients with ventricular arrhythmias. *J. Hypertens.* 22, 1747–1753. doi: 10.1097/00004872-200109000-00010

Grizzo Cucato, G., de Moraes Forjaz, C. L., Kanegusuku, H., da Rocha Chehuen, M., Riani Costa, L. A., Wolosker, N., et al. (2011). Effects of walking and strength training on resting and exercise cardiovascular responses in patients with intermittent claudication. *Vasa* 40, 390–397. doi: 10.1024/0301-1526/a000136

Guzzetti, S., Piccaluga, E., Casati, R., Cerutti, S., Lombardi, F., Pagani, M., et al. (1988). Sympathetic predominance in essential hypertension: a study employing spectral analysis of heart rate variability. *J. Hypertens.* 6, 711–717. doi: 10.1097/00004872-198809000-00004

Heffernan, K. S., Kelly, E. E., Collier, S. R., and Fernhall, B. (2006). Cardiac autonomic modulation during recovery from acute endurance versus resistance exercise. *Eur. J. Cardiovasc. Prev. Rehabil.* 13, 80–86. doi: 10.1097/01.hjr.0000197470.74070.46

Joshua, A. M., D'souza, V., Unnikrishnan, B., Mithra, P., Kamath, A., Acharya, V., et al. (2014). Effectiveness of progressive resistance strength training versus traditional balance exercise in improving balance among the elderly - a randomised controlled trial. *J. Clin. Diagn. Res.* 8, 98–102. doi: 10.7860/jcdr/2014/8217.4119

Kailasam, M. T., Parmer, R. J., Cervenka, J. H., Wu, R. A., Ziegler, M. G., Kennedy, B. P., et al. (1995). Divergent effects of dihydropyridine and phenylalkylamine calcium channel antagonist classes on autonomic function in human hypertension. *Hypertension* 26, 143–149.

Kingsley, J. D., and Figueroa, A. (2014). Acute and training effects of resistance exercise on heart rate variability. *Clin. Physiol. Funct. Imaging.* doi: 10.1111/cpf.12223. [Epub ahead of print].

Malik, M., and Camm, A. J. (1990). Heart rate variability. *Clin. Cardiol.* 13, 570–576. doi: 10.1002/clc.4960130811

Mancia, G., and Grassi, G. (2014). The autonomic nervous system and hypertension. *Circ. Res.* 114, 1804–1814. doi: 10.1161/CIRCRESAHA.114.302524

Mozaffarian, D., Benjamin, E. J., Go, A. S., Arnett, D. K., Blaha, M. J., Cushman, M., et al. (2015). Heart disease and stroke statistics-2015 update: a report from the American Heart Association. *Circulation* 131, e29–e322. doi: 10.1161/CIR.0000000000000157

Niemela, T. H., Kiviniemi, A. M., Hautala, A. J., Salmi, J. A., Linnamo, V., and Tulppo, M. P. (2008). Recovery pattern of baroreflex sensitivity after exercise. *Med. Sci. Sports Exerc.* 40, 864–870. doi: 10.1249/MSS.0b013e3181666f08

Nunan, D., Donovan, G., Jakovljevic, D. G., Hodges, L. D., Sandercock, G. R., and Brodie, D. A. (2009). Validity and reliability of short-term heart-rate variability from the Polar S810. *Med. Sci. Sports Exerc.* 41, 243–250. doi: 10.1249/MSS.0b013e318184a4b1

Pagani, M., Lombardi, F., Guzzetti, S., Rimoldi, O., Furlan, R., Pizzinelli, P., et al. (1986). Power spectral analysis of heart rate and arterial pressure variabilities as a marker of sympatho-vagal interaction in man and conscious dog. *Circ. Res.* 59, 178–193. doi: 10.1161/01.RES.59.2.178

Pagani, M., and Lucini, D. (2001). Autonomic dysregulation in essential hypertension: insight from heart rate and arterial pressure variability. *Auton. Neurosci.* 90, 76–82. doi: 10.1016/S1566-0702(01)00270-3

Queiroz, A. C., Kanegusuku, H., and Forjaz, C. L. (2010). Effects of resistance training on blood pressure in the elderly. *Arq. Bras. Cardiol.* 95, 135–140. doi: 10.1590/S0066-782X2010001100020

Rezk, C. C., Marrache, R. C., Tinucci, T., Mion, D. Jr., and Forjaz, C. L. (2006). Post-resistance exercise hypotension, hemodynamics, and heart rate variability: influence of exercise intensity. *Eur. J. Appl. Physiol.* 98, 105–112. doi: 10.1007/s00421-006-0257-y

Rondon, M. U., Laterza, M. C., de Matos, L. D., Trombetta, I. C., Braga, A. M., Roveda, F., et al. (2006). Abnormal muscle metaboreflex control of sympathetic

activity in never-treated hypertensive subjects. *Am. J. Hypertens.* 19, 951–957. doi: 10.1016/j.amjhyper.2006.02.001

Saul, J. (1990). Beat-to-Beat variations of heart rate reflect modulation of cardiac autonomic outflow. *Physiology* 5, 32–37.

Schlaich, M. P., Lambert, E., Kaye, D. M., Krozowski, Z., Campbell, D. J., Lambert, G., et al. (2004). Sympathetic augmentation in hypertension: role of nerve firing, norepinephrine reuptake, and angiotensin neuromodulation. *Hypertension* 43, 169–175. doi: 10.1161/01.HYP.0000103160.35395.9E

Silva-Batista, C., Kanegusuku, H., Roschel, H., Souza, E. O., Cunha, T. F., Laurentino, G. C., et al. (2014). Resistance training with instability in multiple system atrophy: a case report. *J. Sports Sci. Med.* 13, 597–603.

Singh, J. P., Larson, M. G., Tsuji, H., Evans, J. C., O'donnell, C. J., and Levy, D. (1998). Reduced heart rate variability and new-onset hypertension: insights into pathogenesis of hypertension: the Framingham Heart Study. *Hypertension* 32, 293–297. doi: 10.1161/01.HYP.32.2.293

Smith, L. L., Kukielka, M., and Billman, G. E. (2005). Heart rate recovery after exercise: a predictor of ventricular fibrillation susceptibility after myocardial infarction. *Am. J. Physiol. Heart Circ. Physiol.* 288, H1763–H1769. doi: 10.1152/ajpheart.00785.2004

Tarvainen, M. P., Ranta-Aho, P. O., and Karjalainen, P. A. (2002). An advanced detrending method with application to HRV analysis. *IEEE Trans. Biomed. Eng.* 49, 172–175. doi: 10.1109/10.979357

Task-Force. (1996). Heart rate variability. Standards of measurement, physiological interpretation, and clinical use. Task Force of the European Society of Cardiology and the North American Society of Pacing and Electrophysiology. *Eur. Heart J.* 17, 354–381. doi: 10.1093/oxfordjournals.eurheartj.a014868

Thompson, P. D., Franklin, B. A., Balady, G. J., Blair, S. N., Corrado, D., Estes, N. A. III., et al. (2007). Exercise and acute cardiovascular events placing the risks into perspective: a scientific statement from the American Heart Association Council on Nutrition, Physical Activity, and Metabolism and the Council on Clinical Cardiology. *Circulation* 115, 2358–2368. doi: 10.1161/CIRCULATIONAHA.107.181485

Vechin, F. C., Libardi, C. A., Conceição, M. S., Damas, F. R., Lixandrão, M. E., Berton, R. P., et al. (2015). Comparisons between low-intensity resistance training with blood flow restriction and high-intensity resistance training on quadriceps muscle mass and strength in elderly. *J. Strength Cond. Res.* 29, 1071–1076. doi: 10.1519/JSC.0000000000000703

Williams, M. A., Haskell, W. L., Ades, P. A., Amsterdam, E. A., Bittner, V., Franklin, B. A., et al. (2007). Resistance exercise in individuals with and without cardiovascular disease: 2007 update: a scientific statement from the American Heart Association Council on Clinical Cardiology and Council on Nutrition, Physical Activity, and Metabolism. *Circulation* 116, 572–584. doi: 10.1161/CIRCULATIONAHA.107.185214

Ye, S., Zhong, H., Duong, V. N., and Campese, V. M. (2002). Losartan reduces central and peripheral sympathetic nerve activity in a rat model of neurogenic hypertension. *Hypertension* 39, 1101–1106. doi: 10.1161/01.HYP.0000018590.26853.C7

Conflict of Interest Statement: The authors declare that the research was conducted in the absence of any commercial or financial relationships that could be construed as a potential conflict of interest.

17

Task Failure during Exercise to Exhaustion in Normoxia and Hypoxia Is Due to Reduced Muscle Activation Caused by Central Mechanisms While Muscle Metaboreflex Does Not Limit Performance

Rafael Torres-Peralta[1,2], David Morales-Alamo[1,2], Miriam González-Izal[3], José Losa-Reyna[1,2], Ismael Pérez-Suárez[1,2], Mikel Izquierdo[3] and José A. L. Calbet[1,2]*

[1] Department of Physical Education, University of Las Palmas de Gran Canaria, Las Palmas de Gran Canaria, Spain,
[2] Research Institute of Biomedical and Health Sciences (IUIBS), Las Palmas de Gran Canaria, Spain, [3] Department of Health Sciences, Public University of Navarra, Tudela, Spain

Edited by:
Gregoire P. Millet,
University of Lausanne, Switzerland

Reviewed by:
François Billaut,
Université Laval, Canada
Stuart Goodall,
Northumbria University, UK

*Correspondence:
José A. L. Calbet
lopezcalbet@gmail.com

To determine whether task failure during incremental exercise to exhaustion (IE) is principally due to reduced neural drive and increased metaboreflex activation eleven men (22 ± 2 years) performed a 10 s control isokinetic sprint (IS; 80 rpm) after a short warm-up. This was immediately followed by an IE in normoxia (Nx, P_IO_2:143 mmHg) and hypoxia (Hyp, P_IO_2:73 mmHg) in random order, separated by a 120 min resting period. At exhaustion, the circulation of both legs was occluded instantaneously (300 mmHg) during 10 or 60 s to impede recovery and increase metaboreflex activation. This was immediately followed by an IS with open circulation. Electromyographic recordings were obtained from the *vastus medialis* and *lateralis*. Muscle biopsies and blood gases were obtained in separate experiments. During the last 10 s of the IE, pulmonary ventilation, VO_2, power output and muscle activation were lower in hypoxia than in normoxia, while pedaling rate was similar. Compared to the control sprint, performance (IS-Wpeak) was reduced to a greater extent after the IE-Nx (11% lower $P < 0.05$) than IE-Hyp. The root mean square (EMG_{RMS}) was reduced by 38 and 27% during IS performed after IE-Nx and IE-Hyp, respectively (Nx vs. Hyp: $P < 0.05$). Post-ischemia IS-EMG_{RMS} values were higher than during the last 10 s of IE. Sprint exercise mean (IS-MPF) and median (IS-MdPF) power frequencies, and burst duration, were more reduced after IE-Nx than IE-Hyp ($P < 0.05$). Despite increased muscle lactate accumulation, acidification, and metaboreflex activation from 10 to 60 s of ischemia, IS-Wmean (+23%) and burst duration (+10%) increased, while IS-EMG_{RMS} decreased (-24%, $P < 0.05$), with IS-MPF and IS-MdPF remaining unchanged. In conclusion, close to task failure, muscle activation is lower in hypoxia than in normoxia. Task failure is predominantly caused by central mechanisms, which recover to great extent within 1 min even when the legs remain ischemic. There is dissociation between the recovery of EMG_{RMS} and performance. The reduction of surface electromyogram MPF, MdPF and burst duration due to fatigue is associated but not caused by muscle acidification and lactate accumulation. Despite metaboreflex stimulation, muscle activation and power output recovers partly in ischemia indicating that metaboreflex activation has a minor impact on sprint performance.

Keywords: electromyography, EMG, exhaustion, fatigue, high-intensity, hypoxia, lactate, performance

INTRODUCTION

Muscle fatigue has been defined as "any exercise-induced reduction in the ability to exert muscle force or power, regardless of whether the task can be sustained (Bigland-Ritchie and Woods, 1984), that can be reversed by rest" (Gandevia, 2001). The mechanisms leading to task failure may involve physiological processes at neural (central fatigue) or muscular levels (peripheral fatigue), with failure distal to the neuromuscular junction included in the "peripheral" component. It has been suggested that the rate of muscle fatigue development is regulated by the central nervous system (CNS) with feedback from the type III and IV muscle afferents (Amann and Dempsey, 2008), which sense metabolite accumulation, particularly H^+, lactate, and ATP (Light et al., 2008). Type III/IV muscle afferents have been reported to inhibit corticospinal drive (Amann and Dempsey, 2008; Rossman et al., 2012; Kennedy et al., 2015), with greater inhibitory effect on extensor than flexor muscles (Martin et al., 2006). However, whether metabolite accumulation and the expected metaboreflex stimulation impair muscle activation and limit peak power during whole-body sprint exercise remains unknown.

During whole-body exercise in severe acute hypoxia ($F_IO_2 <$ 0.115, or altitude above 4500 m) the level of peripheral fatigue at exhaustion seems lower, indicating that central mechanisms, likely linked to reduced brain oxygenation (Rasmussen et al., 2010), predominate over local mechanisms in determining the cessation of exercise (Amann et al., 2007). In agreement with this hypothesis, an instantaneous increase of the inspired O_2 fraction (F_IO_2) from 0.21 to 1.00 does not eliminate muscle fatigue at the end of an incremental exercise test performed at sea level (Calbet et al., 2003a). In contrast, during constant-intensity or incremental exercise to exhaustion in severe hypoxia ($P_IO_2 \approx 75$ mmHg), muscle fatigue is swiftly relieved by mild hyperoxic gas or room air (Kayser et al., 1994; Calbet et al., 2003a,b; Amann et al., 2007). These findings led to the concept that during incremental exercise to exhaustion in normoxia, task

failure is most likely caused by peripheral mechanisms while central mechanisms prevail in severe hypoxia (Calbet et al., 2003a; Amann et al., 2007). In support, peripheral fatigue, as assessed via decreases in potentiated quadriceps twitch force 2 min after constant-intensity exercise to exhaustion, was lower when the exercise was performed in severe hypoxia than in normoxia (Amann et al., 2007). Nevertheless, this observation was not accompanied by an assessment of muscle metabolites and obviates the fact that reduced potentiated quadriceps twitch force may occur without reduction of peak power output (Fernandez-del-Olmo et al., 2013; Hureau et al., 2014). Moreover, the recovery process starts as early as muscle contraction ceases, and given the fast kinetics of phosphocreatine re-synthesis at the end of exercise (Bogdanis et al., 1996; Dawson et al., 1997; Yoshida et al., 2013), most of the recovery has already occurred within the first 2 min post-exercise (Sargeant and Dolan, 1987; Froyd et al., 2013). Also, muscle fatigue is task-specific (Gandevia, 2001), implying that a procedure using a similar pattern of movement, and hence recruitment of neural pathways, is expected to be more sensitive to detect fatigue.

In this context, every possible combination of effects and interpretation of results has been reported in regard to the contribution of central and peripheral mechanisms to muscle fatigue after dynamic contractions in normoxia (Sidhu et al., 2009, 2012; Marcora and Staiano, 2010; Fernandez-del-Olmo et al., 2013) and hypoxia (Amann et al., 2007; Goodall et al., 2010; Millet et al., 2012). Some of these discrepancies can be attributed to the fact that neural mechanisms of muscle fatigue are task-specific (Sidhu et al., 2012), to different levels of input from type III and IV muscle afferents (Sidhu et al., 2012), and to methodological limitations (Rodriguez-Falces et al., 2013; Héroux et al., 2015; Bachasson et al., 2016). Although the inhibition of type III and IV muscle afferents has been shown to attenuate muscle fatigue in certain exercise models (Sidhu et al., 2014), whether type III and IV muscle afferent input contributes to reduce exercise performance by a central mechanism remains controversial (Millet et al., 2009, 2012; Marcora, 2010; Amann et al., 2013a; Kennedy et al., 2015). Part of the discrepancies may be due to the fact that type III and IV muscle afferent discharge cannot be directly measured during whole-body exercise in humans, combined with the difficulty in interpreting the effects of intrathecal fentanyl when this drug differently alters ventilation, arterial O_2 content, arterial $PaCO_2$, heart rate and mean arterial blood pressure, depending on the exercise intensity, exercise duration, and the study population (Dempsey et al., 2014; Olson et al., 2014; Poon and Song, 2015). Thus, we decided to explore the role of III/IV muscle afferents on exercise performance (peak power output) using a completely different experimental approach.

Abbreviations: ADP, Adenosine diphosphate; ATP, Adenosine triphosphate; CNS, Central nervous system; d.w., Dry weight; DEXA, Dual-energy x-ray absorptiometry; EMG, Surface electromyogram; EMG_{RMS}, Root mean square of the EMG; F_IO_2, Inspired oxygen fraction; HR, Heart rate; HRmax, Maximal heart rate; Hyp, Hypoxia; Hypb, session in hypoxia with biopsies taken; IE, Incremental exercise to exhaustion; IS, Isokinetic sprint; MPF, Mean power frequency; MdPF, Median power frequency; MVC, Maximal voluntary contraction; Nx, Normoxia; Nxb, Session in normoxia with biopsies taken; PaO_2, Arterial oxygen pressure; PCr, Phosphocreatine; P_IO_2, Inspired O_2 pressure; RMS, root mean square; RMSNz, Normalized root mean square; V_E, Minute ventilation; VO_2, Oxygen consumption; VO_2max, Maximal oxygen uptake; VO_2peak, Peak oxygen uptake; Wpeak-i, Instantaneous peak power output; Wmax, Peak power output at exhaustion during the incremental exercise test; Wmean, mean power output during the 10 s sprints; w.w., wet weight; TAI, Total activation index.

The main aim of this investigation was to determine whether task failure during an incremental exercise to exhaustion is principally due to central mechanisms that cause a reduction in neural activation, modulated by the level of oxygenation. This hypothesis has been previously examined but with different procedures (Kayser et al., 1994; Amann et al., 2007, 2013b) which did not include measurements of muscle metabolites or performance immediately after exhaustion. Another aim was to determine if increased afferent feedback from metabolite accumulation in an exhausted muscle has a negative influence on sprint performance by reducing neural activation, as assessed through electromyogram (EMG) recordings.

We aimed to test these two hypotheses: (i) task failure during incremental exercise to exhaustion in hypoxia occurs with lower levels of muscle activation compared to normoxia, and (ii) increased afferent feedback from III and IV muscle afferents impairs sprint performance.

METHODS

Subjects

Eleven healthy men (age: 21.5 ± 2.0 years, height: 174 ± 8 cm, body mass: 72.3 ± 9.3 kg, body fat: $16.1 \pm 4.9\%$, VO_2max: 51 ± 5 mL.kg^{-1}.min^{-1}) agreed to participate in this investigation. Before volunteering, subjects received full oral and written information about the experiments and possible risks associated with participation. Written consent was obtained from each subject. The study was performed by the Helsinki Declaration and was approved by the Ethical Committee of the University of Las Palmas de Gran Canaria (CEIH-2010-01 and CEIH-2009-01).

General Overview

This study was a part of a larger project that included several experiments designed to address the mechanisms limiting whole-body exercise performance in humans. The results focusing on O_2 transport and muscle metabolism have been published (Calbet et al., 2015; Morales-Alamo et al., 2015). Body composition was determined by dual-energy x-ray absorptiometry (DEXA) (Hologic QDR-1500, Hologic Corp., software version 7.10, Waltham, MA) (Calbet et al., 1997), during the familiarization sessions. The leg muscle mass was calculated from the DEXA scans using Wang's et al. model (Wang et al., 1999).

The experimental protocol is summarized in **Figure 1**, and an example of the electromyographic recordings from one subject is given in **Figure 2**. On the experimental days, subjects reported to the laboratory at 08.00 h. after an overnight fast from 22.00 h. The subjects performed an incremental exercise test to exhaustion in normoxia (P_IO_2: ~143 mmHg) or acute hypoxia (P_IO_2: ~73 mmHg, Altitrainer200, SMTEC, Switzerland), in random order and separated by a 120 min rest. Before the exercise test, bilateral cuffs were placed around the thighs and connected to a rapid cuff inflator (SCD10, Hokanson E20 AG101, Bellevue, USA). The test started with a warm-up (2 min at 50 W + 2 min 100 W + 1 min at 160 W) followed by 4.5 min of slow unloaded pedaling. This was followed by a 30 s rest period while the

subjects became ready to sprint at the 5th minute after the end of the warm-up. The volunteers were requested to sprint as hard and fast as possible during 10 s with the ergometer set in isokinetic mode and at 80 rpm (Excalibur Sport 925900, Lode, Groningen, The Netherlands). This sprint was used as a control sprint and was always performed in normoxia. Five minutes later, the incremental exercise began. For the test in normoxia, the load was increased by 30 W every 2 min until exhaustion, starting from an initial load of 80 W. In hypoxia, the incremental test started from 60 W, and the load was increased by 20 W every 2 min until exhaustion. Exhaustion during the incremental exercise tests was defined by the subject stopping pedaling or dropping pedaling rate below 50 rpm during 5 s, despite strong verbal encouragement. At exhaustion, the cuffs were inflated at maximal speed and pressure (i.e., 300 mmHg) to completely and instantaneously occlude the circulation (ischemia). This prevented any increase of oxygenation during the recovery and caused anoxia within 3–5 s of the application of the occlusion as reported elsewhere (Morales-Alamo et al., 2015). A limitation of previous studies was that the impact of the early recovery could not be accounted for (Marcora and Staiano, 2010; Coelho et al., 2015), and certainly some recovery occurs during the time elapsed between the end of the exercise and the start of the sprint. To circumvent this limitation we applied complete ischemia during the recovery and we used short (10 s) and long (60 s) ischemia periods. We surmised that peripheral fatigue would be exacerbated by the prolonged ischemia at the end of an incremental exercise to exhaustion.

The incremental exercise test in normoxia and hypoxia ended with two different periods of ischemia of 10 or 60 s, during which the subjects breathed normoxic gas. Following a countdown, the subject performed a 10 s isokinetic sprint as hard and fast as possible while the ergometer was set at 80 rpm. The cuffs were always instantaneously deflated at the beginning of the post-ischemia sprints. In the unfatigued state, peak power increases with pedaling rate, but peak power is less affected by pedaling rate in the fatigued state (Beelen and Sargeant, 1991). Importantly, the difference in peak power between the fatigued and unfatigued state increases the higher the pedaling rate used in the control sprint (unfatigued) (Beelen and Sargeant, 1991). Thus, to avoid the limitations associated with varying pedaling rates sprints were performed in isokinetic mode at 80 rpm, a pedaling rate that allows maximal power output in the fatigued state (Beelen and Sargeant, 1991).

A few weeks later, the IEs were repeated in two additional experimental sessions; 1 day in normoxia (Nxb, P_IO_2: ~143 mmHg) and the other in hypoxia (Hypb, P_IO_2: ~73 mmHg; "b" indicates biopsy session). In the Nxb session, after 10 min rest in the supine position, a muscle biopsy was obtained from the m. *vastus lateralis* with local anesthesia (lidocaine 2%, 2 ml), using the Bergstrom technique with suction (Bergstrom, 1962). This biopsy was obtained with the needle pointing distally with 45° inclination (Guerra et al., 2011). An additional incision was performed before the beginning of the exercise in the contralateral leg. Afterward, the incisions were covered with a transient plaster, and a cuff was placed around the left leg. The subjects then sat on the cycle ergometer and resting

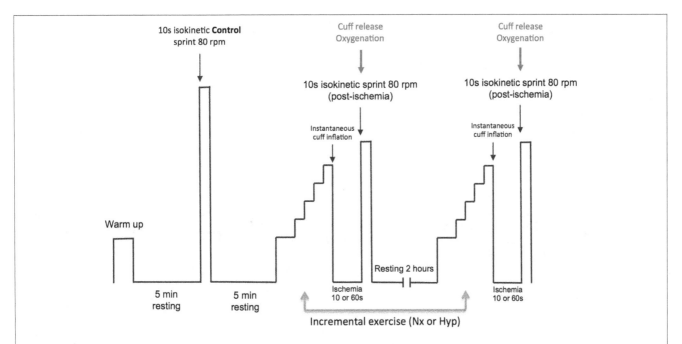

FIGURE 1 | Experimental protocol. The experimental day started with a warm-up followed by 4.5 min of slow unloaded pedaling and a 30 s resting phase, while the subjects became ready to perform the first sprint (isokinetic, 10 s at 80 rpm) at the 5th minute after the end of the warm-up. This sprint was used as a control sprint and was always performed in normoxia. Five minutes later, an incremental exercise to exhaustion began in normoxia (P_IO_2: ~143 mmHg) or acute hypoxia (P_IO_2: ~73 mmHg). The order of the incremental exercise test was randomized. Between the two incremental exercise tests, the subjects were allowed to rest during 120 min. At the end of the incremental exercise test, bilateral cuffs were inflated at maximal speed and pressure (i.e., 300 mmHg) to occlude completely and instantaneously the circulation (ischemia) of the legs. The incremental exercise test in normoxia and hypoxia ended with an ischemia period of 10 s on one experimental day and 60 s on another day. The order of the duration of the ischemia period was randomized. At the end of the ischemia period, the subjects performed a 10 s isokinetic sprint as hard and fast as possible (80 rpm) while the cuffs were always instantaneously deflated at the beginning of the post-ischemia sprints.

measurements were performed. Two minutes later, the IE was begun as described above. At exhaustion, the cuff was inflated instantaneously at 300 mmHg, and a biopsy was taken exactly 10 s after the end of the incremental exercise test. The biopsy needle was introduced perpendicular to the thigh. This biopsy was followed by a final biopsy at 60 s with the needle pointing proximally (45° inclination). In the Hypb session, essentially the same procedures were applied. All biopsies were immediately frozen in liquid nitrogen and stored at −80°C. Hypb and Nxb sessions were performed in random order.

Power Output, Oxygen Uptake and Hemoglobin Oxygen Saturation

Power output during the sprint was reported as instantaneous peak power output (Wpeak-i) and mean power output (Wmean) during the 10 s duration of the sprint. Oxygen uptake was measured with a metabolic cart (Vmax N29; Sensormedics, Yorba Linda, California, USA), calibrated before each test according to the manufacturer instructions, with high-grade calibration gasses (Carburos Metálicos, Las Palmas de Gran Canaria, Spain). Respiratory variables were analyzed breath-by-breath and averaged every 20 s during the incremental exercise tests. The highest 20-s averaged VO_2 recorded in normoxia was taken as the VO_2max. The same criterion was applied to determine the VO_2peak in hypoxia. Hemoglobin oxygen

saturation (SpO_2) was determined with a finger pulse oximeter (OEM III module, 4549-000, Plymouth, MN).

Muscle Metabolites

From each muscle biopsy, 30 mg of wet tissue were freeze-dried, cleaned and powdered with a manual mortar on ice. Subsequently, the samples were suspended in 0.5 M $HClO_4$ and centrifuged at 15,000 g at 4°C for 15 min. The supernatant was neutralized with $KHCO_3$ 2.1M. ATP, phosphocreatine (PCr), creatine, pyruvate and lactate concentrations were enzymatically determined in neutralized extracts by fluorometric analysis (Lowry and Passonneau, 1972; Morales-Alamo et al., 2013).

Electromyography

Electrical muscle activation was monitored using surface electromyography (EMG). EMG signals were continuously recorded from the *vastus medialis* and *vastus lateralis*. Before the application of the EMG electrodes the skin surface was carefully shaved and wiped with alcohol to reduce skin impedance. Bipolar single differential electrodes were placed longitudinally on the muscles following the SENIAM recommendations (Merletti and Hermens, 2000) and taped to the skin to minimize movement artifacts. The reference electrode was placed on the skin over the acromion. The position of the electrodes was marked on the skin with indelible ink, and these references were used for precise electrode placement on repeated experiments.

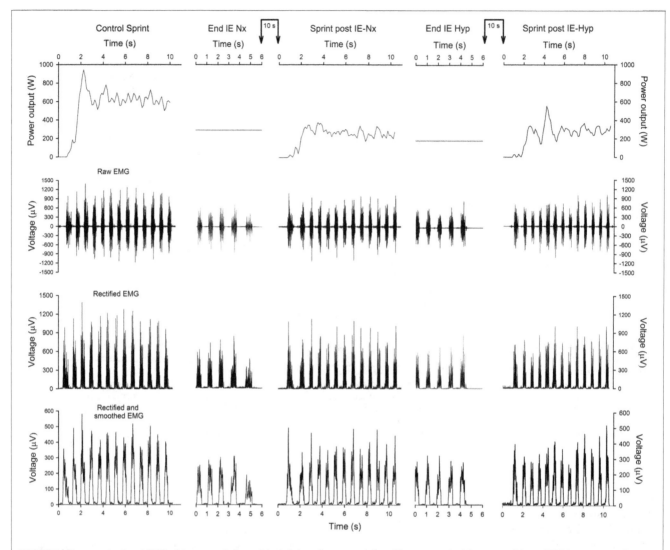

FIGURE 2 | Power output and EMG of a representative subject. Schematic representation of the power output (upper panels), raw EMG (2nd row), rectified EMG (3rd row) and rectified and smoothed EMG (lower panels), during the control sprint, last 6 s of the incremental exercise (IE) in normoxia (Nx), subsequent 10-s isokinetic sprint at 80 rpm (normoxia), IE in hypoxia (Hyp) and subsequent 10-s isokinetic sprint at 80 rpm (normoxia). The connected vertical arrows indicate the duration of the ischemia period, which in this example was 10 s.

The EMG signals were acquired using a 16-channel recording system (Myomonitor IV, Delsys Inc., Boston, MA) at a sampling rate of 1000 Hz using rectangular shaped (19.8 mm wide and 35 mm long) bipolar surface electrodes with 1×10 mm 99.9% Ag conductors, and with an inter-conductor distance of 10 mm (DE-2.3 Delsys Inc.). The EMG data were filtered with a high-pass filter of 20 Hz and a low-pass filter of 450 Hz using a fifth-order Butterworth filter. The system has an input impedance of $> 10^{15} \Omega$ per 0.2pF of input capacitance, a common mode rejection ratio of >80 dB, signal-to-noise ratio <1.2 μV, and a pre-amplifier gain 1000 V/V ±1%. Each pedal revolution was detected using an electrogoniometer (Goniometer Biosignal Sensor S700 Joint Angle Shape Sensor; Delsys Inc. Boston) fixed on the left knee and sampled at 500 Hz. EMG and joint movement were simultaneously recorded by a portable device (Myomonitor

IV, Delsys Inc. Boston) and wirelessly transmitted to a computer (EMGWorks Wireless application and EMGWorks Acquisition 3.7.1.3; Delsys, Inc. Boston).

The EMG signal corresponding to each muscle contraction was analyzed using code developed "in house" (Matlab R2012b, MathWorks, Natick, MA, USA). The EMG recordings were full-wave rectified and to provide an index of muscle activation, the amplitude characteristics were analyzed via average RMS of a 25-ms moving window for the duration of the burst. Burst onset and offset detection were determined using 20% of the maximal EMG$_{RMS}$ activity of each burst as a reference (Baum and Li, 2003; Hug and Dorel, 2009; Torres-Peralta et al., 2014), rather than a mean threshold value from 15 consecutive bursts (Ozgünen et al., 2010). This approach yielded the same result as direct simple visual discrimination with 100% detection of all bursts. The EMG_{RMS} recorded during the last minute of a 2 min 80 W load (in normoxia) was used to normalize the remaining EMG_{RMS} data. Besides, we defined a total activity index during the sprint (TAI) as TAI = EMG_{RMS} × burst duration (ms) × number of pedal strokes during the sprint. The total activity index is similar to the integrated EMG signal, but was computed separately for each burst and excluded the baseline EMG between burst (Torres-Peralta et al., 2014). The TAI recorded during the last minute of a 2 min 80 W load (in normoxia) was used to normalize the rest of the TAI values.

The mean (MPF) and median (MdPF) power spectrum frequencies were calculated using the Fast Fourier Transform (Solomonow et al., 1990). All variables were reported as the mean values of the pedal strokes recorded during the last 10 s of the incremental exercise or the 10 s sprints. EMG variables responded similarly during the four control sprints. Therefore, to reduce EMG variability the four control sprints were averaged. EMG data are reported separately for *vastus medialis* and *lateralis*, and also as the average of the two muscles. Since the incremental exercise tests in normoxia and hypoxia were repeated, the mean of each pair was used in further analysis to represent either normoxia or hypoxia.

Statistics

Normal distribution of variables was checked with the Shapiro-Wilks test. A repeated-measures ANOVA with F_IO_2 condition (normoxia vs. hypoxia) and occlusion duration (10 vs. 60 s) was used to analyze the responses observed during the sprints. Pairwise comparisons at specific time points were performed with Student t-tests, and adjusted for multiple comparisons using the Holm–Bonferroni method. Values are reported as the mean ± standard deviation (unless otherwise stated). $P \leq 0.05$ was considered statistically significant. All statistical analyses were performed using SPSS v.15.0 for Windows (SPSS Inc., Chicago, IL) and Excel 2011 (Microsoft, Redmond, WA, USA).

RESULTS

Incremental Exercise

Compared to normoxia, Wmax, pulmonary ventilation, respiratory rate, heart rate and VO_2peak were reduced during the last 10 s of exercise in hypoxia. Additional information regarding the respiratory and cardiovascular responses to the IE can be found elsewhere (Calbet et al., 2015; Morales-Alamo et al., 2015). The ergospirometric variables corresponding to the last 10 s of incremental exercise are reported in **Table 1**, together with the corresponding electromyographic responses.

Muscle Fatigue

Compared to the control sprints, post-IE sprint performance was reduced (32–46%, $P < 0.05$; **Figure 3**) as previously reported (Morales-Alamo et al., 2015). Sprint Wpeak-i was 11% lower following post-IE in normoxia than hypoxia. Similar effects were observed in Wmean. Sprint performance was improved after ischemic recovery. Wpeak-i and Wmean were 11 and 23% higher, respectively, following 60 than 10 s of occlusion ($P < 0.05$), as previously reported (Morales-Alamo et al., 2015).

TABLE 1 | Ergospirometric and electromyographic responses during the last 10 s of the incremental exercise to exhaustion in normoxia ($P_IO_2 \approx$ 143 mmHg) and severe hypoxia ($P_IO_2 \approx$ 73 mmHg).

	Normoxia	Hypoxia	P
F_IO_2 (%)	20.8 ± 0.1	10.8 ± 0.1	<0.001
SpO_2 (%)	93.1 ± 4.4	64.6 ± 4.6	<0.001
Wmax (W)	259.2 ± 32.0	170.1 ± 21.0	<0.001
VO_2peak (l.min^{-1})	3.62 ± 0.37	2.41 ± 0.29	<0.001
V_E (l.min^{-1})	143.5 ± 19.5	123.8 ± 22.5	<0.001
RR (breaths.min^{-1})	60.2 ± 7.6	53.8 ± 7.0	<0.001
HR (beats.min^{-1})	185.4 ± 6.0	175.1 ± 9.0	<0.001
$P_{ET}O_2$ (mmHg)	113.2 ± 2.3	58.6 ± 2.8	<0.001
$P_{ET}CO_2$ (mmHg)	32.1 ± 2.6	27.5 ± 2.1	<0.001
RER	1.15 ± 0.03	1.35 ± 0.11	<0.001
VCO_2 (l.min^{-1})	4.12 ± 0.49	3.23 ± 0.41	<0.001
Pedaling rate (rpm)	56.7 ± 7.4	55.4 ± 5.9	0.5
VM RMSraw (μV)	134.2 ± 60.1	113.3 ± 48.9	<0.05
VL RMSraw (μV)	103.0 ± 30.9	88.9 ± 30.9	0.12
Average RMSraw (μV)	121.0 ± 37.7	101.1 ± 33.7	<0.01
VM RMSNz (A.U.)	219.1 ± 77.6	182.3 ± 45.5	<0.05
VL RMSNz (A.U.)	193.7 ± 76.4	165.0 ± 62.4	0.07
Average RMSNz (A.U.)	206.4 ± 61.2	173.7 ± 41.8	<0.05
VM TAINz (A.U.)	289.5 ± 109.6	222.6 ± 88.1	<0.001
VL TAINz (A.U.)	246.5 ± 102.2	187.5 ± 73.1	<0.05
Average TAINz (A.U.)	268.0 ± 80.1	205.0 ± 68.2	<0.001
VM MPF (Hz)	84.2 ± 18.4	89.6 ± 18.0	0.13
VL MPF (Hz)	84.1 ± 18.6	89.6 ± 17.8	0.13
Average MPF (Hz)	84.2 ± 18.5	89.6 ± 17.9	0.13
VM MdPF (Hz)	68.6 ± 12.3	73.3 ± 14.8	<0.05
VL MdPF (Hz)	68.5 ± 12.5	73.0 ± 14.6	<0.05
Average MdPF (Hz)	68.6 ± 12.4	73.1 ± 14.7	<0.05
VM Burst (ms)	401.9 ± 51.7	362.5 ± 55.9	0.12
VL Burst (ms)	401.4 ± 55.2	368.3 ± 55.7	0.10
Average Burst (ms)	401.7 ± 49.4	365.4 ± 52.8	0.10

F_IO_2, inspiratory oxygen fraction; SpO_2, hemoglobin saturation in capillary blood measured by pulse oximetry; Wmax, power output at exhaustion; VO_2, oxygen consumption; V_E, pulmonary ventilation; RR, respiratory rate; HR, heart rate; $P_{ET}O_2$, end-tidal O_2 pressure; $P_{ET}CO_2$, end-tidal CO_2 pressure; RER, respiratory exchange ratio, VCO_2, CO_2 production; rpm, revolutions per minute; VL, vastus lateralis; VM, vastus medialis; RMSraw, raw root mean square; RMSNz, normalized root mean square; TAINz, Normalized total activation index (arbitrary units, A.U.); MPF, mean power frequency; MdPF, median power frequency; Burst, burst duration; Average, mean of VM and VL.

EMG responses

Vastus Lateralis EMGs

Figure 2 depicts an example of the EMG recordings during one experimental day. During the last 10 s of the incremental exercise to exhaustion the raw (average of the two muscles) and normalized RMS were 16% lower in hypoxia than in normoxia ($P < 0.05$) (**Table 1**). The average normalized TAI was also lower (23%) in hypoxia than in normoxia ($P < 0.001$). The median frequency was 6% lower in normoxia than hypoxia ($P < 0.05$). The mean and median frequencies during the last 10 s of the IE remained at the same level during the subsequent sprints.

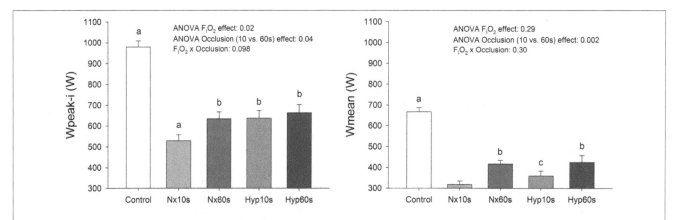

FIGURE 3 | Power output. Peak (Wpeak-i) and mean (Wmean) power output during sprint exercise performed at the end of an incremental exercise to exhaustion in normoxia ($P_IO_2 \approx 143$ mmHg) and severe hypoxia ($P_IO_2 \approx 73$ mmHg), after 10 or 60 s of occlusion of the circulation. [a]$P < 0.05$ compared with the other conditions; [b]$P < 0.05$ compared with Nx10s; [c]$P < 0.05$ compared with Nx60s.

TABLE 2 | *Vastus lateralis* electromyographic variables in response to sprint exercise performed at the end of an incremental exercise to exhaustion in normoxia ($P_IO_2 \approx 143$ mmHg) and severe hypoxia ($P_IO_2 \approx 73$ mmHg), after 10 or 60 s of occlusion of the circulation.

	Control sprint	Nx10s	Nx60s	Hyp10s	Hyp60s	Main Oxy (*P*)	Main Occ (*P*)	Interaction Oxy × Occ (*P*)
RMSraw (μV)	238.1 ± 82.0[a]	153.2 ± 64.7	137.1 ± 53.2	160.2 ± 68.7	161.8 ± 61.8	0.220	0.706	0.429
RMSNz (A.U.)	475.1 ± 155.2[a]	317.3 ± 95.1	254.6 ± 110.0	344.2 ± 126.4[c]	317.0 ± 172.4	0.112	0.059	0.436
Burst (ms)	331.9 ± 24.6[b,d]	299.7 ± 22.7[c]	324.6 ± 27.7	305.5 ± 23.8[c]	337.3 ± 34.4[b,d]	0.026	0.001	0.381
TAINz (A.U.)	1023.1 ± 340.6[a]	600.8 ± 268.8	581.5 ± 244.2	642.9 ± 297.0	715.8 ± 288.2	0.12	0.729	0.326
MPF (Hz)	93.9 ± 9.7[b,c]	81.9 ± 14.2	79.5 ± 16.4	86.3 ± 20.3	89.5 ± 17.2	0.006	0.837	0.212
MdPF (Hz)	80.2 ± 6.0[b,c,d]	66.4 ± 9.4[e]	67.0 ± 13.6	71.4 ± 16.6	74.7 ± 13.9[c]	0.011	0.255	0.500

[a]$P < 0.05$ compared with the other conditions.
[b]$P < 0.05$ compared with Nx10s.
[c]$P < 0.05$ compared with Nx60s.
[d]$P < 0.05$ compared with Hyp10s.
[e]$P < 0.05$ compared with Hyp60s.

RM ANOVA (2 × 2) Main Oxy: main oxygenation effect due to the conditions in which was performed the incremental exercise test (Nx, Normoxia; Hyp, hypoxia); RM ANOVA (2 × 2) Main Occ, Main Occlusion effect due to the duration of the occlusion (10 vs. 60 s); Wpeak-i, instantaneous peak power in the sprint; Wmean, mean power in the 10 s sprint; RMSraw, raw root mean square; RMSNz, Normalized root mean square; Burst, burst duration; TAINz, Normalized total activation index (arbitrary units, A.U.); MPF, mean power frequency; MdPF, median power frequency.

The average RMS, RMSNz, and TAINz were 1.6-, 1.7-, and 2.9-fold higher during the sprints post-IE than during the last 10 s of the IE (all, $P < 0.05$). Compared to the control sprints, the RMSraw and the normalized RMSNz were reduced by 36 and 35%, respectively, in the sprints performed after the IE (**Table 2**). Although the 60 s occlusion caused a 14% lower RMSNz compared to the 10 s occlusion, this difference did not reach statistical significance (Main effect $P = 0.059$). Compared to the control sprints the TAINz was reduced by 42 and 34% during the sprints performed after the incremental test in normoxia and hypoxia, respectively ($P < 0.05$).

Compared to the control sprint, the median frequency was reduced by 18 and 9% in the sprints that followed the IEs in normoxia and hypoxia, respectively (both, $P < 0.05$) (**Table 3**). Thus, the median frequency was 9% lower in the sprints that followed IE in normoxia than in hypoxia (Main effect $P = 0.011$). MPF changes were essentially similar to MdPF (**Tables 1–4**).

Compared to the control sprints, the duration of the bursts was reduced by 9% in the sprints performed after 10 s occlusions.

Nevertheless, after 60 s of occlusion, the duration of burst in the following sprints achieved the same value as in the control sprints (331.9 ± 24.6 and 331.0 ± 29.7 ms, control and 60 s after IE, respectively, $P = 0.91$). The duration of the bursts was 3% longer in the sprints that followed an IE in hypoxia than normoxia ($P = 0.03$). The average contraction time (i.e., burst duration x pedaling rate) was 15% lower during the last 10 s of IE than during the post-IE sprints ($P < 0.001$).

Vastus Medialis EMGs

The *vastus medialis* EMG responses to incremental (**Table 1**) and sprint exercise (**Table 3**) were similar to those described for the *vastus lateralis*. Therefore, we combined both *vastus* EMGs responses to reduce variability (**Table 4**). The combined response was similar to that reported for *vastus lateralis* and *medialis*, but with lower variability, confirming some of the effects that did not reach statistical significance when only analyzed using a single muscle EMG recordings.

TABLE 3 | *Vastus medialis* electromyographic variables in response to sprint exercise performed at the end of an incremental exercise to exhaustion in normoxia and severe hypoxia ($P_IO_2 \approx 73$ mmHg), after 10 or 60 s of occlusion of the circulation.

	Control sprint	Nx10s	Nx60s	Hyp10s	Hyp60s	Main Oxy (P)	Main Occ (P)	Interaction Oxy × Occ (P)
RMSraw (μV)	263.5 ± 115.7[b,c,e]	177.4 ± 95.0[d]	193.9 ± 121.3	204.2 ± 103.1	183.9 ± 81.1	0.333	0.943	0.038
RMSNz (A.U.)	410.4 ± 163.3[a]	284.0 ± 97.1[d]	276.4 ± 126.1	333.0 ± 143.1	279.7 ± 104.8[d]	0.078	0.137	0.098
Burst (ms)	342.2 ± 27.7[b]	309.4 ± 42.5[c]	355.2 ± 49.4[d]	322.0 ± 53.1	347.8 ± 37.9[b]	0.743	0.017	0.154
TAINz (A.U.)	1152.1 ± 463.3[a]	701.1 ± 359.9[d]	809.0 ± 498.6	829.7 ± 397.9	820.7 ± 335.6	0.118	0.638	0.119
MPF (Hz)	94.3 ± 9.9[b,c,d]	81.9 ± 14.0	79.8 ± 15.8	85.8 ± 19.2	89.4 ± 17.4	0.008	0.703	0.241
MdPF (Hz)	80.8 ± 6.7[a]	66.2 ± 9.2	67.1 ± 13.4	71.3 ± 16.6	74.6 ± 14.1[b,c]	0.011	0.218	0.587

[a] $P < 0.05$ compared with the other conditions.
[b] $P < 0.05$ compared with Nx10s.
[c] $P < 0.05$ compared with Nx60s.
[d] $P < 0.05$ compared with Hyp10s.
[e] $P < 0.05$ compared with Hyp60s.
RM ANOVA (2 × 2) Main Oxy, main oxygenation effect due to the conditions in which was performed the incremental exercise test (Nx, Normoxia; Hyp, hypoxia); RM ANOVA (2 × 2) Main Occ, Main Occlusion effect due to the duration of the occlusion (10 vs. 60 s); RMSraw, raw root mean square; RMSNz, Normalized root mean square; Burst, burst duration; TAINz, Normalized total activation index (arbitrary units, A.U.); MPF, mean power frequency; MdPF, median power frequency.

TABLE 4 | Electromyographic variables (average of *vastus medialis* and *lateralis*) in response to sprint exercise performed at the end of an incremental exercise to exhaustion in normoxia ($P_IO_2 \approx 143$ mmHg) and severe hypoxia ($P_IO_2 \approx 73$ mmHg), after 10 or 60 s of occlusion of the circulation.

	Control	Nx10s	Nx60s	Hyp10s	Hyp60s	Main Oxy (P)	Main Occ (P)	Interaction Oxy × Occ (P)
RMSraw (μV)	250.8 ± 89.1[a]	165.3 ± 69.6[d]	165.5 ± 76.5	182.2 ± 79.8	172.9 ± 50.7	0.164	0.793	0.536
RMSNz (A.U.)	442.7 ± 141.9[a]	300.6 ± 88.9[d]	265.5 ± 93.9[d]	338.6 ± 122.7	298.3 ± 117.7[d]	0.042	0.043	0.835
Burst (ms)	337.1 ± 23.9[b,d]	304.5 ± 29.8[c]	339.9 ± 36.0[d]	313.7 ± 36.0	342.6 ± 35.3[b,d]	0.305	0.005	0.754
TAINz (A.U.)	1089.7 ± 355.0	653.1 ± 274.8[d]	720.1 ± 323.5	739.6 ± 331.4	769.7 ± 238.9	0.082	0.510	0.575
MPF (Hz)	94.1 ± 9.8[b,c,d]	81.9 ± 14.1	79.6 ± 16.1	86.0 ± 19.7	89.5 ± 17.3[b,c]	0.007	0.769	0.221
MdPF (Hz)	80.5 ± 6.3[b,c,d]	66.3 ± 9.2	67.0 ± 13.5	71.3 ± 16.6	74.6 ± 14.0[b,c]	0.011	0.234	0.543

[a] $P < 0.05$ compared with the other conditions.
[b] $P < 0.05$ compared with Nx10s.
[c] $P < 0.05$ compared with Nx60s.
[d] $P < 0.05$ compared with Hyp10s.
RM ANOVA (2 × 2) Main Oxy, main oxygenation effect due to the conditions in which was performed the incremental exercise test (Nx, Normoxia; Hyp, hypoxia); RM ANOVA (2 × 2) Main Occ, Main Occlusion effect due to the duration of the occlusion (10 vs. 60 s); RMSraw, raw root mean square; RMSNz, Normalized root mean square; Burst, burst duration; TAINz, Normalized total activation index (arbitrary units, A.U.); MPF, mean power frequency; MdPF, median power frequency.

Muscle Metabolites

Muscle metabolites and the aerobic and anaerobic energy yield during the sprints have been reported elsewhere (Morales-Alamo et al., 2015). Briefly, ATP and PCr concentrations were reduced to a similar extent both in normoxia and hypoxia (ANOVA time effect: $P < 0.05$). From the 10th to 60th s of ischemic recovery ATP concentration remained unchanged while PCr declined an additional ~5% (ANOVA time effect: $P < 0.05$ compared to Post and $P < 0.001$, compared to PRE). Muscle lactate concentration was increased to similar values 10 s after both incremental exercise tests (93.5 ± 24.3 and 88.3 ± 26.6 mmol kg d.w.$^{-1}$, in normoxia and hypoxia, respectively (ANOVA time effect: $P < 0.001$). From the 10th to 60th s of ischemia muscle lactate was increased by 24.0 ± 20.7 and 21.6 ± 24.5 mmol kg d.w.$^{-1}$, and muscle pH reduced by 0.102 ± 0.040 and 0.109 ± 0.041 units, after the IE in normoxia and hypoxia, respectively (ANOVA time effect: $P < 0.01$).

DISCUSSION

This investigation confirms, in agreement with previous studies using constant intensity (Marcora and Staiano, 2010) and incremental exercise to exhaustion in normoxia (Coelho et al., 2015), that task failure during incremental exercise in normoxia is not caused by muscle fatigue. The present study extends these findings to whole-body incremental exercise in severe hypoxia. We have also shown that muscle activation during the last 10 s of an incremental exercise to exhaustion is lower in severe hypoxia than in normoxia. This reduction in muscle activation cannot be explained by differences in metabolite accumulation between hypoxia and normoxia, and likely reflects central mechanisms of fatigue, which recovered, at least partly, during the next 10 or 60 s of ischemia, as reflected by the greater activation of the muscles during the subsequent sprint. The latter occurred despite the lower energy availability and the greater accumulation of metabolites after the ischemic recoveries. We have shown that neuromuscular performance, as assessed by a sprint test, at the end of an incremental exercise to exhaustion, is greater when the incremental exercise has been performed in severe acute hypoxia than in normoxia despite similar muscle metabolite accumulation. This is also compatible with the incremental exercise in hypoxia ending by central mechanism/s acting earlier, i.e., with a lower amount of peripheral fatigue in hypoxia than in normoxia. This reduction in sprint performance is accompanied by a greater reduction in muscle activation (as reflected by the EMG_{RMS} changes) in the sprints carried out after IE in normoxia than hypoxia. This could also be interpreted as indicative of slower recovery of central mechanisms of fatigue during the 10 s of ischemic recovery that followed the IE performed in normoxia compared to the sprint performed after the IE in hypoxia.

Strikingly, following 60 s of recovery with complete occlusion of the circulation sprint performance was higher than that observed immediately following 10 s of occlusion, as previously reported (Morales-Alamo et al., 2015). This improvement in performance was achieved with lower EMG_{RMS} compared to the sprints executed after 10 s of ischemia. Thus, this investigation demonstrates dissociation between the recovery of the EMG_{RMS} and the recovery of power output. Since occlusion resulted in an increase of muscle lactate and H^+ accumulation from 10 to 60 s of occlusion (Morales-Alamo et al., 2015), the present experiments support the concept that muscle acidification contributes to reduce EMG_{RMS}. In addition, we have demonstrated that despite similar muscle concentrations of lactate and H^+ at the beginning of the respective sprints, the MPF and MdPF during sprint exercise are reduced by muscle fatigue when the sprint is performed after an incremental exercise in normoxia, but not in hypoxia. MPF and MdPF did not recover from the end of the incremental exercise to the start of the sprints, or from the 10th to the 60th second of ischemia, despite cessation of neural activation and appropriate oxygenation of the brain. These results point to peripheral mechanisms being primarily responsible for the reduction of MPF and MdPF during the sprints post-IE (Juel, 1988; Brody et al., 1991). Moreover, despite greater lactate and H^+ accumulation after 60 s of ischemic recovery, sprint exercise MPF and MdPF were not further reduced; therefore these two metabolites do not seem to account for the observed reduction of MPF and MdPF with muscle fatigue (Vestergaard-Poulsen et al., 1995). We have also shown that the duration of the bursts is reduced in fatigued muscles contracting under isokinetic conditions, recovering to non-fatigued levels within 60 s, regardless of the muscular concentrations of lactate and H^+. We lastly provided evidence for a minor impact, if any, of increased group III/IV afferent feedback on sprint exercise performance.

Surface EMG Changes are More Sensitive to Central than Peripheral Fatigue

To demonstrate the existence of central fatigue it is necessary to show that during a maximal voluntary contraction, direct stimulation of motor neural pathways or cortical motoneurons results in greater levels of force than elicited voluntarily (Merton, 1954; Gandevia et al., 1996). These procedures have several constraints limiting their application to complex tasks, such

as pedaling. To circumvent these problems, a commonly used approach has been to carry out potentiated and interpolated twitch assessments at exhaustion as fast as possible, i.e., 1–2 min after the task failure, when most of the reduction in power output has already been recovered (Sargeant and Dolan, 1987; Fernandez-del-Olmo et al., 2013; Froyd et al., 2013; Coelho et al., 2015). Another limitation of stimulation techniques is that muscle fatigue is task-specific (Gandevia, 2001). Stimulation techniques cannot reproduce the complexity of motor orders involving thousands of motor units from different muscles firing at different rates, which are recruited with specific timings to achieve a coordinated movement. Also, in fatigued muscles, the increase in force elicited by an interpolated twitch may be due in part to intracellular mechanisms (i.e., a peripheral mechanism that is likely related to the force/$[Ca^{2+}]_i$ relationship) (Gandevia et al., 2013), not necessarily reflecting increased central fatigue.

An alternative approach for assessing muscle fatigue is to measure the maximal power that can be generated during the task that elicits muscle fatigue (Cairns et al., 2005; Marcora and Staiano, 2010; Coelho et al., 2015). However, during whole-body exercise on the cycle ergometer, pedaling frequency slows down close to task failure (Torres-Peralta et al., 2014). Given the dependency of power on muscle contraction velocity, fatigue should ideally be tested under similar muscle contraction velocities as during isokinetic pedaling (Sargeant and Dolan, 1987).

In the present experiments, the sprints were performed in isokinetic conditions, i.e., the duration of each pedaling cycle was always the same, regardless of the state of muscle fatigue (**Figure 2**). This isokinetic approach was possible because the cycle ergometer servo-control instantaneously varied the resistance applied to the pedals depending on the force exerted resulting in a constant pedaling rate of 80 rpm. These conditions allowed us to examine the impact of fatigue on certain components of the EMG signal without the variability induced by the speed of movement.

At a given pedaling rate, the duration of contraction bursts increases with the intensity of exercise, reaching maximal values at intensities close to Wmax (Torres-Peralta et al., 2014). In all conditions and every subject, the mean intensity achieved during the 10 s sprints was above the intensity reached at exhaustion during the IEs. This result implies that concerning intensity, burst duration should have been maximal during all sprints. However, burst duration during the sprints performed after 10 s of ischemic recovery was reduced, meaning that muscles were activated during a shorter fraction of the pedaling cycle compared to the control sprints. This effect might have been caused by reduced sarcolemmal excitability as a consequence of fatigue (Sejersted and Sjogaard, 2000; Sidhu et al., 2012). Reduced sarcolemmal excitability during hand grip exercise has been associated with lactic acidosis in blood (Hilbert et al., 2012). However, if present at exhaustion, sarcolemmal excitability appears to recover in less than 60 s after a fatiguing sprint exercise (Fernandez-del-Olmo et al., 2013). In agreement, burst duration recovered within the 60 s of ischemic rest after both IEs. Despite the observed recovery of burst duration, the EMG_{RMS} was further reduced following 60 s of ischemia. Since the reduction in EMG_{RMS}

was accompanied by increased power output and normal burst duration, it seems unlikely that the lower sprint EMG_{RMS} after 60 s of ischemia originates from a failure of the muscle cells to respond to neural activation.

During high-intensity contractions, the myosin ATPase and ion pumps account for most of the energy expenditure in muscles because no energy can be diverted to biosynthetic processes as the required enzymes are blocked (Morales-Alamo and Calbet, 2014). In our experimental conditions, upon cessation of incremental exercise the ion pumps are expected to be maximally activated, particularly the Na^+-K^+ pump, which has a critical role in restoring sarcolemmal excitability (Pedersen et al., 2003; Hostrup et al., 2014). During ischemia, the energy needed to maintain the activity of the ion pumps was provided by the glycolysis and to a lesser extent by the minute amount of remaining PCr (Morales-Alamo et al., 2015). The O_2 that still remained bound to myoglobin at the end of incremental exercise was rapidly used upon occlusion due to the strong activation of mitochondrial respiration by the increased ADP concentration at task failure (Morales-Alamo et al., 2015). Femoral vein and mean capillary PO_2 were lower at exhaustion after the incremental exercise test in severe hypoxia than in normoxia (Calbet et al., 2015). Therefore, the potential contribution of the small amount of O_2 trapped in the occluded leg (or remaining bound to myoglobin) to ATP re-synthesis should have been lower in hypoxia than in normoxia. However, although more O_2 was available at exhaustion for the initial recovery in normoxia, i.e., within the first 10 s of occlusion, performance was more impaired in the sprint performed after 10 s of ischemic recovery that followed the normoxic rather than the hypoxic IEs. This result concurs with task failure occurring with a lower level of peripheral fatigue during IE in hypoxia than normoxia, as our results indicate.

Studies in cats (Hill et al., 1992; Lagier-Tessonnier et al., 1993) and rabbits (Arbogast et al., 2000) have shown increased baseline discharge frequency of group III and IV muscle afferents by PO_2 close to the values observed in the femoral vein in the present investigation (Calbet et al., 2015). Thus, lower interstitial PO_2 values in hypoxia than normoxia could have enhanced III/IV afferent feedback to cause increased inhibition of the corticospinal drive during exercise in severe acute hypoxia, as previously suggested (Calbet et al., 2015). Muscle III and IV afferent, and perhaps other sensory endings in joints and tendons, have been postulated to contribute to central fatigue (Reid, 1927; Bigland-Ritchie et al., 1986; Garland, 1991; Amann et al., 2008, 2013a). Animal studies have shown that when motoneurons are stimulated repetitively many neurons reduce their discharge frequency or stop firing (Kernell and Monster, 1982a,b; Spielmann et al., 1993). This phenomenon is likely accentuated by hypoxia. Consequently, reduced responsiveness of some motoneurons pools (central fatigue) combined with increased III/IV muscle afferent feedback and increased ventilatory demand at any given absolute intensity might have increased the perception of effort (Marcora, 2009), leading to task failure at the end of IE in hypoxia with a lower level of peripheral fatigue than in normoxia (Pierrefiche et al., 1997). Oxygenation upon exhaustion might have restored faster

central fatigue at the end of the IE in hypoxia than normoxia, by reinstating within seconds normoxic interstitial PO_2 levels in the CNS. In agreement, with altitude acclimatization, oxygen delivery at VO_2max is almost restored to sea level values (Calbet and Lundby, 2009), improving brain oxygenation compared to acute hypoxia and reducing supraspinal fatigue (Goodall et al., 2014a,b).

The absolute exercise intensity at task failure was lower in hypoxia than normoxia. However, metabolite accumulation was similar regardless of F_IO_2 and, hence, differences in absolute exercise intensity do not seem to account for the differences in peripheral fatigue.

Group III and IV Muscle Afferent Stimulation does not Limit Peak Power Output during Whole-Body Sprint Exercise in Healthy Humans

Group III/IV muscle afferent neurons include a complex family of afferent endings some of which act as nociceptors while others respond to thermal, mechanical or chemical stimulation (Light et al., 2008; McCord and Kaufman, 2010; Jankowski et al., 2013). Metabolic products of muscle contraction like H^+ (Rotto and Kaufman, 1988; Light et al., 2008), lactate (Light et al., 2008), adenosine (Middlekauff et al., 1997), ATP (Light et al., 2008), nitric oxide (Arbogast et al., 2001), and inflammation mediators may also increase III/IV muscle afferent discharge (Light et al., 2008; McCord and Kaufman, 2010). It is particularly important that the response to the isolated increase of H^+, ATP and lactate is much lower than observed to the combination of the three (Light et al., 2008). Some metaboreceptive III and IV muscle afferents seem specialized in detecting innocuous levels of metabolites, while others respond to noxious levels and contribute to muscle pain (Kniffki et al., 1978; Mense, 1996). It is thought that both low and high concentration responding-endings could contribute to sympathetic reflexes and to increase the perception of effort (Light et al., 2008).

Using lumbar intrathecal fentanyl administration before exercise to block μ-opioid receptor-sensitive group, Amann and co-workers (Amann et al., 2009, 2011) studied the influence of group III and IV afferents on voluntary activation (assessed by the twitch-interpolation technique) after constant-intensity bicycling exercise. After 3 min of recovery, voluntary activation was reduced by 1.2% during the placebo trial (non-significant) and 1.7% during the fentanyl trial (Amann et al., 2011). Moreover, 3 min after a time trial that caused fatigue in 7.5 min, voluntary activation was reduced by 1.6% (compared to 0.8% in the placebo trial) (Amann et al., 2009). These results further emphasize that any potentially negative influence of III and IV muscle afferents on voluntary activation is likely small after whole-body exercise or that voluntary activation capacity recovers rather quickly (Bigland-Ritchie et al., 1986; Kennedy et al., 2015; Pageaux et al., 2015).

Amann et al. (2011) reported that despite the inhibition of III and IV muscle afferents, fentanyl markedly reduced performance (from 8.7 to 6.8 min) during a constant-intensity trial to exhaustion. In another study by the same group

(Amann et al., 2009), where the subjects performed a time trial, performance was similar in the fentanyl and placebo experiments. The reason for these discrepant effects of III/IV muscle afferents inhibition on performance is not clear (Marcora, 2010). In the case of the constant-intensity trial, there was a substantial impairment in O_2 transport in the fentanyl trial, an effect caused by reduced ventilation, leading to lower hemoglobin saturation and VO_2 with fentanyl than placebo. A slightly lower impairment of O_2 transport was reported in the time trial experiments, which could have been compensated for by increased involvement of the anaerobic metabolism (Amann et al., 2009). Marcora (2010) have suggested that during the time trial, the "belief effect" induced by reducing leg muscle pain with fentanyl-induced a fast start, which compensated for the negative effect of fentanyl on cardiorespiratory responses. As a result, exercise performance was unchanged during the time trial. During the constant-intensity trial, the "belief effect" could not induce a fast start and consequently exercise performance was reduced.

Interestingly, in both experiments with fentanyl the reduction of quadriceps potentiated twitch forces elicited by magnetic neural stimulation were greater than in the control trials (Amann et al., 2009, 2011). Assuming that a reduction in the force elicited by potentiated twitches indicates a greater level of peripheral fatigue and that the subjects exercised to their limits in all trials, Amann and co-workers studies give support to the concept that III/IV afferent feedback is used to set the limit of peripheral fatigue that is permitted. However, these experiments, combined with the present findings, show that task failure at the end of an IE to exhaustion (current study), or at the end of constant-intensity (Marcora and Staiano, 2010; Bosio et al., 2012) or a simulated time-trial competition (Amann and co-workers studies) is not due to a peripheral failure. Both types of experiments show that greater levels of peripheral fatigue are possible, but not reached because the exercise ends due to central mechanisms of fatigue (Kayser, 2003). The critical question is whether peripheral fatigue causes central fatigue and task failure through a central mechanism by activating the metaboreflex. If the latter is the main mechanism causing central fatigue and task failure a reduction in sprint performance under conditions with increased metaboreflex activation will be expected. However, our results show that this is not the case.

Metabolite accumulation at task failure and during ischemia should have promoted a sustained discharge of III/IV muscle afferents (Darques and Jammes, 1997; Darques et al., 1998; Light et al., 2008; McCord and Kaufman, 2010), an effect that would be expected to be greater after 60 than 10 s occlusions in the present investigation. Nevertheless, sprint exercise power output was higher after 60 than 10 s of ischemia. Increased metaboreflex activation should exacerbate the ventilatory response to exercise (Amann et al., 2010), as observed during the sprints performed following 60 s of ischemia in the present investigation (Morales-Alamo et al., 2015). Thus, despite increased metaboreflex activation during the sprints after 60 s of ischemia, and a theoretically worsened metabolic situation, peak and mean power output was higher during the sprints after 60 than 10 s of ischemia. Our findings appear to be at odds with the recent study by Kennedy et al. (2015), in which the occlusion of the circulation during 2 min after a 2-min sustained MVC of the knee extensors resulted in a progressive reduction of the maximal voluntary contraction (MVC) (see Figure 3A of Kennedy et al., 2015). This effect was accompanied by a progressive reduction of maximal voluntary activation indicative of increasing central fatigue (see Figure 3B of Kennedy et al., 2015). In agreement with our results, Kennedy et al. (2015) observed a fast recovery of voluntary activation upon release of the cuff, indicating that the negative influence of III/IV afferent discharge on voluntary activation was also relieved very rapidly. This quick response could be due to (i) the release of the direct compression on the femoral nerve, (ii) the washout of metabolites combined with oxygenation due to reactive hyperemia, or (iii) the combination of these effects. In our experimental conditions, the hyperemic response to the release of the cuff was likely much greater than in Kennedy et al. (2015) as reflected by the rapid increase of pulmonary VO_2 and the elevated heart rate at the beginning of the sprint (Morales-Alamo et al., 2015). Another interesting aspect of the study by Kennedy et al. (2015) is that the level of peripheral fatigue as assessed by potentiated twitches remained at the same level during the 2 min of ischemia, despite 5×2-s long MVC maneuvers (i.e., 10 s of maximal contractile activity with occlusion of the circulation). Thus, the 2 min of post-exercise ischemia did not worsen peripheral fatigue (Kennedy et al., 2015). Although Kennedy et al. (2015) did not measure muscle metabolites, 10 s of maximal contractile activity during the 2 min of ischemia, in combination with increased metabolic demand due to the preceding MVC (sustained during 2 min), should have increased peripheral fatigue according to the prevailing paradigm.

The present investigation strongly suggests that the inhibitory role of muscle afferent discharge on the corticospinal motor drive during maximal intensity whole-body exercise is either small or counteracted by a strong corticospinal drive (central command). Otherwise, the III/IV muscle afferent feedback due to ischemia (PO_2 close to 0 mmHg in our experimental conditions) and the metabolites accumulated during the IEs should have decreased Wpeak and Wmean during the 10 or 60 s post-ischemia sprints below the Wmax achieved at task failure in the IEs. This finding contrasts with experiments using single joint (Gandevia et al., 1996; Kennedy et al., 2015) or handgrip dynamic contractions (Broxterman et al., 2015), where a clear inhibition of voluntary activation is consistently shown.

In the present investigation, increased III/IV muscle afferent feedback could explain why the observed EMG_{RMS} were lower in the sprints performed after 60 s than after 10 s of ischemia. Likewise, that MPF and MdPF remained at task failure levels during the post-IE sprints is also consistent with an on-going negative feedback reducing motoneurons firing frequencies (Broxterman et al., 2015). However, the power output achieved during the sprints after 60 s of ischemia is close to the maximal power attainable by our subjects without phosphagens (Morales-Alamo et al., 2015), leaving little room for central mechanisms to limit sprint performance after 60 s of ischemia. Thus, it seems that 60 s of ischemic recovery allows for restoration of the central mechanisms of fatigue, despite the discharge from the III/IV muscle afferents. The latter was likely counteracted by a strong central command and a rapid reperfusion of the muscle upon the release of the cuff during the post-IE sprints. In agreement with this interpretation, Amann et al. (2009) reported no effect of intrathecal fentanyl on time trial performance, although the power output profile was dramatically changed.

Reduced Sprint EMG$_{RMS}$ But Increased Power Output after 60 than 10 s Post-Exercise Ischemia

In vitro experiments have shown that lactate and H^+ accumulation may facilitate peripheral recovery by increasing chloride conductance (Nielsen et al., 2001; Pedersen et al., 2003; Karelis et al., 2004). Thus, an elevated glycolytic rate combined with a progressive rise of muscle temperature due to flow arrest during ischemic recovery could have exerted two opposing actions. Positively, increased glycolysis may have facilitated peripheral recovery by enhancing sarcolemmal excitability (Pedersen et al., 2003), which was likely depressed immediately after the IEs. Negatively, increased glycolysis and the subsequent metabolite accumulation may have increased III/IV muscle afferent discharge, interfering with muscle activation. The combination of both mechanisms could explain the lower EMG$_{RMS}$ values observed during the sprints performed 60 s compared to 10 s after the IEs. If we assume that the normalized EMG$_{RMS}$ is a valid index of corticospinal motor output, only reduced when the corticospinal motor drive is lower, a greater reduction in sprint EMG$_{RMS}$ after prolonged (60 s) compared to shorter (10 s) ischemia would lead to the untenable conclusion that all of the improvement in Wpeak and Wmean observed from 10 to 60 s of ischemic recovery is due to peripheral mechanisms. Moreover, this peripheral-based improvement would have to be sufficient to counteract the reduced motor command. A more plausible explanation is that for a given level of neural activation, EMG$_{RMS}$ is reduced by metabolite accumulation; i.e., EMG$_{RMS}$ does not faithfully reflect the level of neural activation (Vestergaard-Poulsen et al., 1995). In agreement with this interpretation, it has been shown that central fatigue recovers rapidly upon cessation of contractile activity, even when peripheral fatigue remains at the same level (Bigland-Ritchie et al., 1986; Gandevia et al., 1996). Therefore, the observed reduction in sprint EMG$_{RMS}$ after 60 s compared to 10 s of ischemic recovery is unlikely to be caused only by increased central mechanisms of fatigue.

Fatigue Reduces the Duration of the Burst during Isokinetic Sprints

The duration of the burst was similarly decreased in the sprints performed 10 s after the incremental exercise in hypoxia and normoxia. However, sprint power output was greater after the incremental exercise in hypoxia. To generate greater power, more

mechanical impulse must be produced. As the duration of the bursts (a surrogate of contraction time) was similar in the sprints performed 10 s after both IEs, the subjects must have applied a greater force on the pedals after the hypoxic IE. Therefore, greater motor cortical drive was required in the sprint that occurred after hypoxia. In agreement, with this conclusion, the MPF and MdPF were higher in the sprints preceded by IE in hypoxia than normoxia, suggesting greater firing rates (Solomonow et al., 1990; Gerdle and Fugl-Meyer, 1992; Sbriccoli et al., 2003) and a lower degree of central fatigue during the sprint 10 s after the IE in hypoxia. Alternatively, central fatigue could have recovered more rapidly after the IE in hypoxia, likely due to a direct effect of oxygenation on the CNS, as previously postulated (Kayser et al., 1994; Calbet et al., 2003a,b; Amann et al., 2007; Goodall et al., 2014a).

Limitations

At the end of the incremental exercise muscle activation was much lower than during the subsequent sprints, despite the fact muscles remained ischemic and that metabolite accumulation reduces EMG$_{RMS}$. This finding indicates that task failure was not due to muscle fatigue; it was caused by reduced muscle activation. However, this conclusion is not based on genuine assessments of central fatigue and peripheral fatigue with stimulation techniques. Nonetheless, there is not an ideal method to quantify the extent of change in neuromuscular function (Cairns et al., 2005). Current methods based on stimulation techniques have also limitations. For example, the response of fatigued muscles to potentiated twitches depends on the method of stimulation (Froyd et al., 2013). Moreover, methods based on electrical or magnetic stimulation may give results different from those obtained using voluntary dynamic contractions. Few minutes after a 30 s all out sprint exercise (Wingate test) potentiated quadriceps twitches indicate substantial peripheral fatigue, when at the same time peak power output has completely recovered (Fernandez-del-Olmo et al., 2013).

In summary, task failure at the end of an incremental exercise to exhaustion depends more on central than peripheral mechanisms, as indicated by the fact that the level of muscle activation observed during the last 10 s of the incremental exercise was much lower than that reached 10 s later during a 10 s sprint, despite the fact that muscle remained ischemic from the end of exercise to the start of the sprint. The central components of fatigue appear to recover to a greater extent, during the first 10 s following an incremental exercise to exhaustion in hypoxia than in normoxia, concomitant with a rapid change to normoxic breathing during the recovery. We have also shown that ischemic recovery after incremental exercise to exhaustion allows for a partial restoration of power output despite increased acidification and reduced EMG$_{RMS}$. Moreover, this study demonstrates that MPF, MdPF and the duration of the bursts during isokinetic sprints are reduced with fatigue. Lastly, this investigation indicates that increased group III/IV muscle afferent discharge has a minor, if any, negative impact on sprint exercise performance in healthy humans.

AUTHOR CONTRIBUTIONS

Conception and design of the experiments: JC; pre-testing, experimental preparation, data collection and analysis: RT, DM, JL, IP, and JC; EMG analysis: RT, MG, and MI. The first version of the manuscript was written by RT and JC. All co-authors read, contributed comments and approved the final version of the manuscript.

ACKNOWLEDGMENTS

This study was supported by a grant from the Ministerio de Educación y Ciencia of Spain (DEP2009-11638 and FEDER) and VII Convocatoria de Ayudas a la Investigación Cátedra Real Madrid-Universidad Europea de Madrid (2015/04RM). Especially thanks are given to José Navarro de Tuero for his excellent technical assistance.

REFERENCES

Amann, M., Blain, G. M., Proctor, L. T., Sebranek, J. J., Pegelow, D. F., and Dempsey, J. A. (2010). Group III and IV muscle afferents contribute to ventilatory and cardiovascular response to rhythmic exercise in humans. *J. Appl. Physiol.* 109, 966–976. doi: 10.1152/japplphysiol.00462.2010

Amann, M., Blain, G. M., Proctor, L. T., Sebranek, J. J., Pegelow, D. F., and Dempsey, J. A. (2011). Implications of group III and IV muscle afferents for high-intensity endurance exercise performance in humans. *J. Physiol.* 589, 5299–5309. doi: 10.1113/jphysiol.2011.213769

Amann, M., and Dempsey, J. A. (2008). Locomotor muscle fatigue modifies central motor drive in healthy humans and imposes a limitation to exercise performance. *J. Physiol.* 586, 161–173. doi: 10.1113/jphysiol.2007.141838

Amann, M., Goodall, S., Twomey, R., Subudhi, A. W., Lovering, A. T., and Roach, R. C. (2013b). AltitudeOmics: on the consequences of high-altitude acclimatization for the development of fatigue during locomotor exercise in humans. *J. Appl. Physiol. (1985)* 115, 634–642. doi: 10.1152/japplphysiol.00606.2013

Amann, M., Proctor, L. T., Sebranek, J. J., Eldridge, M. W., Pegelow, D. F., and Dempsey, J. A. (2008). Somatosensory feedback from the limbs exerts inhibitory influences on central neural drive during whole body endurance exercise. *J. Appl. Physiol.* 105, 1714–1724. doi: 10.1152/japplphysiol.90456.2008

Amann, M., Proctor, L. T., Sebranek, J. J., Pegelow, D. F., and Dempsey, J. A. (2009). Opioid-mediated muscle afferents inhibit central motor drive and limit peripheral muscle fatigue development in humans. *J. Physiol.* 587, 271–283. doi: 10.1113/jphysiol.2008.163303

Amann, M., Romer, L. M., Subudhi, A. W., Pegelow, D. F., and Dempsey, J. A. (2007). Severity of arterial hypoxaemia affects the relative contributions of peripheral muscle fatigue to exercise performance in healthy humans. *J. Physiol.* 581, 389–403. doi: 10.1113/jphysiol.2007.129700

Amann, M., Venturelli, M., Ives, S. J., McDaniel, J., Layec, G., Rossman, M. J., et al. (2013a). Peripheral fatigue limits endurance exercise via a sensory feedback-mediated reduction in spinal motoneuronal output. *J. Appl. Physiol.* 115, 355–364. doi: 10.1152/japplphysiol.00049.2013

Arbogast, S., Darques, J. L., Bregeon, F., and Jammes, Y. (2001). Effects of endogenous nitric oxide in activation of group IV muscle afferents. *Muscle Nerve* 24, 247–253. doi: 10.1002/1097-4598(200102)24:2<247::AID-MUS100>3.0.CO;2-T

Arbogast, S., Vassilakopoulos, T., Darques, J. L., Duvauchelle, J. B., and Jammes, Y. (2000). Influence of oxygen supply on activation of group IV muscle afferents after low-frequency muscle stimulation. *Muscle Nerve* 23, 1187–1193. doi: 10.1002/1097-4598(200008)23:8<1187::AID-MUS5>3.0.CO;2-9

Bachasson, D., Temesi, J., Gruet, M., Yokoyama, K., Rupp, M., Millet, G. Y., et al. (2016). Transcranial magnetic stimulation intensity affects exercise-induced changes in corticomotoneuronal excitability and inhibition and voluntary activation. *Neuroscience* 314, 125–133. doi: 10.1016/j.neuroscience.2015.11.056

Baum, B. S., and Li, L. (2003). Lower extremity muscle activities during cycling are influenced by load and frequency. *J. Electromyogr. Kinesiol.* 13, 181–190. doi: 10.1016/S1050-6411(02)00110-4

Beelen, A., and Sargeant, A. J. (1991). Effect of fatigue on maximal power output at different contraction velocities in humans. *J. Appl. Physiol.* 71, 2332–2337.

Bergstrom, J. (1962). Muscle electrolytes in man. *Scand. J. Clin. Lab. Invest. Suppl.* 68, 1–110.

Bigland-Ritchie, B., and Woods, J. J. (1984). Changes in muscle contractile properties and neural control during human muscular fatigue. *Muscle Nerve* 7, 691–699. doi: 10.1002/mus.880070902

Bigland-Ritchie, B. R., Dawson, N. J., Johansson, R. S., and Lippold, O. C. (1986). Reflex origin for the slowing of motoneurone firing rates in fatigue of human voluntary contractions. *J. Physiol.* 379, 451–459. doi: 10.1113/jphysiol.1986.sp016263

Bogdanis, G. C., Nevill, M. E., Boobis, L. H., and Lakomy, H. K. (1996). Contribution of phosphocreatine and aerobic metabolism to energy supply during repeated sprint exercise. *J. Appl. Physiol.* 80, 876–884.

Bosio, A., de Morree, H. M., Rampinini, E., and Marcora, S. M. (2012). "Is exercise tolerance limited by muscle fatigue in humans?" in *The Biomedical Basis of Elite Performance* (London: The Physiological Society), PC98.

Brody, L. R., Pollock, M. T., Roy, S. H., De Luca, C. J., and Celli, B. (1991). pH-induced effects on median frequency and conduction velocity of the myoelectric signal. *J. Appl. Physiol.* 71, 1878–1885.

Broxterman, R. M., Ade, C. J., Craig, J. C., Wilcox, S. L., Schlup, S. J., and Barstow, T. J. (2015). Influence of blood flow occlusion on muscle oxygenation characteristics and the parameters of the power-duration relationship. *J. Appl. Physiol.* 118, 880–889. doi: 10.1152/japplphysiol.00875.2014

Cairns, S. P., Knicker, A. J., Thompson, M. W., and Sjøgaard, G. (2005). Evaluation of models used to study neuromuscular fatigue. *Exerc. Sport. Sci. Rev.* 33, 9–16.

Calbet, J. A., Boushel, R., Rådegran, G., Søndergaard, H., Wagner, P. D., and Saltin, B. (2003a). Determinants of maximal oxygen uptake in severe acute hypoxia. *Am. J. Physiol. Regul.* 284, R291–R303. doi: 10.1152/ajpregu.00155.2002

Calbet, J. A., Boushel, R., Radegran, G., Sondergaard, H., Wagner, P. D., and Saltin, B. (2003b). Why is VO$_2$max after altitude acclimatization still reduced despite normalization of arterial O$_2$ content? *Am. J. Physiol. Regul.* 284, R304–R316. doi: 10.1152/ajpregu.00156.2002

Calbet, J. A., Chavarren, J., and Dorado, C. (1997). Fractional use of anaerobic capacity during a 30- and a 45-s Wingate test. *Eur. J. Appl.* 76, 308–313. doi: 10.1007/s004210050253

Calbet, J. A., Losa-Reyna, J., Torres-Peralta, R., Rasmussen, P., Ponce-González, J. G., Sheel, A. W., et al. (2015). Limitations to oxygen transport and utilization during sprint exercise in humans: evidence for a functional reserve in muscle O$_2$ diffusing capacity. *J. Physiol.* 593, 4649–4664. doi: 10.1113/JP270408

Calbet, J. A., and Lundby, C. (2009). Air to muscle O$_2$ delivery during exercise at altitude. *High. Alt. Med. Biol.* 10, 123–134. doi: 10.1089/ham.2008.1099

Coelho, A. C., Cannon, D. T., Cao, R., Porszasz, J., Casaburi, R., Knorst, M. M., et al. (2015). Instantaneous quantification of skeletal muscle activation, power production, and fatigue during cycle ergometry. *J. Appl. Physiol.* 118, 646–654. doi: 10.1152/japplphysiol.00948.2014

Darques, J. L., Decherchi, P., and Jammes, Y. (1998). Mechanisms of fatigue-induced activation of group IV muscle afferents: the roles played by lactic acid and inflammatory mediators. *Neurosci. Lett.* 257, 109–112. doi: 10.1016/S0304-3940(98)00816-7

Darques, J. L., and Jammes, Y. (1997). Fatigue-induced changes in group IV muscle afferent activity: differences between high- and low-frequency electrically induced fatigues. *Brain Res.* 750, 147–154. doi: 10.1016/S0006-8993(96)01341-8

Dawson, B., Goodman, C., Lawrence, S., Preen, D., Polglaze, T., Fitzsimons, M., et al. (1997). Muscle phosphocreatine repletion following single and repeated short sprint efforts. *Scand. J. Med. Sci. Sports* 7, 206–213. doi: 10.1111/j.1600-0838.1997.tb00141.x

Dempsey, J. A., Blain, G. M., and Amann, M. (2014). Are type III-IV muscle afferents required for a normal steady-state exercise hyperpnoea in humans? *J. Physiol.* 592, 463–474. doi: 10.1113/jphysiol.2013.261925

Fernandez-del-Olmo, M., Rodriguez, F. A., Marquez, G., Iglesias, X., Marina, M., Benitez, A., et al. (2013). Isometric knee extensor fatigue following a Wingate test: peripheral and central mechanisms. *Scand. J. Med. Sci. Sports* 23, 57–65. doi: 10.1111/j.1600-0838.2011.01355.x

Froyd, C., Millet, G. Y., and Noakes, T. D. (2013). The development of peripheral fatigue and short-term recovery during self-paced high-intensity exercise. *J. Physiol.* 591, 1339–1346. doi: 10.1113/jphysiol.2012.245316

Gandevia, S. C. (2001). Spinal and supraspinal factors in human muscle fatigue. *Physiol. Rev.* 81, 1725–1789.

Gandevia, S. C., Allen, G. M., Butler, J. E., and Taylor, J. L. (1996). Supraspinal factors in human muscle fatigue: evidence for suboptimal output from the motor cortex. *J. Physiol.* 490(Pt 2), 529–536. doi: 10.1113/jphysiol.1996.sp021164

Gandevia, S. C., McNeil, C. J., Carroll, T. J., and Taylor, J. L. (2013). Twitch interpolation: superimposed twitches decline progressively during a tetanic contraction of human adductor pollicis. *J. Physiol.* 591, 1373–1383. doi: 10.1113/jphysiol.2012.248989

Garland, S. J. (1991). Role of small diameter afferents in reflex inhibition during human muscle fatigue. *J. Physiol.* 435, 547–558. doi: 10.1113/jphysiol.1991.sp018524

Gerdle, B., and Fugl-Meyer, A. R. (1992). Is the mean power frequency shift of the EMG a selective indicator of fatigue of the fast twitch motor units? *Acta Physiol. Scand.* 145, 129–138.

Goodall, S., Ross, E. Z., and Romer, L. M. (2010). Effect of graded hypoxia on supraspinal contributions to fatigue with unilateral knee-extensor contractions. *J. Appl. Physiol.* 109, 1842–1851. doi: 10.1152/japplphysiol.00458.2010

Goodall, S., Twomey, R., and Amann, M. (2014a). Acute and chronic hypoxia: implications for cerebral function and exercise tolerance. *Fatigue Biomed. Health Behav.* 2, 73–92. doi: 10.1080/21641846.2014.909963

Goodall, S., Twomey, R., Amann, M., Ross, E. Z., Lovering, A. T., Romer, L. M., et al. (2014b). AltitudeOmics: exercise-induced supraspinal fatigue is attenuated in healthy humans after acclimatization to high altitude. *Acta Physiol. (Oxf.)* 210, 875–888. doi: 10.1111/apha.12241

Guerra, B., Gomez-Cabrera, M. C., Ponce-Gonzalez, J. G., Martinez-Bello, V. E., Guadalupe-Grau, A., Santana, A., et al. (2011). Repeated muscle biopsies through a single skin incision do not elicit muscle signaling, but IL-6 mRNA and STAT3 phosphorylation increase in injured muscle. *J. Appl. Physiol.* 110, 1708–1715. doi: 10.1152/japplphysiol.00091.2011

Héroux, M. E., Taylor, J. L., and Gandevia, S. C. (2015). The use and abuse of transcranial magnetic stimulation to modulate corticospinal excitability in humans. *PLoS ONE* 10:e0144151. doi: 10.1371/journal.pone.0144151

Hilbert, M., Shushakov, V., and Maassen, N. (2012). The influence of respiratory acid-base changes on muscle performance and excitability of the sarcolemma during strenuous intermittent hand grip exercise. *J. Appl. Physiol. (1985)* 112, 571–579. doi: 10.1152/japplphysiol.00869.2010

Hill, J. M., Pickar, J. G., Parrish, M. D., and Kaufman, M. P. (1992). Effects of hypoxia on the discharge of group III and IV muscle afferents in cats. *J. Appl. Physiol.* 73, 2524–2529.

Hostrup, M., Kalsen, A., Ortenblad, N., Juel, C., Mørch, K., Rzeppa, S., et al. (2014). beta2-adrenergic stimulation enhances Ca^{2+} release and contractile properties of skeletal muscles, and counteracts exercise-induced reductions in Na^+-K^+-ATPase Vmax in trained men. *J. Physiol.* 592, 5445–5459. doi: 10.1113/jphysiol.2014.277095

Hug, F., and Dorel, S. (2009). Electromyographic analysis of pedaling: a review. *J. Electromyogr. Kinesiol.* 19, 182–198. doi: 10.1016/j.jelekin.2007.10.010

Hureau, T. J., Olivier, N., Millet, G. Y., Meste, O., and Blain, G. M. (2014). Exercise performance is regulated during repeated sprints to limit the development of peripheral fatigue beyond a critical threshold. *Exp. Physiol.* 99, 951–963. doi: 10.1113/expphysiol.2014.077974

Jankowski, M. P., Rau, K. K., Ekmann, K. M., Anderson, C. E., and Koerber, H. R. (2013). Comprehensive phenotyping of group III and IV muscle afferents in mouse. *J. Neurophysiol.* 109, 2374–2381. doi: 10.1152/jn.01067.2012

Juel, C. (1988). Muscle action potential propagation velocity changes during activity. *Muscle Nerve* 11, 714–719. doi: 10.1002/mus.880110707

Karelis, A. D., Marcil, M., Péronnet, F., and Gardiner, P. F. (2004). Effect of lactate infusion on M-wave characteristics and force in the rat plantaris muscle during repeated stimulation *in situ*. *J. Appl. Physiol.* 96, 2133–2138. doi: 10.1152/japplphysiol.00037.2004

Kayser, B. (2003). Exercise starts and ends in the brain. *Eur. J. Appl.* 90, 411–419. doi: 10.1007/s00421-003-0902-7

Kayser, B., Narici, M., Binzoni, T., Grassi, B., and Cerretelli, P. (1994). Fatigue and exhaustion in chronic hypobaric hypoxia: influence of exercising muscle mass. *J. Appl. Physiol.* 76, 634–640.

Kennedy, D. S., Fitzpatrick, S. C., Gandevia, S. C., and Taylor, J. L. (2015). Fatigue-related firing of muscle nociceptors reduces voluntary activation of ipsilateral but not contralateral lower limb muscles. *J. Appl. Physiol.* 118, 408–418. doi: 10.1152/japplphysiol.00375.2014

Kernell, D., and Monster, A. W. (1982a). Motoneurone properties and motor fatigue. An intracellular study of gastrocnemius motoneurones of the cat. *Exp. Brain Res.* 46, 197–204.

Kernell, D., and Monster, A. W. (1982b). Time course and properties of late adaptation in spinal motoneurones of the cat. *Exp. Brain Res.* 46, 191–196.

Kniffki, K. D., Mense, S., and Schmidt, R. F. (1978). Responses of group IV afferent units from skeletal muscle to stretch, contraction and chemical stimulation. *Exp. Brain Res.* 31, 511–522. doi: 10.1007/BF00239809

Lagier-Tessonnier, F., Balzamo, E., and Jammes, Y. (1993). Comparative effects of ischemia and acute hypoxemia on muscle afferents from tibialis anterior in cats. *Muscle Nerve* 16, 135–141. doi: 10.1002/mus.880160203

Light, A. R., Hughen, R. W., Zhang, J., Rainier, J., Liu, Z., and Lee, J. (2008). Dorsal root ganglion neurons innervating skeletal muscle respond to physiological combinations of protons, ATP, and lactate mediated by ASIC, P2X, and TRPV1. *J. Neurophysiol.* 100, 1184–1201. doi: 10.1152/jn.01344.2007

Lowry, O. H., and Passonneau, J. V. (1972). *A Flexible System of Enzymatic Analysis.* New York, NY: Academic Press.

Marcora, S. (2009). Perception of effort during exercise is independent of afferent feedback from skeletal muscles, heart, and lungs. *J. Appl. Physiol.* 106, 2060–2062. doi: 10.1152/japplphysiol.90378.2008

Marcora, S. (2010). Counterpoint: afferent feedback from fatigued locomotor muscles is not an important determinant of endurance exercise performance. *J. Appl. Physiol.* 108, 454–456. discussion: 456–457. doi: 10.1152/japplphysiol.00976.2009a

Marcora, S. M., and Staiano, W. (2010). The limit to exercise tolerance in humans: mind over muscle? *Eur. J. Appl.* 109, 763–770. doi: 10.1007/s00421-010-1418-6

Martin, P. G., Smith, J. L., Butler, J. E., Gandevia, S. C., and Taylor, J. L. (2006). Fatigue-sensitive afferents inhibit extensor but not flexor motoneurons in humans. *J. Neurosci.* 26, 4796–4802. doi: 10.1523/JNEUROSCI.5487-05.2006

McCord, J. L., and Kaufman, M. P. (2010). "Reflex autonomic responses evoked by group III and IV muscle afferents," in *Translational Pain Research: From Mouse to Man*, eds L. Kruger and A. R. Light (Light Boca Raton, FL: CRC Press; Taylor and Francis Group), 283–298.

Mense, S. (1996). Group III and IV receptors in skeletal muscle: are they specific or polymodal? *Prog. Brain Res.* 113, 83–100. doi: 10.1016/S0079-6123(08)61082-1

Merletti, R., and Hermens, H. (2000). Introduction to the special issue on the SENIAM European Concerted Action. *J. Electromyogr. Kinesiol.* 10, 283–286. doi: 10.1016/S1050-6411(00)00019-5

Merton, P. A. (1954). Voluntary strength and fatigue. *J. Physiol.* 123, 553–564. doi: 10.1113/jphysiol.1954.sp005070

Middlekauff, H. R., Nitzsche, E. U., Nguyen, A. H., Hoh, C. K., and Gibbs, G. G. (1997). Modulation of renal cortical blood flow during static exercise in humans. *Circ. Res.* 80, 62–68. doi: 10.1161/01.RES.80.1.62

Millet, G. Y., Aubert, D., Favier, F. B., Busso, T., and Benoît, H. (2009). Effect of acute hypoxia on central fatigue during repeated isometric leg contractions. *Scand. J. Med. Sci. Sports* 19, 695–702. doi: 10.1111/j.1600-0838.2008.00823.x

Millet, G. Y., Muthalib, M., Jubeau, M., Laursen, P. B., and Nosaka, K. (2012). Severe hypoxia affects exercise performance independently of afferent feedback and peripheral fatigue. *J. Appl. Physiol.* 112, 1335–1344. doi: 10.1152/japplphysiol.00804.2011

Morales-Alamo, D., and Calbet, J. A. (2014). Free radicals and sprint exercise in humans. *Free Radic. Res.* 48, 30–42. doi: 10.3109/10715762.2013.825043

Morales-Alamo, D., Losa-Reyna, J., Torres-Peralta, R., Martin-Rincon, M., Perez-Valera, M., Curtelin, D., et al. (2015). What limits performance during whole-body incremental exercise to exhaustion in humans? *J. Physiol.* 593, 4631–4648. doi: 10.1113/JP270487

Morales-Alamo, D., Ponce-Gonzalez, J. G., Guadalupe-Grau, A., Rodriguez-Garcia, L., Santana, A., Cusso, R., et al. (2013). Critical role for free radicals on sprint exercise-induced CaMKII and AMPKalpha phosphorylation in human skeletal muscle. *J. Appl. Physiol.* 114, 566–577. doi: 10.1152/japplphysiol.01246.2012

Nielsen, O. B., de Paoli, F., and Overgaard, K. (2001). Protective effects of lactic acid on force production in rat skeletal muscle. *J. Physiol.* 536, 161–166. doi: 10.1111/j.1469-7793.2001.t01-1-00161.x

Olson, T. P., Joyner, M. J., Eisenach, J. H., Curry, T. B., and Johnson, B. D. (2014). Influence of locomotor muscle afferent inhibition on the ventilatory response to exercise in heart failure. *Exp. Physiol.* 99, 414–426. doi: 10.1113/expphysiol.2013.075937

Ozgünen, K. T., Celik, U., and Kurdak, S. S. (2010). Determination of an optimal threshold value for muscle activity detection in EMG analysis. *J. Sports Sci. Med.* 9, 620–628.

Pageaux, B., Angius, L., Hopker, J. G., Lepers, R., and Marcora, S. M. (2015). Central alterations of neuromuscular function and feedback from group III-IV muscle afferents following exhaustive high-intensity one-leg dynamic exercise. *Am. J. Physiol. Regul.* 308, R1008–R1020. doi: 10.1152/ajpregu.00280.2014

Pedersen, T. H., Clausen, T., and Nielsen, O. B. (2003). Loss of force induced by high extracellular [K+] in rat muscle: effect of temperature, lactic acid and beta2-agonist. *J. Physiol.* 551, 277–286. doi: 10.1113/jphysiol.2003.041418

Pierrefiche, O., Bischoff, A. M., Richter, D. W., and Spyer, K. M. (1997). Hypoxic response of hypoglossal motoneurones in the *in vivo* cat. *J. Physiol.* 505(Pt 3), 785–795.

Poon, C. S., and Song, G. (2015). Type III-IV muscle afferents are not required for steady-state exercise hyperpnea in healthy subjects and patients with COPD or heart failure. *Respir. Physiol. Neurobiol.* 216, 78–85. doi: 10.1016/j.resp.2015.04.007

Rasmussen, P., Nielsen, J., Overgaard, M., Krogh-Madsen, R., Gjedde, A., Secher, N. H., et al. (2010). Reduced muscle activation during exercise related to brain oxygenation and metabolism in humans. *J. Physiol.* 588, 1985–1995. doi: 10.1113/jphysiol.2009.186767

Reid, C. (1927). The mechanism of voluntary muscular fatigue. *Br. Med. J.* 2, 545–546. doi: 10.1136/bmj.2.3481.545

Rodriguez-Falces, J., Maffiuletti, N. A., and Place, N. (2013). Twitch and M-wave potentiation induced by intermittent maximal voluntary quadriceps contractions: differences between direct quadriceps and femoral nerve stimulation. *Muscle Nerve* 48, 920–929. doi: 10.1002/mus.23856

Rossman, M. J., Venturelli, M., McDaniel, J., Amann, M., and Richardson, R. S. (2012). Muscle mass and peripheral fatigue: a potential role for afferent feedback? *Acta Physiol. (Oxf.)* 206, 242–250. doi: 10.1111/j.1748-1716.2012.02471.x

Rotto, D. M., and Kaufman, M. P. (1988). Effect of metabolic products of muscular contraction on discharge of group III and IV afferents. *J. Appl. Physiol.* 64, 2306–2313.

Sargeant, A. J., and Dolan, P. (1987). Effect of prior exercise on maximal short-term power output in humans. *J. Appl. Physiol.* 63, 1475–1480.

Sbriccoli, P., Bazzucchi, I., Rosponi, A., Bernardi, M., De Vito, G., and Felici, F. (2003). Amplitude and spectral characteristics of biceps Brachii sEMG depend upon speed of isometric force generation. *J. Electromyogr. Kinesiol.* 13, 139–147. doi: 10.1016/S1050-6411(02)00098-6

Sejersted, O. M., and Sjøgaard, G. (2000). Dynamics and consequences of potassium shifts in skeletal muscle and heart during exercise. *Physiol. Rev.* 80, 1411–1481.

Sidhu, S. K., Bentley, D. J., and Carroll, T. J. (2009). Locomotor exercise induces long-lasting impairments in the capacity of the human motor cortex to voluntarily activate knee extensor muscles. *J. Appl. Physiol.* 106, 556–565. doi: 10.1152/japplphysiol.90911.2008

Sidhu, S. K., Cresswell, A. G., and Carroll, T. J. (2012). Motor cortex excitability does not increase during sustained cycling exercise to volitional exhaustion. *J. Appl. Physiol.* 113, 401–409. doi: 10.1152/japplphysiol.00486.2012

Sidhu, S. K., Weavil, J. C., Venturelli, M., Garten, R. S., Rossman, M. J., Richardson, R. S., et al. (2014). Spinal mu-opioid receptor-sensitive lower limb muscle afferents determine corticospinal responsiveness and promote central fatigue in upper limb muscle. *J. Physiol.* 592, 5011–5024. doi: 10.1113/jphysiol.2014.275438

Solomonow, M., Baten, C., Smit, J., Baratta, R., Hermens, H., D'Ambrosia, R., et al. (1990). Electromyogram power spectra frequencies associated with motor unit recruitment strategies. *J. Appl. Physiol.* 68, 1177–1185.

Spielmann, J. M., Laouris, Y., Nordstrom, M. A., Robinson, G. A., Reinking, R. M., and Stuart, D. G. (1993). Adaptation of cat motoneurons to sustained and intermittent extracellular activation. *J. Physiol.* 464, 75–120. doi: 10.1113/jphysiol.1993.sp019625

Torres-Peralta, R., Losa-Reyna, J., González-Izal, M., Perez-Suarez, I., Calle-Herrero, J., Izquierdo, M., et al. (2014). Muscle activation during exercise in severe acute hypoxia: role of absolute and relative intensity. *High. Alt. Med. Biol.* 15, 472–482. doi: 10.1089/ham.2014.1027

Vestergaard-Poulsen, P., Thomsen, C., Sinkjaer, T., and Henriksen, O. (1995). Simultaneous 31P-NMR spectroscopy and EMG in exercising and recovering human skeletal muscle: a correlation study. *J. Appl. Physiol.* 79, 1469–1478.

Wang, W., Wang, Z., Faith, M. S., Kotler, D., Shih, R., and Heymsfield, S. B. (1999). Regional skeletal muscle measurement: evaluation of new dual-energy X-ray absorptiometry model. *J. Appl. Physiol.* 87, 1163–1171.

Yoshida, T., Abe, D., and Fukuoka, Y. (2013). Phosphocreatine resynthesis during recovery in different muscles of the exercising leg by 31P-MRS. *Scand. J. Med. Sci. Sports* 23, e313–e319. doi: 10.1111/sms.12081

Conflict of Interest Statement: The authors declare that the research was conducted in the absence of any commercial or financial relationships that could be construed as a potential conflict of interest.

18

Preparation of Paralympic Athletes; Environmental Concerns and Heat Acclimation

Mike J. Price *

Faculty of Health and Life Sciences, School of Life Sciences, Applied Biology and Exercise Science Research Centre, Coventry University, Coventry, UK

Keywords: spinal cord injury, paraplegia, tetraplegia, exercise, performance, heat, humidity

High ambient temperature and relative humidity (rh) are of great importance when considering athletic performance. Such factors are of particular interest when considering that the majority of Paralympic Games have been hosted at locations with potentially challenging environmental conditions (e.g., Atlanta, Sydney, Athens, Beijing) and a range of Paralympic athletes exhibit conditions manifesting thermal dysfunction. Prior to the Atlanta Games in 1996, Nielsen (1996) considered the "fight against physics" with respect to high ambient temperature (30–38°C) and relative humidity (rh; 40–80%) on endurance performance for able-bodied athletes. It was noted that with such potentially severe conditions outdoor endurance based performances could be severely reduced, especially in spells of high humidity. Strategies to prevent heat illness were recommended including events being scheduled at times of lower thermal stress or re-scheduled if temperatures were above 35°C. However, how these conditions may affect Paralympic athletes has not yet been reported. This article will consider what is known regarding enhancing (or maintaining) performance in the heat in athletes with motor disabilities in preparation for Rio 2016.

Edited by:
*Pierre-Marie Leprêtre,
Université de Picardie Jules Verne,
Lab. APERE, EA-3300, UFR-STAPS,
France*

Reviewed by:
*Sebastien Racinais,
Aspetar, Qatar Orthopaedic and
Sports Medicine Hospital, Qatar*

*Correspondence:
*Mike J. Price
aa5969@coventry.ac.uk*

LIKELY CONDITIONS FOR RIO, 2016

Average daily environmental temperatures expected for Rio during August are ∼28°C. However, at the time of writing (August, 2015), peak daily environmental temperatures at the four Paralympic venues (Deodoro, Maracana, Copacabana, and Barra) were between 32 and 36°C (35 50% rh) at 12:00–15:00 h. Furthermore, peak humidity rose to 70–75% during early to late evening (18:00–21:00 h) with some early morning humidity values reaching 100% (Worldwideweather, August 2015)[1]. As optimal environmental temperatures for endurance performance in those with intact thermoregulatory systems are between 6–10°C (Galloway and Maughan, 1997) and uncompensable heat stress occurs at environmental temperatures of ∼35°C and >60% rh (Nielsen, 1996) these conditions are challenging at best. For Paralympic athletes with thermal dysfunction performance, as well as daily activities and health, may well be negatively affected.

PARALYMPIC POPULATIONS AT RISK

Paralympic classifications for competition include spinal cord impairment, visual impairment, cerebral palsy, amputees, and Les Autres. Athletes with motor disabilities are reflected across a number of classifications. Contributing causes of motor disabilities include traumatic (spinal cord injury or loss of limbs) and disease or congenital conditions (cerebral palsy, muscular dystrophy,

---

[1]Worldweatheronline (2015). Available online at: http://www.worldweatheronline.com/Rio-De-Janeiro-weather-averages/Rio-De-Janeiro/BR.aspx (Accessed August 16, 2015).

multiple sclerosis, or spina bifida). The greatest amount of literature pertaining to thermoregulatory responses during exercise for any group of Paralympic related conditions is for athletes with spinal cord injury (SCI) who demonstrate both motor and neurological deficits. This body of literature most likely reflects the clear thermal dysfunction of this population in proportion to the level of spinal cord injury (For review see Price, 2006). Literature concerning thermoregulatory responses of other Paralympic conditions is unfortunately lacking.

Spinal cord injury results in a loss of motor function and neurological innervation below the level of injury (Price, 2006). In general, athletes with paraplegia (i.e., thoracic and lumbar spinal injuries) demonstrate reduced recruitable muscle mass and a sympathetic nervous system in proportion to the level of lesion. Those athletes with tetraplegia (i.e., cervical spinal injuries) demonstrate the smallest amount of recruitable muscle mass, characterized by upper limb dysfunction due to the injury occurring at a level within the brachial plexus which serves the upper limb. Athletes with tetraplegia also generally demonstrate no sympathetic nervous system innervation due to the level of injury also being above the thoracolumbar sympathetic outflow. As the key thermoregulatory effectors for heat dissipation, namely sweating, and changes in cutaneous blood flow, are sympathetically driven athletes with tetraplegia demonstrate an absent or much reduced sweating capacity. As the imbalance between rate of heat production and heat dissipation determines the magnitude of heat storage and increases in core temperature (Kenny and Jay, 2013) athletes with tetraplegia demonstrate continual increases in body temperature during continuous submaximal exercise in both cool and warm conditions (Price and Campbell, 1999, 2006). For athletes with paraplegia, the reduced sweating capacity appears reasonably matched by the reduction in metabolic heat production as evidenced by similar increases in body temperature for athletes with high level lesion paraplegia (T1–T6) and lower level paraplegia (T7 and below) (Price and Campbell, 2003). Athletes with tetraplegia are thus considered to be at a greater risk of heat injury when compared to athletes with paraplegia who, in turn, have a greater risk of heat injury when compared to able-bodied athletes.

CLASSICAL APPROACHES TO REDUCE HEAT STRAIN

In preparation for competition in hot conditions, athletes generally consider heat acclimation (HA) or various cooling techniques to reduce heat strain and the subsequent risk of heat injury. Although HA is the key method recommended to optimize performance in hot conditions (Racinais et al., 2015) recommendations for reducing exertional heat injury for athletes with SCI are brief (Binkley et al., 2002) with no update in recent years (National Athletic Trainers' Association (NATA), 2014). Conversely, Griggs et al. (2015) recently reviewed cooling strategies in athletes with SCI concluding that due to the athletes reduced heat dissipation potential, using water sprays and cooling garments may be of great benefit. Furthermore, the majority of studies had not simulated true competitive situations

and factors to optimize cooling potential within the constraints of competitive regulations have yet to be established. This is also true for cold slurry ingestion which may provide a useful heat sink for this population. Therefore, this article will focus on heat acclimation.

Heat acclimation refers to procedures to elicit favorable physiological adaptations to heat stress using artificial conditions whereas heat acclimatization involves natural conditions. Heat acclimation usually occurs as part of the athlete's preparation prior to traveling to holding camps where the more natural heat acclimatization can be undertaken prior to the competitive event. Heat acclimation (and heat acclimatization) classically occurs from repeated exposure to exercise in the heat over 5–14 days (Armstrong and Maresh, 1991). More recently, intermittent and shorter duration heat acclimation procedures as well as a "thermal clamp" method, where core temperature is increased during heat stress trials and maintained at a desired level, have been considered (Garrett et al., 2009; Chen et al., 2013). Nevertheless, whichever methods are utilized, HA and acclimatization result in a number of key physiological adaptations to improve heat dissipation (Armstrong and Maresh, 1991). In able-bodied athletes with an unaffected thermoregulatory system HA adaptations typically include; reduced deep body ("core") temperature at rest as well as reduced deep body temperature, reduced skin temperature (and therefore reduced heat storage), increased skin blood flow and increased sweat rates at a given exercise intensity (Armstrong and Maresh, 1991; Armstrong, 2000; Lorenzo and Minson, 2010).

Sweating capacity and dynamic skin blood flow changes are well-known to be reduced or absent below the level of lesion in persons with SCI (Hopman, 1994; Price, 2006). Furthermore, similar deep body temperature and whole body sweat losses have been observed for both able-bodied upper body trained athletes and athletes with SCI during 60–90 min of arm crank exercise at the same relative exercise intensity ($\sim$60% peak oxygen uptake) in cool conditions (Price and Campbell, 1997, 1999). As these athletes with SCI would have had $\sim$50% of their body surface area available for sweating these data suggest a greater sweat output per gland under the same exercise conditions and thermal strain. Subsequently, maximal sweat rates are potentially being achieved during exercise in cool environmental conditions by athletes with SCI (Price and Campbell, 2006). Alternatively, persons with SCI could demonstrate increased sweat gland activity and local sweat rates with heat acclimation. However, those persons with higher lesions levels (and lower whole body sweat rates) may not be able elicit a great enough increase in whole body sweat rate to affect core temperature responses. An athlete's remaining sweating capacity may subsequently be of key importance to heat acclimation success in this population.

HEAT ACCLIMATION STUDIES IN PERSONS WITH SCI

Two studies have reported the responses of persons with SCI to a period of HA. Although it is difficult to conclude any specific HA outcomes in this population from such a small body of literature it is important to consider what is currently known to stimulate future research. Castle et al. (2013) examined a 7 day period of HA (33°C, 65% rh) in a mixed group of Paralympic shooters ($n = 5$) comprising of one athlete with tetraplegia (C4/5) two athletes with paraplegia (T9/10), one athlete with spina bifida (T6), and one athlete with Polio. Each day athletes undertook 60 min of heat exposure including 20 min of arm crank ergometry at 50 W followed by passive heat exposure or simulated shooting practice. Heat acclimation was partially evidenced as a reduction in resting and exercising aural temperature on day 7 compared to day 1 as well as decreased perceptions of effort, thermal strain, and increased plasma volume, thus supporting expected able-bodied adaptations.

Conversely, observations from our laboratory (Price et al., 2011) observed no typical HA responses for participants with tetraplegia ($n = 5$; C5–C7) or paraplegia ($n = 5$; T7-L1) also undertaking 7 days of HA, The protocol was similar to Castle et al. (2013) consisting of daily exercise in the heat (35°C, 40% rh) for 30 min at 50% peak aerobic power output followed by 30 min of passive recovery in the heat. Although the expected differences between groups for aural temperature were observed during exercise in the heat (Price and Campbell, 2003) no changes in aural temperature were observed between day 1 and day 7 for either group. A lack of HA may have been expected for the persons with tetraplegia with an absence of sweating, but not for the persons with paraplegia who demonstrated visible sweating capacity. It is possible that the exercise intensity, and thus body temperature stimulus, was not great enough to elicit heat acclimation however, the intensity was comparable to that of Castle et al. In addition both studies reported aural temperature as the deep body temperature estimate, with similar magnitudes of increase, so differences in deep body temperature site cannot solely explain the difference in results. Inter- and intra-individual variation in thermal responses, which are known to be large in the SCI population, along with differing lesion levels and disabilities may be key contributing factors between these studies observations.

Interestingly, reductions in perceived thermal strain on day 7 compared to day 1 with no change in aural temperature were observed for the group with paraplegia (Price et al., 2011). Such a response though may not be an advantageous adaptation as those individuals who cannot accurately assess their thermal status may be at a greater risk of heat injury (Goosey-Tolfrey et al., 2008). The group with tetraplegia showed no change in perceptions of thermal strain between day 1 and day 7, although thermal strain values were perceived at a similar level to the group with paraplegia even though aural temperatures during exercise were consistently greater. These responses suggest differences in the perception of thermal stimuli to those individuals with paraplegia and may potentially be due

to much reduced surface area for afferent thermal information with tetraplegia when compared to paraplegia. Such responses should be examined in further detail. Although our data were collected from predominantly recreationally active, non-athlete participants such a population may represent athletes in sports where aerobic capacity and associated partial acclimation (as observed in able-bodied athletes; Piwonka et al., 1965) are not fully developed, coaches, or spectators. All of whom may be exposed to environmental stressors.

In addition to outdoor performances, indoor performances such as wheelchair basketball, rugby, and fencing may be of concern for some athletes. For example, a number of athletes, particularly those with tetraplegia, are unaware of the magnitude of rising body temperature during competitions undertaken in air-conditioned venues. Elevated "on court" body temperatures for some such players have been reported anecdotally by support staff and are similar to those observed during exercise in the heat or indeed the safety limits utilized in laboratory based thermoregulation studies. As heat acclimation has been shown to improve performance in cool conditions in able-bodied athletes (Lorenzo et al., 2010) this procedure may be of value for those athletes with lower level SCI and a significant sweating area, competing in indoor venues. However, the potential of reduced perceived thermal strain with no change in deep body temperature should always be considered. It should also be noted that other authors have observed no effect of heat acclimation on performance in cool conditions (Karlsen et al., 2015).

PRACTICAL CONSIDERATIONS

As can be gleaned from the above review, our knowledge of heat acclimation in athletes with SCI is considerably lacking. In addition, the wide range of individual responses to exercise in the heat, including skin temperature and sweating (Goosey-Tolfrey et al., 2008), makes general heat acclimation recommendations for this population difficult. It is possible that if athletes are educated regarding awareness of their thermal state during repeated exposure to heat and, importantly, have access to temperature monitoring devices for enhanced thermal safety assessment, such procedures may have performance benefits. As yet, few studies have considered performance aspects of thermal physiology in athletes with SCI so we are unfortunately unable to determine the efficacy of heat acclimation in this population with confidence. The same can also be stated for other groups of Paralympic athletes. As with most aspects of performance optimization, a considered individual approach needs to be taken with respect to environmental challenges. Appropriate medical back up and monitoring should always to available in such instances.

REFERENCES

Armstrong, L. E. (2000). *Performance in Extreme Environments*. Champaign, IL: Human Kinetics.

Armstrong, L. E., and Maresh, C. M. (1991). The induction and decay of heat acclimatisation in trained athletes. *Sports Med.* 12, 302–312. doi: 10.2165/00007256-199112050-00003

Binkley, H. M., Beckett, J., Casa, D. J., Kleiner, D. M., and Plummer, P. E. (2002). National athletic trainers' association position statement: exertional heat illnesses. *J. Athl. Train.* 37, 329–334.

Castle, P. C., Kularatne, B. P., Brewer, J., Mauger, A. R., Austen, R. A., Tuttle, J. A., et al. (2013). Partial heat acclimation of athletes with spinal cord lesion. *Eur. J. Appl. Physiol.* 113, 109–111. doi: 10.1007/s00421-012-2417-6

Chen, T.-I., Tsai, P.-H., Lin, J.-H., Lee, N.-Y., and Liang, M. T. C. (2013). Effect of short-term heat acclimation on endurance time and skin blood flow in trained athletes. *Open Access J. Sports Med.* 4, 161–170. doi: 10.2147/OAJSM.S45024

Galloway, S. D., and Maughan, R. J. (1997). Effects of ambient temperature on the capacity to perform prolonged cycle exercise in man. *Med. Sci. Sports Exerc.* 29, 1240–1249. doi: 10.1097/00005768-199709000-00018

Garrett, A. T., Goosens, N. G., Rehrer, N. J., Patterson, M. J., and Cotter, J. D. (2009). Induction and decay of short-term heat acclimation. *Eur. J. Appl. Physiol.* 107, 659–670. doi: 10.1007/s00421-009-1182-7

Goosey-Tolfrey, V. L., Diaper, N. J., Crosland, J., and Tolfrey, K. (2008). Fluid intake during wheelchair exercise in the heat: Effects of localized cooling garments. *Int. J. Sports Physiol. Perf.* 3, 145–156.

Griggs, K. E., Price, M. J., and Goosey-Tolfrey, V. L. (2015). Cooling athletes with a spinal cord injury: physiological responses and future directions. *Sports Med.* 45, 9–21. doi: 10.1007/s40279-014-0241-3

Hopman, M. T. E. (1994). Circulatory responses during arm exercise in individuals with paraplegia. *Int. J. Sports Med.* 15, 156–131. doi: 10.1055/s-2007-1021033

Karlsen, A., Racinais, S., Jensen, M. V., Nørgaard, S. J., Bonne, T., and Nybo, L. (2015). Heat acclimatization does not improve VO2max or cycling performance in a cool climate in trained cyclists. *Scand. J. Med. Sci. Sports* 25(Suppl. 1), 269–276. doi: 10.1111/sms.12409

Kenny, G. P., and Jay, O. (2013). Thermometry, calorimetry, and mean body temperature during heat stress. *Compr. Physiol.* 3, 1689–1719. doi: 10.1002/cphy.c130011

Lorenzo, S., Halliwill, J. R., Michael, N., Sawka, M. N., and Minson, C. T. (2010). Heat acclimation improves exercise performance. *J. Appl. Physiol.* 109, 1140–1147. doi: 10.1152/japplphysiol.00495.2010

Lorenzo, S., and Minson, C. T. (2010). Heat acclimation improves cutaneous vascular function and sweating in trained cyclists. *J. Appl. Physiol.* 109, 1736–1743. doi: 10.1152/japplphysiol.00725.2010

National Athletic Trainers' Association (NATA) (2014). *Executive Summary of National Athletic Trainers' Association Position Statement on Exertional Heat Illnesses: An update to the 2002 NATA Guideline*. Available online at: http://www.nata.org/sites/default/files/Heat-Illness-Executive-Summary.pdf (Accessed November 11, 2015).

Nielsen, B. (1996). Olympics in Atlanta: a fight against physics. *Med. Sci. Sports Exerc.* 28, 665–668. doi: 10.1097/00005768-199606000-00004

Piwonka, R. W., Robinson, S., Gay, V. L., and Manalis, R. S. (1965). Preacclimatization of men to heat by training. *J. Appl. Physiol.* 20, 379–384.

Price, M. J. (2006). Thermoregulation during exercise in individuals with spinal cord injuries. *Sports Med.* 36, 863–879. doi: 10.2165/00007256-200636100-00005

Price, M. J., and Campbell, I. G. (1997). Thermoregulatory responses of able-bodied and paraplegic athletes to prolonged upper body exercise. *Europ. J. Appl. Physiol.* 76, 552–560. doi: 10.1007/s004210050289

Price, M. J., and Campbell, I. G. (1999). Thermoregulatory responses of able-bodied, paraplegic and a tetraplegic athlete at rest, during prolonged upper body exercise and during passive recovery. *Spinal Cord* 37, 772–779. doi: 10.1038/sj.sc.3100907

Price, M. J., and Campbell, I. G. (2003). Effects of spinal cord lesion level upon thermoregulation during exercise in the heat. *Med. Sci. Sports Exerc.* 35, 1100–1107. doi: 10.1249/01.MSS.0000074655.76321.D7

Price, M. J., and Campbell, I. G. (2006). "Thermoregulatory responses of athletes with a spinal cord injury to prolonged wheelchair exercise in cool and warm conditions," in *Focus on Exercise and Health Research*, ed T. B. Selkirk (New York, NY: Nova Science Publications), 203–220.

Price, M. J., Kiratli, J., and Brand, M. (2011). "The effects of a 7-day heat acclimation protocol in persons with paraplegia and tetraplegia," *Proceedings of the 14th International Conference on Environmental Ergonomics, Nafplio, Greece, July 2011* (Nafplio).

Racinais, S. S., Alonso, J.-M., Coutts, A. J., Flouris, A. D., Girard, O., González-Alonso, J., et al. (2015). Consensus recommendations on training and competing in the heat. *Sports Med.* 45, 925–938. doi: 10.1007/s40279-015-0343-6

Conflict of Interest Statement: The author declares that the research was conducted in the absence of any commercial or financial relationships that could be construed as a potential conflict of interest.

19

The "Abdominal Circulatory Pump": An Auxiliary Heart during Exercise?

Barbara Uva[1,2], Andrea Aliverti[2], Dario Bovio[2] and Bengt Kayser[1]*

[1] Institute of Sport Sciences and Department of Physiology, Faculté de Biologie et de Médecine, Université de Lausanne, Lausanne, Switzerland, [2] Dipartimento di Elettronica, Informazione e Bioingegneria, Politecnico di Milano, Milano, Italy

Apart from its role as a flow generator for ventilation the diaphragm has a circulatory role. The cyclical abdominal pressure variations from its contractions cause swings in venous return from the splanchnic venous circulation. During exercise the action of the abdominal muscles may enhance this circulatory function of the diaphragm. Eleven healthy subjects (25 ± 7 year, 70 ± 11 kg, 1.78 ± 0.1 m, 3F) performed plantar flexion exercise at ~4 METs. Changes in body volume (ΔV_b) and trunk volume (ΔV_{tr}) were measured simultaneously by double body plethysmography. Volume of blood shifts between trunk and extremities (V_{bs}) was determined non-invasively as ΔV_{tr}-ΔV_b. Three types of breathing were studied: spontaneous (SE), rib cage (RCE, voluntary emphasized inspiratory rib cage breathing), and abdominal (ABE, voluntary active abdominal expiration breathing). During SE and RCE blood was displaced from the extremities into the trunk (on average 0.16 ± 0.33 L and 0.48 ± 0.55 L, $p < 0.05$ SE vs. RCE), while during ABE it was displaced from the trunk to the extremities (0.22 ± 0.20 L $p < 0.001$, $p < 0.05$ RCE and SE vs. ABE respectively). At baseline, V_{bs} swings (maximum to minimum amplitude) were bimodal and averaged 0.13 ± 0.08 L. During exercise, V_{bs} swings consistently increased (0.42 ± 0.34 L, 0.40 ± 0.26 L, 0.46 ± 0.21 L, for SE, RCE and ABE respectively, all $p < 0.01$ vs. baseline). It follows that during leg exercise significant bi-directional blood shifting occurs between the trunk and the extremities. The dynamics and partitioning of these blood shifts strongly depend on the relative predominance of the action of the diaphragm, the rib cage and the abdominal muscles. Depending on the partitioning between respiratory muscles for the act of breathing, the distribution of blood between trunk and extremities can vary by up to 1 L. We conclude that during exercise the abdominal muscles and the diaphragm might play a role of an "auxiliary heart."

Keywords: exercise, cardiac output, venous return, splanchnic circulation, inferior vena cava

Edited by:
J. A. Taylor,
Harvard University, USA

Reviewed by:
Yu-Chieh Tzeng,
University of Otago, New Zealand
Samuel Verges,
Université Joseph Fourier, France

*Correspondence:
Bengt Kayser
bengt.kayser@unil.ch

INTRODUCTION

The cyclical swings in intrathoracic and abdominal pressures caused by breathing influence cardiovascular function at rest and during exercise. The effects on venous return and blood redistribution from and to the limbs have been described qualitatively, both in humans and in animal models (Harms et al., 1997; Aliverti and Macklem, 2001; Aliverti et al., 2004, 2010; Miller et al., 2005a). The splanchnic region contains a large venous reservoir capable of rapidly delivering blood toward the right heart upon increases in transdiaphragmatic pressure, such as during exercise or expulsive maneuvers (Flamm et al., 1990; Aliverti et al., 2009). Flamm et al. (1990) estimated a reduction of splanchnic blood volume by 20% from rest to exercise and a corresponding increase in rib cage blood volume.

Aliverti et al. quantified the dynamics of blood shifting between the trunk and the extremities during quiet breathing and voluntary expulsive maneuvers, consisting of simultaneous contraction of the diaphragm and the abdominal muscles (Aliverti et al., 2009, 2010). The diaphragm, acting both on abdominal and pleural pressures, clearly had a circulatory function in addition to its ventilatory one. Through its effects on abdominal pressure it produced breath-by-breath oscillation of inferior vena cava blood flow, confirming the cyclical effect of intrathoracic and abdominal pressure swings on venous return, as shown before (Miller et al., 2005b).

The variations in abdominal pressure during quiet diaphragmatic breathing at rest, result in a blood volume of ~50–75 ml to be shifted in and out of the splanchnic reservoir during each breath (Aliverti et al., 2009). With expulsive maneuvers, which increased abdominal pressure up to 140 cmH_2O, more than 600 ml of blood was shifted out of the splanchnic venous compartment while femoral venous return was halted (Aliverti et al., 2009). The splanchnic region may thus play the role of an auxiliary heart, and it was hypothesized that such a role might be of even greater importance during physical exercise, when metabolic demand leads to an increase in cardiac output and larger abdominal and transdiaphragmatic pressure swings impact on venous return (Aliverti et al., 2010).

We therefore studied 11 healthy subjects during exercise, while breathing in 3 different ways: (a) spontaneously (hereafter referred to as "spontaneous mode"); (b) predominantly using the inspiratory rib cage muscles ("rib cage mode"); and (c) predominantly using the abdominal muscles during expiration and the diaphragm during inspiration ("abdominal mode"). We looked at the impact of these breathing modes during moderate exercise, on blood shifts between the trunk and the extremities. The volume of blood shifting between the trunk and the extremities was continuously measured using double body plethysmography (DBP). Changes in body volume (ΔV_b) and trunk volume (ΔV_{tr}) were simultaneously tracked using whole body plethysmography (WBP) and opto-electronic plethysmography (OEP). This allowed quantification of blood shifting between trunk and extremities, calculated as the difference between these two simultaneous measurements ($V_{bs} = \Delta V_{tr} - \Delta V_b$). We hypothesized that during exercise the three breathing modes would differentially impact on

intrathoracic and abdominal pressure variations, and therefore cardiovascular function. In particular, breathing with the diaphragm and the abdominal muscles would primarily act on abdominal pressure, while using the rib cage muscles would primarily act on pleural pressure. We expected that during exercise, compared to resting, the volume of blood displaced in and out the trunk would increase significantly and that the direction and amount of this blood displacement would depend on the relative predominance of the action of diaphragm, rib cage and abdominal muscles during the three breathing modes.

METHODS

Subjects

Eleven healthy subjects (25 ± 7 year, mean ± SD, 70 ± 11 kg, 1.78 ± 0.10 m, 3 women), recruited among laboratory personnel, volunteered for the experiments. Most were experienced in doing complex respiratory maneuvers; all of them were instructed in detail at the beginning of each maneuver. The subjects' characteristics are shown in **Table 1**. The research ethics committee of the INRCA Hospital approved the research protocol and informed written consent was obtained from each participant in accordance with the Declaration of Helsinki.

Volume Measurements

To quantify blood volume shifting between the trunk and the extremities, we used DBP using a WBP with walls made of transparent cast acrylic sheet (20 mm) (Aliverti et al., 2009). WBP allowed monitoring body volume changes (ΔV_b), resulting from the gas flowing in and out of the lungs, and the simultaneous changes in compression and decompression of thoracic gas (Goldman et al., 2005). OEP allowed quantifying the changes of trunk volume (ΔV_{tr}), resulting from the lung volume changes plus any blood shifting between the trunk and the extremities (V_{bs}). By subtracting the two independent measurements of ΔV_{tr} and ΔV_b we thus obtained V_{bs}. ΔV_b was measured continuously with the subjects sitting comfortably in the WBP. The flow in and out of the WBP due to changes in body volume was measured by

TABLE 1 | Subjects' characteristics.

Subj. No	Age (years)	Sex	Weight (kg)	Height (cm)	BMI (kg/m²)	BSA (m²)
1	23	M	58	168	20.55	1.66
2	21	M	62	194	16.47	1.89
3	23	M	77	178	24.30	1.95
4	22	F	62	180	19.14	1.79
5	22	M	70	173	23.39	1.83
6	45	M	75	178	23.67	1.93
7	24	M	83	183	24.78	2.05
8	22	M	83	181	25.34	2.04
9	24	F	50	167	17.93	1.55
10	27	F	58	163	21.83	1.62
11	28	M	80	194	21.26	2.11

Abbreviations: DBP, double body plethysmography; DWT, discrete wavelet transformation; OEP, opto-electronic plethysmography; P_{ab}, abdominal pressure; P_{pl}, pleural pressure; $P_{ET}CO_2$, end-tidal CO_2 pressure; V_b, WBP-measured body volume; V_{bs}, volume of blood shifting between the trunk and the extremities; $V'CO_2$, carbon dioxide expired; V_{ab}, OEP-measured abdominal volume; V_{abEE}, end-expiratory abdominal volume; V_{abEI}, end-inspiratory abdominal volume; V_{cw}, OEP-measured chest wall volume; V_{cwEE}, end-expiratory chest wall volume; V_{cwEI}, end-inspiratory chest wall volume; V_E, minute ventilation; $V'O_2$, oxygen uptake; V_{rc}, OEP-measured rib cage volume; V_{rcEE}, end-expiratory rib cage volume; V_{rcEI}, end-inspiratory rib cage volume; V_T, chest wall tidal volume; V_{tr}, OEP-measured trunk volume; WBP, whole body plethysmography.

a pneumotachometer mounted on the top of the box, connecting the box's interior with the exterior. From this flow signal ΔV_b was obtained by mathematical integration.

ΔV_{tr} was simultaneously measured by OEP, using 89 retro-reflective markers placed on the front and back of the chest wall of the subject (Aliverti et al., 2004). Eight cameras captured the markers' positions at a frequency of 60 Hz and the three-dimensional coordinates of the markers were calculated by stereo-photogrammetry using a 3D calibrated motion analyzer. The chest was modeled in two compartments: the rib cage and the abdomen. The boundary between the rib cage and abdomen was fixed along the lower costal margin, as described in detail in the previous studies (Aliverti et al., 2001, 2003, 2004). Total chest wall volume (V_{cw}) was calculated as the sum of rib cage and abdominal volume (V_{rc} and V_{ab} respectively). Flow at the mouth was measured using a hot wire anemometer, which measured gas velocity in a tube of known cross-sectional area (Sensormedics Vmax, Yorba Linda, USA), connecting the subject to the exterior of the box. Both flow meters were calibrated with a 3 L syringe.

Temperature and humidity inside the box were continuously controlled with a multi-sensor device (SHT11, Sensirion AG, Zuerich, Switzerland) based on a hygroscopic polymer as a humidity sensitive element and a semiconductor as a temperature-sensitive element. Eight Peltier cells (ETH-127-14-15-RS, Global Component Sourcing, Central, Hong Kong, China) were interfaced with a set of finned heat sinks (Hyper Series, Cooler Master Corporation, Zhonghe District, New Taipei City, Taiwan) and placed inside and outside the box. The air conditioning system was placed at the bottom of the body box out of the line of sight between the OEP cameras and the trunk, to allow the correct measurement of V_{tr}, and also to avoid influencing the pneumotachograph placed on the top of the box. Pilot testing in preparation for the experiments showed that this conditioning system allowed keeping temperature quite constant inside the WBP even during exercise, but not relative humidity, which led to integration drift.

Correction for Integration Drift

In clinical practice WBP is routinely used for pulmonary function diagnostic tests that last so short that temperature and humidity changes can be neglected. Conversely, if prolonged volume measurements are needed, for example during an exercise test, increases in temperature and humidity, caused by the subject, cause substantial thermal drift (Goldman et al., 2005). In spite of our air conditioning system, which kept air temperature in the body-box almost constant, a consistent non-linear drift of volume occurred during exercise. We used discrete wavelet transformation (DWT) (von Borries et al., 2005) to remove this drift from the signals, because DWT provides a multi-resolution signal decomposition allowing the analysis of the signal at different frequency bands with different resolutions (Rioul and Vetterli, 1991; Samar et al., 1995). The algorithm used is based on a discrete wavelet transformation using high-pass and low-pass filters (scaling function) applied iteratively to the signal, which is progressively down sampled. The low-pass filter gives the new scaling coefficients while the high-pass filter gives the wavelet coefficients in two orthogonal subspaces. The scaling and

wavelet coefficient correspond to the low and high frequency components of the input. The decomposition is then repeated with the analysis filter over the scaling coefficient a number of times depending on the bandwidth of the baseline drift (Rioul and Vetterli, 1991; Samar et al., 1995; von Borries et al., 2005). We used a second order discrete biohortogonal function as mother wavelet, because it best fit our signal, and because it was linear in phase, symmetrical, and had good local properties. After decomposition the input signal was then reconstructed using the same family of wavelets but forcing to zero the low frequency coefficient, representing the thermal drift. This allowed removing the thermal drift without introducing distortion and protecting the shape of the original signal. In order to choose the correct level of wavelet decomposition and to verify if the resulting volume signal was well filtered, we did a linear regression between the first phase of quiet breathing of the filtered signal and the same part of quiet breathing of the chest wall volume, acquired by OEP, which was by definition not affected by thermal drift. During spontaneous quiet breathing these two signals should be aligned and in phase (Aliverti et al., 2009, 2010). For each trial the level with the highest R^2 resulting from this procedure was then used.

Exercise Testing

The subjects were studied while sitting inside the WBP during pre-exercise baseline and submaximal constant workload exercise. We used a custom-made stepper, the only possible exercise solution because of the dimensions of the WBP. It consisted of an electric motor used as a generator, connected to two pedals via a chain-sprocket system to transfer the movement of the pedals to the axis of the motor. The current generated was used to calculate the instantaneous power developed by the subject measuring the voltage drop over a known resistance using the formula $P = V^2/R$. Subjects were asked to step at a frequency of about 30 cycles/min, which provided an average workload of about 64 W.

Oxygen uptake ($V'O_2$), carbon dioxide output ($V'CO_2$) and end-tidal CO_2 pressure ($P_{ET}CO_2$) were continuously measured on a breath-by-breath basis using a respiratory gas analyzer (Sensormedics Vmax, Yorba Linda, USA). O_2 and CO_2 concentrations at the mouth were measured by paramagnetic and infrared gas analyzers, integral part of the system, calibrated with gases of known composition. The flow meter was calibrated with a 3 L syringe. For each subject, data are presented as the mean of at least 10 breaths collected pre-exercise and the last part of the three exercise bouts.

Protocol

The subjects were asked to breathe during the exercise tests using the three prescribed different modes: "spontaneous," "rib cage," and "abdominal," performed in separate trials. In spontaneous mode, after 1 min of sitting baseline (quiet breathing during rest, while sitting in the WBP), they engaged in 5 min of stepping exercise while breathing spontaneously, followed by 4 min of recovery (no exercise) (see **Figure 1**). After instructions and some practice runs they then performed several different trials for each breathing mode. Rib cage breathing mode consisted

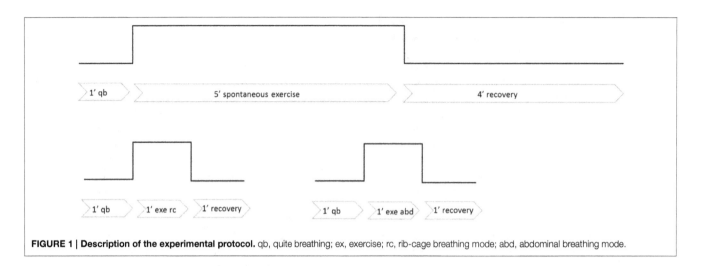

FIGURE 1 | Description of the experimental protocol. qb, quite breathing; ex, exercise; rc, rib-cage breathing mode; abd, abdominal breathing mode.

of voluntary emphasizing inspiratory rib cage breathing, which, when effectuated correctly, resulted in ribcage volume changes over a breathing cycle while keeping abdominal volume constant. Abdominal breathing mode consisted of voluntary abdominal expiration, resulting in a decrease of abdominal volume accompanied by a simultaneous increase of abdominal pressure, followed by diaphragm contraction for inspiration, while keeping the rib cage configuration invariant. Since abdominal and rib cage breathing modes were difficult to sustain, we shortened these to 1 min, long enough for the larger initial cardiovascular and metabolic changes to occur, while short enough to allow the subjects to correctly perform the exercise. Thus, after 1 min of quiet breathing at rest, rib cage or abdominal mode exercise were executed for 1 min, followed by 1 min of recovery. Subjects did each exercise trial a minimum of one time, recovering between trials. The WBP was opened in between trials to reestablish the initial thermodynamic conditions. The order of the three breathing modes was randomized within and between subjects.

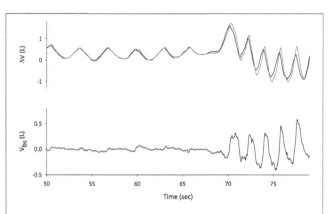

FIGURE 2 | Traces during spontaneous pre-exercise breathing. Top Panel: changes in Lungs volume, measured with WBP (V_L, red line) and Trunk volume derived from OEP (V_{tr}, black line). The difference between V_{tr} and V_L gives the volume of the blood shifted between the splanchnic vasculature and the extremities (**bottom panel**).

Data Analysis

Pre-exercise and exercise phases were analyzed in terms of volume changes and blood shifts. The analysis of V_{bs}, obtained by subtracting the ΔV_{tr} and ΔV_b (see **Figure 2**), focused on two different parameters: V_{bs} swings, defined as the difference of maximum and minimum values within each breath, averaged over at least 10 breaths, pre-exercise and during the three exercise conditions, and ΔV_{bs}-mean, i.e., the difference between average V_{bs} pre-exercise and during exercise (see **Figure 3**). The effects of different exercise breathing patterns on blood shift and volume changes were assessed by a generalized linear mixed-model (repeated measurements analysis of variance) since the missing values for some of the subjects participating to the study precluded the use of simple ANOVA. When the outcome data were not normally distributed, we used the inverse Gaussian distribution, the closest available theoretical distribution to fit the sample. The breathing modes (spontaneous, rib cage, and abdominal), the phase of exercise (quiet breathing vs. exercise) and their interactions were defined as fixed effects in the model. The subjects' variability was used as random effect. Pairwise

comparisons were carried out with Holm Sidak's *post-hoc* test. The significance level was set at $P < 0.05$. All statistical analyses were carried out using SPSS, version 21 (IBM Corp., Armonk, NY, USA). Data are expressed as mean $\pm$ SD unless otherwise specified.

RESULTS

Exercise

The square-wave submaximal stepping exercise was performed at about 30 cycles/min and an average power output of 64 W. Individual metabolic equivalent of task (MET) values were calculated by dividing the $V'O_2$, reached during exercise between the third and fourth minute while breathing spontaneously, by 3.5 ml kg^{-1} min^{-1}. The exercise intensity corresponded to an average of 4.3 METs, indicating low to moderate intensity exercise (3–6 METs). Even though the stepping effort was equivalent in the three modes, because of the shorter durations of rib cage and abdominal breathing modes compared to

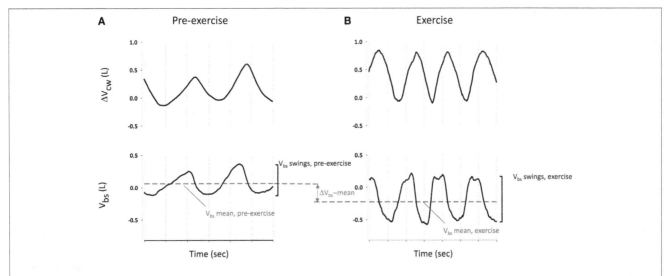

FIGURE 3 | Blood shift volume and chest wall volume variation during pre-exercise breathing (A) and an example of spontaneous breathing mode during exercise (B). ΔV_{bs}-mean was calculated as difference between V_{bs} mean (red dashed line) during exercise and pre-exercise. V_{bs} swings were calculated as difference between the maximum and the minim values during each breathing of quiet breathing and exercise respectively.

spontaneous mode, steady state gas exchange was not reached in rib cage and abdominal modes (duration of exercise 1 min).

Ventilatory parameters for pre-exercise and exercise are shown in **Table 2**. Exercise significantly increased $V'O_2$ and $V'CO_2$ compared to pre-exercise condition. $V'O_2$ increased from pre-exercise by $11.1 \pm 3.9, 8.5 \pm 2.4$, and $6.8 \pm 2.6 \, \mathrm{ml \, kg^{-1} \, min^{-1}}$ (all $p < 0.001$), for spontaneous, rib cage and abdominal mode, respectively. $V'CO_2$ increased during exercise ($p < 0.001$) mostly during spontaneous breathing mode; $12.8 \pm 3.6, 7.5 \pm 1.4, 6.0 \pm 1.9 \, \mathrm{ml \, kg^{-1} \, min^{-1}}$ for spontaneous, rib cage and abdominal mode, respectively ($p < 0.001, p < 0.01$, spontaneous vs. abdominal and rib cage exercise, respectively). $P_{ET}CO_2$ during spontaneous breathing was higher compared to pre-exercise, rib cage mode and abdominal mode ($33.7 \pm 3.8, 40 \pm 4.3, 31.1 \pm 6.0, 33.3 \pm 4.6 \, \mathrm{mmHg}$, for pre-exercise, spontaneous, rib cage and abdominal modes, respectively. $p < 0.001$ for pre-exercise and rib cage, $p < 0.01$ for abdominal). The baseline ventilation, $P_{ET}CO_2$ and RQ indicated some hyperventilation related to the experimental conditions.

Exercise significantly increased ventilation, which passed from 14.4 ± 4.3 L/min at pre-exercise baseline to $31.5 \pm 7.8, 42.2 \pm 15.1$, and 37.7 ± 13 L/min (all $p < 0.001$), during spontaneous, rib cage, and abdominal mode, respectively.

Representative traces of spontaneous, rib cage, and abdominal breathing modes during exercise are shown in **Figure 4**. From top to bottom are depicted rib cage volume (V_{rc}), abdominal volume (V_{ab}), and trunk volume (V_{tr}), all three obtained with OEP (black lines). Superimposed in red on V_{tr} is shown WBP-measured body volume (V_b), the difference with V_{tr} representing blood shifting (V_{bs}), shown in the bottom panels.

When the subject inspired using predominantly her/his rib cage muscles—i.e., during rib cage breathing mode—end-inspiratory rib cage volume increased, while abdominal volume remained approximately constant. This resulted in blood being

displaced from the extremities to the trunk, presumably to the rib cage, as illustrated by negative values of V_{bs} (**Figure 4B**). Conversely, during exercise while in abdominal breathing mode, end-expiratory abdominal volume decreased while the blood shifted from the trunk to the extremities, as indicated by the positive values of V_{bs} (**Figure 4C**).

Chest Wall Volumes

Figure 5 depicts the rib cage, abdominal and total chest wall end-expiratory volumes (black circles) and end-inspiratory volumes (white circles), at baseline and during exercise for each of the breathing modes. Exercise induced an increase in chest wall tidal volume (V_T), defined as the difference of end-inspiratory volume and end-expiratory volume, for all breathing modes ($0.66 \pm 0.45, 0.76 \pm 0.73$, and 0.65 ± 0.63 L, $p < 0.001, p < 0.01, p < 0.01$, for spontaneous rib cage and abdominal mode respectively) as shown in **Figure 5**. In spontaneous mode, the increase in V_T was reached by an increase of end-inspiratory rib cage volume (V_{rcEI}) and a concomitant decrease in end-expiratory abdominal volume (V_{abEE}). V_{rcEI} increased on average by 0.37 ± 0.28 L ($p < 0.01$) while V_{abEE} decreased on average by 0.21 ± 0.20 L ($p < 0.05$) compared with pre-exercise baseline.

In rib cage breathing mode chest wall tidal volume significantly increased ($p < 0.01$), mostly due to an increase in end-inspiratory rib cage volume (0.88 ± 0.39 L, $p < 0.001$), while end-expiratory abdominal volume was kept nearly constant (0.09 ± 0.2 L, $p =$ n.s.). No significant differences were found in V_{cwEE} and V_{cwEI} during abdominal exercise. The increase in tidal volume was due to a decrease in V_{abEE} (0.41 ± 0.16 L, $p < 0.05$), while V_{rcEI} was kept approximately constant (0.15 ± 0.27 L, $p =$ n.s.).

Rib cage breathing mode significantly increased V_{rcEI} (0.84 ± 0.39 L) during exercise compared to spontaneous and abdominal

TABLE 2 | Ventilatory parameters at pre-exercise baseline and during exercise, calculated at the same relative intensity for 5′ spontaneous breathing, rib cage breathing, and abdominal breathing respectively.

	Pre-exercise	Exercise		
		5′ spontaneous breathing	1′ rib cage breathing	1′ abdominal breathing
V′O$_2$/kg (ml/Kg/min)	4.0 ± 1.5	$15.2 \pm 3.9^*$	$12.2 \pm 2.5^*$	$11.6 \pm 2.0^*$
V′CO$_2$/kg (ml/Kg/min)	4.3 ± 1.8	$17.4 \pm 4.1^*$	$11.1 \pm 2.5^{*\#}$	$11.2 \pm 2.0^{*\#}$
RQ	1.0 ± 0.2	0.9 ± 0.1	$1.2 \pm 0.2^{\#}$	1.1 ± 0.2
VE (L/min)	14.4 ± 4.3	$31.5 \pm 7.8^*$	$42.2 \pm 15.1^*$	$37.7 \pm 13^*$
PETCO$_2$ (mmHg)	33.7 ± 3.8	$40 \pm 4.3^*$	$31.1 \pm 6.0^{\#}$	$33.3 \pm 4.6^{\#}$

Values are presented as mean ± SD; *$p < 0.05$ vs. pre-exercise; $^{\#}p < 0.05$ vs. 5′ spontaneous breathing mode. V′O$_2$ and V′CO$_2$ individual values are given in the text.

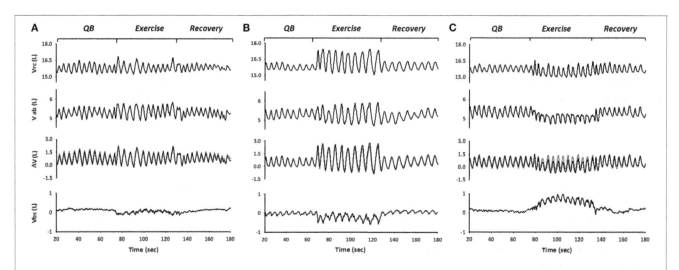

FIGURE 4 | The figure shows the three different breathing modes during exercise performed by the subjects, spontaneous (A), rib cage (B), and abdominal mode (C) respectively. From top to bottom: OEP measured Rib cage volume (V$_{rc}$), abdominal volume (V$_{ab}$), derived from OEP, WBP measured changes in body volume variation and thus in lung volume variations (V$_b$), superimposed in red on V$_{cw}$ variations and blood shifts between trunk and extremities (V$_{bs}$) calculated as the differences between ΔV$_{cw}$ and ΔV$_b$.

breathing modes (0.41 ± 0.26, 0.16 ± 0.27 L, $p < 0.05$ and $p < 0.01$, respectively).

Blood Shifts

Within-breath V$_{bs}$ swings and variations of average V$_{bs}$ values (ΔV$_{bs}$-mean) during spontaneous, rib cage and abdominal breathing modes are presented in **Figures 6, 7**, respectively. Mean V$_{bs}$ swings, were calculated as the mean difference between maximum and minimum values for each series of breaths analyzed, for quiet breathing and exercise respectively. During exercise, each subject showed a consistent increase in within-breath V$_{bs}$ swings compared to pre-exercise (0.26 ± 0.26, 0.28 ± 0.25, 0.33 ± 0.22 L, respectively during spontaneous, ribcage and abdominal modes, $p < 0.05$, $p < 0.01$, and $p < 0.001$). On average, ΔV$_{bs}$-mean decreased by 0.19 ± 0.31 L and 0.53 ± 0.51 L (p = n.s., $p < 0.01$) respectively during spontaneous and rib cage modes, indicating blood shifts from the extremities into the trunk. Conversely during abdominal exercise ΔV$_{bs}$-mean tended to increase in average by 0.23 ± 0.16 L ($p < 0.01$), indicating blood shifting from the trunk to the extremities (**Figure 7**) and showing complex

V$_{bs}$ patterns, resulting from the specific breathing patterns used by the subjects. This led to significant differences in blood redistribution. On average 0.16 ± 0.33 L and 0.48 ± 0.55 L were drawn into the trunk, presumably into the rib cage, in spontaneous and rib cage breathing mode, respectively (p = n.s., spontaneous vs. rib cage mode) while during abdominal mode 0.22 ± 0.20 L of blood ($p < 0.01$, both rib cage and spontaneous vs. abdominal) was pushed out of the trunk.

DISCUSSION

We investigated how changes in breathing mode, during exercise, by acting on intrathoracic and abdominal pressure variations, influence blood shifting between different body compartments, and in particular in and out of the trunk. We expected that during exercise, compared to rest, splanchnic venous blood would be mobilized, that the amount of blood displaced within each breathing cycle would increase, and that the direction and amount of this blood displacement would depend on the relative contributions of the actions of the

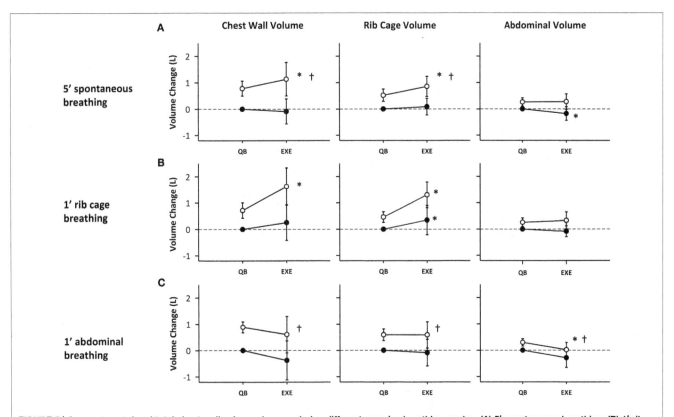

FIGURE 5 | Compartmental and total chest wall volume changes during different exercise breathing modes: (A) 5′ spontaneous breathing; (B) 1′ rib cage breathing; (C) 1′ abdominal breathing mode. White circles: end-inspiration volume; Black circles: end-expiration volume; Mean values and standard deviation bars are shown. $*p < 0.05$ vs. pre-exercise; $^{†}p < 0.05$ vs. rib cage breathing mode.

diaphragm, the rib cage and abdominal muscles. The main results can be summarized as follows: (a) for the first time the extent of blood volume shifting between the trunk and the extremities was non-invasively quantified during a form of leg exercise; (b) compared to pre-exercise baseline conditions, during exercise, while in spontaneous breathing mode, on average 160 ml of blood were pulled into the trunk from the extremities; (c) during abdominal mode, when the subjects breathed predominantly using the diaphragm and the abdominal muscles, about 225 ml was shifted out of the trunk to the extremities; (d) conversely, during rib cage mode, when the subjects voluntary emphasized the use of inspiratory rib cage muscles, about 478 ml was pulled into the trunk from the extremities; (e) at baseline, intra-breath V_{bs} amounted to 134 ml on average, slightly higher as reported before, probably because of slight hyperventilation, while during exercise it increased to about 420 ml, independently of the breathing mode, increasing inferior vena cava venous return from 2.5 L/min at baseline to 11.4 L/min during exercise. It follows that depending on the partitioning between respiratory muscles for the act of breathing, the distribution of blood between trunk and extremities can vary by up to 1 L and that during exercise the abdominal muscles together with the diaphragm might play a role of an "auxiliary heart."

Measuring Blood Shifting

Other studies examined the influence of the mechanics of breathing on the circulatory system, mainly qualitatively, evaluating the effects of within-breath changes of intrathoracic and abdominal pressures on venous return and blood redistribution from the splanchnic region (Flamm et al., 1990; Miller et al., 2005a,b). Aliverti et al. (2009) were the first to quantify this blood redistribution. They demonstrated that the increase in abdominal pressure during the descent of the diaphragm leads to substantial quantities of blood (V_{bs}) shifted from the trunk and presumably the splanchnic venous reservoir, to the extremities. These observations support the notion of a circulatory role for the diaphragm, as also illustrated by the effects of phrenic pacing of the diaphragm on blood shifting reported by Roos et al. (2009).

We now quantified the effects of different breathing modes on blood volume redistribution between the trunk and the extremities during physical activity of moderate intensity. Three breathing patterns were chosen deliberately to vary the contribution of different muscles groups, in order to attain various combinations of breath-by-breath changes in intra-thoracic and abdominal pressures. We chose this approach to complement the results from Aliverti et al. (2010) who measured blood redistribution during expulsive maneuvers while sitting at

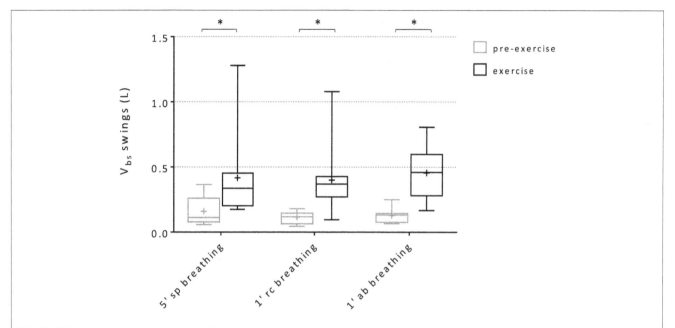

FIGURE 6 | Box-and-whisker plot displaying V$_{bs}$ swings during the three breathing modes. Black boxes: pre-exercise; Gray boxes: exercise. Central line, box and whisker limits represent median, interquartile range and minimum and maximum values of the data, respectively. $^+$ represents the mean value $^*p < 0.01$ vs. pre-exercise.

rest. They found that the circulatory effect of the diaphragm was enhanced when supported by the action of abdominal muscles, and resulted in a consistent "stroke volume" of V$_{bs}$ (on average 350 ml), corresponding to blood coming from the splanchnic circulation (presumably mostly from the liver), through the hepatic vein into the inferior vena cava downstream toward the heart.

In the present study, the three breathing modes, by acting differently on breath-by-breath changes in intra-thoracic and abdominal pressures, affected V$_{bs}$ in two ways. According to Aliverti et al. (2009, 2010), during abdominal mode breathing and expulsive maneuvers, V$_{bs}$ represents blood coming from the splanchnic vascular bed returning to the right heart to be then injected into the systemic circulation, since the venous return between the femoral vein and the inferior vena cava at the inlet of hepatic vein is temporarily stopped by the disappearance of the pressure gradient between those points (Miller et al., 2005b; Uva et al., 2010). Conversely, during rib cage mode breathing, a decrease in esophageal pressure decreases right atrial pressure, thus increasing the pressure gradient between the femoral veins and the right heart, facilitating venous return from the lower extremities. In this case what we measured as ΔV$_{bs}$-mean is mostly venous return from the extremities. In this perspective our results complete and extend previous reports by others (Miller et al., 2005b; Aliverti et al., 2010).

Respiratory Modulation of Splanchnic Blood Shifting

In our study, most subjects, when switching from pre-exercise baseline to exercise while breathing spontaneously, predominantly recruited their inspiratory ribcage muscles, which resulted in an increase in end-inspiratory rib cage volume, while

end-expiratory abdominal volume did not differ significantly from that at pre-exercise baseline (see **Figure 5**). The breathing patterns used by the subjects during this breathing mode, led to substantial variation in V$_{bs}$ (see **Figure 6**) but the prevailing effect with regard to V$_{bs}$-mean was a drop. This result indicates that blood was being pulled into the trunk, suggesting increased venous return toward the right heart. During rib cage mode exercise, when the subjects emphasized the use of inspiratory rib cage muscles, while relaxing the diaphragm and abdominal muscles, this effect was amplified (ΔV$_{bs}$-mean amounted to 0.19 ± 0.31 L (p = n.s.) and 0.53 ± 0.51 L ($p < 0.01$), for spontaneous and rib cage exercise, respectively). The stronger contraction of the inspiratory rib cage muscles, by lowering intra-thoracic pressure during inspiration likely resulted in a more pronounced right atrial to inferior vena cava pressure difference, thus facilitating venous return, confirming earlier observations (Guyton et al., 1955; Miller et al., 2005a,b). This more pronounced effect during rib cage mode breathing in our set-up could be explained by a moderate degree of chest wall hyperinflation, likely due to a persistent contraction of the inspiratory muscles during the expiratory phase of the breathing cycle (see **Figure 5**), that would have led to a decreased P$_{pl}$ for a more prolonged time. These findings during rib cage mode and also somewhat during spontaneous mode are qualitatively similar to what Flamm et al. (1990) found in their study, demonstrating a consistent blood volume shift from the splanchnic reservoir and the lower extremities to the pulmonary circulation during zero load spontaneous upright exercise.

By contrast, during abdominal mode breathing the situation was reversed. When the subjects activated their abdominal expiratory muscles, tidal volume increased due to a decrease of end-expiratory abdominal volume, while rib cage end-inspiratory

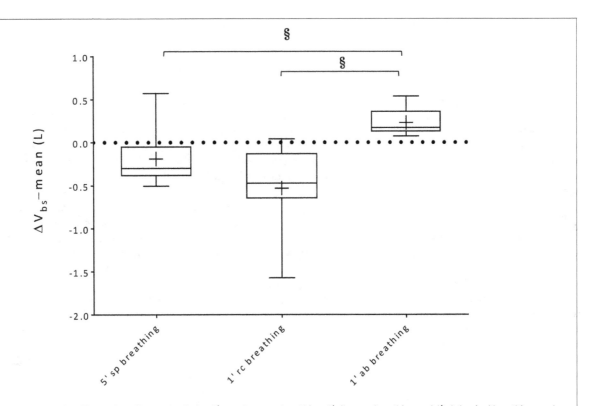

FIGURE 7 | Box-and-whisker plots illustrating ΔV$_{bs}$-mean during 5′ spontaneous breathing, 1′ rib cage breathing and 1′ abdominal breathing mode exercise respectively. Central line, box and whisker limits represent median, interquartile range and minimum and maximum values of the data, respectively. + represents the mean value; [§]$p < 0.05$ vs. abdominal breathing mode.

volume remained nearly constant (see **Figure 5**). The contraction of the diaphragm and of the abdominal muscles, respectively during inspiration and expiration, presumably increased baseline abdominal pressures and pressure swings, while average pleural pressure remained rather invariant. This led to a significant increase both in V$_{bs}$ swings and in the amount of blood displaced out of the trunk, since the femoral venous return toward the trunk was likely stopped by the increase in abdominal pressure (Willeput et al., 1984; Miller et al., 2005a). The source of the V$_{bs}$ must then have been the splanchnic venous reservoir (Aliverti et al., 2009).

We acquired esophageal and abdominal pressures in three of our subjects but do not present the results in detail because of the small number of observations and the variability between subjects. But although abdominal and pleural pressure patterns differed between subjects during the various breathing modes, it appeared that the V$_{bs}$ bimodal shape uniquely tracked the individual changes in abdominal and pleural pressures. In particular, when breathing in abdominal mode during stepping exercise, in all three an increase in abdominal pressure swings was found while pleural pressure swings remained similar to those during pre-exercise baseline breathing, which led to a series of repeated expulsive-like maneuvers. This cyclical increase in abdominal pressure (~20 cmH$_2$O on average) led to a tidal blood volume of 460 ml, presumably through the hepatic vein, and a global splanchnic output of about ~12 L/min.

Conversely, when the subjects started to exercise while breathing in rib cage mode, a marked increase in pleural swings was evident, while the abdominal pressure swings were determined by the passive movement of the diaphragm, which transmitted pleural pressure variations to the abdominal content. In this case, as demonstrated by Miller et al. (2005b), augmenting the inspiratory negative intrathoracic pressure excursions resulted in a more negative right atrial pressure. The greater inspiratory facilitation of venous return resulted in an average 470 ml of blood pulled into the rib cage for each breath, which led a total flow drawn from the extremities of about ~11 L/min.

The intra-breath increase in V$_{bs}$ swings during exercise was found during all three breathing modes, suggesting a dynamic impact on venous return through the inferior vena cava to the heart. A "stroke volume" of about 420 ml during all breathing modes was found in agreement of what has been previously published by Aliverti et al. during intermittent expulsive maneuvers (Aliverti et al., 2010). A further bimodal time course of V$_{bs}$ was found during all breathing modes. During abdominal exercise it seemed tracked only by the changes in abdominal pressure, suggesting that the V$_{bs}$ pattern was driven mostly by the diaphragm, which is the only muscle acting on the abdominal compartment during inspiration, and by the abdominal muscle contraction during expiration. By contrast, during rib cage breathing mode, the biphasic V$_{bs}$ pattern was determined by the large pleural pressure swings, while abdominal pressure variations were kept similar to those at pre-exercise baseline.

These results support previous findings, which suggest that the respiratory muscles, acting on abdominal and pleural pressure dynamics, have an important cardiovascular function. Based on our oxygen uptake measurements we can estimate (Beck et al., 2006) that cardiac output while sitting in the body box at baseline was 6.4 ± 0.6 L/min and during exercise in spontaneous breathing mode increased to 10.2 ± 1.4 L/min, suggesting that the above mentioned 11 L/min somewhat overestimates inferior venous cava venous return, since superior venous cava return obviously was not nil.

Rib Cage, Abdominal, and Lower Limb Blood Volume Redistribution

Our results contribute quantitative evidence for important respiratory modulation of V_{bs} partitioning during exercise. As previously described, we believe that what we report as V_{bs} is the volume of blood moved between the splanchnic vascular bed, rib cage, lungs and extremities. Since with our set-up we measured the variation in the total chest wall volume, we cannot precisely estimate the blood that during exercise is shifting between the splanchnic bed, and thus the abdomen, and the pulmonary circulation and the rib cage, because they belong to the same compartment.

Upon starting the stepping activity, while breathing in abdominal mode, we measured a positive blood shift from baseline, indicating that blood was shifted out of the trunk to the extremities. Aliverti et al. (2010) measured cardiac output and blood pressure during expulsive maneuvers and demonstrated that V_{bs} is of splanchnic venous compartment origin. In the present study we therefore believe that the V_{bs} we measured must be the result of splanchnic vascular outflow toward the heart minus concomitant arterial outflow toward the extremities. Within each breath the splanchnic blood reservoir would not be completely refilled, resulting into a significant redistribution of blood between splanchnic bed, exercising muscles (i.e., leg muscles and respiratory muscles) and lungs (Harms et al., 1997).

This hypothesis is consistent with previous studies which proposed the splanchnic vascular bed as a significant venous reservoir for blood redistribution during exercise (Rowell, 1974). During rib cage mode breathing, we found on average 478 ml of blood coming into the trunk from the extremities. Contraction of the rib cage inspiratory muscles, by making average pleural pressure more negative, thus increased venous return to the right heart. Our data do not permit partitioning of where exactly this extra venous return then went. Presumably part was used for lung capillary recruitment (Johnson et al., 1960; Flamm et al., 1990) while part of it left the trunk through the big arteries into the extremities. This effect, which is expected to be more important during rib cage breathing mode, might contribute in part to the increase in rib cage blood volume compared with the other breathing modes. Part of the blood may have gone to the respiratory muscles, which require an increase in blood flow because of increased activity. In our study rib cage mode exercise led to an increase in ventilation and a decrease in $P_{ET}CO_2$ indicating increased breathing workload compared to

abdominal breathing mode. This would be consistent with data obtained in an animal model showing an increase in perfusion of the respiratory muscles (diaphragm and intercostal muscles) and a decrease in intestinal blood flow (Fixler et al., 1976). In several animal studies this redistribution of cardiac output seems to reflect the increase in peripheral vascular resistance related to the concomitant decrease in respiratory vascular resistance (Fixler et al., 1976; Robertson et al., 1977; Sheel et al., 2001).

The Role of Skeletal and Respiratory Muscle Pumps

It is thought that lower limb muscle contraction contributes to venous return (Laughlin, 1987; Hamann et al., 2003; Tschakovsky and Sheriff, 2004) facilitating the propulsion of the blood from the skeletal muscle vasculature. In the present study, we have no data on changes in blood flow by the action of the skeletal muscle pump and its relative role with respect to the respiratory muscle pump. During mild calf contraction exercise, Miller et al. (2005b) found a biphasic within-breath modulation of femoral venous blood flow, which seemed to be in phase with the rhythmic muscular contraction (**Figure 4** of their paper). Likewise the biphasic within-breath V_{bs} shape we observed might be attributed to the cyclical contraction of the skeletal muscle pump during the exercise. But since the legs were exercised in the same manner in all breathing modes exercise and the biphasic V_{bs} pattern seemed to be determined by the individual variation of abdominal and esophageal pressure variations, we assume that the large variations in blood flow partitioning that we found between abdominal and rib cage modes should be mainly attributed to the action of the different respiratory muscles involved.

Our study thus lends support to what previously was found by Miller et al. who demonstrated that the respiratory muscle pump has a prevailing effect during exercise rather than the skeletal muscle pump (Miller et al., 2005b). The respiratory muscle pump, enhancing negative intrathoracic pressure, draws blood toward the heart and increases venous return, stroke volume and cardiac output, corroborating its importance in enhancing systemic circulation and vital organ perfusion, also during critical conditions such as hemorrhage (Hodges et al., 2001; Convertino et al., 2004; Yannopoulos et al., 2006; Poh et al., 2014).

Potential Implications of Blood Redistribution during Whole Body Exercise

Our findings open interesting perspectives on the role of the "abdominal pump" during various types of physical activity, for example during walking or running, when the diaphragm and the abdominal muscles contribute to postural control of the trunk through elevation of the intra-abdominal pressure and the skeletal muscle pump forces blood centrally. In this study we have expanded the findings reported by Aliverti et al. (2010) during expulsive maneuvers and Miller et al. (2005b) during light exercise, demonstrating that during submaximal upright exercise, the respiratory muscles acting on pleural and abdominal pressure swings, are able to partition blood flow between the rib cage and pulmonary circulation, the working muscles, and the abdominal venous compartment.

These results have important implications in whole-body exercise, as for example walking or running when also the upper limb will be involved in the exercise and the abdominal pressure would increase in order to increase the lumbar spine stability (Cholewicki et al., 1999a,b; Hodges and Gandevia, 2000). Ainsworth and colleagues demonstrated in exercising horses a locomotory-associated modulation of the abdominal and intrathoracic pressure (Ainsworth et al., 1996). It remains to be investigated if also during human running such phase-coupling relationships between limb movement and breathing will influence the circulatory function of respiratory muscles and thus the subsequent blood volume partition between different compartments.

LIMITATIONS

When interpreting the results of our study one should keep in mind some limitations. First, because of the complexity of our experimental setup we decided to refrain from measuring cardiac output (heart rate and stroke volume), which precludes any strong conclusions on the effects of the observed blood shifts on cardiac function. Second, what was measured in this study as V_{bs} was considered to represent liquid (mainly blood) moved between the trunk and the extremities. Since we measured the total V_{cw} using OEP, we could not determine the amount of blood shifted between the rib cage and the abdominal compartments, limiting our assertions on splanchnic blood volume recruitment. Third, in this study we have not investigated the effect of the specific breathing modes at rest in comparison to during exercise in the same subject. Fourth we do not report gastric and esophageal pressures since these were only acquired in 3 subjects and equivocal. Fifth, because of the complexity of thermodynamic control inside the body box exercise duration had to be kept short. Even though our conditioning system was able to keep temperature quite stable during exercise, it did not allow complete control of humidity. We had to develop a mathematical method to correct for this drift. In order to avoid all the possible problems related to the influence of filtering on the signal baseline, we therefore analyzed the blood shifts only in terms of variations of baseline and tidal volumes respectively. Sixth, the respiratory maneuvers were difficult to perform. Several of the subjects had difficulties in performing the complex respiratory maneuvers by changing their breathing modes correctly during exercise. The various attempts were classified according to the variations in compartmental volumes, which led to various numbers of repetitions between breathing modes for some subjects. Finally, because of the complexity of the maneuvers there were missing values precluding the use of simple ANOVA. We therefore chose generalized linear mixed modeling, but in the worst case the proportion of missing values was one third, limiting the robustness of the statistical analysis.

CONCLUSIONS

In summary, for the first time the volume of blood redistributed between the trunk and the extremities was quantified non-invasively and continuously during exercise. The amount and the partial redistribution of this blood depended on the activation of rib cage, diaphragm and abdominal muscles on a breath-by-breath basis. In particular we found that during abdominal exercise the action of the diaphragm and abdominal muscles, increasing the abdominal pressure can shift blood from the extremities, while the rib cage inspiratory muscles' action facilitates blood shifting toward the pulmonary circulation. Depending on the partitioning between respiratory muscles for the act of breathing, the distribution of blood between trunk and extremities can vary by up to 1 L. We conclude that during exercise the abdominal muscles assist the diaphragm in its role of an "auxiliary heart."

REFERENCES

Ainsworth, D. M., Eicker, S. W., Nalevanko, M. E., Ducharme, N. G., Hackett, R. P., and Snedden, K. (1996). The effect of exercise on diaphragmatic activation in horses. *Respir. Physiol.* 106, 35–46. doi: 10.1016/0034-5687(96)00058-8

Aliverti, A., Bovio, D., Fullin, I., Dellaca, R. L., Lo Mauro, A., Pedotti, A., et al. (2009). The abdominal circulatory pump. *PLoS ONE* 4:e5550. doi: 10.1371/journal.pone.0005550

Aliverti, A., Dellacà, R., Pelosi, P., Chiumello, D., Gatihnoni, L., and Pedoti, A. (2001). Compartmental analysis of breathing in the supine and prone positions by optoelectronic plethysmography. *Ann. Biomed. Eng.* 29, 60–70. doi: 10.1114/1.1332084

Aliverti, A., Ghidoli, G., Dellacà, R. L., Pedotti, A., and Macklem, P. T. (2003). Chest wall kinematic determinants of diaphragm length by optoelectronic plethysmography and ultrasonography. *J. Appl. Physiol. (1985)* 94, 621–630. doi: 10.1152/japplphysiol.00329.2002

Aliverti, A., and Macklem, P. T. (2001). How and why exercise is impaired in COPD. *Respiration* 68, 229–239. doi: 10.1159/000050502

Aliverti, A., Stevenson, N., Dellacà, R. L., Lo Mauro, A., Pedotti, A., and Calverley, P. M. (2004). Regional chest wall volumes during exercise in chronic obstructive pulmonary disease. *Thorax* 59, 210–216. doi: 10.1136/thorax.2003.011494

Aliverti, A., Uva, B., Laviola, M., Bovio, D., Lo Mauro, A., Tarperi, C., et al. (2010). Concomitant ventilatory and circulatory functions of the diaphragm and abdominal muscles. *J. Appl. Physiol. (1985)* 109, 1432–1440. doi: 10.1152/japplphysiol.00576.2010

Beck, K. C., Randolph, L. N., Bailey, K. R., Wood, C. M., Snyder, E. M., and Johnson, B. D. (2006). Relationship between cardiac output and oxygen consumption during upright cycle exercise in healthy humans. *J. Appl. Physiol. (1985)*, 101, 1474–1480. doi: 10.1152/japplphysiol.00224.2006

Cholewicki, J., Juluru, K., and McGill, S. M. (1999a). Intra-abdominal pressure mechanism for stabilizing the lumbar spine. *J. Biomech.* 32, 13–17. doi: 10.1016/S0021-9290(98)00129-8

Cholewicki, J., Juluru, K., Radebold, A., Panjabi, M. M., and McGill, S. M. (1999b). Lumbar spine stability can be augmented with an abdominal belt and/or increased intra-abdominal pressure. *Eur. Spine J.* 8, 388–395. doi: 10.1007/s005860050192

Convertino, V. A., Ratliff, D. A., Ryan, K. L., Doerr, D. F., Ludwig, D. A., Muniz, G. W., et al. (2004). Hemodynamics associated with breathing through an inspiratory impedance threshold device in human volunteers. *Crit. Care Med.* 32, S381–386. doi: 10.1097/01.CCM.0000134348.69165.15

Fixler, D. E., Atkins, J. M., Mitchell, J. H., and Horwitz, L. D. (1976). Blood flow to respiratory, cardiac, and limb muscles in dogs during graded exercise. *Am. J. Physiol.* 231(Pt 1), 1515–1519.

Flamm, S. D., Taki, J., Moore, R., Lewis, S. F., Keech, F., Maltais, F., et al. (1990). Redistribution of regional and organ blood volume and effect on cardiac function in relation to upright exercise intensity in healthy human subjects. *Circulation* 81, 1550–1559. doi: 10.1161/01.CIR.81.5.1550

Goldman, M., Smith, H. J., and Ulmer, W. T. (2005). "Whole-body plethysmography," in *Lung Function Testing*, eds R. Gosselink and H. Stam (Wakefield: European Respiratory Society) 15–39.

Guyton, A. C., Lindsey, A. W., and Kaufmann, B. N. (1955). Effect of mean circulatory filling pressure and other peripheral circulatory factors on cardiac output. *Am. J. Physiol.* 180, 463–468.

Hamann, J. J., Valic, Z., Buckwalter, J. B., and Clifford, P. S. (2003). Muscle pump does not enhance blood flow in exercising skeletal muscle. *J. Appl. Physiol. (1985)* 94, 6–10. doi: 10.1152/japplphysiol.00337.2002

Harms, C. A., Babcock, M. A., McClaran, S. R., Pegelow, D. F., Nickele, G. A., Nelson, W. B., et al. (1997). Respiratory muscle work compromises leg blood flow during maximal exercise. *J. Appl. Physiol. (1985)* 82, 1573–1583.

Hodges, P. W., and Gandevia, S. C. (2000). Changes in intra-abdominal pressure during postural and respiratory activation of the human diaphragm. *J. Appl. Physiol. (1985)* 89, 967–976. Available online at: http://jap.physiology.org/content/89/3/967

Hodges, P. W., Heijnen, I., and Gandevia, S. C. (2001). Postural activity of the diaphragm is reduced in humans when respiratory demand increases. *J. Physiol.* 537, 999–1008. doi: 10.1113/jphysiol.2001.012648

Johnson, R. L. Jr., Spicer, W. S., Bishop, J. M., and Forster, R. E. (1960). Pulmonary capillary blood volume, flow and diffusing capacity during exercise. *J. Appl. Physiol.* 15, 893–902.

Laughlin, M. H. (1987). Skeletal muscle blood flow capacity: role of muscle pump in exercise hyperemia. *Am. J. Physiol.* 253(Pt 2), H993–1004.

Miller, J. D., Pegelow, D. F., Jacques, A. J., and Dempsey, J. A. (2005a). Effects of augmented respiratory muscle pressure production on locomotor limb venous return during calf contraction exercise. *J. Appl. Physiol. (1985)* 99, 1802–1815. doi: 10.1152/japplphysiol.00278.2005

Miller, J. D., Pegelow, D. F., Jacques, A. J., and Dempsey, J. A. (2005b). Skeletal muscle pump versus respiratory muscle pump: modulation of venous return from the locomotor limb in humans. *J. Physiol.* 563(Pt 3), 925–943. doi: 10.1113/jphysiol.2004.076422

Poh, P. Y., Carter, R. 3rd, Hinojosa-Laborde, C., Mulligan, J., Grudic, G. Z., and Convertino, V. A. (2014). Respiratory pump contributes to increased physiological reserve for compensation during simulated haemorrhage. *Exp. Physiol.* 99, 1421–1426. doi: 10.1113/expphysiol.2014.081208

Rioul, O., and Vetterli, M. (1991). Wavelets and signal processing. *IEEE Signal Process. Mag.* 8, 14–38. doi: 10.1109/79.91217

Robertson, C. H. Jr., Foster, G. H., and Johnson, R. L. Jr. (1977). The relationship of respiratory failure to the oxygen consumption of, lactate production by, and distribution of blood flow among respiratory muscles during increasing inspiratory resistance. *J. Clin. Invest.* 59, 31–42. doi: 10.1172/JCI108619

Roos, M., Kobza, R., Jamshidi, P., Bauer, P., Resink, T., Schlaepfer, R., et al. (2009). Improved cardiac performance through pacing-induced diaphragmatic stimulation: a novel electrophysiological approach in heart failure management? *Europace* 11, 191–199. doi: 10.1093/europace/eun377

Rowell, L. B. (1974). Human cardiovascular adjustments to exercise and thermal stress. *Physiol. Rev.* 54, 75–159.

Samar, V. J., Swartz, K. P., and Raghuveer, M. R. (1995). Multiresolution analysis of event-related potentials by wavelet decomposition. *Brain Cogn.* 27, 398–438. doi: 10.1006/brcg.1995.1028

Sheel, A. W., Derchak, P. A., Morgan, B. J., Pegelow, D. F., Jacques, A. J., and Dempsey, J. A. (2001). Fatiguing inspiratory muscle work causes reflex reduction in resting leg blood flow in humans. *J. Physiol.* 537(Pt 1), 277–289. doi: 10.1111/j.1469-7793.2001.0277k.x

Tschakovsky, M. E., and Sheriff, D. D. (2004). Immediate exercise hyperemia: contributions of the muscle pump vs. rapid vasodilation. *J. Appl. Physiol. (1985)* 97, 739–747. doi: 10.1152/japplphysiol.00185.2004

Uva, B., Aliverti, A., Laviola, M., Bovio, D., Lo Mauro, A., Colombo, E., et al. (2010). Inferior vena caval flow modulation by abdominal pressure. *Eur. Respir. J.* 36(Suppl. 54), 1002.

von Borries, R., Pierluissi, J., and Nazeran, H. (2005). Wavelet transform-based ECG baseline drift removal for body surface potential mapping. *Conf. Proc. IEEE Eng. Med. Biol. Soc.* 4, 3891–3894. doi: 10.1109/iembs.2005.1615311

Willeput, R., Rondeux, C., and De Troyer, A. (1984). Breathing affects venous return from legs in humans. *J. Appl. Physiol. Respir. Environ. Exerc. Physiol.* 57, 971–976.

Yannopoulos, D., Metzger, A., McKnite, S., Nadkarni, V., Aufderheide, T. P., Idris, A., et al. (2006). Intrathoracic pressure regulation improves vital organ perfusion pressures in normovolemic and hypovolemic pigs. *Resuscitation* 70, 445–453. doi: 10.1016/j.resuscitation.2006.02.005

Conflict of Interest Statement: The authors declare that the research was conducted in the absence of any commercial or financial relationships that could be construed as a potential conflict of interest.

20

Change of Direction Ability Performance in Cerebral Palsy Football Players According to Functional Profiles

Raúl Reina[1]*, Jose M. Sarabia[1], Javier Yanci[2], María P. García-Vaquero[1] and María Campayo-Piernas[1]

[1] *Sports Research Centre, Miguel Hernández University, Elche, Spain,* [2] *Faculty of Physical Activity and Sports Science, University of the Basque Country, UPV/EHU, Vitoria-Gasteiz, Spain*

Edited by:
Igor B. Mekjavic,
Jozef Stefan Institute, Slovenia

Reviewed by:
Pierre-Marie Leprêtre,
Université de Picardie Jules Verne,
France
Miroljub Jakovljevic,
University of Ljubljana, Slovenia

*Correspondence:
Raúl Reina
rroina@goumh.es

The aims of the present study were to evaluate the validity and reliability of the two different change of direction ability (CODA) tests in elite football players with cerebral palsy (CP) and to analyse the differences in performance of this ability between current functional classes (FT) and controls. The sample consisted of 96 international cerebral palsy football players (FPCP) and 37 football players. Participants were divided into four different groups according to the International Federation of Cerebral Palsy Football (IFCPF) classes and a control group (CG): FT5 ($n = 8$); FT6 ($n = 12$); FT7 ($n = 62$); FT8 ($n = 14$); and CG ($n = 37$). The reproducibility of Modified Agility Test (MAT) and Illinois Agility Test (IAT) (ICC = 0.82–0.95, SEM = 2.5–5.8%) showed excellent to good values. In two CODA tests, CG performed faster scores compared with FPCP classes ($p < 0.01$, $d = 1.76$–3.26). In IAT, FT8 class comparisons regarding the other classes were: FT5 ($p = 0.047$, $d = 1.05$), FT6 ($p = 0.055$, $d = 1.19$), and FT7 ($p = 0.396$, $d = 0.56$). With regard to MAT, FT8 class was also compared with FT5 ($p = 0.006$, $d = 1.30$), FT6 ($p = 0.061$, $d = 0.93$), and FT7 ($p = 0.033$, $d = 1.01$). No significant differences have been found between FT5, FT6, and FT7 classes. According to these results, IAT and MAT could be useful and reliable and valid tests to analyse CODA in FPCP. Each test (IAT and MAT) could be applied considering the cut point that classifiers need to make a decision about the FT8 class and the other FT classes (FT5, FT6, and FT7).

Keywords: agility, classification, impairment, performance, paralympics

INTRODUCTION

Football for people with cerebral palsy (CP) is a 7-a-side game with two 30 min halves (Kloyiam et al., 2011; Cámara et al., 2013). This is one of the 23 sports included in the programme of the next Paralympic Games in Rio 2016. The Fédération Internationale de Football Association (FIFA) laws of the game apply with some exceptions made by the new (1 January 2015) International Federation of Cerebral Palsy Football (IFCPF). Some of the changes include a smaller pitch and goal posts, no offside rule and players rolling the ball into play instead of a throw in (IFCPF, 2015a). This sport became independent on, under the umbrella of the IFCPF. On the field, teams are made up of seven ambulant CP players.

All players participating in official events must have an IFCPF classification. IFCPF has a classification system which allows all ambulant athletes with CP and related neurological conditions to take part. Paralympic classification systems aim to promote participation in sport by people with disabilities by controlling for the impact of impairment on the outcome of competition (Tweedy et al., 2014). The language and structure of the International Classification of Functioning, Disability, and Health (World Health Organization, 2012) is central to Paralympic classification, and the concepts of impairment and activity limitation are particularly important (Tweedy and Vanlandewijck, 2011). The International Paralympic Committee (IPC) recognizes eight eligible physical impairments in Paralympic sport: five impairments of function (i.e., impaired strength, impaired range of movement, hypertonia, ataxia, and athetosis) and three impairments of structure (i.e., limb deficiency, leg length difference, and short stature). In addition, the activities of focus are the Paralympic sports in which athletes compete. It is not mandatory for Paralympic sports to provide classification systems that cater to all eight physical impairment types (Tweedy et al., 2014). For example, CP Football is for athletes with hypertonia, ataxia, or athetosis of cerebral origin (e.g., cerebral palsy, traumatic brain injury, or stroke). Although this sport is governed by an international federation which includes cerebral palsy in its definition, the classification unit in Paralympic sport is the impairment, and it is related to several health conditions, not only cerebral palsy.

Based on these eligible impairments, CP Football has four classes based on the traditional Cerebral Palsy International Sports and Recreation Association (CPISRA) classification system, that is, four classes (C1–C4) for wheelchair athletes and the other four (C5–C8) for ambulant athletes (Reina, 2014). Applied to CP-football, the last four classes (FT) appear in the rules as: "(a) Class FT5: Diplegia, asymmetric diplegia, double hemiplegic, or dystonic. It includes moderate involvement with spasticity grade 2–3; involvement of both legs which may require orthotics/splints for walking; an asymmetric diplegia or double hemiplegic athlete with involvement on both sides with the lower limbs more affected than the upper extremities; or athletes with dystonia where the lower limbs are more affected than the upper extremities. (b) Class FT6: Athetosis, dystonic, ataxic or mixed cerebral palsy or related neurological conditions. It includes moderate involvement in all four limbs; the athlete ambulates without assistive devices but might require orthotics/splints; athetosis, dystonia, or ataxia is typically the most prevalent factor but some athletes can have problems with athetosis or ataxia mixed with spasticity; athletes with dystonic athetosis in all four limbs belong in this classification unless the impairment is minimal. (c) Class FT7. Hemiplegic, including spasticity grade 2–3 in one half of the body (on the frontal plane); athletes walk/run with a clearly noticeable limp due to spasticity in the lower limb; hemi gait pattern 2, 3, or 4 as per grouping described in gait patterns in spastic hemiplegia in children and young adults. They usually have a good functional ability on the other side of the body. (d) Class FT8. Diplegia, asymmetric diplegia, double hemiplegia,

and/or dystonia. It includes hemiplegia with spasticity grade 1–2; monoplegia with spasticity grade 1 or 2 in a major joint in the lower limbs; athetosis, dystonia, ataxia or mixed cerebral palsy or other neurological conditions."

In Paralympic sport, an evidence-based system of classification is one in which the system has a clearly stated purpose, and methods used for assigning class will achieve the stated purpose (Tweedy and Vanlandewijck, 2011). Although evidence-based methods for classifying impairments must primarily use valid and reliable measures of impairment, such measures cannot be the sole basis of classification (Beckman and Tweedy, 2009). This is because, although eligible impairments are permanent, many types of impairment are, to varying degrees, responsive to training. In most circumstances, current best practice requires classification panels to assign a class by collectively considering outcomes from the impairment assessment, together with three other forms of assessment [International Paralympic Committee (IPC), 2015]:(a) novel motor tasks, which are tasks that are unlikely to have been practiced by the athlete in the usual course of training for his or her sport; (b) sport-specific activities that are likely to have been frequently practiced by athletes training for the sport; and (c) a detailed training history and other personal and environmental factors likely to affect sports proficiency.

Football players are required to turn, sprint and change pace during matches (Stølen et al., 2005). Indeed, frequent variation in activities has been reported during a competitive match in elite football players (Bloomfield et al., 2007). During a football game, ~1300 changes in activity are undertaken in off-the-ball conditions (Stølen et al., 2005). Therefore, due to the relevance of change of direction ability (CODA) in this sport, the examination of the nature of this activity and its evaluation is one of the objectives of this study. Evaluating CODA in football has entailed the use of many different tests including T-test (Sporis et al., 2010; Chaouachi et al., 2012) T-test modifications (Sassi et al., 2009) and Illinois test (Miller et al., 2006). However, despite the fact that CODA has been evaluated in football players (Sporis et al., 2010; Chaouachi et al., 2012) children and adolescents with CP (Verschuren et al., 2009, 2010) and can be a determining performance component in CP Football, to our knowledge, no scientific articles have been published to determine the CODA in elite football players eligible for CP football, and its relationships with current classification profiles.

The aims of the present study were, firstly, to evaluate the reliability of the CODA measured by modified agility test (MAT) and Illinois agility test (IAT) in international football players with cerebral palsy (FPCP); secondly, to evaluate the validity of both CODA tests to check activity limitation of cerebral palsy football players (FPCP) regarding controls; and thirdly, to analyse the differences in this ability between different current IFCPF functional classes. Due to the different CP motor alterations (Unnithan et al., 1998) and that different types of tests used may determine the performance (Chaouachi et al., 2012) our working hypothesis is that there may be differences in the CODA between CPISRA functional classes, and also between FPCP and football players.

MATERIALS AND METHODS

Participants

Ninety-nine international FPCP and 37 football players took part in this study ($n = 136$). Written informed consent was obtained from the participants and their coaches, and data collection was conducted during 2013 CPISRA Intercontinental Cup (ICUP) qualifying tournament for the World Championships in 2015, while the control group was measured 1 month before the end of the regular league. Sixteen teams took part in the CPISRA ICUP, and players from 10 national teams voluntarily participated in the data collection. Reported competition experience indicated that 24.7% of players from FPCP group participated in the last Paralympics Games (London 2012). Football players had national level competition, and this control group (CG) was built up considering the mean age and training activity (**Table 1**). The study was approved by the institutional review committee (DPS.RRV.01.14) of the Miguel Hernández University (Elche, Spain) and conformed to the recommendations of the Declaration of Helsinki.

Procedures

A standardized warm-up was performed, consisting of a 5 min self-paced low-intensity run, skipping exercises, strides and two 15 m sprints with and without changes of direction. Information about the protocols was sent in advance to the teams, and participants practiced test protocols twice before data collection. Each participant performed anthropometric measures and two trials of two agility tests: IAT and MAT. A 3 min rest period was given between each trial (Mayhew et al., 1995). The best score in each test was used for data analysis.

Anthropometric Measurements

The players' heights were measured using a stadiometer with an accuracy of ±1 mm (Harpenden, Holtain® Ltd., Crosswell, UK). Electronic scales (Oregon Scientific®, GR101, Portland, USA) with an accuracy of ± 0.01 kg were used to measure the body mass.

Illinois Agility Test

The IAT is set up with four cones forming the agility area (**Figure 1**). On command, (1) the athlete sprints 10 m, turns and (2) returns to the starting line. After returning to the starting line, (3) he swerves in and out of four cones (4, 5)

completing two 10 m sprints to finish the agility course (Miller et al., 2006). Performances were recorded using an electronic timing system (Globus®, Codogne, Italy). The infrared timing gates were positioned at the start and the finish lines at a height of 1 m. No technical advice was given as to the most effective movement technique. Subjects were only instructed to complete the test as quickly as possible. Subjects were instructed not to jump over the markers; they were to run around them, and the trial was not valid if they touched or toppled a marker.

Modified Agility Test

This test was originally described as a measure of four-directional agility and body control that evaluates the ability to change directions rapidly while maintaining balance without loss of speed (Semenick, 1990). The MAT was proposed by Sassi et al. (2009) and Pauole et al. (2000), and recently adapted by Yanci et al. (2013). This is considered a short duration test where linear movement in the antero-posterior and medio-lateral directions is required (Sassi et al., 2009). A previous study conducted with football players showed excellent MAT test reproducibility values (CV = 2.3%) (Yanci et al., 2014). The participants' movements during the MAT were as follows (**Figure 2**): (i) A–B movement (5 m): participants sprinted forward to cone B and touched the top of it with the right hand; (ii) B–C movement (2.5 m): moving laterally without crossing the feet, participants ran to cone C and touched the top of it with the left hand; (iii) C–D movement (5 m): participants ran laterally to cone D and touched the top of it with the right hand; (iv) D–B movement (2.5 m): participants moved back to cone B and touched the top of it with the left hand; (v) B–A movement (5 m): participants ran backward to line A. Start position was standardized, with the preferred foot close to the start line. The test was repeated if the athlete crossed one foot in front of the other, did not touch the cone and failed to face forward throughout. MAT performances test were recorded using an electronic timing system (Globus®, Codogne, Italy) positioned at the start line at a height of 1 m.

Data Analysis

Results are presented as mean ± standard deviation (SD), and coefficient of variation (CV) was also calculated using next formula: $CV = (SD/Mean \cdot 100)$ (Atkinson and Nevill, 1998). Reliability among two trials in each agility test was assessed using intra-class correlations (ICC) and Standard Error Measurement (SEM). ICC > 0.90 were considered excellent, 0.75–0.90 good

TABLE 1 | Descriptive data of elite football players with cerebral palsy (FPCP) and football players (CG).

Class	n	Age (yr)	Mass (kg)	Height (cm)	BMI (kg·m^{-2})	Sport experience	Football sessions	Gym sessions
FT5	8	23.2 ± 6.4	67.0 ± 7.5	175.9 ± 6.1	21.7 ± 2.7	11.4 ± 5.2	4.6 ± 1.2	3.0 ± 1.3
FT6	12	27.1 ± 8.9	65.6 ± 6.5	175.3 ± 4.7	21.5 ± 1.5	11.0 ± 3.6	2.6 ± 1.2	2.7 ± 1.1
FT7	64	24.8 ± 6.2	68.3 ± 8.5	175.1 ± 7.6	22.5 ± 2.9	9.8 ± 6.9	3.2 ± 1.3	2.7 ± 1.5
FT8	15	26.5 ± 7.6	73.2 ± 7.9	176.7 ± 8.9	23.5 ± 2.2	13.6 ± 9.6	3.1 ± 0.9	3.5 ± 1.7
CG	37	19.6 ± 3.4	72.6 ± 7.8	178.0 ± 5.9	22.9 ± 1.7	10.2 ± 5.1	3.4 ± 0.5	1.7 ± 0.9
Sample	136	23.7 ± 6.6	69.8 ± 8.2	176.0 ± 7.1	22.6 ± 2.5	10.5 ± 6.5	3.3 ± 1.1	2.5 ± 1.5

BMI, Body Mass Index; Sport experience expressed in years; Football and Gym (strength) sessions expressed by times/week.

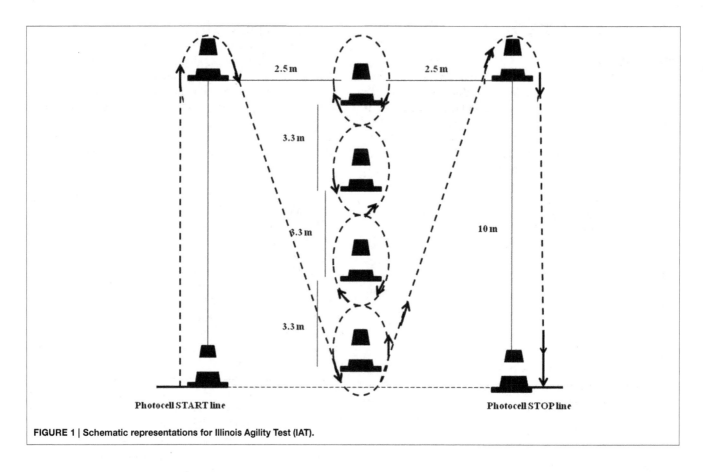

FIGURE 1 | Schematic representations for Illinois Agility Test (IAT).

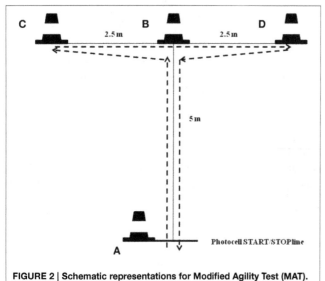

FIGURE 2 | Schematic representations for Modified Agility Test (MAT).

and <0.75 as poor to moderate (Portney and Watkins, 2008). The SEM was calculated by using the following formula: $SEM = SD \cdot \sqrt{1 - ICC}$. Strength of association between two agility tests used in this study was assessed using a Pearson correlation (r). To interpret those results the threshold values for Pearson product-moment used by Salaj and Markovic (2011) were used: low ($r \leq 0.3$), moderate ($0.3 < r \leq 0.7$) to high ($r > 0.7$). A spreadsheet

designed by Hopkins (2015) was used to evaluate changes in scores (bias) between testing repetitions.

Kolmogorov test was applied to evaluate the normal data distribution. All analyzed variables had a normal distribution, and parametric statistic was used. Atypical scores were evaluated for those players scoring above 95% interval of confidence, and one player from the class FT6 and two players from the class FT7 have been removed from the data analysis. A One-way analysis of variance (ANOVA) with least significant difference *post-hoc* comparison (Scheffé correction) was used to examine the mean differences between groups and FPCP sub-groups. Cohen's effect sizes (*d*) between groups were also calculated (Cohen, 1988). Interpretation of effect sizes for highly trained athletes was: above 1.0, between 0.5 and 1.0, between 0.25 and 0.5 and lower than 0.25 were considered as large, moderate, small and trivial, respectively (Rhea, 2004). Data analysis was performed using the Statistical Package for Social Sciences (version 21.0 for Windows, SPSS Inc, Chicago, IL, USA). Statistical significance was set at an alpha level of $p < 0.05$.

RESULTS

Due to the different classification profiles about the players who took part in the study, a within-group correlation analysis was conducted between two CODA tests. Within-session reliability for each player was evaluated among two trials performed. IAT reliability was ICC = 0.96 (0.91, 0.98) and SEM = 2.5% (2.23,

2.86) for the FPCP group, and ICC = 0.84 (0.73, 0.91) and SEM = 1.88% (1.57, 2.38) for CG. CV for CG was 4.21%, and higher in the FPCP classes: FT8 = 7.01%, FT7 = 9.48%, FT6 = 6.85%, and FT5 = 10.37%. The change in mean scores (bias) were −0.14 s (−0.26, −0.02) for FPCP group and 0.01 s (−0.12, −0.14) for CG respectively. On the other hand, FPCP group showed a reliability in MAT of ICC = 0.82 (0.75, 0.87) and SEM = 5.84% (5.20, 6.68), while CG was ICC = 0.76 (0.61, 0.86) and SEM = 3.02% (2.53, 3.78). Similar results were obtained regarding CV: CG = 6%, FT8 = 10.01%, FT7 = 11.43%, FT6 = 17.09%, and FT5 = 16.81%. The bias for this test was −0.25 s (−0.37, −0.12) for FPCP group and −0.17 s (−0.24, −0.09) for CG respectively.

Overall correlation analysis between two CODA tests showed a significant and positive relationship ($r = 0.736$, $p < 0.001$); both FPCP ($r = 0.555$, $p < 0.001$) and CG ($r = 0.453$, $p < 0.01$). However, if we analyse this relationship between the different classes in the FPCP group, correlation is not significant for classes FT5 ($r = 0.359$, $p = 0.383$), while it is significant for classes FT6 ($r = 0.838$, $p < 0.01$), FT7 ($r = 0.517$, $p < 0.001$), and FT8 ($r = 0.641$, $p < 0.01$).

Mean, standard deviations, maximum and minimum scores for each group and overall are reported in **Figures 3, 4**. In IAT, CG performed faster scores (15.91 ± 0.67 s), compared with FT8 (17.75 ± 1.24 s; $d = 1.84$, large), FT7 (18.67 ± 1.77 s; $d = 2.06$, large), FT6 (19.34 ± 1.32 s; $d = 3.27$, large), and FT5 (19.49 ± 2.02 s; $d = 2.38$, large) respectively. Similar results were obtained for MAT: CG (5.99 ± 0.36 s), FT8 (7.09 ± 0.71 s; $d = 1.95$, large), FT7 (7.94 ± 0.91 s; $d = 2.82$, large), FT6 (8.22 ± 1.41 s; $d = 2.17$, large), and FT5 (8.59 ± 1.44 s; $d = 2.48$, large).

One-way ANOVA showed significant differences between groups, both IAT [$F_{(4, 128)} = 36.93$; $p < 0.001$] and MAT [$F_{(4, 129)} = 26.30$; $p < 0.001$]. Pair comparisons also report significant differences between CG and all FPCP classes ($p < 0.001$ regarding FT7, FT6, and FT5; $p < 0.01$ regarding FT8; $d > 1.0$, large).

In IAT, FT8 class comparisons regarding the other classes were: FT5 ($p = 0.128$; $d = 1.03$, large), FT6 ($p = 0.124$; $d = 1.23$, large), and FT7 ($p = 0.325$; $d = 0.60$, moderate). With regard to MAT, FT8 players showed significant differences regarding all the other FPCP groups: FT5 ($p = 0.005$; $d = 1.32$, large), FT6 ($p = 0.034$; $d = 1.01$, large), and FT7 ($p = 0.026$; $d = 1.04$, large). No significant differences have been found between FPCP classes FT5, FT6 and FT7.

DISCUSSION

The aim of this study was to compare the performance of FPCP and football players in two CODA tests, and analyse its relationship with current functional classification profiles in CP-football. To our knowledge, there is no study in the literature of the CODA in football players with CP and other related neurological conditions eligible for CP-football. According to IPC's Classification Policy, the development of evidence-based classification procedures is necessary, and tis check the activity limitation in sporting skills due to eligible impairment.

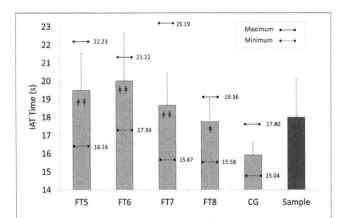

FIGURE 3 | Descriptive scores for each group in Illinois Agility test (IAT): FT5, FT6, FT7, and FT8, Football Players with Cerebral Palsy Classes; CG, control group; ‡‡, CG vs. FT5, FT6, or FT7, $p < 0.001$; ‡, CG vs. FT8, $p < 0.01$.

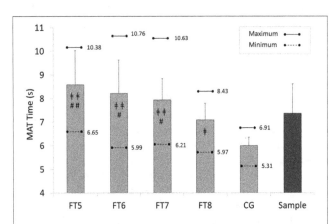

FIGURE 4 | Descriptive scores for each group in Modified Agility test (MAT); FT5, FT6, FT7, and FT8, Football Players with Cerebral Palsy Classes; CG, control group; ‡‡, CG vs. FT5, FT6, or FT7, $p < 0.001$; ‡, CG vs. FT8, $p < 0.01$; ##, FT8 vs. FT5, $p < 0.01$; #, FT8 vs. FT6-FT7, $p < 0.05$.

The analysis of the reproducibility of MAT and IAT showed excellent to good values, as other studies which used T-design CODA tests (Pauole et al., 2000; Sassi et al., 2009; Yanci et al., 2014) and IAT (Miller et al., 2006; Lockie et al., 2013). Also, high to moderate correlations have been obtained between both tests. However, FPCP groups showed CVs in MAT higher than 10% (FT8 = 10.01%, FT7 = 11.43%, FT6 = 17.09%, and FT5 = 16.81%). Future studies could include three trials of the test to improve CV, although SEM and ICC values were good. On the other hand, this test could be considered a "novel" task for the players (International Paralympic Committee (IPC), 2015).

A test that assesses linear acceleration, in addition to the ability to make several sharp cuts while continuing to sprint forward over specific distances, has value for field sports (Lockie et al., 2013). IAT involves acceleration, as well as directional changes when sprinting in a linear fashion. In the same way, CODA is considered a determinant for successful performance in football (Chaouachi et al., 2012, 2014) and the response to different, short and rapid movements is essential in football players. For this reason, CODA has been tested in order to assess football players' conditioning (Chaouachi et al., 2012; Yanci et al., 2014; Reilly et al., 2000). In spite of the fact difficulty in turning and stopping are characteristics of IFCPF (2015a) to the best of our knowledge, this is the first study of such ability in international FPCP. Both IAT and MAT tests showed that best score in CG is better than the best score in FPCP classes, and both tests could be valid and reliable to evaluate CODA activity limitation due to eligible impairments.

Current CP Football rules state that at least one player from the classes FT5 or FT6 should be on the field of play during the game, and teams cannot play with more than one player of class FT8. This rule is expected to change after the Rio Paralympic Games, and the IFCPF Board have suggested increasing to two FT5 or FT6 players in the lineup. This rule change will have an impact on team management and training, because these two classes are colloquially named "lower classes." Then, the general performance of a team could be influenced by the classification of its players. In other words, a player with "moderate" or "mild" spastic diplegia could be classified as FT5 or FT8, with a major impact on team play or team squad (Reina, 2014). According to Tweedy et al. (2014), to assess the relative strength of association between valid measures of impairment and measures of performance, development of valid measures of impairment must be complemented by the development of standardized, sport-specific measures of performance, and tests applied in this study could be helpful in CP Football classification.

In our study, FT8 ("mild impairment" regarding the other three classes) showed significant differences with FT5, FT6, and FT7 in IAT (large effect sizes); but not in MAT, but with large (FT5 and FT6) and moderate (FT7) effect sizes. Players from class FT5 (e.g., spastic diplegia) presented the worst scores in both tests. Spastic diplegia manifests as high and constant "tightness" or "stiffness" in the muscles of the lower extremities, usually on the legs, hips, and pelvis. The abnormally high muscle tone that results creates lifelong difficulty with all voluntary and passive movement in the legs, such as ankle rotational anomalies, identified as the most frequent cause of lower limb torsional deviations followed by pelvic malalignment (Simon et al., 2015). The consequence of this impairment is shorter strides and difficulties performing rapid changes of direction, which explains the lower scores in both CODA tests.

Class FT6 players showed also significant differences with regard to FT8 players in MAT but not IAT, but both comparisons with large effect sizes ($d = 1.01 - 1.23$). We should consider the eligible impairments for class FT6: ataxia (impaired control of voluntary movement), athetosis (involuntary contractions of the muscles), or dystonia (sustained muscle contractions that cause twisting and repetitive movements or abnormal postures). FT6 players may have good dynamic balance compared with static balance (IFCPF, 2015b). Athletes with dystonia, athetosis and ataxia, in particular, usually have problems with balance and starting, stopping and turning when running. They also have varying degrees of difficulty with balance while hopping

and jumping; with many postural body adjustments for static/dynamic balance. If we compare the CV within each class in the two CODA tests, we observe that MAT test has higher scores. Particularly, FT6 class exhibits a CV of 6.85% in IAT and 17.09% in MAT (10.24% difference between tests), higher than the other FPCP classes (FT5 = 6.45%; FT7 = 1.94%; FT8 = 3%). The main activity limitation in these players is the coordination and movement control, and MAT requires displacements in several directions (frontwards, backwards, and lateral). Their CV is lower than other classes as FT5 or FT7 in IAT, because this athlete usually demonstrates better running mechanics or running pace (IFCPF, 2015b). However, because three different impairments are eligible for this class, large variability is also expected among players within this functional profile.

With regard to class FT7, we should consider again the functional profile of this class: spastic hemiplegia. These athletes usually have activity limitations in gait/running both in stance and swing phase on the impaired side. Foot placement is affected by either weakness in dorsiflexion muscles and/or over-activity in plantar flexor muscles. Knee and hip control are also affected by spasticity and possible loss of range of motion due to contracture. The kinematics of walking in youth and adults with CP (e.g., increased limb asymmetry, reduced stride length, and increased stride time) has been linked to their reduced walking economy (Unnithan et al., 1996). Although the athlete usually walks with a noticeable limp, he may appear to have a smoother stride when running but may not have a consistent heel strike. Asymmetry in the angle of touch down during landing probably resides within a compensation for unilateral neurological impairment of the individual (Kloyiam et al., 2011).

Larger angle of touch down (increased plantar flexion) may result from the fact that the affected limb is less able to conserve energy and stabilize the joints during movement. In MAT test, lateral displacements (toward right and left sides) were required, and these athletes exhibited difficulties in pivoting and balancing on the impaired side. In comparison, no differences between FT7 and FT8 classes in IAT could be explained because displacement is forwards, and a higher degree of plantar flexion allows greater energy conservation in the tendon, and the plantar flexed foot acts like a vertical (Fonseca et al., 2004) contributing to greater joint stability. IPC Athletics (2015) classification rulebook states that in T37 athletes, with similar profile to FT7 in CP Football, a limp may disappear almost totally while they run. The reason is that when walking the leg support during stance phase begins with a heel strike, and this is the most difficult action for athletes with a spastic paresis. When running only the forefoot hits the ground, providing support and push off, and a tight calf muscle facilitates the push off. Therefore, MAT appears here as a better CODA test for the cut-point FT7 vs. FT8 than IAT.

CONCLUSIONS

The IPC is continually developing and refining evidence-based classifications for all sports. No research has systematically investigated the relationship between the CP Football players' functional profiles and their ability to perform CODA tests. The present study makes the following suggestions:

a) IAT and MAT could be useful, reliable and valid tests to analyse CODA performance in FPCP, because activity limitation in test performance has been demonstrated compared with controls.

b) Comparing between current FPCP classes (IFCPF, 2015b), each test (IAT and MAT) could be applied considering the cut point that classifiers need to make a decision about the FT8 class and other FT classes (FT5, FT6, and FT7).

According to Tweedy et al. (2014) future research should focus on the assessment of the relative strength of association between valid measures of impairment and measures of performance. It is vital that athletes who have positively influenced their impairment scores through effective training are not competitively disadvantaged by being placed in a class for athletes with less severe impairments (Tweedy and Vanlandewijck, 2011). Since CPISRA classification system is based on a functional approach, more research is necessary to develop a sport-specific and evidence-classification system.

Our results can improve the current classification process in CP Football under the new International Federation (IFCPF), and contribute to the description of the current classification profiles, which will be modified and redefined after Rio 2016 Paralympic Games.

AUTHOR CONTRIBUTIONS

RR: design of the work, data acquisition, analysis, interpretation of data, drafting the work, revising, final approval of the version to be published. JS: design of the work, analysis, interpretation of data, drafting the work, revising. JY: analysis, interpretation of data, drafting the work, revising, final approval of the version to be published. MG: data acquisition, interpretation of data, drafting the work. MC: data acquisition, interpretation of data, drafting the work.

ACKNOWLEDGMENTS

The authors thank CPISRA Board members and CPISRA Football Committee for their support in the data collection during the 2013 CPISRA Intercontinental Cup. We also acknowledge players, coaches and team managers who cooperated and participated in the data collection.

REFERENCES

Atkinson, G., and Nevill, A. M. (1998). Statistical methods for assessing measurement error (reliability) in variables relevant to sports medicine. *Sports Med.* 26, 217–238. doi: 10.2165/00007256-199826040-00002

Beckman, E. M., and Tweedy, S. M. (2009). Towards evidence-based classification in Paralympic athletics: evaluating the validity of activity limitation tests for use in classification of Paralympic running events. *Br. J. Sports Med.* 43, 1067–1072. doi: 10.1136/bjsm.2009.061804

Bloomfield, J., Polman, R., and O'Donoghue, P. (2007). Deceleration movements performed during FA premier league soccer matches. *J. Sports Sci. Med.* 10, 6–11.

Cámara, J., Grande, I., Mejuto, G., Los Arcos, A., and Yanci, J. (2013). Jump landing characteristics in elite soccer players with cerebral palsy. *Biol. Sport.* 30, 91–95. doi: 10.5604/20831862.1044223

Chaouachi, A., Chtara, M., Hammami, R., Chtara, H., Turki, O., and Castagna, C. (2014). Multidirectional sprints and small-sided games training effect on agility and change of direction abilities in youth soccer. *J. Strength Cond. Res.* 28, 3121–3127. doi: 10.1519/JSC.0000000000000505

Chaouachi, A., Manzi, V., Chaalali, A., Wong, D. P., Chamari, K., and Castagna, C. (2012). Determinants analysis of change-of-direction ability in elite soccer players. *J. Strength Cond. Res.* 26, 2667–2676. doi: 10.1519/JSC.0b013e318242f97a

Cohen, J. (1988). *Statistical Power Analysis for the Behavioral Sciences.* Hillsdale, NJ: Lawrence Erlbaum Associates.

Fonseca, S. T., Holt, K. G., Fetters, L., and Saltzman, E. (2004). Dynamic resources used in ambulation by children with spastic hemiplegic cerebral palsy: relationship to kinematics, energetics, and asymmetries. *Phys. Ther.* 84, 344–354.

Hopkins, W. G. (2015). Spreadsheets for analysis of validity and reliability. *Sportscience* 19, 36–42.

IFCPF (2015a). *CP-Football Rules and Regulations, 2015.* Available online at: http://www.ifcpf.com/library (Accessed December 20, 2015).

IFCPF (2015b). *IFCPF Classification Rulebook, 2015.* Available online at: http://www.ifcpf.com/library (Accessed December 20, 2015).

International Paralympic Committee (IPC) (2015). *Evidence Based Classification: Current Best Practice, 2011.* Available online at: http://www.paralympic.org/sites/default/files/document/120228150200907_11%2B2009_09_12%2BEvidence%2BBased%2BClassification1.pdf (Accessed July 12, 2015).

International Paralympic Committee (IPC Athletics) (2015). *Athletics Classification Rules and Regulations, 2014.* Available online at: http://www.paralympic.org/athletics/classification/rules-and-regulations (Accessed February 2, 2015).

Kloyiam, S., Breen, S., Jakeman, P., Conway, J., and Hutzler, Y. (2011). Soccer-specific endurance and running economy in soccer players with cerebral palsy. *Adapt. Phys. Activ. Q.* 28, 354–367.

Lockie, R. G., Schultz, A. B., Callaghan, S. J., Jeffriess, M. D., and Berry, S. P. (2013). Reliability and validity of a new test of change-of-direction speed for field-based sports: the change-of-direction and acceleration test (CODAT). *J. Sports Sci. Med.* 12, 88–96.

Mayhew, J. L., Prinster, J., Ware, J., Zimmer, D., Arabas, J., and Bemben, M. (1995). Muscular endurance repetitions to predict bench press strength in men of different training levels. *J. Sports Med. Phys. Fitness.* 35, 108–113.

Miller, M. G., Herniman, J. J., Ricard, M. D., Cheatham, C. C., and Michael, T. J. (2006). The effects of a 6-week plyometric training program on agility. *J. Sports Sci. Med.* 5, 459–465.

Pauole, K., Madole, K., Garhammer, J., Lacourse, M., and Rozenek, R. (2000). Reliability and validity of the T-test as a measure of agility, leg power, and leg speed in college-aged men and women. *J. Strength Cond. Res.* 14, 443–450. doi: 10.1519/1533-4287(2000)014<0443:ravott>2.0.co;2

Portney, L., and Watkins, M. (2008). *Foundations of Clinical Research: Applications to Practice.* Upper Saddle River, NJ: Prentice Hall.

Reilly, T., Bangsbo, J., and Franks, A. (2000). Anthropometric and physiological predispositions for elite soccer. *J. Sports Sci.* 18, 669–683. doi: 10.1080/02640410050120050

Reina, R. (2014). Evidence-based classification in paralympic sport: application to football-7-a-side. *Eur. J. Hum. Mov.* 32, 161–185.

Rhea, M. R. (2004). Determining the magnitude of treatment effects in strength training research through the use of the effect size. *J. Strength Cond. Res.* 18, 918–920. doi: 10.1519/14403.1

Salaj, S., and Markovic, G. (2011). Specificity of jumping, sprinting, and quick change-of-direction motor abilities. *J. Strength Cond. Res.* 25, 1249–1255. doi: 10.1519/JSC.0b013e3181da77df

Sassi, R. H., Dardouri, W., Yahmed, M. H., Gmada, N., Mahfoudhi, M. E., and Gharbi, Z. (2009). Relative and absolute reliability of a modified agility T-test and its relationship with vertical jump and straight sprint. *J. Strength Cond. Res.* 23, 1644–1651. doi: 10.1519/JSC.0b013e3181b425d2

Semenick, D. (1990). Tests and measurements: The T-test. *Strength Cond. J.* 12, 36–37. doi: 10.1519/0744-0049(1990)012<0036:TTT>2.3.CO;2

Simon, A. L., Ilharreborde, B., Megrot, F., Mallet, C., Azarpira, R., Mazda, K., et al. (2015). A descriptive study of lower limb torsional kinematic profiles in children with spastic diplegia. *J. Pediatric Orthop.* 35, 576–582. doi: 10.1097/BPO.0000000000000331

Sporis, G., Jukic, I., Milanovic, L., and Vucetic, V. (2010). Reliability and factorial validity of agility tests for soccer players. *J. Strength Cond. Res.* 24, 679–686. doi: 10.1519/JSC.0b013e3181c4d324

Stølen, T., Chamari, K., Castagna, C., and Wisløff, U. (2005). Physiology of soccer. *Sports Med.* 35, 501–536. doi: 10.2165/00007256-200535060-00004

Tweedy, S. M., Beckman, E. M., and Connick, M. J. (2014). Paralympic classification: conceptual basis, current methods, and research update. *PM R.* 6, S11–S17. doi: 10.1016/j.pmrj.2014.04.013

Tweedy, S. M., and Vanlandewijck, Y. C. (2011). International paralympic committee position stand—background and scientific principles of classification in Paralympic sport. *Br. J. Sports Med.* 45, 259–269. doi: 10.1136/bjsm.2009.065060

Unnithan, V. B., Clifford, C., and Bar-Or, O. (1998). Evaluation by exercise testing of the child with cerebral palsy. *Sports Med.* 26, 239–251. doi: 10.2165/00007256-199826040-00003

Unnithan, V. B., Dowling, J. J., Frost, G., and Bar-Or, O. (1996). Role of cocontraction in the O2 cost of walking in children with cerebral palsy. *Med. Sci. Sports Exerc.* 28, 1498–1504. doi: 10.1097/00005768-199612000-00009

Verschuren, O., Bloemen, M., Kruitwagen, C., and Takken, T. (2010). Reference values for anaerobic performance and agility in ambulatory children and adolescents with cerebral palsy. *Dev. Med. Child Neurol.* 52, 222–228. doi: 10.1111/j.1469-8749.2010.03747.x

Verschuren, O., Ketelaar, M., Gorter, J. W., Helders, P. J., and Takken, T. (2009). Relation between physical fitness and gross motor capacity in children and adolescents with cerebral palsy. *Dev. Med. Child Neurol.* 51, 866–871. doi: 10.1111/j.1469-8749.2009.03301.x

World Health Organization (WHO) (2012). *International Classification of Functioning Disability and Health, 2001.* Available online at: http://www.who.int/classifications/icf/en/ (Accessed May 4, 2015).

Yanci, J., Los Arcos, A., Mendiguchia, J., and Brughelli, M. (2014). Relationships between sprinting, agility, one-and two-leg vertical and horizontal jump in soccer players. *Kinesiology.* 46, 194–201.

Yanci, J., Reina, R., Los Arcos, A., and Camara, J. (2013). Effects of different contextual interference training programs on straight sprinting and agility performance of primary school students. *J. Sports Sci. Med.* 12, 601–607.

Conflict of Interest Statement: The authors declare that the research was conducted in the absence of any commercial or financial relationships that could be construed as a potential conflict of interest.

21

Perspective: Does Laboratory-Based Maximal Incremental Exercise Testing Elicit Maximum Physiological Responses in Highly-Trained Athletes with Cervical Spinal Cord Injury?

Christopher R. West [1,2,3*], Christof A. Leicht [4], Victoria L. Goosey-Tolfrey [4] and Lee M. Romer [3]

[1] International Collaboration on Repair Discoveries, University of British Columbia, Vancouver, BC, Canada, [2] School of Kinesiology, University of British Columbia, Vancouver, BC, Canada, [3] Centre for Sports Medicine and Human Performance, Brunel University London, London, UK, [4] School of Sport, Exercise and Health Sciences, The Peter Harrison Centre for Disability Sport, Loughborough University, Loughborough, UK

Edited by:
Olivier Girard,
University of Lausanne, Switzerland

Reviewed by:
Can Ozan Tan,
Harvard Medical School, USA
Masaki Mizuno,
University of Texas Southwestern
Medical Center, USA
Pierre-Marie Leprêtre,
Université de Picardie Jules Verne,
France

*Correspondence:
Christopher R. West
west@icord.org

The physiological assessment of highly-trained athletes is a cornerstone of many scientific support programs. In the present article, we provide original data followed by our perspective on the topic of laboratory-based incremental exercise testing in elite athletes with cervical spinal cord injury. We retrospectively reviewed our data on Great Britain Wheelchair Rugby athletes collected during the last two Paralympic cycles. We extracted and compared peak cardiometabolic (heart rate and blood lactate) responses between a standard laboratory-based incremental exercise test on a treadmill and two different maximal field tests (4 min and 40 min maximal push). In the nine athletes studied, both field tests elicited higher peak responses than the laboratory-based test. The present data imply that laboratory-based incremental protocols preclude the attainment of true peak cardiometabolic responses. This may be due to the different locomotor patterns required to sustain wheelchair propulsion during treadmill exercise or that maximal incremental treadmill protocols only require individuals to exercise at or near maximal exhaustion for a relatively short period of time. We acknowledge that both field- and laboratory-based testing have respective merits and pitfalls and suggest that the choice of test be dictated by the question at hand: if true peak responses are required then field-based testing is warranted, whereas laboratory-based testing may be more appropriate for obtaining cardiometabolic responses across a range of standardized exercise intensities.

Keywords: field tests, aerobic exercise, tetraplegia, cardiovascular system

INTRODUCTION

With the advancement of the Paralympic movement over the last 10–20 years the physiological monitoring of Paralympic athletes, including maximal aerobic and anaerobic exercise testing in both the field and laboratory, is now common practice (Goosey-Tolfrey, 2010). Technological advances in treadmill and wheelchair roller design permit externally valid assessments of physiological parameters during wheelchair propulsion under carefully controlled laboratory conditions. The majority of studies that have assessed maximal exercise responses of elite athletes with cervical spinal cord injury (SCI) during wheelchair propulsion on a treadmill, including our own, have reported peak oxygen uptake values in the range of 0.8–1.6 L/min and maximal heart rate (HR) values in the range of 100–140 bpm, although the mean is typically around 120 bpm (Coutts et al., 1983; Wicks et al., 1983; Lasko-McCarthey and Davis, 1991; Schmid et al., 1998; Leicht et al., 2013; Paulson et al., 2013; West et al., 2014a). The dogmatic pathophysiological explanation for these relatively low values is purported to be loss of descending sympathetic cardiac control along with an attenuated catecholamine response and a decreased active muscle mass (Figoni, 1993; Hopman et al., 1998).

Recently, we reported that field-based exercise testing in elite wheelchair rugby athletes with cervical SCI elicits HR values of 140–180 bpm (West et al., 2014b). These values far exceed those collected in the same athletes during arm-crank ergometry and wheelchair propulsion on a treadmill (West et al., 2013). Further investigation revealed that a large number of these elite tetraplegic athletes (both rugby and hand-cycling) exhibit sparing of descending sympathetic fibers in the face of a motor and sensory compete injury (i.e., autonomic incomplete injury; Currie et al., 2015). Thus, it appears that factors other than disrupted descending sympathetic control may preclude the attainment of true peak physiological responses in the laboratory. To date, no study has specifically compared peak cardiometabolic responses between maximal field- and laboratory-based wheelchair exercise tests in highly-trained athletes with cervical SCI.

We have been collecting physiological data leading into the Beijing and London Paralympic cycles on the Great Britain wheelchair rugby squad. During this time, we have conducted a variety of field- and laboratory-based exercise tests on the same group of athletes, but have never directly compared peak physiological variables between laboratory- and field-based maximal wheelchair exercise tests. In the present study, we retrospectively reviewed our data and compared peak physiological responses between a standard incremental laboratory-based wheelchair treadmill test and two different field testing protocols.

MATERIALS AND METHODS

Data Included

Nine male wheelchair rugby athletes with motor complete traumatic cervical SCI (C6-C7; 28.6 ± 2.6 year, 71 ± 16 kg, 1.80 ± 0.10 m, 7.1 ± 3.7 year post injury) were included into the study. The data were part of other research studies, some of which have been published elsewhere (8 of the present participants' 4 min push data, West et al., 2014b, and 8 of the present participants' maximal incremental test data Leicht et al., 2013; West et al., 2014a). All of the studies were approved by the University research ethics committee. In addition to peak physiological values, we extracted participant demographics and their International Wheelchair Rugby Federation (IWRF) classifications at the time of testing.

Study Design

Data were extracted for three different maximal exercise trials. Trial 1 consisted of a maximal 4 min field-based exercise test on a 110 m long indoor athletics track with a wide turnaround area at each end. Trial 2 ($n = 7$) consisted of a maximal 40 min field-based exercise test in a sports hall. Trial 3 consisted of an incremental wheelchair propulsion test on a treadmill. Athletes were thoroughly familiar with the testing protocols. Each trial was completed with athletes exercising in their own rugby wheelchair with regular strapping and gloves. Prior to each trial, athletes received the same standardized pre-test instructions, namely to void their bladder to minimize the chance of autonomic dysreflexia, and to avoid strenuous exercise for 24 h, caffeine for 4 h and food for 2 h prior to assessment. Trials 1 and 3 were performed between 1 and 8 months apart. Trial 3 was performed approximately 1 month after trial 2.

Experimental Trials

Trial 1

Athletes completed a maximal 4 min push on a 110 m synthetic indoor running track with minimal rolling resistance. Athletes pushed maximally in a straight line and were only required to turn at each end of the track where a wide area was provided to facilitate the maintenance of high speeds. Athletes were encouraged to cover as much distance as they could during 4 min. Environmental temperature ranged from 18.2 to 19.4°C, humidity from 40 to 42%, and barometric pressure from 737 to 739 mmHg.

Trial 2

Athletes completed a maximal 40 min push around a large sports hall. The push consisted of: a straight 40 m push along the first side, a 30 m zigzag push along the second side, a straight 40 m push along the third side and a 30 m backwards zigzag push along the final side. The athletes were encouraged to cover as much distance as possible during 40 min.

Trial 3

Athletes completed a maximal incremental wheelchair test to volitional exhaustion on a motorized treadmill with a moving rail to prevent falls (Saturn 300/125r, HP Cosmos, Nussdorf-Traunstein, Germany). Treadmill speed was kept constant and ranged from 2.0 to 2.8 m·s^{-1}, depending on IWRF classification and previous performance during incremental treadmill exercise. The gradient was set at 1% and was increased gradually by 0.1–0.2% every 40 s. The maximal test was terminated when athletes were unable to maintain the treadmill speed, i.e., when they touched the spring of the safety rail for a third time. Standardized verbal encouragement was given throughout the test and push rate was freely chosen. All athletes underwent a standardized warm up as described elsewhere (Leicht et al., 2013). Environmental temperature ranged from 20.2 to 23.7°C, humidity from 27 to 61%, and barometric pressure from 741 to 758 mmHg.

Methods of Measurement
Heart Rate
For trials 1 and 2, HR was measured beat-by-beat using a team system (Suunto team POD, Suunto Oy, Vantaa, Finland). For trial 3, HR was measured beat-by-beat using an individual HR transmitter coupled to a receiver (Polar Vantage NV, Polar Electro Oy, Kempele, Finland). HR_{peak} was defined for all trials as the highest HR averaged over a 5 s rolling window.

Metabolic
In trials 1 and 3, lactate concentration in haemolysed whole blood ($[L_a^-]_B$) was assessed at rest and immediately post-exercise using an automated analyser [Biosen C-line Sport, EKF Diagnostics, Barleben, Germany (Trial 1) or YSI 1500 SPORT, YSI Incorporated, Yellow Springs, OH, USA (Trial 2)]. In trial 3, oxygen uptake ($\dot{V}o_2$) was assessed using an online system (MetaLyzer 3B, Cortex Biophysik GmbH, Leipzig, Germany). $\dot{V}o_{2peak}$ was defined as the highest $\dot{V}o_2$ over a 30 s rolling window.

Statistics
Between-trial differences in physiological outcomes were assessed using either a one-way repeated-measures ANOVA (HR) or paired sample t-test ($[L_a^-]_B$). Relationships between peak physiological indices from field- and laboratory-based testing were assessed using Pearson's product moment correlation. Statistical analyses were carried out using STATA v12.0, with significance set at $p < 0.05$.

RESULTS

Individual athlete data for all trials are reported in **Table 1**. HR_{peak} was different between trials ($p = 0.0035$) and post-hoc testing revealed HR_{peak} was higher in trial 1 and trial 2 vs. trial 3 ($p = 0.008$ and $p = 0.048$, respectively). There was no difference in HR_{peak} between trial 1 and trial 2 ($p = 0.29$), and the values during both field-based exercise tests were strongly correlated

($r = 0.88$, $p = 0.002$; **Figure 1B**). There were no significant correlations between HR_{peak} achieved during the field-based tests and HR_{peak} achieved in the laboratory ($r = 0.56$–0.61, $p > 0.08$). During field-based testing, HR increased rapidly at the onset of exercise in all athletes and remained elevated throughout (**Figure 1C**). Blood lactate concentration was higher during trial 1 vs. trial 3 ($p = 0.010$; **Figure 1D**).

PERSPECTIVE

For the first time we report that peak heart rate and blood lactate concentration during maximal field-based exercise testing exceed values attained during maximal incremental laboratory-based wheelchair exercise on a treadmill. This suggests that incremental exercise testing in the laboratory, at least using the protocol described herein, does not elicit true peak cardiometabolic responses in highly-trained wheelchair rugby athletes with cervical SCI.

The HR values elicited during our laboratory-based treadmill test typify those reported in previous studies that have used wheelchair ergometry or treadmill exercise to investigate peak exercise responses in tetraplegic athletes (Coutts et al., 1983; Wicks et al., 1983; Lasko-McCarthey and Davis, 1991; Schmid et al., 1998; Paulson et al., 2013; Leicht et al., 2014; West et al., 2014a). An interesting observation from the two field-based trials compared to the laboratory trial was the push technique utilized. In the field-based trial, the athletes favored three small pushes followed by a short break for deep inhalation. During the push-phase many athletes also tended to "lean" into the abdominal strapping used to secure them into their sports chair. Anecdotally, athletes report that this push technique allows them to produce more force (power) with each push stroke. Leaning into the chest strapping likely compresses the abdomen and impairs diaphragmatic descent. In turn, this would be expected to reduce the force generating capacity of the diaphragm and may explain why athletes had to pause every three strokes for

TABLE 1 | Individual peak physiological responses.

| | Level | IWRF | Trial 1 | | Trial 2 | Trial 3 | | | | |
			HR (bpm)	$[L_a^-]_B$ (mmol/L)	HR(bpm)	Duration (min)	HR (bpm)	$[L_a^-]_B$ (mmol/L)	$\dot{V}o_2$ (L/min)	$\dot{V}o_2$ (ml/kg/min)
1	C6	0.5	126	5.6	129	5.83	122	4.2	1.03	18.2
2	C7	1	146	5.5	Not collected	6.66	115	5.8	0.85	17.9
3	C6	1.5	142	6.9	Not collected	16.66	125	4.4	1.45	21.0
4	C7	2	169	5.3	157	13.33	137	5.2	1.47	23.6
5	C7	2.5	172	6.4	171	15.00	178	4.6	2.30	33.7
6	C7	2.5	135	7.2	139	9.41	130	5.9	1.42	21.8
7	C7	2.5	165	8.8	169	9.25	127	5.6	1.87	27.3
8	C7	2.5	148	5.5	150	7.86	119	5.3	1.98	27.3
9	C6	2.5	147	7.5	154	4.83	119	4.1	1.82	18.9
MEAN			150*	6.5*	153*	9.87	130	5.1	1.57	23.3
SD			16	1.2	15	4.19	19	0.7	0.46	5.3

*Trial 1: 4 min field-based maximal exercise test; trial 2: 40 min field-based maximal exercise test; trial 3: maximal laboratory-based incremental wheelchair propulsion test on a treadmill; IWRF, International Wheelchair Rugby Federation; HR, heart rate; $[L_a^-]_B$, blood lactate concentration; $\dot{V}o_2$, oxygen uptake. *Significantly different from trial 3 ($p < 0.05$).*

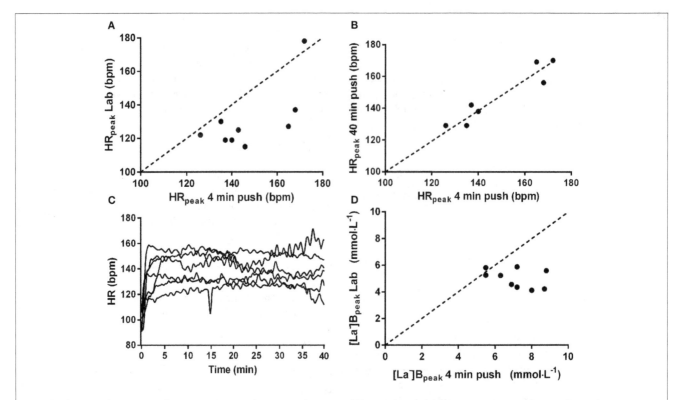

FIGURE 1 | Association between field- and laboratory-based peak heart rate (HR$_{peak}$; A). Association between HR$_{peak}$ during two different field-based assessments **(B)**. Individual HR responses to prolonged field-based exercise **(C)**. Associations between field- and laboratory based peak blood lactate concentration ([L$_a^-$]$_B$peak; **D)**.

deep inhalation. On a treadmill, this technique is impossible to replicate as the wheelchair would roll to the back of the treadmill if pushing were to cease, thereby terminating the test. Thus, different push patterns may have been responsible for the lower cardiometabolic responses during treadmill exercise. To our knowledge, no study has directly compared maximal push mechanics between laboratory- and field-based testing in tetraplegic athletes. In able-bodied individuals, recent research suggests that current treadmill wheelchair propulsion protocols are unable to accurately reproduce the forces applied during field-based (i.e., over ground) propulsion (Mason et al., 2014). It is not yet clear whether these findings translate to highly-trained athletes with cervical SCI. An interesting observation was that the heart rate in three athletes (#1, 5, and 6) was similar between field- and laboratory-based testing. It is unclear why this was the case for these three athletes only. One explanation could be that these three athletes utilize a push technique that can easily be replicated in both the laboratory and field conditions. The idea of "transferability" of different propulsion techniques between laboratory and field settings has to our knowledge never been investigated in elite tetraplegic athletes but may provide important insight as to why some athletes can achieve similar maximal exercise responses in both the laboratory and field settings whilst others cannot.

Lower laboratory-based HR responses may also be a consequence of the inferior metabolic demand of incremental laboratory exercise compared to high-intensity constant load

exercise. Increased acidosis associated with a higher blood lactate concentration in the field would be expected to drive greater peripheral and central chemoreceptor activation and augment central sympathetic outflow (Somers et al., 1989). In cervical SCI athletes with autonomic incomplete injuries, central sympathetic stimulation would elicit a direct and indirect (catecholaminergic) inotropic response. In autonomic complete athletes, it is possible that the sub-lesional sympathetic circuitry can still be activated from chemoreflexes via the pulmonary stretch receptors. Unfortunately, no studies have examined the interactions between chemoreceptor activation and vasomotor outflow after SCI. Moreover, while circulating catecholamines increase marginally during wheelchair ergometry in untrained cervical SCI (Schmid et al., 1998), no study has investigated the catecholaminergic response to field-based exercise. In our opinion, such studies are critical to advance our understanding of the physiological responses to exercise in athletes with cervical SCI.

The field-based measures of physiological performance reported herein are relatively crude, but are typical of those collected by researchers and/or sports physiologists during sports-specific field-based testing. We are yet to conduct field-based assessments of peak oxygen uptake using a portable metabolic cart. Such measures are the next step to confirm that peak cardiometabolic responses during laboratory-based exercise testing are indeed inferior to those obtained in response to field-based exercise testing. Nevertheless, we measured HR values that were considerably higher during both short- and long-duration field-based exercise compared to laboratory testing. Thus, future research should investigate why field-based exercise testing provides superior cardiometabolic responses (at least for most athletes) and seek to optimize maximal treadmill testing protocols. Until such studies are carried out we suggest that sports physiologists working in applied settings continue to use both laboratory and field-based testing and that the choice of test should be dictated by the question at hand as well as the availability of resources. Field-based maximal exercise testing provides superior external validity, the ability to accommodate large groups, and the free choice of push mechanics. Conversely, a laboratory-based exercise test allows for a more detailed physiological assessment under carefully controlled conditions with respect to protocol, temperature, and humidity.

CONSIDERATIONS

We chose to use laboratory-based wheelchair propulsion to investigate peak responses because it is the most externally valid laboratory modality and because peak responses are slightly higher during wheelchair propulsion than during other laboratory modalities such as arm-crank exercise (Gass and Camp, 1984). Our decision to increment grade only was based on previous research that reported no significant differences in peak responses between treadmill protocols which increment speed, gradient, or a combination of both (Hartung et al., 1993). Finally, our participants were highly motivated wheelchair rugby athletes who were well versed in maximal incremental exercise testing. We are confident therefore that the laboratory testing environment was conducive to eliciting peak responses

in the laboratory. That we measured similar HR$_{peak}$ values during both field tests suggests that higher values in the field are indeed a real phenomenon and not an anomaly. Moreover, the mean values reported in the present study are almost identical to our previous field-based assessments of Paralympic hand-cyclists with cervical SCI (West et al., 2015). Finally, environmental conditions were similar between Trial 1 and 3 (not noted for Trial 2), suggesting differences in environmental conditions do not explain between-test differences in physiological responses. Thus, we are confident that the data presented herein represent true differences in physiological responses between laboratory- and field-based exercise testing.

CONCLUDING REMARKS

The present data imply that peak physiological indices measured in response to maximal incremental exercise testing in the laboratory using current protocols may not represent true maximal responses for athletes with tetraplegia. We suggest that future studies should investigate why field-based exercise testing provides superior cardiometabolic responses and seek to optimize maximal treadmill testing protocols to probe true peak responses in elite athletes with cervical SCI.

ACKNOWLEDGMENTS

The authors thank the Great Britain Wheelchair Rugby squad for participating in our research.

REFERENCES

Coutts, K. D., Rhodes, E. C., and McKenzie, D. C. (1983). Maximal exercise responses of tetraplegics and paraplegics. *J. Appl. Physiol.* 55, 479–482.

Currie, K. D., West, C. R., Hubli, M., Gee, C. M., and Krassioukov, A. V. (2015). Peak heart rates and sympathetic function in tetraplegic nonathletes and athletes. *Med. Sci. Sports Exerc.* 47, 1259–1264. doi: 10.1249/MSS.0000000000000514

Figoni, S. F. (1993). Exercise responses and quadriplegia. *Med. Sci. Sports Exerc.* 25, 433–441. doi: 10.1249/00005768-199304000-00005

Gass, G. C., and Camp, E. M. (1984). The maximum physiological responses during incremental wheelchair and arm cranking exercise in male paraplegics. *Med. Sci. Sports Exerc.* 16, 355–359. doi: 10.1249/00005768-198408000-00006

Goosey-Tolfrey, V. (2010). Supporting the paralympic athlete: focus on wheeled sports. *Disabil. Rehabil.* 32, 2237–2243. doi: 10.3109/09638288.2010.491577

Hartung, G. H., Lally, D. A., and Blancq, R. J. (1993). Comparison of treadmill exercise testing protocols for wheelchair users. *Eur. J. Appl. Physiol. Occup. Physiol.* 66, 362–365. doi: 10.1007/BF00237783

Hopman, M. T., Dueck, C., Monroe, M., Philips, W. T., and Skinner, J. S. (1998). Limits to maximal performance in individuals with spinal cord injury. *Int. J. Sports Med.* 19, 98–103. doi: 10.1055/s-2007-971889

Lasko-McCarthey, P., and Davis, J. (1991). Effect of work rate increment on peak oxygen uptake during wheelchair ergometry in men with quadriplegia. *Eur. J. Appl. Physiol. Occup. Physiol.* 63, 349–353. doi: 10.1007/bf00364461

Leicht, C. A., Griggs, K. E., Lavin, J., Tolfrey, K., and Goosey-Tolfrey, V. L. (2014). Blood lactate and ventilatory thresholds in wheelchair athletes with tetraplegia and paraplegia. *Eur. J. Appl. Physiol.* 114, 1635–1643. doi: 10.1007/s00421-014-2886-x

Leicht, C. A., Tolfrey, K., Lenton, J. P., Bishop, N. C., and Goosey-Tolfrey, V. L. (2013). The verification phase and reliability of physiological parameters in peak testing of elite wheelchair athletes. *Eur. J. Appl. Physiol.* 113, 337–345. doi: 10.1007/s00421-012-2441-6

Mason, B., Lenton, J., Leicht, C., and Goosey-Tolfrey, V. (2014). A physiological and biomechanical comparison of over-ground, treadmill and ergometer wheelchair propulsion. *J. Sports Sci.* 32, 78–91. doi: 10.1080/02640414.2013.807350

Paulson, T. A., Goosey-Tolfrey, V. L., Lenton, J. P., Leicht, C. A., and Bishop, N. C. (2013). Spinal cord injury level and the circulating cytokine response to strenuous exercise. *Med. Sci. Sports Exerc.* 45, 1649–1655. doi: 10.1249/MSS.0b013e31828f9bbb

Schmid, A., Huonker, M., Barturen, J. M., Stahl, F., Schmidt-Trucksäss, A., König, D., et al. (1998). Catecholamines, heart rate, and oxygen uptake during exercise in persons with spinal cord injury. *J. Appl. Physiol.* 85, 635–641.

Somers, V. K., Mark, A. L., Zavala, D. C., and Abboud, F. M. (1989). Contrasting effects of hypoxia and hypercapnia on ventilation and sympathetic activity in humans. *J. Appl. Physiol.* 67, 2101–2106.

West, C. R., Campbell, I. G., Goosey-Tolfrey, V. L., Mason, B. S., and Romer, L. M. (2014b). Effects of abdominal binding on field-based exercise responses in Paralympic athletes with cervical spinal cord injury. *J. Sci. Med. Sport* 17, 351–355. doi: 10.1016/j.jsams.2013.06.001

West, C. R., Gee, C. M., Voss, C., Hubli, M., Currie, K. D., Schmid, J., et al. (2015). Cardiovascular control, autonomic function, and elite endurance performance in spinal cord injury. *Scand. J. Med. Sci. Sports.* 25, 476–485. doi: 10.1111/sms.12308

West, C. R., Goosey-Tolfrey, V. L., Campbell, I. G., and Romer, L. M. (2014a). Effect of abdominal binding on respiratory mechanics during exercise in athletes with cervical spinal cord injury. *J. Appl. Physiol.* 117, 36–45. doi: 10.1152/japplphysiol.00218.2014

West, C. R., Romer, L. M., and Krassioukov, A. (2013). Autonomic function and exercise performance in elite athletes with cervical spinal cord injury. *Med. Sci. Sports Exerc.* 45, 261–267. doi: 10.1249/MSS.0b013e31826 f5099

Wicks, J. R., Oldridge, N. B., Cameron, B. J., and Jones, N. L. (1983). Arm cranking and wheelchair ergometry in elite spinal cord-injured athletes. *Med. Sci. Sports Exerc.* 15, 224–231. doi: 10.1249/00005768-198315030-00008

Conflict of Interest Statement: The authors declare that the research was conducted in the absence of any commercial or financial relationships that could be construed as a potential conflict of interest.

22

Hot and Hypoxic Environments Inhibit Simulated Soccer Performance and Exacerbate Performance Decrements When Combined

Jeffrey W. F. Aldous[1], Bryna C. R. Chrismas[2], Ibrahim Akubat[3], Ben Dascombe[4], Grant Abt[5] and Lee Taylor[6,1]*

[1] Department of Sport Science and Physical Activity, Institute of Sport and Physical Activity Research, University of Bedfordshire, Bedford, UK, [2] Sport Science Program, College of Arts and Sciences, Qatar University, Doha, Qatar, [3] Department of Physical Education and Sports Studies, Newman University, Birmingham, UK, [4] Department of Rehabilitation, Nutrition and Sport, School of Allied Health, La Trobe University, Melbourne, VIC, Australia, [5] Department of Sport, Health and Exercise Science, The University of Hull, Hull, UK, [6] ASPETAR, Qatar Orthopedic and Sports Medicine Hospital, Athlete Health and Performance Research Centre, Aspire Zone, Doha, Qatar

Edited by:
Barbara Morgan,
University of Wisconsin-Madison, USA

Reviewed by:
Noah J. Marcus,
Des Moines University, USA
Jerome A. Dempsey,
University of Wisconsin-Madison, USA

*Correspondence:
Lee Taylor
lee.taylor@aspetar.com

The effects of heat and/or hypoxia have been well-documented in match-play data. However, large match-to-match variation for key physical performance measures makes environmental inferences difficult to ascertain from soccer match-play. Therefore, the present study aims to investigate the hot (HOT), hypoxic (HYP), and hot-hypoxic (HH) mediated-decrements during a non-motorized treadmill based soccer-specific simulation. Twelve male University soccer players completed three familiarization sessions and four randomized crossover experimental trials of the intermittent Soccer Performance Test (iSPT) in normoxic-temperate (CON: 18°C 50% rH), HOT (30°C; 50% rH), HYP (1000 m; 18°C 50% rH), and HH (1000 m; 30°C; 50% rH). Physical performance and its performance decrements, body temperatures (rectal, skin, and estimated muscle temperature), heart rate (HR), arterial blood oxygen saturation (S_aO_2), perceived exertion, thermal sensation (TS), body mass changes, blood lactate, and plasma volume were all measured. Performance decrements were similar in HOT and HYP [Total Distance (−4%), High-speed distance (∼−8%), and variable run distance (∼−12%) covered] and exacerbated in HH [total distance (−9%), high-speed distance (−15%), and variable run distance (−15%)] compared to CON. Peak sprint speed, was 4% greater in HOT compared with CON and HYP and 7% greater in HH. Sprint distance covered was unchanged ($p > 0.05$) in HOT and HYP and only decreased in HH (−8%) compared with CON. Body mass (−2%), temperatures (+2–5%), and TS (+18%) were altered in HOT. Furthermore, S_aO_2 (−8%) and HR (+3%) were changed in HYP. Similar changes in body mass and temperatures, HR, TS, and S_aO_2 were evident in HH to HOT and HYP, however, blood lactate ($p < 0.001$) and plasma volume ($p < 0.001$) were only significantly altered in HH. Perceived exertion was elevated ($p < 0.05$) by 7% in all conditions compared with CON. Regression analysis identified that absolute TS and absolute rise in skin and estimated muscle temperature ($r = 0.82$, $r = 0.84$

$r = 0.82$, respectively; $p < 0.05$) predicted the hot-mediated-decrements in HOT. The hot, hypoxic, and hot-hypoxic environments impaired physical performance during iSPT. Future interventions should address the increases in TS and body temperatures, to attenuate these decrements on soccer performance.

Keywords: decrements, football, hot, hypoxia, physical, physiological

INTRODUCTION

Environmental stress in elite soccer is an important consideration for both practitioners and policy makers (Taylor and Rollo, 2014). Indeed, eight of the last 19 Fédération Internationale de Football Association (FIFA) World Cups were hosted by countries located at either low (500–2000 m) or moderate (2001–3000m) altitudes (e.g., 2010 FIFA World Cup, South Africa, 1200–1700 m; Bartsch et al., 2008; Billaut and Aughey, 2013). Specific to the Union of European Football Associations (UEFA) region, fixtures are often played above sea level (e.g., Molde, Norway, 1000 m) and/or in hot environments (e.g., Madrid, Spain, 30°C—Taylor and Rollo, 2014). In relation to heat-stress, temperatures often exceeded 30°C (Maximum: 35°C) in the 2014 FIFA World Cup hosted by Brazil (Nassis et al., 2015). Furthermore, combinations of both high temperature and altitude (hypoxia) can be experienced during elite soccer match-play (e.g., Saint-Etienne, France, 30°C; 1000 m).

Soccer match-play data indicates a decline in physical performance in both heat (Ekblom, 1986; Mohr et al., 2010, 2012; Özgünen et al., 2010) and hypoxia (Aughey et al., 2013; Nassis, 2013; Garvican et al., 2014; Buchheit et al., 2015) due to a complex interplay between peripheral, central and perceptual mechanisms (Nybo and Secher, 2004; Billaut and Aughey, 2013; Goodall et al., 2014; Nybo et al., 2014). However, the combined permutations of heat and hypoxia during match-play have not been investigated, although logically their combination would likely exacerbate physical performance decrements. At 43°C (Mohr et al., 2012), total distance (−7%), and high-speed distance (−26%) covered are reduced, with these changes being attributed to a multitude of proposed mechanisms including increasing body temperatures (Nybo et al., 2014). Furthermore, alterations in tactical behavior (e.g., reduced pressing of the ball) has meant that sprint distance covered is unchanged and peak sprint speed is enhanced during heat-situated soccer match-play (Özgünen et al., 2010; Mohr et al., 2012; Taylor and Rollo, 2014; Flouris and Schlader, 2015). Soccer match-play at low altitudes [1200—(Nassis, 2013); 1600 m—(Garvican et al., 2014) above sea level] leads to a decline in total distance (3.1%) and high-speed distance (15%) covered as recovery from high-speed intermittent activity is prolonged, due to the onset of exercise-induced-arterial-hypoxemia caused by a reduction in partial pressure of oxygen within the atmosphere (Billaut and Aughey, 2013). However, sprint performance is enhanced in hypoxia due to improved aerodynamics and flight time of an athlete through the air (Levine et al., 2008), highlighting that different components of soccer performance (e.g., sprint performance) are likely to respond differently within heat and/or hypoxia (Mohr et al., 2012).

Soccer match-play data, including key physical performance measures (e.g., high-speed distance covered), shows high match-to-match variation due to a plethora of match factors, such as tactics, score, opposition, etc. (Gregson et al., 2010). This variability in key physical performance measures may be exacerbated in both heat (Mohr et al., 2010, 2012; Özgünen et al., 2010; Nassis et al., 2015) and hypoxia (Aughey et al., 2013; Nassis, 2013; Garvican et al., 2014; Buchheit et al., 2015) resulting in an altered "pacing strategy" and exercise intensity (Taylor and Rollo, 2014). Recently, Gregson et al. (2010) suggested that to obtain meaningful inferences from a soccer match-play research design, a minimum sample size of 80 players would be required. Consequently, it appears that the majority of match-play based studies examining environmental influences on soccer performance are underpowered (<25 participants; Özgünen et al., 2010; Mohr et al., 2012; Aughey et al., 2013; Garvican et al., 2014; Buchheit et al., 2015), compared to the sample size ($n = 80$) proposed by Gregson et al. (2010). Only two studies have utilized an appropriate sample size ($>n = 80$) to assess the performance decrements associated with soccer match-play in hypoxia (Nassis, 2013) and heat (Nassis et al., 2015) during the 2010 and 2014 FIFA World Cup's, respectively. In particular, Nassis et al. (2015) revealed that in hot environments, players preserved key physical performance measures (e.g., peak sprint speed) that are associated with the match outcome (Faude et al., 2012), by reducing the number of sprints and high-speed efforts performed during a match. However, irrespective of the environment, players are likely to modulate their physical performance to avoid an earlier onset of fatigue during a tournament (Dellal et al., 2013), making environmental-mediated-inferences difficult to ascertain from the international tournaments data (Nassis, 2013; Nassis et al., 2015).

Recent reviews (Taylor and Rollo, 2014; Roelands et al., 2015) have recommended a solution to this "sample size issue" is to utilize an individualized, valid and reliable soccer-specific simulation to quantify environmentally-mediated performance decrements with greater experimental control. Aldous et al. (2014) demonstrated that the intermittent Soccer Performance Test (iSPT) is a valid, reliable and individualized (i.e., individualized speed thresholds) laboratory and non-motorized treadmill (NMT) based soccer-specific simulation; which can ascertain changes in soccer performance more robustly compared to match-play data with limited sample sizes. By utilizing iSPT, changes in soccer performance between the identified conditions (e.g., hot and/or hypoxic) can be determined in a controlled environment, minimizing match factors (Gregson et al., 2010) and the within game (Mohr et al., 2005, 2010) and tournament (Dellal et al., 2013) enforced pacing strategies (Nybo et al., 2014; Périard and Racinais, 2015; Roelands et al., 2015), unlike previous environmentally-situated match-play derived data (Mohr et al., 2012; Garvican et al., 2014).

Therefore, the aim of this study was to utilize the iSPT to reliably quantify soccer performance in hot (HOT), hypoxic (HYP), and hot-hypoxic (HH) environments (Aldous et al., 2014). The first experimental hypothesis was that physiological strain would be increased in HOT, HYP, and HH compared with CON, causing a significant reduction in physical performance in HOT, HYP, and HH. The second experimental hypothesis expected the hot and hypoxic environments to enhance sprint performance in HOT and HYP. Finally, the third experimental hypothesis was that in HH, physiological strain would be exacerbated compared with HOT and HYP causing a larger decline in physical performance.

METHODS

Participants and Experimental Controls

Twelve male, University level soccer players [median (min-max) age = 23 (18–33) y; mass = 77 (67–93) kg; height = 1.81 (1.68–1.95) m; mean ± SD $\dot{V}O_{2max}$ = 57 ± 2 mL·kg^{-1}·min^{-1}] volunteered for this study. An a priori power calculation (G∗Power 3) was used to determine the number of participants required for this experiment (n = 12) with an alpha level of 0.05 and a statistical power of 99%, using data [(high-speed distance covered)—minimum worthwhile effect = 5 m; SD = 50] from Aldous et al. (2014). All participants were members of the University of Bedfordshire Soccer team who trained at least two times per week and played at least one full 90 min match per week. The study was approved by the University of Bedfordshire Ethics Committee, and conformed to the declaration of Helsinki. All participants were fully informed of the risks associated with this study before they gave full written consent to take part in testing. Participants standardized their food and water consumption (Sawka et al., 2007) and abstained from alcohol, cigarettes, caffeine, and strenuous exercise at least 48 h prior to testing and maintained their normal diet prior to and during the testing sessions (in line with Taylor et al., 2014). Participants refrained from supplementation of ergogenic aids throughout the study and had not been exposed to >30°C and/or >1000 m above sea level three months prior to this study (Taylor et al., 2010). Adherence was assessed by questionnaire, with no violations seen for these control parameters.

Participants were instructed to drink 2–3 L of water 24 h prior to all laboratory visits (Sawka et al., 2007; Taylor et al., 2012) as prior to each experimental trial hydration status was assessed via urine osmolality (Atago-Vitech-Scientific, Pocket-PAL-OSMO, HaB-Direct, Southam). Euhydration was deemed when urine osmolality was below 600 mOsm/l (Hillman et al., 2013). Testing times were held constant for individuals due to the effects of circadian variation upon rectal temperature (T_{re}; Racinais et al., 2012) and physical performance (Drust et al., 2005).

Study Design

All familiarization (FAM), peak speed assessments (PSA), and iSPTs were completed on the same NMT (Force 3.0, Woodway, Cranlea, Birmingham).

Visit 1–3 (FAM$_{1-3}$ and PSA)

The three FAM sessions and one PSA session were completed as per Aldous et al. (2014). FAM$_{1-3}$ robustly familiarized [as demonstrated by Aldous et al. (2014)] participants to iSPT and the running mechanics of NMT locomotion, which compared to "free" running and motorized treadmill running has notable differences (Lakomy, 1987). Familiarized participants (i.e., post FAM$_{1-3}$) subsequently (1 h post-FAM) completed a PSA, which identified each participant's familiarized peak sprint speed. The PSA derived of four 6 s maximal sprints over a 4 min period with equal rest (1 min) between sprints to allow adequate recovery time. For each participant, the peak sprint speed was defined as the fastest speed recorded during the PSA. The peak sprint speed was then utilized to individualize all speed thresholds during iSPT to each participant (Aldous et al., 2014; Coull et al., 2015). So for example, a participant with a peak sprint speed of 24 km·h^{-1}, would have the following speeds to achieve for each movement category across iSPT; stand (0 km·h^{-1}), walk (5 km·h^{-1}), jog (8 km·h^{-1}), run (12 km·h^{-1}), fast run (14 km·h^{-1}), and sprint (24 km·h^{-1}). The percentage of peak sprint, ascertained from the PSA, and how this determines the required speed for each movement category across iSPT is detailed in **Table 1**. These speed thresholds determined the speed (target speed/threshold) participants had to obtain for each movement type (stand, walk, jog, run, fast run, and sprint). The frequency and distribution of these movement types (**Table 1**) were based upon the findings of previous match-play data, and were shown by Aldous et al. (2014) to be valid and reliable. No other physical performance measures were calculated during the FAM and PSA sessions. *Visits 4-7*: A randomized-controlled design was then used with each participant completing four experimental trials of iSPT: CON [0 m; 18°C, 50% Relative Humidity (rH)], HOT (30°C; 50% rH), HYP (1000 m; 18°C 50% rH), and HH (1000 m; 30°C 50% rH). All experimental trials were separated by 7 d and completed within a controlled laboratory environment (Flower-House, Farm-House, Two-Wests and Elliot, Chesterfield) where hot and hypoxic exposures were administered using a portable heater (Bio-Green, Arkansas-3000, Hampshire) and an adjustable hypoxicator (Everest-Summit-II, The Altitude Centre, UK), respectively. The adjustable hypoxicator mask was worn in

TABLE 1 | The percentage of intensity, frequency, and total time spent at each movement category during iSPT (obtained from Aldous et al., 2014).

Movement Category	% of PSS	Frequency	Total Time (s)	Total Time (%)
Stand	0	240	1920	17.8
Walk	20	456	3936	36.4
Jog	35	300	2592	24.0
Run	50	192	1248	11.6
Fast run	60	72	384	3.6
Variable run	Unset	48	288	2.7
Sprint	100	72	432	4.0
Total	—	690	5400	100

PSS, Peak Sprint Speed; s, seconds; %, Percentage.

TABLE 2 | The environmental conditions simulated during this study.

Environmental Condition	Temperature (°C)	rH (%)	Altitude (m)
CON	18.1 ± 0.6	50.8 ± 0.6	0 0 ± 0.0
HOT	30.3 ± 0.5	50.3 ± 0.3	0 0 ± 0.0
HYP	18.2 ± 0.9	50.3 ± 0.6	1.001 ± 10.9
HH	30.5 ± 0.8	50.5 ± 3.6	1.003 ± 10.5

CON, Normoxic-Temperate; HH, Hot-Hypoxic; HOT, Hot; HYP, Hypoxic.

all four experimental trials. Environmental temperature, rH and simulated altitude were measured continuously during all experimental trials (**Table 2**). Prior to completing iSPT, all participants completed a 10 min warm up on the NMT at a speed of 8 km·h^{-1} and including 2 brief sprints (<4 s), as per Oliver et al. (2007). The 10 min warm up took place in the subsequent environment each experimental condition was performed in.

Intermittent Soccer Performance Test

The iSPT consisted of two 45 min halves comprised of three identical 15 min intermittent exercise blocks (**Figure 1**; Aldous et al., 2014), utilizing the movement categories detailed previously (stand, walk, jog, run, fast run, variable run, and sprint). The frequency and durations of these movement categories (and how their respective target speeds/thresholds are calculated) across the iSPT are provided in **Table 1** with an example provided within the previous section. Throughout each 15 min block for all target speeds apart from the variable run, participants interacted with a computer program (Innervation, Pacer Performance System Software, Innervation, Pacer Performance System Software, Lismore, Australia) by following a red line on the screen (which displayed their target speed) and their current (actual) speed (green line). If a discrepancy between target and current speed (i.e., the lines did not closely overlap) was evident participants had to run more quickly, or slowly, accordingly, to realign the lines. Participants were instructed to match their current speed with the target speed as closely as possible throughout iSPT for all target speeds related to each movement type (stand, walk, jog, run, fast run, and sprint) apart from the variable run. Audio cues specific to each movement category (e.g., jog) were also presented. Before each change in speed, three audible tones were played, which were followed by an audible command to inform the subject of the upcoming activity (e.g., "beep," "beep," "beep," "run"). Four self-selected high-speed runs (variable run: 13–14th min of each 15-min block; **Figure 1**) were included, where the participant was instructed to cover as much distance as possible without sprinting.

Physical Performance Measurements

Data for total distance covered was comprised from all movement categories and was calculated between both halves and conditions. High-speed, variable run, and sprint distance covered was computed for each half and entire condition as well as the total amount performed in each 15 min block (Aldous et al., 2014). Peak sprint speed was only obtained as the fastest

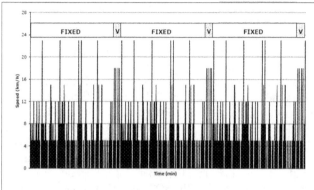

FIGURE 1 | The 45-min activity profile of iSPT for a participant with a peak speed of 23 km·h^{-1} (obtained from Aldous et al., 2014).

speed seen for each 15 min block. Performance decrements for all physical performance measurements were calculated in distance covered (m) and percentage (%) between conditions halves and 15 min blocks.

Physiological Measurements

Prior to the FAM, height (cm) was measured using a Holtain Stationmaster (Stadiometer, Harpenden, HAR 98.602, Holtain). Body Mass (kg) was also measured pre- and post-iSPT using digital scales (Tanita, BWB0800, Allied Weighing) to account for the fluid loss for each player, with the 500 mL of water players consumed during the half-time break accounted for. Heart rate (HR) was recorded beat-by-beat and averaged every 1 min using a telemetric heart rate monitor (Polar, FS1, Polar Electro, Oy). Fingertip blood samples were taken to assess blood lactate (Bla; YSI, 2500 stat plus, YSI) during walking or standing phases of the iSPT at 12, 27, and 45 min of each half (Aldous et al., 2014). All Haematocrit (Hct) samples was collected into heparinised capillary tubes (Hawksley & Sons Ltd, UK) and then centrifuged at 5000 RPM for 3 min (Hawksely, Micro Haematocrit centrifuge, Hawksley & Sons Ltd, UK). The Hct levels were read from the Haematocrit reader (Hawksley, UK). Hemoglobin (Hb) concentration was then collected via micro-cuvettes (Hemocue, Hb 201, Hemocue Ltd, Sweden) and then measured using a B-Hemoglobin photometer (Hemocue, Hb 201$^+$, Hemocue Ltd, Sweden).

Changes in blood plasma volume (%ΔPV) both within/between tests were then estimated from Hb and Hct using the following equation (Dill and Costill, 1974):

$$\%\Delta PV = [(Hb_{preex}/Hb_{postex}) \times [(100 - Hct_{postex})/ (100 - Hct_{preex})] - 1] \times 100$$

Where ΔPV is percent change of PV, subscript a, is pre-iSPT; and subscript b, is post-iSPT.

A single-use rectal thermistor (Henleys, 400H, Henleys Medical, Welwyn Garden City) was used to measure rectal temperature (T_{re}) from a depth of 10 cm past the anal sphincter and read by a connected data logger (Measurement, 4600, Henley-medical, Welwyn Garden City). Skin thermistors (Grant,

EUS-U-VS5-0, Wessex-Power, Dorset) were attached to the right side of the body at the center of the pectoralis major, biceps brachi, rectus femoris, and gastrocnemius to measure skin temperature (T_{sk}) with data recorded separately to a data logger (Eltek/Squirrel, Squirrel Series/model 451, Wessex Power, Dorset).

The following equation was used to calculate T_{sk} (Ramanathan, 1964).

$$T_{sk} = 0.3(T_{chest} + T_{arm}) + 0.2(T_{thigh} + T_{calf})$$

Estimated muscle temperature (T_{mu}) was also calculated using the following equation (Racinais et al., 2005a):

$$T_{mu} = 1.02 \, x \, T_{sk} + 0.89$$

Arterial blood oxygen saturation (S_aO_2) was measured via a finger pulse oximeter (Onyx® II 9550, Nonin-Medical, USA) fixed upon the participant's index finger. All body temperature measures (T_{re}, T_{sk}, and T_{mu}), perceived exertion (RPE; Borg 6–20 scale; Borg, 1998) and thermal sensation (TS; 0–8 scale; Young et al., 1987) were collected in 15 min intervals.

Statistical Analysis

Normality of the observed data was assessed using quantile-quantile (Q—Q) plots and was deemed plausible in all instances with data presented as mean ± standard deviation (SD). Differences between condition, time, and condition x time for all physical and physiological measures were analyzed using linear mixed models (IBM-SPSS statistics for Windows, Version 21, Armonk, NY). This type of analysis was preferred as it (i) allows for missing data, (ii) can accurately model different covariate structures for repeated measures data, and (iii) can model between-subject variability (Vandenbogaerde and Hopkins, 2010; West et al., 2014). Where significance was obtained, Sidak post-hoc tests were used to locate significant pairs on all physical and physiological measures. A step down Hommel adjusted post-hoc pairwise comparisons was calculated for each physical and physiological measure if a significant main effect and/or interaction effect was present (Hommel, 1988). Two-tailed statistical significance was accepted at the $p =< 0.05$ level. The percentage changes between all physical performance measures are also reported and 95% CI presented where necessary. The most appropriate model was chosen using the smallest Hurvich and Tsai's criterion (AICC) in accordance with the principal of parsimony. Second, normality and homogeneity of variance of the residuals were checked using Q—Q plots and scatter plots, respectively, and deemed plausible in each instance. A Stepwise multiple linear regression analysis for each condition was performed in order to investigate which of the "physiological responses" (e.g., Body temperatures, Subjective and Physiological measures) were able to predict the environmentally-induced-decrements in physical performance (e.g., total distance, high-speed distance, sprint distance, and sprint distance covered).

RESULTS

Physical Performance
Overall and Between Halves

A significant main effect for condition ($F = 16.5; p < 0.001$), time ($F = 202.8; p < 0.001$), and an interaction effect for condition x time ($F = 3.6; p = 0.03$) was observed for total distance covered (**Figure 2**). Total distance covered was reduced by 4% in HOT (mean difference = 321 ± 131 m, $p = 0.001$, 95% CI: 65–256 m) and HYP (mean difference = 324 ± 136 m, $p = 0.004$, 95% CI: 44–282 m), and by 9% in HH (mean difference = 756 ± 142 m, $p < 0.001$, 95% CI: 196–560 m), compared to CON. A 5% reduction in total distance covered in HH compared to HOT (mean difference = 431 ± 132 m, $p = 0.01$, 95% CI: 41–395 m) and HYP (mean difference = 431 ± 132 m, $p = 0.01$, 95% CI: 41–395 m) was also evident. Between halves, the performance decrements were greater in HH (4%, mean difference = 164 ± 60 m, $p < 0.001$, 95% CI: 126–202 m), HYP (3%, mean difference = 101 ± 66 m, $p < 0.001$, 95% CI: 59–143 m), and HOT (2%, mean difference = 120 ± 45 m, $p < 0.001$, 95% CI: 91–148 m) compared with CON (1%, mean difference = 81 ± 66 m $p = 0.001$, 95% CI: 39–123 m). Furthermore, total distance covered was 3% (1st half) and 4% (2nd half) greater in CON compared to HOT (1st half: mean difference = 141 ± 53 m $p = 0.007$, 95% CI: 33–249 m, 2nd half: $p = 0.001$, 95% CI: 88–272 m) and HYP (1st half: mean difference = 152 ± 32 m $p = 0.006$, 95% CI: 34–271 m; 2nd half: $p = 0.006$, 95% CI: 41–305 m). Performance decrements in total distance covered were observed in HH compared to CON during the 1st (−8%, mean difference = 336 ± 32 m, $p < 0.001$, 95% CI: 144–529 m) and 2nd half (−10%, mean difference = 420 ± 63 m, $p < 0.001$, 95% CI: 242–597 m). A 4 and 6% reduction in total distance covered was also observed in the 1st and 2nd half in HH compared to HOT (1st half: mean difference = 184 ± 43 m, $p = 0.04$, 95% CI: 10–380 m; 2nd half: mean difference = 240 ± 32 m, $p = 0.004$, 95% CI: 68–412 m) and HYP (1st half: mean difference = 185 ± 33 m, $p = 0.04$, 95% CI: 10–381 m; 2nd half: mean difference = 243 ± 39 m, $p = 0.04$, 95% CI: 73–420 m), respectively (**Figure 2**).

A significant main effect for condition ($F = 39.1; p < 0.001$), time ($F = 22.1; p < 0.001$), and an interaction effect ($F = 3.1; p = 0.04$) was observed for high-speed distance covered (**Figure 2**). High-speed distance covered was reduced in HOT (−7%, mean difference = 160 ± 21 m, $p = 0.001$, 95% CI: 16–78 m), HYP (−9%, mean difference = 203 ± 32 m, $p < 0.001$, 95% CI: 62–81 m), and HH (−15%, mean difference = 340 ± 43 m, $p <0.001$, 95% CI: 91–152 m) compared to CON. An 8% decrement in high-speed distance covered was observed in HH compared to HOT (mean difference = 180 ± 36 m, $p < 0.001$, 95% CI: 44–105 m) and HYP (mean difference = 182 ± 38 m, $p < 0.001$, 95% CI: 28–89 m). The performance decrements between halves was greater in HH (−6%, mean difference = 60 ± 30 m, $p < 0.001$, 95% CI: 126–202 m), HYP (−4%, mean difference = 46 ± 33 m, $p = 0.003$, 95% CI: 59–143 m), and HOT (−4%, mean difference = 48 ± 22 m, $p < 0.001$, 95% CI: 91–148 m) compared with CON (−3%, mean difference = 39 ± 16 m, $p < 0.001$, 95% CI: 39–123 m). Compared to CON, high-speed distance covered was reduced during the 1st half in HOT (−6%, mean difference =

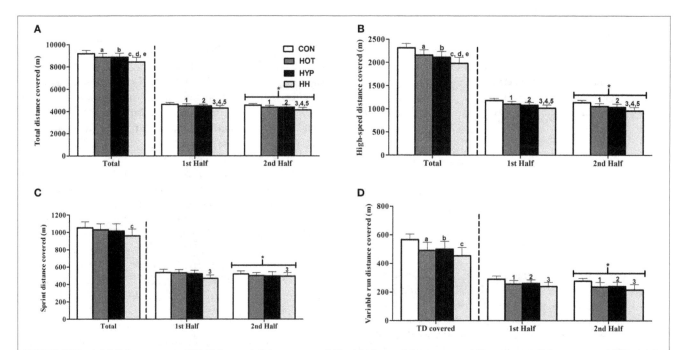

FIGURE 2 | The total distance covered (A), high-speed distance covered (B) variable run distance covered (C) and sprint distance covered (D) in total and in each half at CON, HOT, HYP, and HH. Total, high-speed and variable run distance covered were significantly reduced ($p < 0.05$) in both halves of HOT and HYP compared with CON. These decrements for total and high-speed distance covered were exacerbated in HH compared with HOT and HYP. Sprint distance was significantly reduced ($p < 0.05$) in both halves of HH compared with CON. *Significant difference from the first half;[a]Significant difference between CON and HOT ($p < 0.05$); [b]Significant difference between CON and HYP ($p < 0.05$); [c]Significant difference between CON and HH ($p < 0.05$); [d]Significant difference between HOT and HH ($p < 0.05$); [e]Significant difference between HYP and HH ($p < 0.05$);[1]Significant difference between halves in CON and HOT; [2]Significant difference between halves in CON and HYP; [3]Significant difference between halves in CON and HH [4]Significant difference between halves in HOT and HH; [5]Significant between halves in HYP and HH.

76 ± 36 m, $p = 0.002$, 95% CI: 21–86 m), HYP (−8%, mean difference = 98 ± 64 m, $p < 0.001$, 95% CI: 23–110 m), and HH (−14%, mean difference = 160 ± 58 m, $p < 0.001$, 95% CI: 78–164 m). The high-speed distance covered was also reduced in the 2nd half in HOT (−7%, mean difference = 84 ± 58 m, $p = 0.001$, 95% CI: 7–94 m), HYP (−9%, mean difference = 105 ± 48 m, $p = 0.001$, 95% CI: 41–305 m), and HH (−16%, mean difference = 180 ± 68 m, $p < 0.001$, 95% CI: 78–165 m) compared to CON. Furthermore, a reduction in high-speed distance covered was evident at HH compared to HOT during the 1st (−8%, mean difference = 84 ± 47 m, $p = 0.009$, 95% CI: 35–121 m) and 2nd (−6%, mean difference = 96 ± 54 m, $p = 0.009$, 95% CI: 28–114 m) half. A decrement in high-speed distance covered was observed at HH compared to HYP during the 1st (−9%, mean difference = 61 ± 46 m, $p = 0.007$, 95% CI: 19–106 m) and 2nd (−7%, mean difference = 75 ± 54 m, $p = 0.007$, 95% CI: 12–98 m) half (**Figure 2**).

There was a significant main effect for condition ($F = 4.8$; $p = 0.01$), time ($F = 92.6$; $p < 0.001$), and an interaction effect ($F = 3.7$; $p = 0.03$) for sprint distance covered (**Figure 2**). The sprint distance covered was reduced in HH compared with CON (−8%, mean difference = 93 ± 36 m, $p = 0.009$, 95% CI: 9–83 m) and HOT (−7%, mean difference = 78 ± 46 m, $p = 0.04$, 95% CI: 7–69 m). The performance decrements between halves was greater in HH (−5%, mean difference = 24 ± 19 m, $p = 0.001$, 95% CI: 12–36 m), HYP (−5%, mean difference = 26 ± 24 m, $p = 0.003$,

95% CI: 11–41 m), and HOT (−6%, mean difference = 30 ± 17 m, $p < 0.001$, 95% CI: 20–41 m) compared with CON (−3%, mean difference = 15 ± 9 m, $p < 0.001$, 95% CI: 9–21 m). In CON, the sprint distance covered was greater in both halves (1st: −8%, mean difference = 38 ± 25 m, $p = 0.04$, 95% CI: 1.9, 81.5 m; 2nd: −10%, mean difference = 51 ± 35 m, $p = 0.003$, 95% CI: 14.2, 87.8 m) compared to HH (**Figure 2**).

There was a significant main effect for condition ($F = 28.9$; $p < 0.001$), time ($F = 229.9$; $p < 0.001$), and interaction effect ($F = 5.8$; $p = 0.008$) for variable run distance covered (**Figure 2**). The variable run distance covered was greater in CON compared with HOT (−13%, mean difference = 74 ± 24 m, $p < 0.001$, 95% CI: 22–53 m), HYP (−12%, mean difference = 65 ± 35 m, $p < 0.001$, 95% CI: 17–48 m), and HH (−15%, mean difference = 111 ± 37 m, $p < 0.001$, 95% CI: 34–78 m). The performance decrements between halves was greater in HH (−10%, mean difference = 24 ± 10 m, $p < 0.001$, 95% CI: 18–30 m), HYP (−8%, mean difference = 20 ± 10 m, $p < 0.001$, 95% CI: 14–27 m), and HOT (−7%, mean difference = 19 ± 7 m, $p < 0.001$, 95% CI: 14–23 m) compared with CON (−4%, mean difference = 12 ± 5 m, $p < 0.001$, 95% CI: 9–15 m). Variable run distance covered was greater in both halves of CON compared with HOT (1st: −10%, mean difference = 34 ± 30 m, $p < 0.001$, 95% CI: 20–48 m; 2nd: −15%, mean difference = 41 ± 38 m, $p < 0.001$, 95% CI: 22 59 m), HYP (1st: −9%, mean difference = 29 ± 23 m, $p < 0.001$, 95% CI: 14–43 m; 2nd: −13%, mean difference =

37 ± 25 m, $p < 0.001$, 95% CI: 18–55 m), and HH (1st: -17%, mean difference = 50 ± 35 m, $p < 0.001$, 95% CI: 28–72 m; 2nd: -22%, mean difference = 62 ± 31 m, $p < 0.001$, 95% CI: 38–89 m; **Figure 2**).

Between 15 min Blocks

For high-speed distance covered, the performance decrements between the first and last 15 min blocks for CON (mean difference = 17 ± 6 m, $p = 0.01$, 95% CI: 3–21 m), HOT (mean difference = 31 ± 2 m, $p = 0.001$, 95% CI: 10–51 m), HYP (mean difference = 35 ± 7 m, $p = 0.001$, 95% CI: 11–55 m), and HH (mean difference = 49 ± 5 m, $p = 0.001$, 95% CI: 27–101 m) was -7, -8, -10, and -14%, respectively. The high-speed distance covered was reduced ($p < 0.05$) in all 15 min blocks in HOT [Range (%, m): -6 to -8%, 26–40 m], HYP [Range (%, m): -9 to -11%, 43–51 m], and HH [Range (%, m): -16 to -18%, 45–67 m] compared to CON (**Table 3**).

The performance decrements for sprint distance covered between the first and 15 min block for CON (mean difference = 12 ± 14 m $p = 0.007$, 95% CI: 2–23 m), HOT (mean difference = 18 ± 12 m $p = 0.005$, 95% CI: 1–13 m), HYP (mean difference = 18 ± 12 m, $p = 0.005$, 95% CI: 2–15 m), and HH (mean difference = 22 ± 11 m, $p < 0.001$, 95% CI: -6 to -25 m) was -7, -11, -10, and 13%, respectively. A 6% decrease in sprint distance covered was observed in the final 15 min in CON compared with the identical time point in HOT (mean difference = 10 ± 13 m, $p = 0.03$, 95% CI:

1–20 m) and HYP (mean difference = 12 ± 21 m $p = 0.03$, 95% CI: 1–24 m). In CON compared with HH, the sprint distance covered was also increased by 9% (18 ± 12 m, $p = 0.002$, 95% CI: 6–30 m) and 12% (25 ± 11 m, $p < 0.001$, 95% CI: 9–33 m) in the final two 15 min blocks, respectively (**Table 3**).

The performance decrements between the first and last 15 min block in variable run distance covered for CON (mean difference = 10 ± 8 m, $p = 0.04$, 95% CI: 1–7 m), HOT (mean difference = 14 ± 9 m, $p = 0.001$, 95% CI: 4–18 m), HYP (mean difference = 15 ± 21 m, $p = 0.04$, 95% CI: 1–21 m), and HH (mean difference = 17 ± 21 m $p = 0.04$, 95% CI: 1–17 m) was 7, 8, 10, and 14%, respectively. The variable run distance covered was reduced ($p < 0.05$) in all 15 min blocks by $\sim18\%$ [Range (%, m): 16–18%, 16–23 m] in HH compared to CON. An 8% decrease in variable run distance covered was seen in the final 15 min in CON compared with the identical time points in HOT (mean difference = 16 ± 12 m, $p = 0.009$, 95% CI: 2–17 m) and HYP (mean difference = 16 ± -13 m, $p = 0.01$, 95% CI: 2–17 m; **Table 3**).

The peak sprint speed reached in iSPT was 4% (3 ± 1 km·h^{-1}), 4% (4 ± 1 km·h^{-1}), and 7% (5 ± 1 km·h^{-1}) faster in all 15 min blocks HOT than in CON ($p = 0.03$, 95% CI: 1–2 km·h^{-1}), HYP ($p = 0.03$, 95% CI: 1–3 km·h^{-1}), and HH ($p = 0.03$, 95% CI: 1–3 km·h^{-1}), respectively. Furthermore, there was no significant difference ($p > 0.05$) in peak sprint speed between CON, HYP, and HH (**Table 3**).

TABLE 3 | The HSD, SD, VRD covered and PSS in 15 min blocks during CON, HOT, HYP, and HH.

	0–15 min	15–30 min	30–45 min	45–60 min	60–75 min	75–90 min
HIGH-SPEED DISTANCE COVERED (m)						
CON	400 ± 15	393 ± 17	384 ± 17	388 ± 14	378 ± 18	$373 \pm 21^{*}$
HOT	374 ± 22^{g}	366 ± 20^{g}	362 ± 19^{g}	359 ± 22^{g}	352 ± 23^{g}	$343 \pm 24^{*g}$
HYP	367 ± 20^{h}	362 ± 19^{h}	351 ± 24^{h}	355 ± 23^{h}	347 ± 24^{h}	$332 \pm 27^{*h}$
HH	355 ± 24^{i}	339 ± 26^{i}	324 ± 30^{i}	333 ± 19^{i}	319 ± 20^{i}	$306 \pm 29^{*i}$
SPRINT DISTANCE COVERED (m)						
CON	182 ± 13	177 ± 12	174 ± 12	174 ± 13	175 ± 11	$170 \pm 12^{*}$
HOT	178 ± 14	177 ± 13	174 ± 12	170 ± 11	169 ± 13	$160 \pm 11^{*g}$
HYP	176 ± 13	173 ± 13	171 ± 17	169 ± 17	167 ± 17	$158 \pm 15^{*h}$
HH	171 ± 16	164 ± 17	157 ± 14	162 ± 12	157 ± 12^{i}	$149 \pm 16^{*i}$
VARIABLE RUN DISTANCE COVERED (m)						
CON	100 ± 8	95 ± 7	94 ± 9	95 ± 7	92 ± 7	$90 \pm 7^{*}$
HOT	88 ± 8	85 ± 9	83 ± 11	84 ± 11	79 ± 10	$74 \pm 11^{*g}$
HYP	89 ± 8	86 ± 9	85 ± 9	86 ± 9	80 ± 11	$74 \pm 12^{*h}$
HH	84 ± 10^{i}	80 ± 11^{i}	76 ± 10^{i}	77 ± 11^{i}	71 ± 11^{i}	$67 \pm 10^{*i}$
PEAK SPRINT SPEED (km·h^{-1})						
CON	21.5 ± 1.2	21.1 ± 1.7	20.2 ± 1.6	19.8 ± 1.3	21.1 ± 1.7	21.5 ± 1.8
HOT	$22.1 \pm 1.5^{g,j,k}$	$23.2 \pm 1.4^{g,j,k}$	$23.2 \pm 1.5^{g,j,k}$	$21.1 \pm 1.2^{g,j,k}$	$22.1 \pm 1.3^{g,j,k}$	$22.6 \pm 1.4^{g,j,k}$
HYP	21.1 ± 1.3	22.1 ± 1.2	22.6 ± 1.8	20.7 ± 1.5	21.2 ± 1.5	21.5 ± 1.9
HH	20.4 ± 1.1	20.0 ± 1.6	19.8 ± 1.2	18.1 ± 1.1	19.2 ± 1.5	19.1 ± 2.0

*The HSD, SD, and VRD covered are presented as an overall distance covered during each 15 min period. The PSS is presented as the fastest speed recorded in each 15 min period. CON, Normoxic-Temperate; HH, Hot-Hypoxic; HOT, Hot; HSD, High Speed Distance; Hyp, Hypoxic; PSS, Peak Sprint Speed SD, Sprint Distance; VRD, Variable Run Distance; * Significant difference from the first 15 min; ^{g} Significant difference in 15 min block between CON and HOT; ^{h} Significant difference in 15 min block between CON and HYP; ^{i} Significant difference in 15 min block between CON and HH; ^{j} Significant difference in 15 min block between HOT and HYP; ^{k} Significant difference in 15 min block between HOT and HH.*

Body Temperature

T_{re}

There was a significant main effect for condition ($F = 4576.7$; $p < 0.001$), time ($F = 12.9$; $p < 0.001$), and an interaction effect ($F = 2.2$; $p = 0.007$) for T_{re}. The mean T_{re} in HOT ($38.7 \pm 0.2°C$) was elevated by 2% compared with both CON ($38.3 \pm 0.3°C$, $p < 0.001$, 95% CI: 0.2–0.5°C) and HYP ($38.3 \pm 0.4°C$, $p = 0.001$, 95% CI: 0.1–0.4°C). Furthermore, the mean T_{re} in HH ($38.6 \pm 0.2°C$) was also increased (2%) when compared with both CON ($p = 0.001$, 95% CI: 0.1–0.6°C) and HYP ($p = 0.009$, 95% CI: 0.1–0.4°C). There was no significant difference ($p = 1.000$, 95% CI: −0.2 to 0.2°C) in mean T_{re} between HOT and HH. At all-time points including and after 15 min, T_{re} was significantly increased ($p < 0.001$) in HOT and HH compared with CON and HYP (**Figure 3**).

T_{sk}

There was a significant main effect for condition ($F = 2163.7$; $p < 0.001$), time ($F = 40.9$; $p < 0.001$), and main effect for condition x time ($F = 28.9$; $p < 0.001$) for T_{sk}. The mean T_{sk} in HOT ($34.1 \pm 1.0°C$) was elevated by 5% compared with both CON ($32.5 \pm 1.3 °C$, $p < 0.001$, 95% CI: 1–3°C) and HYP ($32.4 \pm 1.5 °C$, $p < 0.001$, 95% CI: 1–2°C). Furthermore, the mean T_{sk} in HH ($34.5 \pm 1.2°C$) was also increased (5%) when compared with both CON ($p < 0.001$, 95% CI: 1–3°C) and HYP ($p < 0.001$, 95% CI: 1–3°C). There was no significant difference ($p = 1.000$, 95% CI: −1.8 to 0.6°C) in mean T_{sk} between HOT and HH. At all-time points including and after 15 min, T_{sk} was significantly increased ($p < 0.001$) in HOT and HH compared with CON and HYP (**Figure 3**).

Estimated T_{mu}

There was a significant main effect for condition ($F = 2163.7$; $p < 0.001$), time ($F = 40.9$; $p < 0.001$) and an interaction effect ($F = 28.9$; $p < 0.001$) for T_{mu}. The mean estimated T_{mu} in HOT ($35.7 \pm 1.0°C$) was elevated by 5% compared with both CON ($34.1 \pm 1.3 °C$, $p < 0.001$, 95% CI: 1–2 °C) and HYP ($33.9 \pm 1.5°C$, $p < 0.001$, 95% CI: 1–2°C). Furthermore, the mean estimated T_{mu} in HH ($36.1 \pm 1.2°C$) was also increased (5%) when compared with both CON ($p < 0.001$, 95% CI: 1–3°C) and HYP ($p < 0.001$, 95% CI: 1–3°C). There was no significant difference ($p = 1.000$, 95% CI: −1.7 to 0.6°C) in mean estimated T_{mu} between HOT and HH. At all-time points including and after 15 min, estimated T_{mu} was significantly increased ($p < 0.001$) in HOT and HH compared with CON and HYP (**Figure 3**).

Subjective Measures

There was a significant main effect for condition ($F = 20.8$; $p < 0.001$), time ($F = 1140.3$; $p < 0.001$), and an interaction effect ($F = 1.8$; $p = 0.02$) for RPE (**Figure 4**). Perceived Exertion was 7% lower during CON (15 ± 2) compared with HOT (16 ± 2, $p < 0.001$, 95% CI: 0–1), HYP (16 ± 2, $p < 0.001$, 95% CI: 0–1), and HH (17 ± 1, $p < 0.001$, 95% CI: 1–2). Perceived Exertion was greater ($p < 0.05$) in HH compared to CON from all-time points after 15 min, and increased at 45 and 105 min in HOT (*45 min: $p < 0.001$, 95% CI: 1–3, 105 min.*

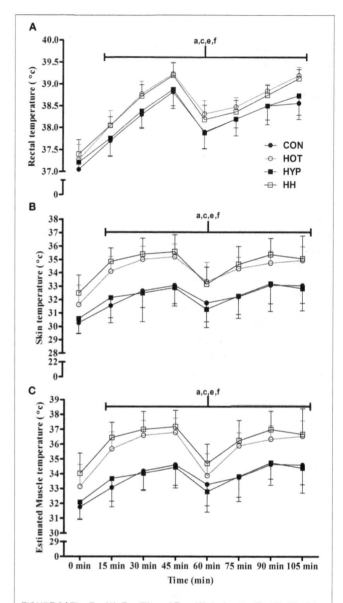

FIGURE 3 | The T_{re} (A), T_{sk} (B), and T_{mu} (C) during the first (0–45 min) and second (60–105 min) half in CON, HOT, HYP, and HH. All body temperatures were significantly increased ($p < 0.05$) in HOT and HH compared with CON and HYP from 15–105 min. [a]Significant difference between CON and HOT ($p < 0.05$); [c]Significant difference between CON and HH ($p < 0.05$); [e]Significant difference between HYP and HH ($p < 0.05$); [f]Significant difference between HOT and HYP ($p < 0.05$).

$p < 0.001$. 95% CI: 1–3) and HYP (*45 min: $p = 0.001$. 95% CI: 1–3; 105 min: $p = 0.006$, 95% CI: 1–3*) compared to CON (**Figure 4**).

Figure 4 reveals a significant main effect for condition ($F = 96.5$; $p < 0.001$), time ($F = 106.2$; $p < 0.001$) and an interaction effect ($F = 1.8$; $p = 0.01$) for TS. The TS was 18% lower during CON (5 ± 1) and HYP (5 ± 1) compared with HOT (6 ± 1) (CON: $p < 0.001$, 95% CI: 1–2; HYP: $p < 0.001$, 95% CI: 1–2) and HH (6 ± 1) (CON: $p < 0.001$, 95% CI: 1–2; HYP: $p < 0.001$, 95% CI: 1–2). A significant increase ($p < 0.05$) in TS during

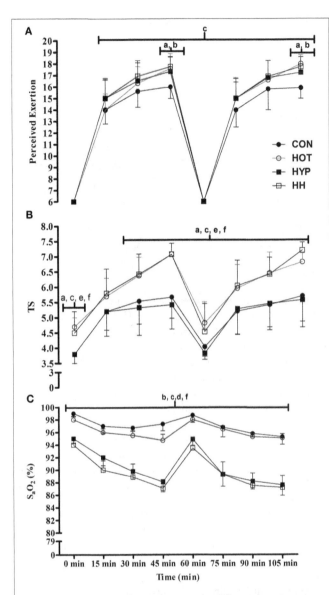

FIGURE 4 | The Perceived Exertion (A) and TS (B) and S_aO_2 (C) during the first (0–45 min) and second (60–105 min) half in CON, HOT, HYP, and HH. Perceived exertion was significantly increased from 30–105 min in HOT, HYP, and HH compared with CON. A significant increase in TS was evident at 0 min and 30–105 min in HOT and HH compared with CON and HYP. Furthermore, S_aO_2 was significantly reduced in from 15–105 min in HYP and HH compared with CON and HOT. [a]Significant difference between CON and HOT ($p < 0.05$); [b]Significant difference between CON and HYP ($p < 0.05$); [c]Significant difference between CON and HH ($p < 0.05$); [d]Significant difference between HOT and HH ($p < 0.05$); [e]Significant difference between HYP and HH ($p < 0.05$); [f]Significant difference between HOT and HYP ($p < 0.05$).

HOT and HH at 0 and 30–105 min compared with CON and HYP (**Figure 4**).

Arterial Blood Oxygen Saturation

There was a significant main effect for condition ($F = 453.8$; $p < 0.001$), time ($F = 133.4$; $p < 0.001$), and an interaction effect ($F = 12.2$; $p < 0.001$) for S_aO_2. Mean S_aO_2 was 97.4, 96.9, 90.5, and 89.4% in CON, HOT, HYP, and HH, respectively. During

HYP and HH a 7% decrease in S_aO_2 was evident compared with CON (HYP: $p < 0.001$, 95% CI: 6–8%; HH: $p < 0.001$, 95% CI: 7–9) and HOT (HYP: $p < 0.001$, 95% CI: 5–6%; HH: $p < 0.001$, 95% CI: 6–7%). A significant reduction ($p < 0.05$) in S_aO_2 was also seen during HYP and HH compared with CON and HOT at all-time points (**Figure 4**).

Heart Rate Response

There was a significant main effect for condition ($F = 5.8$; $p = 0.004$), but there was no significant main effect for time ($F = 1.3$; $p = 0.28$) and no interaction effect ($F = 0.1$; $p = 0.99$) for HR. Mean HR during CON, HOT, HYP, and HH was 161 ± 10, 163 ± 3, 165 ± 7, and 168 ± 8 b·min⁻¹, respectively. In HH, a significant increase (7 ± 11 b·min⁻¹, $p < 0.001$, 95% CI: 1–13 b·min⁻¹) by 4% was seen compared with CON. Furthermore, The HR was also increased (4 ± 9 b·min⁻¹, $p = 0.002$, 95% CI: 2–13 b·min⁻¹) by 3% in HYP compared with CON. No significant change (2 ± 9 b·min⁻¹, $p = 0.30$, 95% CI: −2 to 8 b·min⁻¹) in HR was seen between CON and HOT.

Body Mass Changes

There was a significant main effect for condition ($F = 10.8$; $p < 0.001$), time ($F = 162.5$; $p < 0.001$), and an interaction effect ($F = 2.9$; $p = 0.04$) for body mass. Body mass was significantly reduced post-iSPT by 2% (2 ± 1 kg) in both HOT (HOT vs. CON: 75 ± 12 kg, $p < 0.001$, 95% CI: 1–2 kg; HOT vs. HYP: $p < 0.001$, 95% CI: 1–2 kg) and HH (HH vs. CON: 75.6 ± 11.2 kg, $p = 0.005$, 95% CI: 0–2 kg; HH vs. HYP: $p = 0.005$, 95% CI: 0–2 kg) compared to CON (77 ± 11 kg) and HYP (77 ± 11 kg).

Blood Lactate And Plasma Volume Changes
Bla Concentration

There was a significant main effect for condition ($F = 18.4$; $p < 0.001$) and time ($F = 90.1$; $p < 0.001$), for Bla. However, no interaction effect ($F = 0.7$; $p = 0.77$) was evident between halves and individual time points for Bla. Between conditions, the Bla concentration at HH was only significantly increased (1.5 mmol⁻¹, $p < 0.001$, 95% CI: 1–2 mmol⁻¹) compared with CON. No significant difference ($p < 0.05$) in Bla concentration was evident between CON, HOT, and HYP (**Table 4**).

Plasma Volume Change

There was also a significant main effect for condition ($F = 20.2$; $p < 0.001$), time ($F = 88.6$; $p < 0.001$), and interaction effect ($F = 0.9$; $p = 0.04$) for plasma volume change. Between pre- and post-iSPT, there was a significant reduction in plasma volume change in CON ($p = 0.001$, 95% CI = −1 to −3%), HOT ($p < 0.001$, 95% CI = −1 to −5%), HYP ($p < 0.001$, 95% CI = −1 to −4%), and HH ($p < 0.001$, 95% CI = −3 to −11%), between pre- and post-iSPT. In HH, a significantly greater reduction ($p < 0.001$, 95% CI: −3 to −7%) in plasma volume change was evident compared with CON (**Table 4**).

Regression Analysis

A stepwise regression analysis identified that absolute TS at the end of HOT was a predictor of the total distance ($r = 0.82$,

TABLE 4 | The Bla concentration and plasma volume changes at each individual time point, half and total during CON, HOT, HYP, and HH. The Bla concentration is presented in mmol^{-1}.

	0 min	12 min	27 min	45 min	1st half	57 min	72 min	90 min	2nd half	Total
BLA CONCENTRATION (mmol^{-1})										
CON	0.9 ± 0.3	4.8 ± 1.0	4.6 ± 1.0	4.7 ± 1.1	4.6 ± 1.0	4.3 ± 1.4	4.0 ± 1.5	3.3 ± 1.3	3.9 ± 1.3	4.3 ± 1.3
HOT	0.9 ± 0.3	5.1 ± 1.8	5.4 ± 1.4	4.1 ± 1.7	5.1 ± 1.5	3.9 ± 1.6	4.7 ± 2.0	3.3 ± 1.5	4.0 ± 1.3	4.4 ± 1.9
HYP	0.8 ± 0.2	5.3 ± 1.0	5.3 ± 1.1	4.4 ± 1.7	5.1 ± 1.1	4.0 ± 1.9	4.3 ± 1.5	3.3 ± 0.9	3.8 ± 1.2	4.5 ± 1.6
HH	0.9 ± 0.3	6.7 ± 1.1	6.0 ± 1.4	5.5 ± 1.5	6.0 ± 1.0	5.7 ± 1.2	5.7 ± 1.3	5.0 ± 1.3	5.6 ± 1.0	5.8 ± 1.8[c]
PLASMA VOLUME CHANGE (%)										
CON	0 ± 0	–	–	–	–	–	–	–	–	−2.3 ± 1.2
HOT	0 ± 0	–	–	–	–	–	–	–	–	−3.1 ± 1.5
HYP	0 ± 0	–	–	–	–	–	–	–	–	−3.1 ± 1.7
HH	0 ± 0	–	–	–	–	–	–	–	–	−7.2 ± 2.2[c]

Plasma volume change is presented as a percentage (%) change between pre- and post-iSPT. Bla, Blood lactate; CON, Normoxic-Temperate; HH, Hot-Hypoxic; HOT, Hot; Hyp, Hypoxic; [c]Significant difference between CON and HH (p < 0.05).

$p = 0.05$) and high-speed distance covered ($r = 0.82$, $p = 0.05$) during the HOT condition. The absolute rise from the start to end of HOT for T_{mu} ($r = 0.84$, $p = 0.02$) and T_{sk} ($r = 0.82$, $p = 0.02$) was also a predictor for the total distance and high-speed distance covered at HOT. The absolute TS during HOT was also a predictor of the percentage reduction (5%) for the total distance covered ($r = 0.82$, $p = 0.02$) from CON to HOT. No other physiological measures were found to be significant predictors of the physical performance decrements seen in HYP and HH.

DISCUSSION

The present study examined the changes in simulated soccer performance in HOT, HYP, and HH conditions compared with CON, by utilizing the recently validated iSPT (Aldous et al., 2014). The main finding revealed a marked decline in total distance, high-speed distance, and variable run distance covered during HOT, HYP, and HH conditions when compared to CON (**Figure 2**), supporting the first experimental hypothesis. A secondary finding was that peak sprint speed, was increased in HOT compared with CON, HYP, and HH and that sprint distance covered was unchanged in HOT and HYP, supporting the second experimental hypothesis (**Figure 2** and **Table 3**). Furthermore, a greater decline in physical performance was seen in HH even though physiological changes in body mass and temperatures (**Figure 3**), HR, subjective measures (**Figure 4**) and S_aO_2 (**Figure 4**) were not exacerbated compared to HOT and HYP. This change in physical performance was likely due to alterations in Bla concentration and plasma volume which were only present in HH, supporting the third experimental hypothesis.

The data from this study reveals a 4% reduction in total distance and high-speed distance covered in both HOT and HYP compared with CON, which agrees with previous match-play studies in the heat (43°C; Mohr et al., 2012) and at low altitudes (1600 m; Garvican et al., 2014). The performance decrements for total distance, high-speed distance and variable

run distance covered between halves (**Figure 2**) were greater in HOT (8–11%), HYP (10%), and HH (13–14%) compared to CON (7%). In contrast to our results, Mohr et al. (2012) reported the performance decrements between halves was greater in temperate (21°C) compared to hot (43°C) conditions during match-play. This increased performance decrement is indicative of an adaptive match-play-specific pacing strategy which is postulated to preserve technical skill execution (Mohr et al., 2012; Nassis, 2013; Nassis et al., 2015). The environmental stress may likely reduce the "willingness" of an athlete to perform physical exercise during match-play (Mohr et al., 2012; Aughey et al., 2013). The iSPT (Aldous et al., 2014) prevents adoption of these pacing strategies (i.e., match factors; Gregson et al., 2010) with the same exercise performed in each half due to the individualized and externally-controlled speed thresholds. Therefore, players cannot preserve their sprinting characteristics during iSPT by minimizing their high-speed activity as observed during soccer match play (Nassis et al., 2015).

A participants "willingness" to perform high-speed exercise at a self-paced speed was measured during iSPT, via the variable run component, which is designed to quantify high-speed running without an external cue (Aldous et al., 2014). However, when these external cues are removed in the variable run, participants choose a lower running speed in HOT, HYP, and HH compared to CON, which might be indicative of the environment-mediated performance decrements observed in soccer match play (Mohr et al., 2012; Garvican et al., 2014). Furthermore, significant reductions in variable run distance covered in HOT, HYP, and HH both between halves (**Figure 2**) and in the final 15 min compared with CON (**Table 3**) were observed. Conversely to soccer match-play at 43°C (Mohr et al., 2012) the performance decrements (high-speed distance, sprint distance, and variable run distance) between the first and last 15 min block was increased in HOT, HYP, and HH when compared with CON (**Table 3**); likely due to iSPT controlling pacing and match factors (Aldous et al., 2014). This decline in variable run distance supports the notion that the individualized externally-controlled movement patterns employed by iSPT prevented participants adopting an altered pacing strategy. However, previous soccer match-play data has identified that soccer players can preserve key physical performance measures (e.g., sprint distance covered) in hot and hypoxic environments (Nassis, 2013; Nassis et al., 2015), yet decrements in high-speed and sprint distance covered still occur in the final 15 min of match-play (76–90 min) when compared to the first 15 min (0–15 min; (Mohr et al., 2010, 2012)). These performance impairments may influence the match outcome as a number of studies have revealed more goals are scored/conceded in the final 15 min (76–90 min) of match-play (Abt et al., 2002; Armatas et al., 2007). This phenomenon in goals scored/conceded is likely due to an inability to maintain repeated sprint exercise or discrete episodes of non-fatigued maximal physical performance [central to match outcome (Faude et al., 2012)], within the final 15 min of match-play (Gregson et al., 2010; Faude et al., 2012) as supported by the presented data (**Figure 2**).

A further finding from the present study was that sprint distance covered was unchanged in HYP and HOT, however, peak sprint speed was also improved in HOT compared with CON, showing synergy with previous match-play data (Mohr et al., 2012; Nassis, 2013; Nassis et al., 2015). In HOT, the increase in peak sprint speed could be explained by an increase in estimated T_{mu} which has been shown to improve muscle contractile properties (Racinais et al., 2004), leading to a higher power production and in turn a better sprint performance (Racinais et al., 2005b). However, improvements in sprint performance during soccer match-play in hot environments has been only shown to occur when T_{re} is below 39°C (Mohr et al., 2012). Therefore, this could explain the significant reduction in sprint distance covered in the last 15 min in HOT (**Table 3**). Furthermore, Nassis (2013) identified that elite soccer players in the 2010 FIFA World Cup were able to preserve their peak sprint speed across match-play at low altitudes due to the altered composition to the atmosphere (i.e., air being thinner) which improves the aerodynamics and flight time of an athlete through the air (Levine et al., 2008). However, a hypobaric chamber was not available during this study, so a hypoxicator mask was used to simulate a low altitude environment despite the larger energy cost required when these types of masks are worn (Coppel et al., 2015). The mask was worn in all four experimental conditions to control for this potential confounding factor. Previous research has identified single and repeated sprint performance is maintained at altitude due to a greater anaerobic energy release (Calbet et al., 2003; Morales-Alamo et al., 2012). This is due to several metabolic pathways being stimulated to supplement energy production when aerobic metabolism is not capable of matching aerobic ATP production to consumption, especially the splitting of phosphocreatine (PCr) and glycolysis (Calbet et al., 2003). However, this is likely to manifest itself as a greater and earlier onset of fatigue toward the end of prolonged high-speed exercise as an increase in muscle lactate accumulation would account for a reduction in aerobic ATP production (Balsom et al., 1994; Billaut and Smith, 2010). Therefore, this could explain the exacerbated decline in sprint distance covered during the final 15 min in HYP (**Table 3**).

Despite similar decrements in physical performance in both HOT and HYP compared to CON, the physiological underpinning of such responses differ. Elevated T_{re}, T_{sk}, and estimated T_{mu} (**Figure 2**) in HOT and HH were seen from 15 min onwards compared with CON and HYP, showing parity with previous soccer match-play research (Mohr et al., 2010, 2012; Özgünen et al., 2010). In HOT, the absolute rise in T_{sk} and estimated T_{mu} predicted total and high-speed distance covered, with end TS predicting the decrement in total distance. As both T_{sk} and TS have a strong relationship (Sawka et al., 2012), thermal comfort is likely central to the physical performance decrements seen in HOT. Interventions should target these specific factors (T_{sk}, estimated T_{mu} and TS) in an attempt to maintain "temperate-like" match play soccer performance.

An increase in HR at HYP when compared with CON, shows synergy with previous soccer match-play data at 1600 m above sea level (Garvican et al., 2014). The rise in HR seen in HYP can be attributed to a hemodynamic response arising from a reduction in S_aO_2 which drives a compensatory increase in cardiac output (Mazzeo, 2008; Stembridge et al., 2015a,b). However, during high-speed exercise bouts at altitude a decrease in stroke volume can decrease O_2 delivery to the active muscles as it cannot match the muscle demand, manifesting as a decline to physical performance in HYP (Mazzeo, 2008). A reduction in S_aO_2 by ~8% compared to CON was also apparent by the end of iSPT in both HYP and HH which indicates the onset of exercise induced arterial hypoxemia had occurred causing a plethora of detrimental physiological responses (Billaut and Aughey, 2013), driving the exacerbated performance decrements seen in HYP and HH (**Figure 2**). Indeed, reduced phosphocreatine re-synthesis at altitude is due to sub-optimal re-oxygenation of the active skeletal muscle elongating the recovery time between high-speed exercise bouts (Garvican et al., 2014). Changes in high-speed running are important for maintaining match-play physical performance, due to its association with game defining moments (Gregson et al., 2010), possibly impacting upon the match result (Taylor and Rollo, 2014). Furthermore, the employed design cannot distinguish precisely between whether the changes in S_aO_2 were apparent due to exercise and/or environmentally-induced-arterial-hypoxemia, highlighting that future work should look to explore these complex phenomena within an appropriate design. Data by Billaut and Smith (2010) indicates that intermittent running based exercise can induce exercise-induced-arterial-hypoxemia in University level soccer players. Therefore, although the employed design cannot distinguish precisely between exercise and environmentally-mediated-arterial-hypoxemia future work should look to explore these complex phenomena within an appropriate design.

In HH, the largest performance decrement both between halves (**Figure 2**) and 15 min blocks was evident (**Table 3**). However, all changes in TS (**Figure 4**), body mass and temperature (**Figure 3**) were similar compared with HOT. Furthermore, all changes to both S_aO_2 (**Figure 4**) and HR were comparable with HYP. This is despite a greater decline in total distance and high-speed distance covered, as well as an additional reduction in sprint distance covered in HH which were not present in HOT and HYP (**Figure 2**). This exacerbated reduction to physical performance in HH may have been due to a significant increase in Bla concentration which may indicate a greater anaerobic energy release compared with CON, HOT, and HYP (Amann et al., 2006). Furthermore, a 5% reduction in plasma volume (**Table 3**) which coincided with a 2% change in body mass post-iSPT in HH may have meant that the participants finished iSPT in a hypo-hydrated state, (Cheuvront et al., 2003) causing an increase to the rate of heat storage and sweat output which in turn can impair prolonged high-speed activities in hot environments (Cheuvront and Kenefick, 2014). Additionally, HR was also increased during HH, showing parity with previous research in a hot and low altitude environment (30°C; 1900 m; Buono et al., 2012). This augmented HR response in HH likely stemmed from an impaired stroke volume and/or cardiac output, previously seen during prolonged exercise bouts in heat (González-Alonso et al., 2008) and hypoxia (Mazzeo, 2008). Thus, the exacerbated decline in performance was likely caused by a combination of both hot and hypoxic-mediated fatigue mechanisms. It is already acknowledged that both heat and hypoxia induce performance decrements via these mechanisms during soccer match-play likely influencing match outcome (Taylor and Rollo, 2014). Therefore, the number of game defining moments may be further decreased within HH.

The use of recreationally active male volunteers, rather than elite soccer players, is a limitation of this study; so any generalization of the results to such populations should be considered cautiously. However, our sample included participants with a $\dot{V}O_{2max} > 55$ mL·kg^{-1}·min^{-1}, demonstrating some parity with elite soccer (Tonnessen et al., 2013). The assessment of technical skills and multi-directional movements were unable to be quantified by iSPT (Aldous et al., 2014). Therefore, to assess these within a similarly valid soccer-specific simulation, match factors and protective adaptive pacing strategies must be controlled, in order to robustly assess whether technical skills would remain unchanged in line with previous match-play data (Mohr et al., 2012; Nassis, 2013; Nassis et al., 2015).

The data from this study can be utilized to ascertain the efficacy of any ergogenic intervention to offset the environmentally-induced-decrements. For example, pre- and/or half-time-cooling has been reported to have an ergogenic effect upon both aerobic (Duffield et al., 2010) and repeated-sprint performance in the heat (Castle et al., 2006). Dietary nitrate has also been shown to improve muscle oxygenation during sub-maximal and maximal exercise in acute severe hypoxia (Masschelein et al., 2012; Wylie et al., 2013; Thompson et al., 2015). Furthermore, key physical performance measures (e.g., high-speed distance and sprint distance covered) associated with the match outcome in soccer (Gregson et al., 2010; Faude et al., 2012) are impaired in hot, hypoxic and hot-hypoxic environments, potentially decreasing the number of game defining events during match-play (Taylor and Rollo,

2014). Therefore, the efficacy of these interventions may be important for practitioners and governing bodies to attenuate these decrements present for key physical performance measures during soccer match-play in hot and hypoxic environments.

In conclusion, the present study shows that during simulated soccer performance, total distance, high-speed distance and variable run distance covered are significantly impaired within hot (30°C), hypoxic (1000 m above sea level), and hot-hypoxic (30°C; 1000 m above sea level) conditions when compared to a normoxic-temperate environment. Furthermore, peak sprint speed, was increased in HOT compared with CON, HYP, and HH. However, sprint distance covered was unchanged in HOT and HYP and only decreased in HH compared with CON. It is also revealed that the reduction in soccer physical performance is exacerbated in HH, compared to HOT and HYP alone. The heat-induced-decrements in HOT stem from increasing body temperatures, TS and the 2% reduction in body mass. The hypoxic-induced-decrements in HYP were most likely initiated by a decrease in SaO2 and increase in HR. Similar changes in TS, body mass and temperatures were seen in HOT compared with HH, whilst similar changes in HR and SaO2 were evident in HH compared to HYP. Furthermore, both Bla and plasma volume change alterations were only seen in HH compared with CON, highlighting that both these measures may play a role in the exacerbated decrements seen in HH. However, a deductive design to assess whether simulated soccer performance would still decrease in HH if plasma volume was maintained is needed to understand the mechanistic cause of these findings. The aforementioned physiological changes seen in the present study may influence the decrements to physical performance seen in HOT, HYP, and HH. Therefore, a detrimental effect on the match outcome may be seen in soccer match-play in these environments, which would be important to practitioners within soccer.

AUTHOR CONTRIBUTIONS

Conceived and designed the experiments JA, BC, IA, BD, GA, and LT. Performed the experiments JA, BC, IA, BD, GA, and LT. Analyzed the data JA, BC, IA, BD, GA, and LT. Contributed reagents/materials/analysis tools JA, BC, IA, BD, GA, and LT. Wrote the paper JA, BC, IA, BD, GA, and LT.

FUNDING

This research was funded by the João Havelange Research Scholarship on behalf of the Fédération Internationale de Football Association (FIFA). No commercial or financial incentives were provided that can have caused any potential conflict of interest. The authors would like to thank the participants for their involvement in this study. There was no conflict of interest for any author in this study.

REFERENCES

Abt, G., Dickson, G., and Mummery, W. (2002). "Goal scoring patterns over the course of a match: an analysis of the Australian National Soccer League," in *Science and Football IV*, eds W. Spinks, T. Reilly, and A. Murphy (London: Routledge), 106–111.

Aldous, J. W. F., Akubat, I., Chrismas, B. C. R., Watkins, S. L., Mauger, A. R., Midgley, A. W., et al. (2014). The reliability and validity of a soccer-specific non-motorised treadmill simulation (Intermittent Soccer Performance Test). *J. Strength Cond. Res.* 28, 1971–1980. doi: 10.1519/JSC.0000000000000310

Amann, M., Eldridge, M. W., Lovering, A. T., Stickland, M. K., Pegelow, D. F., and Dempsey, J. A. (2006). Arterial oxygenation influences central motor output and exercise performance via effects on peripheral locomotor muscle fatigue in humans. *J. Physiol.* 575, 937–952. doi: 10.1113/jphysiol.2006.113936

Armatas, V., Yiannakos, A., and Sileloglou, P. (2007). Relationship between time and goal scoring in soccer games: analysis of three World Cups. *Int. J. Perform. Anal. Sport* 7, 48–58.

Aughey, R. J., Hammond, K., Varley, M. C., Schmidt, W. F., Bourdon, P. C., Buchheit, M., et al. (2013). Soccer activity profile of altitude versus sea-level natives during acclimatisation to 3600 m (ISA3600). *Br. J. Sports Med.* 47(Suppl. 1), i107–i113. doi: 10.1136/bjsports-2013-092776

Balsom, P. D., Gaitanos, G. C., Ekblom, B., and Sjödin, B. (1994). Reduced oxygen availability during high intensity intermittent exercise impairs performance. *Acta Physiol. Scand.* 152, 279–285. doi: 10.1111/j.1748-1716.1994.tb09807.x

Bartsch, P., Saltin, B., and Dvorak, J. (2008). Consensus statement on playing football at different altitude. *Scand. J. Med. Sci. Sports* 18(Suppl. 1), 96–99. doi: 10.1111/j.1600-0838.2008.00837.x

Billaut, F., and Aughey, R. J. (2013). Update in the understanding of altitude-induced limitations to performance in team-sport athletes. *Br. J. Sports Med.* 47, i22–i25. doi: 10.1136/bjsports-2013-092834

Billaut, F., and Smith, K. (2010). Prolonged repeated-sprint ability is related to arterial O2 desaturation in men. *Int. J. Sports Physiol. Perform.* 5, 197–209.

Borg, G. (1998). *Borg's Perceived Exertion and Pain Scales.* Champaign, IL: Human Kinetics.

Buchheit, M., Hammond, K., Bourdon, P. C., Simpson, B. M., Garvican-Lewis, L. A., Schmidt, W. F., et al. (2015). Relative match intensities at high altitude in highly-trained young soccer players (ISA3600). *J. Sports Sci. Med.* 14, 98–102.

Buono, M. J., Green, M., Jones, D., and Heaney, J. H. (2012). Increases in heart rate and RPE are additive during prolonged exercise in heat and hypoxia [Abstract 2912]. *Med. Sci. Sports Exerc.* 44, 759–760.

Calbet, J. A., De Paz, J. A., Garatachea, N., Cabeza de Vaca, S., and Chavarren, J. (2003). Anaerobic energy provision does not limit Wingate exercise performance in endurance-trained cyclists. *J. Appl. Physiol. (1985)* 94, 668–676. doi: 10.1152/japplphysiol.00128.2002

Castle, P. C., MacDonald, A. L., Philp, A., Webborn, A., Watt, P. W., and Maxwell, N. S. (2006). Precooling leg muscle improves intermittent sprint exercise performance in hot, humid conditions. *J. Appl. Physiol.* 100, 1377–1384. doi: 10.1152/japplphysiol.00822.2005

Cheuvront, S. N., Carter, R. III., and Sawka, M. N. (2003). Fluid balance and endurance exercise performance. *Curr. Sports Med. Rep.* 2, 202–208. doi: 10.1249/00149619-200308000-00006

Cheuvront, S. N., and Kenefick, R. W. (2014). Dehydration: physiology, assessment, and performance effects. *Compr. Physiol.* 4, 257–285. doi: 10.1002/cphy.c130017

Coppel, J., Hennis, P., Gilbert-Kawai, E., and Grocott, M. P. (2015). The physiological effects of hypobaric hypoxia versus normobaric hypoxia: a systematic review of crossover trials. *Extrem. Physiol. Med.* 4, 2. doi: 10.1186/s13728-014-0021-6

Coull, N. A., Watkins, S. L., Aldous, J. W., Warren, L. K., Chrismas, B. C., Dascombe, B., et al. (2015). Effect of tyrosine ingestion on cognitive and physical performance utilising an intermittent soccer performance test (iSPT) in a warm environment. *Eur. J. Appl. Physiol.* 115, 373–386. doi: 10.1007/s00421-014-3022-7

Dellal, A., Lago-Peñas, C., Rey, E., Chamari, K., and Orhant, E. (2013). The effects of a congested fixture period on physical performance, technical activity and injury rate during matches in a professional soccer team. *Br. J. Sports Med.* 49, 390–394. doi: 10.1136/bjsports-2012-091290

Dill, D. B., and Costill, D. L. (1974). Calculation of percentage changes in volumes of blood, plasma, and red cells in dehydration. *J. Appl. Physiol. (1985)* 37, 247–248.

Drust, B., Waterhouse, J., Atkinson, G., Edwards, B., and Reilly, T. (2005). Circadian rhythms in sports performance-an update. *Chronobiol. Int.* 22, 21–44. doi: 10.1081/CBI-200041039

Duffield, R., Green, R., Castle, P., and Maxwell, N. (2010). Precooling can prevent the reduction of self-paced exercise intensity in the heat. *Med. Sci. Sports Exerc.* 42, 577–584. doi: 10.1249/MSS.0b013e3181b675da

Ekblom, B. (1986). Applied physiology of soccer. *Sports Med.* 3, 50–60. doi: 10.2165/00007256-198603010-00005

Faude, O., Koch, T., and Meyer, T. (2012). Straight sprinting is the most frequent action in goal situations in professional football. *J. Sports Sci.* 30, 625–631. doi: 10.1080/02640414.2012.665940

Flouris, A. D., and Schlader, Z. J. (2015). Human behavioral thermoregulation during exercise in the heat. *Scand. J. Med. Sci. Sports* 25(Suppl. 1), 52–64. doi: 10.1111/sms.12349

Garvican, L. A., Hammond, K., Varley, M. C., Gore, C. J., Billaut, F., and Aughey, R. J. (2014). Lower running performance and exacerbated fatigue in soccer played at 1600 m. *Int. J. Sports Physiol. Perform.* 9, 397–404. doi: 10.1123/IJSPP.2012-0375

González-Alonso, J., Crandall, C. G., and Johnson, J. M. (2008). The cardiovascular challenge of exercising in the heat. *J. Physiol. (Lond).* 586, 45–53. doi: 10.1113/jphysiol.2007.142158

Goodall, S., Twomey, R., and Amann, M. (2014). Acute and chronic hypoxia: implications for cerebral function and exercise tolerance. *Fatigue* 2, 73–92. doi: 10.1080/21641846.2014.909963

Gregson, W., Drust, B., Atkinson, G., and Di Salvo, V. (2010). Match-to-match variability of high speed activities in premier league soccer. *Int. J. Sports Med.* 31, 237–242. doi: 10.1055/s-0030-1247546

Hillman, A. R., Turner, M. C., Peart, D. J., Bray, J. W., Taylor, L., McNaughton, L. R., et al. (2013). A comparison of hyperhydration versus ad libitum fluid intake strategies on measures of oxidative stress, thermoregulation, and performance. *Res. Sports Med.* 21, 305–317. doi: 10.1080/15438627.2013.825796

Hommel, G. (1988). A stagewise rejective multiple test procedure based on a modified Bonferroni test. *Biometrika* 75, 383–386. doi: 10.1093/biomet/75.2.383

Lakomy, H. K. A. (1987). The use of a non-motorized treadmill for analysing sprint performance. *Ergonomics* 30, 627–637. doi: 10.1080/00140138708969756

Levine, B. D., Stray-Gundersen, J., and Mehta, R. D. (2008). Effect of altitude on football performance. *Scand. J. Med. Sci. Sports* 18, 76–84. doi: 10.1111/j.1600-0838.2008.00835.x

Masschelein, E., Van Thienen, R., Wang, X., Van Schepdael, A., Thomis, M., and Hespel, P. (2012). Dietary nitrate improves muscle but not cerebral oxygenation status during exercise in hypoxia. *J. Appl. Physiol.* 113, 736–745. doi: 10.1152/japplphysiol.01253.2011

Mazzeo, R. (2008). Physiological responses to exercise at altitude. *Sports Med.* 38, 1–8. doi: 10.2165/00007256-200838010-00001

Mohr, M., Krustrup, P., and Bangsbo, J. (2005). Fatigue in soccer: a brief review. *J. Sports Sci.* 23, 593–599. doi: 10.1080/02640410400021286

Mohr, M., Mujika, I., Santisteban, J., Randers, M. B., Bischoff, R., Solano, R., et al. (2010). Examination of fatigue development in elite soccer in a hot environment: a multi-experimental approach. *Scand. J. Med. Sci. Sports* 20, 125–132. doi: 10.1111/j.1600-0838.2010.01217.x

Mohr, M., Nybo, L., Grantham, J., and Racinais, S. (2012). Physiological responses and physical performance during football in the heat. *PLoS ONE* 7:e39202. doi: 10.1371/journal.pone.0039202

Morales-Alamo, D., Ponce-González, J. G., Guadalupe-Grau, A., Rodríguez-García, L., Santana, A., Cusso, M. R., et al. (2012). Increased oxidative stress and anaerobic energy release, but blunted Thr172-AMPKalpha phosphorylation, in response to sprint exercise in severe acute hypoxia in humans. *J. Appl. Physiol. (1985)* 113, 917–928. doi: 10.1152/japplphysiol.00415.2012

Nassis, G. P. (2013). Effect of altitude on football performance: analysis of the 2010 FIFA World Cup data. *J. Strength Cond. Res.* 27, 703–707. doi: 10.1519/JSC.0b013e31825d999d

Nassis, G. P., Brito, J., Dvorak, J., Chalabi, H., and Racinais, S. (2015). The association of environmental heat stress with performance: analysis of the 2014

FIFA World Cup Brazil. *Br. J. Sports Med.* 49, 609–613. doi: 10.1136/bjsports-2014-094449

Nybo, L., Rasmussen, P., and Sawka, M. N. (2014). Performance in the heat-physiological factors of importance for hyperthermia-induced fatigue. *Compr. Physiol.* 4, 657–689. doi: 10.1002/cphy.c130012

Nybo, L., and Secher, N. H. (2004). Cerebral perturbations provoked by prolonged exercise. *Prog. Neurobiol.* 72, 223–261. doi: 10.1016/j.pneurobio.2004.03.005

Oliver, J. L., Armstrong, N., and Williams, C. A. (2007). Reliability and validity of a soccer-specific test of prolonged repeated-sprint ability. *Int. J. Sports Physiol. Perform.* 2, 137.

Özgünen, K. T., Kurdak, S. S., Maughan, R. J., Zeren, Ç., Korkmaz, S., Yazıcı, L, Z., et al. (2010). Effect of hot environmental conditions on physical activity patterns and temperature response of football players. *Scand. J. Med. Sci. Sports* 20, 140–147. doi: 10.1111/j.1600-0838.2010.01219.x

Périard, J. D., and Racinais, S. (2015). Training and competing in the heat. *Scand. J. Med. Sci. Sports* 25, 2–3. doi: 10.1111/sms.12448

Racinais, S., Blonc, S., and Hue, O. (2005a). *Med. Sci. Sports Exerc.* 37, 2134–2139. doi: 10.1249/01.mss.0000179099.81706.11

Racinais, S., Blonc, S., Jonville, S., and Hue, O. (2005b). Time of day influences the environmental effects on muscle force and contractility. *Med. Sci. Sports Exerc.* 37, 256–261. doi: 10.1249/01.MSS.0000149885.82163.9F

Racinais, S., Fernandez, J., Farooq, A., Valciu, S., and Hynes, R. (2012). Daily variation in body core temperature using radio-telemetry in aluminium industry shift-workers. *J. Therm. Biol.* 37, 351–354. doi: 10.1016/j.jtherbio.2011.08.006

Racinais, S., Hue, O., and Blonc, S. (2004). Time-of-day effects on anaerobic muscular power in a moderately warm environment. *Chronobiol. Int.* 21, 485–495. doi: 10.1081/CBI-120038632

Ramanathan, N. L. (1964). A new weighting system for mean surface temperature of the human body. *J. Appl. Physiol.* 19, 531–533.

Roelands, B., De Pauw, K., and Meeusen, R. (2015). Neurophysiological effects of exercise in the heat. *Scand. J. Med. Sci. Sports* 25, 65–78. doi: 10.1111/sms.12350

Sawka, M. N., Burke, L. M., Eichner, E. R., Maughan, R. J., Montain, S. J., and Stachenfeld, N. S. (2007). Exercise and fluid replacement. *Med. Sci. Sports Exerc.* 39, 377–390. doi: 10.1249/mss.0b013e31802ca597

Sawka, M. N., Cheuvront, S. N., and Kenefick, R. W. (2012). High skin temperature and hypohydration impair aerobic performance. *Exp. Physiol.* 97, 327–332. doi: 10.1113/expphysiol.2011.061002

Stembridge, M., Ainslie, P. N., Hughes, M. G., Stöhr, E. J., Cotter, J. D., Tymko, M. M., et al. (2015a). Impaired myocardial function does not explain reduced left ventricular filling and stroke volume at rest or during exercise at high altitude. *J. Appl. Physiol. (1985)* 119, 1219–1227. doi: 10.1152/japplphysiol.00995.2014

Stembridge, M., Ainslie, P. N., and Shave, R. (2015b). Short–term adaptation and chronic cardiac remodelling to high altitude in lowlander natives and Himalayan Sherpa. *Exp. Physiol.* 100, 1242–1246. doi: 10.1113/expphysiol.2014.082503

Taylor, L., Fitch, N., Castle, P., Watkins, S., Aldous, J., Sculthorpe, N., et al. (2014). Exposure to hot and cold environmental conditions does not affect the decision making ability of soccer referees following an intermittent sprint protocol. *Front. Physiol.* 5:185. doi: 10.3389/fphys.2014.00185

Taylor, L., Hillman, A. R., Midgley, A. W., Peart, D. J., Chrismas, B., and McNaughton, L. (2012). Hypoxia-mediated prior induction of monocyte-expressed HSP72 and HSP32 provides protection to the disturbances to redox balance associated with human sub-maximal aerobic exercise. *Amino Acids* 43, 1933–1944. doi: 10.1007/s00726-012-1265-3

Taylor, L., Midgley, A. W., Chrismas, B., Madden, L. A., Vince, R. V., and McNaughton, L. (2010). The effect of acute hypoxia on heat shock protein 72 expression and oxidative stress *in vivo*. *Eur. J. Appl. Physiol.* 109, 849–855. doi: 10.1007/s00421-010-1430-x

Taylor, L., and Rollo, I. (2014). *Impact of Altitude and Heat on Football Performance*. Gatorade Sport Science Institute (GSSI) - Sports Science Exchange (SSE). 27. Available online at: http://www.gssiweb.org/Article/sse-131-impact-of-altitude-and-heat-on-football-performance

Thompson, C., Wylie, L. J., Fulford, J., Kelly, J., Black, M. I., McDonagh, S. T., et al. (2015). Dietary nitrate improves sprint performance and cognitive function during prolonged intermittent exercise. *Eur. J. Appl. Physiol.* 115, 1825–1834. doi: 10.1007/s00421-015-3166-0

Tonnessen, E., Hem, E., Leirstein, S., Haugen, T., and Seiler, S. (2013). VO2 max characteristics of male professional soccer players 1989-2012. *Int. J. Sports Physiol. Perform.* 8, 323–329.

Vandenbogaerde, T. J., and Hopkins, W. G. (2010). Monitoring acute effects on athletic performance with mixed linear modeling. *Med. Sci. Sports Exerc.* 42, 1339–1344. doi: 10.1249/MSS.0b013e3181cf7f3f

West, B. T., Welch, K. B., and Galecki, A. T. (2014). *Linear Mixed Models: A Practical Guide Using Statistical Software*. Boca Raton, FL: CRC Press.

Wylie, L. J., Mohr, M., Krustrup, P., Jackman, S. R., Ermıdis, G., Kelly, J., et al. (2013). Dietary nitrate supplementation improves team sport-specific intense intermittent exercise performance. *Eur. J. Appl. Physiol.* 113, 1673–1684. doi: 10.1007/s00421-013-2589-8

Young, A. J., Sawka, M. N., Epstein, Y., Decristofano, B., and Pandolf, K. B. (1987). Cooling different body surfaces during upper and lower body exercise. *J. Appl. Physiol.* 63, 1218–1223.

Conflict of Interest Statement: The authors declare that the research was conducted in the absence of any commercial or financial relationships that could be construed as a potential conflict of interest.

23

Recovery from exercise: vulnerable state, window of opportunity, or crystal ball?

Meredith J. Luttrell and John R. Halliwill *

Department of Human Physiology, University of Oregon, Eugene, OR, USA

Why should we study the recovery from exercise as a discrete phenomenon from exercise itself? We identify three distinct (but not mutually exclusive) rationales that drive the need to investigate the physiology of recovery from exercise. (1) Some individuals are at a heightened risk of clinical outcomes in the immediate post-exercise period; thus the potential negative outcomes of this "vulnerable state" must be weighed against the numerous benefits of exercise training, and may be mitigated to reduce risk. (2) Many of the signaling mechanisms responsible for the beneficial effects of exercise training remain amplified during the exercise recovery period, and may present a "window of opportunity" that can be exploited by interventions to enhance the beneficial adaptations to exercise training, especially in clinical populations. (3) On an individual level, exercise recovery responses may provide investigators with a "crystal ball" ability to predict future clinical outcomes even in apparently healthy individuals. In short, the physiology of recovery is a multi-faceted and complex process, likely involving systems and pathways that are distinct from the physiology of exercise itself. For these reasons, it merits ongoing study.

Keywords: exercise, recovery, athletic performance, regional blood flow, post-exercise, post-exercise hypotension

Edited by:
Sergej Ostojic,
University of Novi Sad, Serbia

Reviewed by:
Can Ozan Tan,
Harvard Medical School, USA
Naoto Fujii,
University of Ottawa, Canada
Claudia Lucia De Moraes Forjaz,
University of São Paulo, Brazil

*Correspondence:
John R. Halliwill,
Department of Human Physiology,
University of Oregon, 1525 University
Ave., Eugene, OR 97403-1240, USA
halliwil@uoregon.edu

Introduction

Traditionally, the field of exercise physiology has been devoted to researching the physiological changes that occur during an acute bout of exercise, and the long-term adaptations to exercise training. More recently, the "physiology of recovery" has emerged as a sub-discipline focused on the time period between the end of a bout of exercise and the subsequent return to what is considered a "resting" or "recovered" state.

Precisely defining "recovery from exercise" is a challenging task due to the varied meanings of recovery. Recovery can refer to a distinct time frame. Depending on the physiological system or pathway of interest, this temporal definition of recovery may range from minutes (e.g., the return of heart rate to near-resting levels) to weeks (e.g., restoration of force-generating capacity after muscle damaging exercise). Additionally, these time frames vary with individual phenotype; for example, trained athletes and individuals with chronic diseases often display altered recovery time courses relative to healthy individuals. Recovery can also refer to specific physiological processes or states, which are distinct from exercise itself and resting physiological states. As a representation of what occurs during the transition from an exercising state to a resting state, we may ask, how do we enhance recovery in athletes? Lastly, recovery can refer to an end-point, e.g., having reached a state of recovery after a bout of exercise, or a starting-point, e.g., an athlete has recovered from prior training and is physiologically ready for additional training stress, or an injured athlete has recovered and can return to play.

This emerging research area, the physiology of recovery, encompasses multiple physiological systems, and is ripe for rigorous study by integrative physiologists with an interest in generating novel insights related to exercise and physical activity. Translating the basic science of recovery from exercise into practical applications related to human health and performance drives much of the interest in pursuing this intriguing (but often overlooked) aspect of exercise physiology. In this perspective, we identify three distinct (but not mutually exclusive) paradigms that drive the need to investigate the human physiology of recovery from exercise.

Recovery from Exercise: A Vulnerable State?

There is substantial evidence that regular endurance and resistance exercise training reduces vulnerability to a number of chronic diseases and conditions (Booth et al., 2000). However, despite the countless beneficial effects of exercise on health and well-being, some individuals may be vulnerable to negative health outcomes (ranging from minor to life threatening) during recovery from exercise.

A dramatic example of this is the significant risk of sudden cardiac death in the 30 min following a bout of vigorous activity in men free from overt cardiovascular disease, as reported in the Physicians' Health Study (Albert et al., 2000). While this data appears alarming, these authors also note that the overall absolute risk of sudden cardiac death after exercise is quite low, with estimates of 1 death occurring for every 1.5 million bouts of exercise in men, and is even more rare in women, with 1 death for every 36.5 million hours (the difference between bouts of exercise in men and hours of exercise in women are reflective of the measurements reported in the respective studies) (Albert et al., 2000; Whang et al., 2006). The physiological mechanisms underpinning these adverse events are varied, but are likely due to cardiac abnormalities in structure or function in young individuals that lead to fatal arrhythmias, and to the disruption of unstable atherosclerotic plaques resulting in myocardial infarction in adults, particularly in previously sedentary individuals (Thompson et al., 2007). Recommended screening that includes information about previous episodes of exercise-related syncope and screening for cardiac abnormalities can identify individuals at high risk of exercise-related sudden cardiac death, especially in young athletes who are unlikely to have atherosclerotic cardiovascular disease (Maron et al., 1996; Bille et al., 2006).

Although it can be a predictor of sudden cardiac death, post-exercise syncope in the absence of structural or functional cardiac abnormalities is most often benign. An obvious example is that of prolonged dynamic exercise in warm weather, which generates a combination of blood volume loss/dehydration and elevated cutaneous blood flow that contribute to reduced venous return, predisposing individuals to orthostatic intolerance (heat syncope) during or after exercise (Hayes et al., 2000;

González-Alonso, 2007). However, even in the absence of heat stress and hypovolemia, between 50 and 80% of otherwise healthy adults develop pre-syncopal signs and symptoms when subjected to head-up tilt following exercise, as recently reviewed (Halliwill et al., 2014). Both prolonged endurance and brief intense exercise predispose individuals to syncope or pre-syncopal symptoms by reducing orthostatic tolerance, a manifestation of an altered physiological state which is distinct from both the exercising state and the resting state (Bjurstedt et al., 1983; Halliwill, 2001; Halliwill et al., 2013). Briefly, post-exercise syncope (in individuals without underlying cardiac or vascular dysfunction, and in the absence of heat stress and hypovolemia) is multifactorial, involving centrally mediated sympatho-inhibition, local sustained release of a post-exercise vasodilator substance within the previously active skeletal muscle, loss of the muscle pump, and in some cases, hyperventilation induced cerebral vasoconstriction (Halliwill et al., 1996; VanNess et al., 1996; Carter et al., 1999; Kulics et al., 1999; MacDonald, 2002; Moynes et al., 2013). Research into this post-exercise phenomenon has provided insight into effective countermeasures against pre-syncopal symptoms (McCord et al., 2008; Lacewell et al., 2014). Wieling et al. (2015) have identified physical countermeasures, such as bending and contracting lower body muscles, that engage the skeletal muscle pump to augment venous return after exercise. External countermeasures, such as the impedance threshold device, which generate negative intrathoracic pressure to enhance venous return, also protect against pre-syncopal symptoms post-exercise (Lacewell et al., 2014). Lower limb compression garments, which have recently become popular among elite and recreational athletes, may also reduce pre-syncopal signs and symptoms after exercise (Privett et al., 2010).

Another vulnerable state is that of delayed-onset muscle soreness (DOMS), a common occurrence among individuals performing unfamiliar or strenuous exercise that can occur with either endurance or resistance exercise (Armstrong, 1984; Cheung et al., 2003). The muscle fiber and connective tissue damage caused by novel exercise results in a temporary decrement in muscle force development, in addition to the pain and muscle tenderness that is characteristic of this condition. The inflammatory process occurring over the following 48 h after the damaging exercise bout results in macrophage infiltration and edema which is implicated as critical in resolving the muscle damage associated with DOMS, but it is also responsible for the pain and discomfort associated with this condition (Armstrong, 1984; Smith, 1991). Complete recovery from DOMS may take weeks, but this phenomenon is complex and specific components of recovery may vary in duration. Whether this vulnerable state can be mitigated by interventions during recovery is a vibrant area of research, particularly among coaches and athletic training staff who are concerned about returning athletes to full capacity for training and competition. A number of recent articles have investigated the impact of common treatments used to prevent or attenuate soreness, including post-exercise cryotherapy and non-steroidal anti-inflammatory drugs (NSAIDs), on exercise recovery characteristics. The current consensus appears to be that cryotherapy has a negligible impact on alleviating discomfort, but may hinder the skeletal muscle repair and recovery process (Isabell et al., 1992; Paddon-Jones and Quigley, 1997; Sellwood et al., 2007). Likewise, NSAIDs may also hinder the repair and recovery, but can alleviate some of the discomfort (Urso, 2013). Support for alternative modalities such as massage or light exercise on DOMS-associated pain remains largely inconclusive, but they potentially exert a mild analgesic effect without hindering repair and recovery.

Recovery from Exercise: A Window of Opportunity?

For many physiological systems, recovery from exercise provides a window of opportunity to maximize or even exploit the altered physiology of the recovery period. Many of the responses we discuss here occur anywhere from 2 to 3 h immediately following exercise (e.g., post-exercise hypotension), but may last up to 48 h or more (e.g., altered blood lipids). Athletes have been taking advantage of the physiology of recovery to improve training and athletic performance during competition, by strategically consuming macronutrients during recovery. In the context of clinical populations, recovery from exercise can be exploited to mitigate the negative effects of some chronic diseases. In this section, we discuss just a few situations where recovery from exercise provides a window of opportunity to maximize the benefits of exercise.

Exercise training is a common intervention for many chronic diseases and conditions, both for the long-term training benefits, but also for the acute effects of a single bout of exercise. A bout of dynamic exercise transiently increases insulin sensitivity, decreases blood lipid levels, and reduces blood pressure after exercise, making exercise and the subsequent recovery period an ideal time for therapeutic intervention in individuals with these cardiovascular risk factors (Braun et al., 1995; Crouse et al., 1997, 1995; Grandjean et al., 2000; Holloszy, 2005; Halliwill et al., 2013). In fact, repeated bouts of exercise at least every other day have been suggested as a treatment for high cholesterol (Crouse et al., 1997). The post-exercise "window of opportunity" could be used to exploit these transient changes associated with exercise; for example, this may be a time when pharmacological interventions may act synergistically with enhanced insulin sensitivity and blunted blood lipid levels. Ideally, these interventions would slow or reverse the progression of chronic diseases, thus reducing the need for pharmacological interventions and improving quality of life in these individuals.

Our research group and others have documented the phenomenon of sustained post-exercise hypotension in young healthy adults, and the exaggerated post-exercise hypotensive response in individuals with hypertension (Rueckert et al., 1996; Pescatello et al., 1999; Forjaz et al., 2000; Halliwill, 2001; Halliwill et al., 2013). As with hypercholesterolemia, exercise training (and a single bout of dynamic exercise in particular) induced post-exercise hypotension is a proposed therapy to treat hypertension in some individuals (Hamer, 2006). Evidence from hypertensive animals models suggests that this effect may be at least partially mediated by altered gamma-aminobutyric acid

(GABA) signaling in the rostral ventrolateral medulla (RVLM) and nucleus tractus solitarii (NTS), ultimately reducing the gain and range of baroreceptor activity post-exercise (Kajekar et al., 2002; Chen et al., 2009). Further exploiting this mechanism with additional interventions, pharmacological or otherwise, may be a viable treatment option in hypertensive individuals who are resistant to exercise training alone. Pro-angiogenic factors (including vascular endothelial growth factor-a, angiopoietin-2, matrix metalloproteinases) are transiently elevated after an acute exercise bout (Breen et al., 1996; Gustafsson and Kraus, 2001; Hoier et al., 2012), and may also be of therapeutic interest for patients with limited exercise capacity or impaired limb blood flow (e.g., peripheral artery disease, spinal cord injury, or muscular dystrophies). Hypoxic and blood flow restricted exercise have both been hypothesized to enhance the angiogenic adaptation to endurance exercise, although little is known about their effects on angiogenic factors when applied in the post-exercise time period (Esbjörnsson et al., 1993; Minchenko et al., 1994; Richardson et al., 1999; Olfert et al., 2001).The recovery period, when angiogenic factors are already increased, may be a window in which additional therapeutic interventions could prove more potent. It may be possible that reducing blood flow or oxygen delivery post-exercise can have an additive effect on angiogenic signaling induced by exercise alone, although to our knowledge, this has not been experimentally tested in humans.

For athletes concerned with optimizing training and performance, macronutrient intake during recovery may be a key component of their training regimen. The metabolic changes associated with both endurance and resistance exercise and recovery may be enhanced with appropriate nutrient timing strategies. In endurance athletes, maximizing skeletal muscle glycogen storage by ingesting carbohydrates in recovery has a significant effect on subsequent performance. This is taking advantage of the physiology of recovery related to glucose transporters, insulin sensitivity, and perhaps elevations in blood flow (Emhoff et al., 2011). For power and strength athletes, as well as endurance athletes, there is an analogous window of opportunity based on the elevated rate of protein synthesis in recovery, so that this time period is ripe for protein ingestion (Levenhagen et al., 2001; Areta et al., 2013). Optimization of macronutrient intake during recovery is a large area of research related to human performance, and may translate to clinical populations and older adults (Esmarck et al., 2001).

Recent evidence also suggests that interventions such as muscle cooling, applied during recovery from exercise, can enhance skeletal muscle expression of transcription factor PGC-1α, potentially promoting mitochondrial biogenesis beyond levels observed without this intervention (Ihsan et al., 2014). This finding provides a contrast to the use of cryotherapy for mitigating muscle soreness and inflammation, which was discussed above, and leads to the interesting possibility that common interventions may have divergent effects on muscle recovery, depending on the outcome variable of interest (i.e., acute inflammation vs. skeletal muscle mitogenesis). Obviously, more research focused on unraveling these complex and interconnected pathways is necessary, and may provide valuable insight into the unique physiology of recovery from exercise and how it can be exploited to improve athletic or clinical outcomes.

Recovery from Exercise: A Crystal Ball?

In clinical settings, exercise testing has clear and proven prognostic value, providing insight into future disease risk. Among apparently healthy and clinical populations, the physiology of recovery can also predict an individual's risk of an adverse health outcome. For example, heart rate recovery between 1 and 5 min after a moderate intensity bout of dynamic exercise is an independent predictor of all-cause mortality (Johnson and Goldberger, 2012). Both heart rate and blood pressure recovery can provide non-invasive clinical indicators related to autonomic function, making these simple measurements highly informative (Terziotti et al., 2001; Buchheit et al., 2007; Cahalin et al., 2013). In fact, measurements in recovery can non-invasively be used to assess future clinical risks that would otherwise not be apparent in a typical health screening (Cole et al., 2000; Shetler et al., 2001).

Beyond general screening functions, blood pressure recovery and post-exercise hypotension after a single bout of exercise are predictive of an individual's blood pressure response to chronic exercise training (Liu et al., 2012; Hecksteden et al., 2013). This simple, minimally invasive test could make effective use of resources in a clinical setting to identify individuals who are responsive to blood pressure reductions with training, and individuals who may require additional pharmacological intervention. In these cases, recovery from exercise provides researchers and clinicians clues to patient cardiovascular health. This concept aligns with current interest in identifying "responders" and "nonresponders" to exercise and exercise training (Karavirta et al., 2011; Timmons, 2011). With additional research in this area, it may soon be possible to identify individuals who may reap more health or performance benefits from one type of training (e.g., endurance vs. resistance training), or may also identify individuals for whom exercise would be contra-indicated (e.g., hypertrophic cardiomyopathy) (Keller et al., 2011). To our knowledge, there are currently no studies that have identified recovery from exercise variables as a means to identify responders vs. non-responders to specific exercise interventions, but this may be an interesting future direction for the physiology of recovery.

Can these notions be generalized beyond the realm of the cardiovascular and autonomic nervous systems? Relatively little is currently known about how other major organ systems recover from exercise, or how other recovery phenotypes could provide clues about either future health or even future athletic performance. For example, are there individual differences in recovery of skeletal muscle function and force development that could predict development or loss of muscle strength or function with age or training? Or could metabolic recovery predict adaptations in substrate utilization that may identify individuals for whom exercise training may prevent insulin resistance? These questions may appear far-fetched, but given what we now understand about individual responses to exercise

and exercise training, it would not be surprising to discover that individual recovery from exercise is heterogeneous, phenotype-sensitive, and can be exploited for prediction of health or athletic performance benefits. It is also conceivable that the results of a simple recovery test which predicts an individual's mortality risk could provide sufficient motivation for some individuals to make lifestyle improvements to mitigate this risk. Given the relative ease of tracking heart rate and blood pressure, these recovery measurements could be made on an individual level to monitor exercise effectiveness or track health outcomes. Ideally, this information will inform future patient care through personalized medication and exercise prescription (i.e., precision exercise training). As research on the physiology of recovery expands, there is great potential for studies to find new "crystal ball" forecasters of future health.

The Trifecta of Recovery

As evidenced by the diversity of systems engaged during recovery from exercise, this field of research has implications for both human health and athletic performance, and can be useful to researchers and healthcare professionals alike. From what is currently known about the physiology of recovery, the three paradigms we have outlined in this perspective all likely overlap within an individual after a single bout of exercise. For example, our personal interest in the sustained post-exercise vasodilation crosses all three paradigms, creating vulnerabilities and opportunities, and providing prognostic implications, as depicted in **Figure 1**. Such responses allow for potentially different pathways of intervention, depending on the health and goals of the individual. For example, an athlete vulnerable to post-exercise syncope may choose

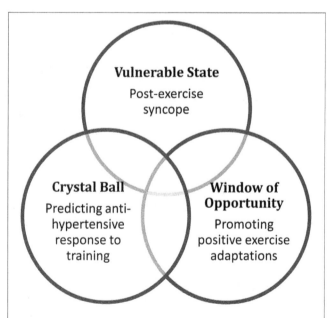

FIGURE 1 | Recovery from exercise can be conceptualized as creating vulnerable states, windows of opportunity, and providing crystal ball prognostic value.

to perform physical counter-maneuvers to prevent syncopal symptoms, rather than pursue a pharmacological intervention that may close the window of opportunity after exercise for beneficial exercise training effects. By conceptualizing the physiology of recovery as this balance of vulnerable state,

window of opportunity, and crystal ball paradigms provides a way to frame lines of inquiry and help broaden the field of exercise physiology in exciting directions for the benefit of the clinical patient, elite athlete, and weekend warrior alike.

References

Albert, C. M., Mittleman, M. A., Chae, C. U., Lee, I. M., Hennekens, C. H., and Manson, J. E. (2000). Triggering of sudden death from cardiac causes by vigorous exertion. *N. Engl. J. Med.* 343, 1355–1361. doi: 10.1056/NEJM200011093431902

Areta, J. L., Burke, L. M., Ross, M. L., Camera, D. M., West, D. W. D., Broad, E. M., et al. (2013). Timing and distribution of protein ingestion during prolonged recovery from resistance exercise alters myofibrillar protein synthesis. *J. Physiol.* 591, 2319–2331. doi: 10.1113/jphysiol.2012.244897

Armstrong, R. B. (1984). Mechanisms of exercise-induced delayed onset muscular soreness: a brief review. *Med. Sci. Sport. Exerc.* 16, 529–538. doi: 10.1249/00005768-198412000-00002

Bille, K., Figueiras, D., Schamasch, P., Kappenberger, L., Brenner, J. I., Meijboom, F. J., et al. (2006). Sudden cardiac death in athletes: the Lausanne Recommendations. *Eur. J. Cardiovasc. Prev. Rehabil.* 13, 859–875. doi: 10.1097/01.hjr.0000238397.50341.4a

Bjurstedt, H., Rosenhamer, G., Balldin, U., and Katkov, V. (1983). Orthostatic reactions during recovery from exhaustive exercise of short duration. *Acta Physiol. Scand.* 119, 25–31. doi: 10.1111/j.1748-1716.1983.tb07301.x

Booth, F. W., Gordon, S. E., Carlson, C. J., and Hamilton, M. T. (2000). Waging war on modern chronic diseases: primary prevention through exercise biology. *J. Appl. Physiol.* 88, 774–787.

Braun, B., Zimmermann, M. B., and Kretchmer, N. (1995). Effects of exercise intensity on insulin sensitivity in women with non-insulin-dependent diabetes mellitus. *J. Appl. Physiol.* 78, 300–306.

Breen, E. C., Johnson, E. C., Wagner, H., Tseng, H. M., Sung, L. A., and Wagner, P. D. (1996). Angiogenic growth factor mRNA responses in muscle to a single bout of exercise. *J. Appl. Physiol.* 81, 355–361.

Buchheit, M., Papelier, Y., Laursen, P. B., and Ahmaidi, S. (2007). Noninvasive assessment of cardiac parasympathetic function: postexercise heart rate recovery or heart rate variability? *Am. J. Physiol. Heart Circ. Physiol.* 293, H8–H10. doi: 10.1152/ajpheart.00335.2007

Cahalin, L. P., Forman, D. E., Chase, P., Guazzi, M., Myers, J., Bensimhon, D., et al. (2013). The prognostic significance of heart rate recovery is not dependent upon maximal effort in patients with heart failure. *Int. J. Cardiol.* 168, 1496–1501. doi: 10.1016/j.ijcard.2012.12.102

Carter, R. I., Watenpaugh, D. E., Wasmund, W. L., Wasmund, S. L., and Smith, M. L. (1999). Muscle pump and central command during recovery from exercise in humans. *J. Appl. Physiol.* 87, 1463–1469.

Chen, C.-Y., Bechtold, A. G., Tabor, J., and Bonham, A. C. (2009). Exercise reduces GABA synaptic input onto nucleus tractus solitarii baroreceptor second-order neurons via NK1 receptor internalization in spontaneously hypertensive rats. *J. Neurosci.* 29, 2754–2761. doi: 10.1523/JNEUROSCI.4413-08.2009

Cheung, K., Hume, P. A., and Maxwell, L. (2003). Delayed onset muscle soreness. *Sport. Med.* 33, 145–164. doi: 10.2165/00007256-200333020-00005

Cole, C. R., Foody, J. M., Blackstone, E. H., and Lauer, M. S. (2000). Heart rate recovery after submaximal exercise testing as a predictor of mortality in a cardiovascularly healthy cohort. *Ann. Intern. Med.* 132, 552–555. doi: 10.7326/0003-4819-132-7-200004040-00007

Crouse, S. F., O'Brien, B. C., Grandjean, P. W., Lowe, R. C., Rohack, J. J., and Green, J. S. (1997). Effects of training and a single session of exercise on lipids and apolipoproteins in hypercholesterolemic men. *J. Appl. Physiol.* 83, 2019–2028.

Crouse, S. F., O'Brien, B. C., Rohack, J. J., Lowe, R. C., Green, J. S., Tolson, H., et al. (1995). Changes in serum lipids and apolipoproteins after exercise in men with high cholesterol: influence of intensity. *J. Appl. Physiol.* 79, 279–286.

Emhoff, C. A., Barrett-O'Keefe, Z., Padgett, R. C., Hawn, J. A., and Halliwill, J. R. (2011). Histamine-receptor blockade reduces blood flow but not muscle

glucose uptake during postexercise recovery in humans. *Exp. Physiol.* 96, 664–673. doi: 10.1113/expphysiol.2010.056150

Esbjörnsson, M., Jansson, E., Sundberg, C. J., Sylvén, C., Eiken, O., Nygren, A., et al. (1993). Muscle fibre types and enzyme activities after training with local leg ischaemia in man. *Acta Physiol. Scand.* 148, 233–241. doi: 10.1111/j.1748-1716.1993.tb09554.x

Esmarck, B., Andersen, J. L., Olsen, S., Richter, E. A., Mizuno, M., and Kjaer, M. (2001). Timing of postexercise protein intake is important for muscle hypertrophy with resistance training in elderly humans. *J. Physiol.* 535, 301–311. doi: 10.1111/j.1469-7793.2001.00301.x

Forjaz, C. L., Tinucci, T., Ortega, K. C., Santaella, D. F., Mion, D., and Negrão, C. E. (2000). Factors affecting post-exercise hypotension in normotensive and hypertensive humans. *Blood Press. Monit.* 5, 255–262. doi: 10.1097/00126097-200010000-00002

González-Alonso, J. (2007). Separate and combined influences of dehydration and hyperthermia on cardiovascular responses to exercise. *Int. J. Sports Med.* 19, S111–S114. doi: 10.1055/s-2007-971972

Grandjean, P. W., Crouse, S. F., and Rohack, J. J. (2000). Influence of cholesterol status on blood lipid and lipoprotein enzyme responses to aerobic exercise. *J. Appl. Physiol.* 89, 472–480.

Gustafsson, T., and Kraus, W. E. (2001). Exercise-induced angiogenesis-related growth and transcription factors in skeletal muscle, and their modification in muscle pathology. *Front. Biosci.* 6, D75–D89. doi: 10.2741/gustafss

Halliwill, J. R. (2001). Mechanisms and clinical implications of post-exercise hypotension in humans. *Exerc. Sport Sci. Rev.* 29, 65–70. doi: 10.1097/00003677-200104000-00005

Halliwill, J. R., Buck, T. M., Lacewell, A. N., and Romero, S. A. (2013). Postexercise hypotension and sustained postexercise vasodilation: what happens after we exercise? *Exp. Physiol.* 98, 7–18. doi: 10.1113/expphysiol.2011.058065

Halliwill, J. R., Sieck, D. C., Romero, S. A., Buck, T. M., and Ely, M. R. (2014). Blood pressure regulation X: what happens when the muscle pump is lost? Post-exercise hypotension and syncope. *Eur. J. Appl. Physiol.* 114, 561–578. doi: 10.1007/s00421-013-2761-1

Halliwill, J. R., Taylor, J. A., and Eckberg, D. L. (1996). Impaired sympathetic vascular regulation in humans after acute dynamic exercise. *J. Physiol.* 495, 279–288. doi: 10.1113/jphysiol.1996.sp021592

Hamer, M. (2006). The anti-hypertensive effects of exercise: integrating acute and chronic mechanisms. *Sport. Med* 36, 109–116. doi: 10.2165/00007256-200636020-00002

Hayes, P. M., Lucas, J. C., and Shi, X. (2000). Importance of post-exercise hypotension in plasma volume restoration. *Acta Physiol. Scand.* 169, 115–124. doi: 10.1046/j.1365-201x.2000.00728.x

Hecksteden, A., Grütters, T., and Meyer, T. (2013). Association between postexercise hypotension and long-term training-induced blood pressure reduction: a pilot study. *Clin. J. Sport Med.* 23, 58–63. doi: 10.1097/JSM.0b013e31825b6974

Hoier, B., Nordsborg, N., Andersen, S., Jensen, L., Nybo, L., Bangsbo, J., et al. (2012). Pro- and anti-angiogenic factors in human skeletal muscle in response to acute exercise and training. *J. Physiol.* 590, 595–606. doi: 10.1113/jphysiol.2011.216135

Holloszy, J. O. (2005). Exercise-induced increase in muscle insulin sensitivity. *J. Appl. Physiol.* 99, 338–343. doi: 10.1152/japplphysiol.00123.2005

Ihsan, M., Watson, G., Choo, H. C., Lewandowski, P., Papazzo, A., Cameron-Smith, D., et al. (2014). Postexercise muscle cooling enhances gene expression of PGC-1α. *Med. Sci. Sport. Exerc.* 46, 1900–1907. doi: 10.1249/MSS.0000000000000308

Isabell, W. K., Durrant, E., Myer, W., and Anderson, S. (1992). The effects of ice massage, ice massage with exercise, and exercise on the prevention and treatment of delayed onset muscle soreness. *J. Athl. Train.* 27, 208–217.

Johnson, N. P., and Goldberger, J. J. (2012). Prognostic value of late heart rate recovery after treadmill exercise. *Am. J. Cardiol.* 110, 45–49. doi: 10.1016/j.amjcard.2012.02.046

Kajekar, R., Chen, C.-Y., Mutoh, T., and Bonham, A. C. (2002). GABA(A) receptor activation at medullary sympathetic neurons contributes to postexercise hypotension. *Am. J. Physiol. Heart Circ. Physiol.* 282, H1615–H1624. doi: 10.1152/ajpheart.00725.2001

Karavirta, L., Häkkinen, K., Kauhanen, A., Arija-Blázquez, A., Sillanpää, E., Rinkinen, N., et al. (2011). Individual responses to combined endurance and strength training in older adults. *Med. Sci. Sports Exerc.* 43, 484–490. doi: 10.1249/MSS.0b013e3181f1bf0d

Keller, P., Vollaard, N. B. J., Gustafsson, T., Gallagher, I. J., Sundberg, C. J., Rankinen, T., et al. (2011). A transcriptional map of the impact of endurance exercise training on skeletal muscle phenotype. *J. Appl. Physiol.* 110, 46–59. doi: 10.1152/japplphysiol.00634.2010

Kulics, J. M., Collins, H. L., and DiCarlo, S. E. (1999). Postexercise hypotension is mediated by reductions in sympathetic nerve activity. *Am. J. Physiol. Hear. Circ Physiol.* 276, H27–H32.

Lacewell, A. N., Buck, T. M., Romero, S. A., and Halliwill, J. R. (2014). Post-exercise syncope: wingate syncope test and effective countermeasure. *Exp. Physiol.* 99, 172–186. doi: 10.1113/expphysiol.2013.075333

Levenhagen, D. K., Gresham, J. D., Carlson, M. G., Maron, D. J., Borel, M. J., and Flakoll, P. J. (2001). Postexercise nutrient intake timing in humans is critical to recovery of leg glucose and protein homeostasis. *Am. J. Physiol. Endocrinol. Metab.* 280, E982–E993.

Liu, S., Goodman, J., Nolan, R., Lacombe, S., and Thomas, S. G. (2012). Blood pressure responses to acute and chronic exercise are related in prehypertension. *Med. Sci. Sport. Exerc.* 44, 1644–1652. doi: 10.1249/MSS.0b013e318 25408fb

MacDonald, J. R. (2002). Potential causes, mechanisms, and implications of post exercise hypotension. *J. Hum. Hypertens.* 16, 225–236. doi: 10.1038/sj.jhh.1001377

Maron, B. J., Thompson, P. D., Puffer, J. C., McGrew, C. A., Strong, W. B., Douglas, P. S., et al. (1996). Cardiovascular preparticipation screening of competitive athletes: a statement for health professionals from the Sudden Death Committee (clinical cardiology) and Congenital Cardiac Defects Committee (cardiovascular disease in the young), American Heart As. *Circulation* 94, 850–856. doi: 10.1161/01.CIR.94.4.850

McCord, J. L., Pellinger, T. K., Lynn, B. M., and Halliwill, J. R. (2008). Potential benefit from an H1-receptor antagonist on postexercise syncope in the heat. *Med. Sci. Sport. Exerc.* 40, 1953–1961. doi: 10.1249/MSS.0b013e31817f1970

Minchenko, A., Bauer, T., Salceda, S., and Caro, J. (1994). Hypoxic stimulation of vascular endothelial growth factor expression *in vitro* and *in vivo. Lab. Invest.* 71, 374–379.

Moynes, J., Bentley, R. F., Bravo, M., Kellawan, J. M., and Tschakovsky, M. E. (2013). Persistence of functional sympatholysis post-exercise in human skeletal muscle. *Front. Physiol.* 4:131. doi: 10.3389/fphys.2013.00131

Olfert, I. M., Breen, E. C., Mathieu-Costello, O., and Wagner, P. D. (2001). Skeletal muscle capillarity and angiogenic mRNA levels after exercise training in normoxia and chronic hypoxia. *J. Appl. Physiol.* 91, 1176–1184.

Paddon-Jones, D. J., and Quigley, B. M. (1997). Effect of cryotherapy on muscle soreness and strength following eccentric exercise. *Int. J. Sports Med.* 18, 588–593. doi: 10.1055/s-2007-972686

Pescatello, L. S., Miller, B., Danias, P. G., Werner, M., Hess, M., Baker, C., et al. (1999). Dynamic exercise normalizes resting blood pressure in mildly hypertensive premenopausal women. *Am. Heart J.* 138, 916–921. doi: 10.1016/S0002-8703(99)70017-7

Privett, S. E., George, K. P., Whyte, G. P., and Cable, N. T. (2010). The effectiveness of compression garments and lower limb exercise on post-exercise blood pressure regulation in orthostatically intolerant athletes. *Clin. J. Sport Med.* 20, 362–367. doi: 10.1097/JSM.0b013e3181f20292

Richardson, R. S., Wagner, H., Mudaliar, S. R. D., Henry, R., Noyszewski, E. A., and Wagner, P. D. (1999). Human VEGF gene expression in skeletal muscle: effect of acute normoxic and hypoxic exercise. *Am. J. Physiol. Hear. Circ Physiol.* 277, H2247–H2252.

Rueckert, P. A., Slane, P. R., lillis, D. L., and Hanson, P. (1996). Hemodynamic patterns and duration of post-dynamic exercise hypotension in hypertensive humans. *Med. Sci. Sport. Exerc.* 28, 24–32. doi: 10.1097/00005768-199601000-00010

Sellwood, K. L., Brukner, P., Williams, D., Nicol, A., and Hinman, R. (2007). Ice-water immersion and delayed-onset muscle soreness: a randomised controlled trial. *Br. J. Sports Med.* 41, 392–397. doi: 10.1136/bjsm.2006.033985

Shetler, K., Marcus, R., Froelicher, V. F., Vora, S., Kalisetti, D., Prakash, M., et al. (2001). Heart rate recovery: validation and methodologic issues. *J. Am. Coll. Cardiol.* 38, 1980–1987. doi: 10.1016/S0735-1097(01)01652-7

Smith, L. L. (1991). Acute inflammation: the underlying mechanism in delayed onset muscle soreness? *Med. Sci. Sport. Exerc.* 23, 542–551. doi: 10.1249/00005768-199105000-00006

Terziotti, P., Schena, F., Gulli, G., and Cevese, A. (2001). Post-exercise recovery of autonomic cardiovascular control: a study by spectrum and cross-spectrum analysis in humans. *Eur. J. Appl. Physiol.* 84, 187–194. doi: 10.1007/s004210170003

Thompson, P. D., Franklin, B. A., Balady, G. J., Blair, S. N., Corrado, D., Estes, N. A. M., et al. (2007). Exercise and acute cardiovascular events placing the risks into perspective: a scientific statement from the American Heart Association Council on Nutrition, Physical Activity, and Metabolism and the Council on Clinical Cardiology. *Circulation* 115, 2358–2368. doi: 10.1161/CIRCULATIONAHA.107.181485

Timmons, J. A. (2011). Variability in training-induced skeletal muscle adaptation. *J. Appl. Physiol.* 110, 846–853. doi: 10.1152/japplphysiol.00934.2010

Urso, M. L. (2013). Anti-inflammatory interventions and skeletal muscle injury: benefit or detriment? *J. Appl. Physiol.* 115, 920–928. doi: 10.1152/japplphysiol.00036.2013

VanNess, J. M., Takata, H. J., and Overton, J. M. (1996). Attenuated blood pressure responsiveness during post-exercise hypotension. *Clin. Exp. Hypertens.* 18, 891–900. doi: 10.3109/10641969609097906

Whang, W., Manson, J. E., Hu, F. B., Chae, C. U., Rexrode, K. M., Willett, W. C., et al. (2006). Physical exertion, exercise, and sudden cardiac death in women. *JAMA* 295, 1399–1403. doi: 10.1001/jama.295.12.1399

Wieling, W., van Dijk, N., Thijs, R. D., de Lange, F. J., Krediet, C. T. P., and Halliwill, J. R. (2015). Physical countermeasures to increase orthostatic tolerance. *J. Int. Med.* 277, 69–82. doi: 10.1111/joim.12249

Conflict of Interest Statement: This research was funded by National Institutes of Health Grant HL115027. The authors declare that the research was conducted in the absence of any commercial or financial relationships that could be construed as a potential conflict of interest.

Permissions

List of Contributors

Jihong Xing
Department of Emergency Medicine, The First Hospital of Jilin University, Changchun, Jilin, China

Jian Lu and Jianhua Li
Pennsylvania State Heart and Vascular Institute, The Pennsylvania State University College of Medicine, Hershey, PA, USA

Ibai Garcia-Tabar, José F. Aramendi and Esteban M. Gorostiaga
Studies, Research and Sports Medicine Center, Government of Navarre, Pamplona, Spain

Jean P. Eclache
Laboratory of Performance, Sport-Occupational Activities-Biology-Association, Lyon-Chassieu, France

Thomas Abel, Barbara Thees, Stefan Schneider, and Heiko K. Strüder
Institute of Movement and Neurosciences, German Sport University Cologne, Cologne, Germany

Brendan Burkett and Christopher D. Askew
Faculty of Science, Health, Education and Engineering, School of Health and Sport Sciences, University of the Sunshine Coast, Maroochydore, QLD, Australia

Olivier Girard
Department of Physiology, Faculty of Biology and Medicine, Institute of Sport Sciences, University of Lausanne, Lausanne, Switzerland
Athlete Health and Performance Research Center, Aspetar, Qatar Orthopaedic and Sports Medicine Hospital, Doha, Qatar

Franck Brocherie and Grégoire P. Millet
Department of Physiology, Faculty of Biology and Medicine, Institute of Sport Sciences, University of Lausanne, Lausanne, Switzerland

Jean-Benoit Morin
Laboratory of Human Motricity, Education Sport and Health, University of Nice Sophia Antipolis, Nice, France

Gaël Guilhem, Christine Hanon and Nicolas Gendreau
Laboratory Sport, Expertise and Performance (EA7370), Research Department, French National Institute of Sport (INSEP), Paris, France

Dominique Bonneau
Laboratory Sport, Expertise and Performance (EA7370), Research Department, French National Institute of Sport (INSEP), Paris, France
Fatigue and Vigilance Unit (EA7330), Neurosciences and Operational Constraints Department, French Armed Forces Biomedical Research Institute (IRBA), Paris Descartes University, Brétigny-sur-Orge, France

Arnaud Guével
Laboratory "Movement, Interactions, Performance" (EA4334), University of Nantes, Nantes, France

Mounir Chennaoui
Fatigue and Vigilance Unit (EA7330), Neurosciences and Operational Constraints Department, French Armed Forces Biomedical Research Institute (IRBA), Paris Descartes University, Brétigny-sur-Orge, France

Laurent Schmitt
Centre National de Ski Nordiqueet de Moyenne Montagne, Ecole Nationale des Sports de Montagne, Prémanon, France
Faculty of Biology and Medicine, Institute of Sport Sciences, University of Lausanne, Lausanne, Switzerland

Grégoire P. Millet
Faculty of Biology and Medicine, Institute of Sport Sciences, University of Lausanne, Lausanne, Switzerland

Jacques Regnard
Unité de Recherche EA 3920, Marqueurs Pronostiqueset Facteurs de Régulations des Pathologies Cardiaqueset Vasculaires, Hôpital Universitaire de Besançon, Université de Franche-Comté, Besançon, France

Tomasz Tomiak and Viktor S.Mishchenko
Unit of the Theory of Sport and Motorics, Chair of Individual Sports, Gdansk University of Physical Education and Sport, Gdańsk, Poland

Andriy V. Gorkovenko, Arkadii N. Tal'nov, Tetyana I. Abramovych , Inna V. Vereshchaka and Alexander I. Kostyukov
Department of Movement Physiology, Bogomoletz Institute of Physiology, National Academy of Sciences, Kiev, Ukraine

Andrea Dennis, Nancy B. Rawlings, Stuart Clare and Heidi Johansen-Berg
Oxford Centre for Functional MRI of the Brain (FMRIB), Nuffield Department of Clinical Neurosciences, University of Oxford, Oxford, UK

Adam G. Thomas
Oxford Centre for Functional MRI of the Brain (FMRIB), Nuffield Department of Clinical Neurosciences, University of Oxford, Oxford, UK
Section on Functional Imaging Methods, National Institute of Mental Health, National Institutes of Health, Department of Health and Human Services, Bethesda, MD, USA

Jamie Near
Oxford Centre for Functional MRI of the Brain (FMRIB), Nuffield Department of Clinical Neurosciences, University of Oxford, Oxford, UK
Douglas Mental Health University Institute and Department of Psychiatry, Mc Gill University, Montreal, QC, Canada

Thomas E. Nichols
Oxford Centre for Functional MRI of the Brain (FMRIB), Nuffield Department of Clinical Neurosciences, University of Oxford, Oxford, UK
Department of Statistics and Warwick Manufacturing Group, University of Warwick, Coventry, UK

Charlotte J. Stagg
Oxford Centre for Functional MRI of the Brain (FMRIB), Nuffield Department of Clinical Neurosciences, University of Oxford, Oxford, UK
Physiological Neuroimaging Group, Oxford Centre for Human Brain Activity (OHBA), University of Oxford, Oxford, UK

Annika Willems, Thomas A. W. Paulson and Victoria L. Goosey-Tolfrey
The Peter Harrison Centre for Disability Sport, School of Sport, Exercise and Health Sciences, Loughborough University, Loughborough, UK

Mhairi Keil
Lilleshall National Sport Centre, English Institute of Sport, Sheffield, UK

Katherine Brooke-Wavell
School of Sport, Exercise and Health Sciences, Loughborough University, Loughborough, UK

Shu Fang Cui, Chen Yu Zhang and Xi Chen
State Key Laboratory of Pharmaceutical Biotechnology, NJU Advanced Institute for Life Sciences (NAILS), School of Life Sciences, Nanjing University, Nanjing, China
Jiangsu Engineering Research Center for Micro RNA Biology and Biotechnology, Nanjing University, Nanjing, China

Wei Li and Jie Niu
The Lab of Military Conditioning and Motor Function Assessment, The PLA University of Science and Technology, Nanjing, China

Ji Zheng Ma
State Key Laboratory of Pharmaceutical Biotechnology, NJU Advanced Institute for Life Sciences (NAILS), School of Life Sciences, Nanjing University, Nanjing, China
Jiangsu Engineering Research Center for Micro RNA Biology and Biotechnology, Nanjing University, Nanjing, China
The Lab of Military Conditioning and Motor Function Assessment, The PLA University of Science and Technology, Nanjing, China

Thomas A. W. Paulson, Barry Mason, James Rhodes and Victoria L. Goosey-Tolfrey
The Peter Harrison Centre for Disability Sport, School of Sport, Exercise and Health Sciences, Loughborough University, Loughborough, UK

Brianna Larsen
School of Exercise and Nutrition Sciences, Faculty of Health, Deakin University, Melbourne, VIC, Australia

Rod Snow and Brad Aisbett
School of Exercise and Nutrition Sciences, Faculty of Health, Deakin University, Melbourne, VIC, Australia
Centrefor Physical Activity and Nutrition Research, Faculty of Health, Deakin University, Melbourne, VIC, Australia

Michael Williams-Bell
Faculty of Health Sciences, University of Ontario Institute of Technology, Oshawa, ON, Canada

Thierry Weissland
Laboratoire de Recherche Adaptations Physiquesà L'exerciceet RéadaptationàL' effort, EA-3300, UFR-STAPS, Université de Picardie Jules Verne, Amiens, France
Institut d'Ingénierie dela Santé, UFR de Médecine, Université de Picardie Jules Verne, Amiens, France

Arnaud Faupin
Laboratoire Motricité Humaine Education Sport Santé, EA-6312, UFR-STAPS, Université de Toulon, La Garde, France
Laboratoire Motricité Humaine Education Sport Santé, EA-6312, Université Nice Sophia Antipolis, Nice, France

Benoit Borel
Laboratoire Handicap, Activité, Vieillissement, Autonomie, Environnement, EA-6310, Département STAPS, Université de Limoges, Limoges, France

Pierre-Marie Leprêtre
Laboratoire de Recherche Adaptations Physiologiquesà L'exercice et Réadaptationà L'effort, EA-3300, UFR-STAPS, Université de Picardie Jules Verne, Amiens, France

Irineu Loturco, Ronaldo Kobal, Cesar C. Cal Abad, Katia Kitamura, Amaury W. Veríssimo and Lucas A. Pereira
Nucleus of High Performance in Sport, São Paulo, Brazil

Ciro Winckler
Brazilian Paralympic Committee, Brasília, Brazil

Fábio Y. Nakamura
Nucleus of High Performance in Sport, São Paulo, Brazil
Department of Physical Education, State University of Londrina, Londrina, Brazil

Tiziana Pietrangelo and Stefania Fulle
Department of Neuroscience, Imaging and Clinical Sciences, University "G.d'Annunzio" Chieti-Pescara, Chieti, Italy
Laboratory of Functional Evaluation, "G.d'Annunzio" University of Chieti-Pescara, Chieti, Italy
Centre for Aging Sciences, d'Annunzio Foundation, Chieti, Italy
Department of Neuroscience, Imaging and Clinical Sciences, Interuniversity Institute of Myology, Chieti, Italy

Ester S. Di Filippo and Rosa Mancinelli
Department of Neuroscience, Imaging and Clinical Sciences, University "G.d'Annunzio" Chieti-Pescara, Chieti, Italy
Centre for Aging Sciences, d'Annunzio Foundation, Chieti, Italy
Department of Neuroscience, Imaging and Clinical Sciences, Interuniversity Institute of Myology, Chieti, Italy

Christian Doria
Department of Neuroscience, Imaging and Clinical Sciences, University "G.d'Annunzio" Chieti-Pescara, Chieti, Italy
Laboratory of Functional Evaluation, "G.d'Annunzio" University of Chieti-Pescara, Chieti, Italy
Department of Neuroscience, Imaging and Clinical Sciences, Interuniversity Institute of Myology, Chieti, Italy

Alessio Rotini
Department of Neuroscience, Imaging and Clinical Sciences, University "G.d'Annunzio" Chieti-Pescara, Chieti, Italy
Department of Neuroscience, Imaging and Clinical Sciences, Interuniversity Institute of Myology, Chieti, Italy

Giorgio Fanò-Illic
Laboratory of Functional Evaluation, "G.d'Annunzio" University of Chieti-Pescara, Chieti, Italy
Centre for Aging Sciences, d'Annunzio Foundation, Chieti, Italy
Department of Neuroscience, Imaging and Clinical Sciences, Interuniversity Institute of Myology, Chieti, Italy

Gabriela A. Trevizani, Olivassé Nasario-Junior and Jurandir Nadal
Biomedical Engineering Program COPPE, Universidade Federaldo Riode Janeiro, Riode Janeiro, Brazil

Tiago Peçanha
Exercise Hemodynamic Laboratory, School of Physical Education and Sport, Universidade de São Paulo, São Paulo, Brazil

Jeferson M. Vianna
Faculty of Physical Education and Sports, Universidade Federal de Juizde Fora, Juizde Fora, Brazil

Lilian P. Silva
Faculty of Physiotheraphy, Universidade Federal de Juizde Fora, Juizde Fora, Brazil

Rafael Torres-Peralta, David Morales-Alamo, José Losa-Reyna, Ismael Pérez-Suárez and José A. L. Calbet
Department of Physical Education, University of Las Palmas de Gran Canaria, Las Palmas de Gran Canaria, Spain
Research Institute of Biomedical and Health Sciences (IUIBS), Las Palmas de Gran Canaria, Spain

Miriam González-Izal and Mikel Izquierdo
Department of Health Sciences, Public University of Navarra, Tudela, Spain

Mike J. Price
Faculty of Health and Life Sciences, School of Life Sciences, Applied Biology and Exercise Science Research Centre, Coventry University, Coventry, UK

Barbara Uva and Bengt Kayser
Institute of Sport Sciences and Department of Physiology, Faculté de Biologieet de Médecine, Université de Lausanne, Lausanne, Switzerland

Andrea Aliverti and Dario Bovio
Dipartimento di Elettronica, Informazionee Bioingegneria, Politecnico di Milano, Milano, Italy

Raúl Reina, Jose M. Sarabia, María P. García-Vaquero and María Campayo-Piernas
Sports Research Centre, Miguel Hernández University, Elche, Spain

Javier Yanci
Faculty of Physical Activity and Sports Science, University of the Basque Country, UPV/EHU, Vitoria-Gasteiz, Spain

Christopher R. West
International Collaboration on Repair Discoveries, University of British Columbia, Vancouver, BC, Canada
School of Kinesiology, University of British Columbia, Vancouver, BC, Canada
Centre for Sports Medicine and Human Performance, Brunel University London, London, UK

Christof A. Leicht and Victoria L. Goosey-Tolfrey
School of Sport, Exercise and Health Sciences, The Peter Harrison Centre for Disability Sport, Loughborough University, Loughborough, UK

Lee M. Romer
Centre for Sports Medicine and Human Performance, Brunel University London, London, UK

Jeffrey W. F. Aldous
Department of Sport Science and Physical Activity, Institute of Sport and Physical Activity Research, University of Bedfordshire, Bedford, UK

Bryna C. R. Chrismas
Sport Science Program, College of Arts and Sciences, Qatar University, Doha, Qatar

Ibrahim Akubat
Department of Physical Education and Sports Studies, Newman University, Birmingham, UK

Ben Dascombe
Department of Rehabilitation, Nutrition and Sport, School of Allied Health, La Trobe University, Melbourne, VIC, Australia

Grant Abt
Department of Sport, Health and Exercise Science, The University of Hull, Hull, UK

Lee Taylor
ASPETAR, Qatar Orthopedic and Sports Medicine Hospital, Athlete Health and Performance Research Centre, Aspire Zone, Doha, Qatar

Meredith J. Luttrell and John R. Halliwill
Department of Human Physiology, University of Oregon, Eugene, OR, USA